ASSOCIATION OF AMERICAN MEDICAL COLLEGES

Medical School Admission Requirements
United States and Canada
2001-2002

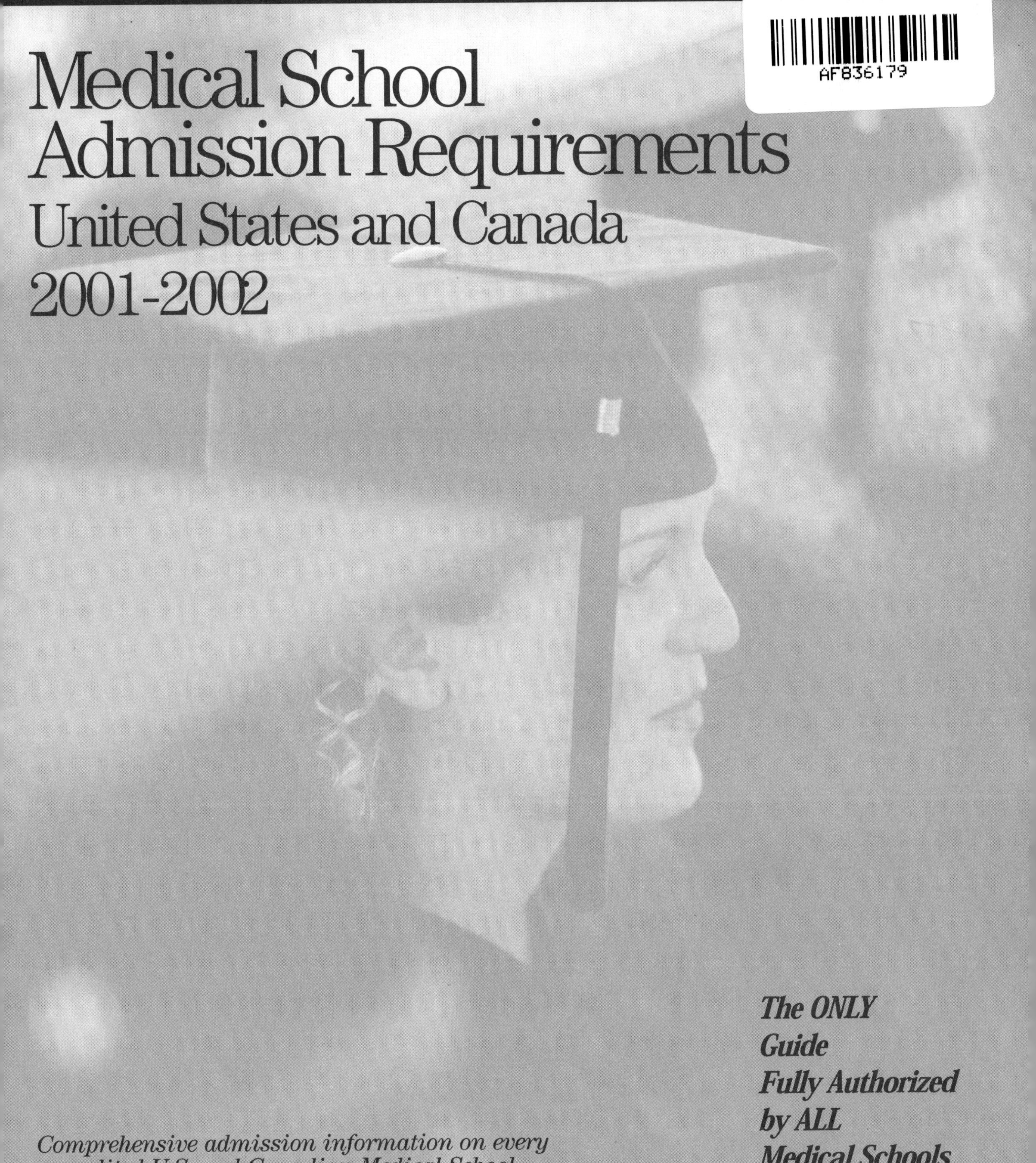

Comprehensive admission information on every accredited U.S. and Canadian Medical School

The ONLY Guide Fully Authorized by ALL Medical Schools

www.tomorrowsdoctors.org

MSAR AAMC
MEDICAL SCHOOL ADMISSION REQUIREMENTS

AAMC Staff for the
Medical School Admission Requirements, 2001–2002, United States and Canada

Editor
Cari L. Coleman

Staff Associate
M. LaVerne Alexander

Consultants
Susan K. Neely, Senior Vice President for Communications
Frances R. Hall, Associate Vice President for Student Programs

The assistance of other AAMC staff members and the admission officers and other representatives of the medical schools is noted with appreciation.

Revised annually; new edition available in April.

To order additional copies of this publication, please contact:

Association of American Medical Colleges
Section for Publication Orders
2450 N Street, NW
Washington, DC 20037
Phone: 202-828-0416
Fax: 202-828-1123

Price: $25.00, plus $5 shipping (single copy)

ISBN 1-57754-014-X

Printed in the United States of America

GROUP ON STUDENT AFFAIRS (GSA) STEERING COMMITTEE, 1999–2000

ASSOCIATION OF AMERICAN MEDICAL COLLEGES

The Association of American Medical Colleges (AAMC) has as its purpose the advancement of medical education and the nation's health. In pursuing this purpose, the Association works with many national and international organizations, institutions, and individuals interested in strengthening the quality of medical education at all levels, the search for biomedical knowledge, and the application of these tools to providing effective health care.

As an educational association representative of members having similar purposes, the primary role of the AAMC is to assist those members by providing services at the national level that will facilitate the accomplishment of their mission. Such activities may include collecting data and conducting studies on issues of major concern, evaluating the quality of educational programs through the accreditation process, providing consultation and technical assistance to institutions as needs are identified, synthesizing the opinions of an informed membership for consideration at the national level, and improving communication among those concerned with medical education and the nation's health. Other activities of the Association reflect the expressed concerns and priorities of the officers and governing bodies.

The AAMC represents all 125 accredited U.S. medical schools; the 16 accredited Canadian medical schools; some 400 major teaching hospitals, including 75 Veterans Affairs medical centers; 88 academic and professional societies representing 92,000 faculty members; and the nation's 67,000 medical students and 103,000 residents.

In addition to the types of activities listed above, the AAMC is responsible for the Medical College Admission Test (MCAT) and the American Medical College Application Service (AMCAS) and provides detailed admissions information to the medical schools and to undergraduate premedical advisers.

Important Notice

The information in this book is based on the most recent data provided at the request of the Association of American Medical Colleges (AAMC) by its member schools prior to publication deadlines. The material so supplied has been edited by the staff of the publication and in some instances condensed to meet limitations of space. In compiling this edition, the AAMC made every reasonable effort to assure the accuracy and timeliness of the information included in it, and, except where noted, the data and estimates were updated as of January 1999. All information contained herein, however, especially figures on tuition and expenses, is subject to change, and nothing included in this edition will be binding upon any of the medical schools listed or the AAMC. All the medical schools listed in this edition, like other educational institutions, are also subject to the requirements of federal and state laws prohibiting discrimination on the basis of race, color, religion, sex, age, handicap, or national origin. Such laws include Title VI of the Civil Rights Act of 1964, Title IX of the Education Amendments of 1972, Section 504 of the Rehabilitation Act of 1973, and the Age Discrimination Act of 1975, as amended. For the most current and complete information regarding costs, official policies, procedures, and other matters, the particular school in which the applicant is interested should be contacted.

In applying to U.S. or foreign medical schools, it is not necessary to go through any commercial agencies. The AAMC neither endorses nor has any relationship with commercial agencies.

Contents

List of Tables

Part 1 • Admission Information

Part 2 • School Entries

List of Figures

Alphabetical Listing of Medical Schools

Part 2 • Chapter 11
U.S. Medical Schools

Part 2 • Chapter 12
Canadian Medical Schools

Geographical Listing of Medical Schools

Part 2 • Chapter 11 • U.S. Medical Schools

Foreword

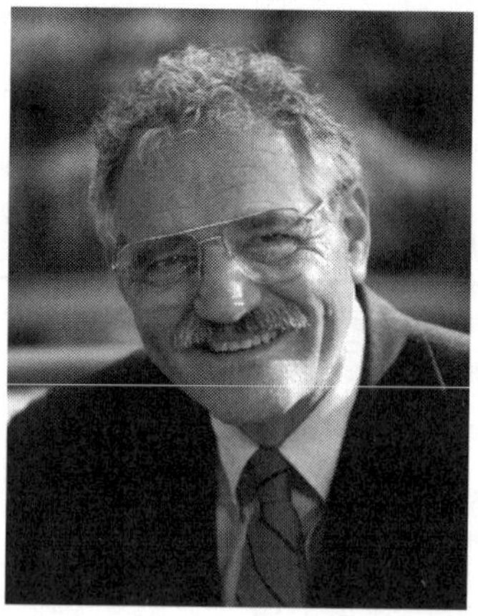

The landscape of the medical profession has changed dramatically in the half century since the Association of American Medical Colleges (AAMC) first published the *Medical School Admission Requirements* (MSAR). But one important thing hasn't changed over that time: deciding to become a doctor is still one of the most momentous decisions one can ever hope to make. And let me be among the first to congratulate you on your decision. In my opinion, admittedly biased by my own gratifying experiences as a physician, no other profession offers as many challenges, as many chances to be of service to others, and as many opportunities for a satisfying and rewarding career.

More than that, I can't imagine a more exciting time to begin medical school. Just think of what you have to look forward to. Tomorrow's doctors will be at the forefront of the most dramatic developments in medical science in all of history. They will be armed with unimaginably powerful tools to relieve human suffering and prevent the ravages of disease. They will help shape technological improvements that will revolutionize both the way doctors conduct research and the way they diagnose and treat patients. And they will be in a position to help reshape the way the health care delivery system provides affordable services of high quality to everyone who needs them.

Yet despite this wealth of opportunity, I know that many aspiring medical school applicants are advised by some well-meaning friends and family members not to pursue their dream of becoming a doctor. It seems to me that those who proffer such advice are overly influenced by the current anxieties about the rising costs of medical care and by the prospects for a major restructuring of the way health care is organized and financed. What they fail to take fully into account, however, is a fundamental truth about the human condition: people get sick and, when they do, they need help. And that's what medicine is all about. Caring for and about people has always been, and always will be, the essence of the medical profession and the principal reason students continue to study medicine.

Which is not to say that the study of medicine is a simple matter. Far from it! The path to becoming a doctor is undeniably long, and the many requirements students must meet just to apply to medical school often appear confusing, if not daunting. To help aspiring students understand and prepare for medical school requirements, recent volumes of the *Medical School Admission Requirements*, have evolved and expanded to serve as a comprehensive and authoritative guide to premedical preparation and admission to medical school. This book is more than a listing of prerequisites and courses offered at each school; it also is a general reference manual for the medical education experience itself. Because medical school is ultimately not for everybody, the guide is designed to assist those committed to a career in medicine to approach their goals realistically and to assess their personal commitment for meeting the many challenges ahead.

We like to think of the *Medical School Admission Requirements* as a first contact in a long relationship between AAMC and future medical students. We hope it will allow individuals considering careers in medicine to be better informed about the opportunities available and more capable of realistically assessing their potential for admission to medical school. And we hope it serves as a springboard for a long, rewarding career in medicine.

JORDAN J. COHEN, M.D.
AAMC

Accredited U.S. Medical Schools*

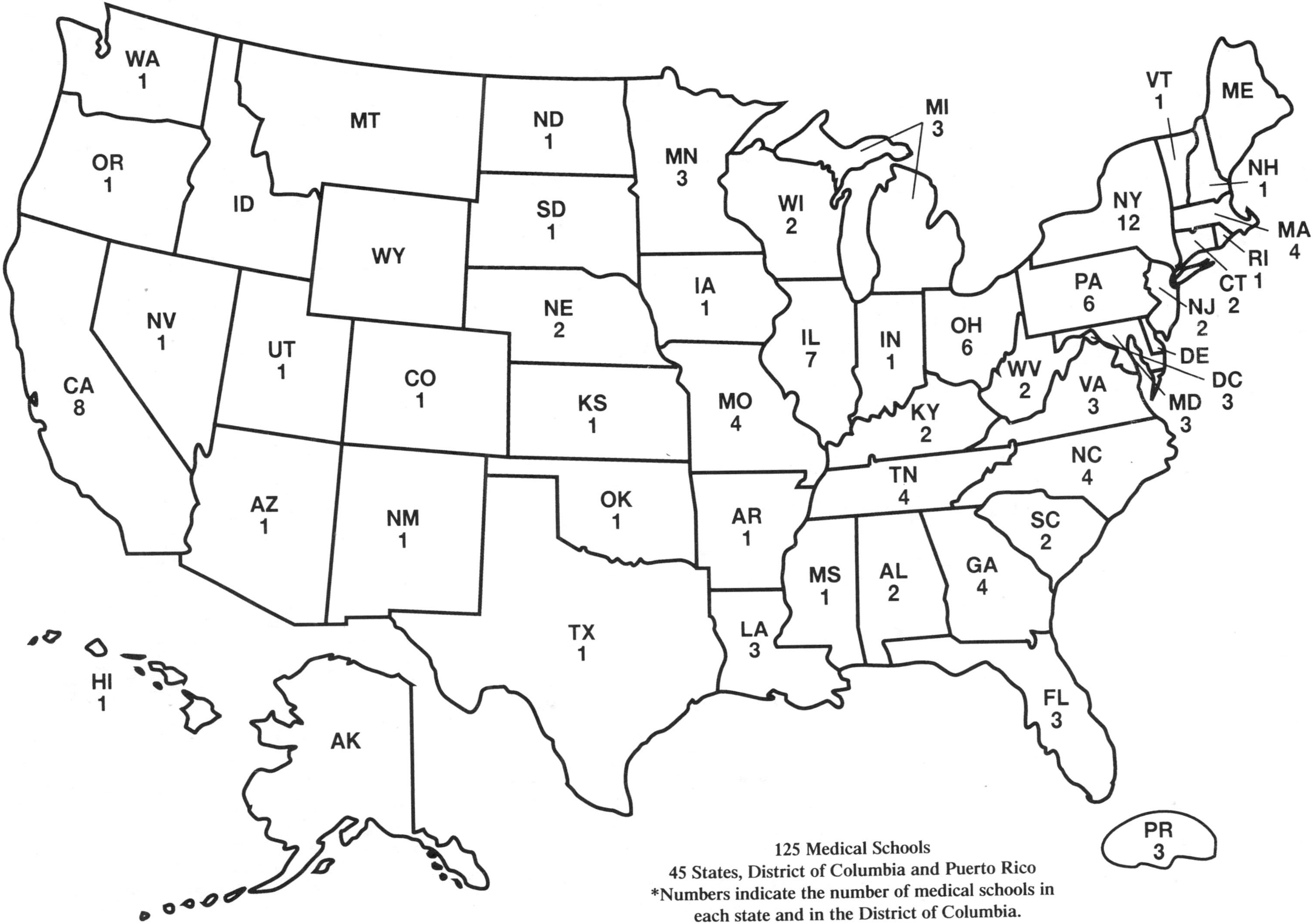

125 Medical Schools
45 States, District of Columbia and Puerto Rico
*Numbers indicate the number of medical schools in each state and in the District of Columbia.

ASSOCIATION OF AMERICAN MEDICAL COLLEGES

Admission Information

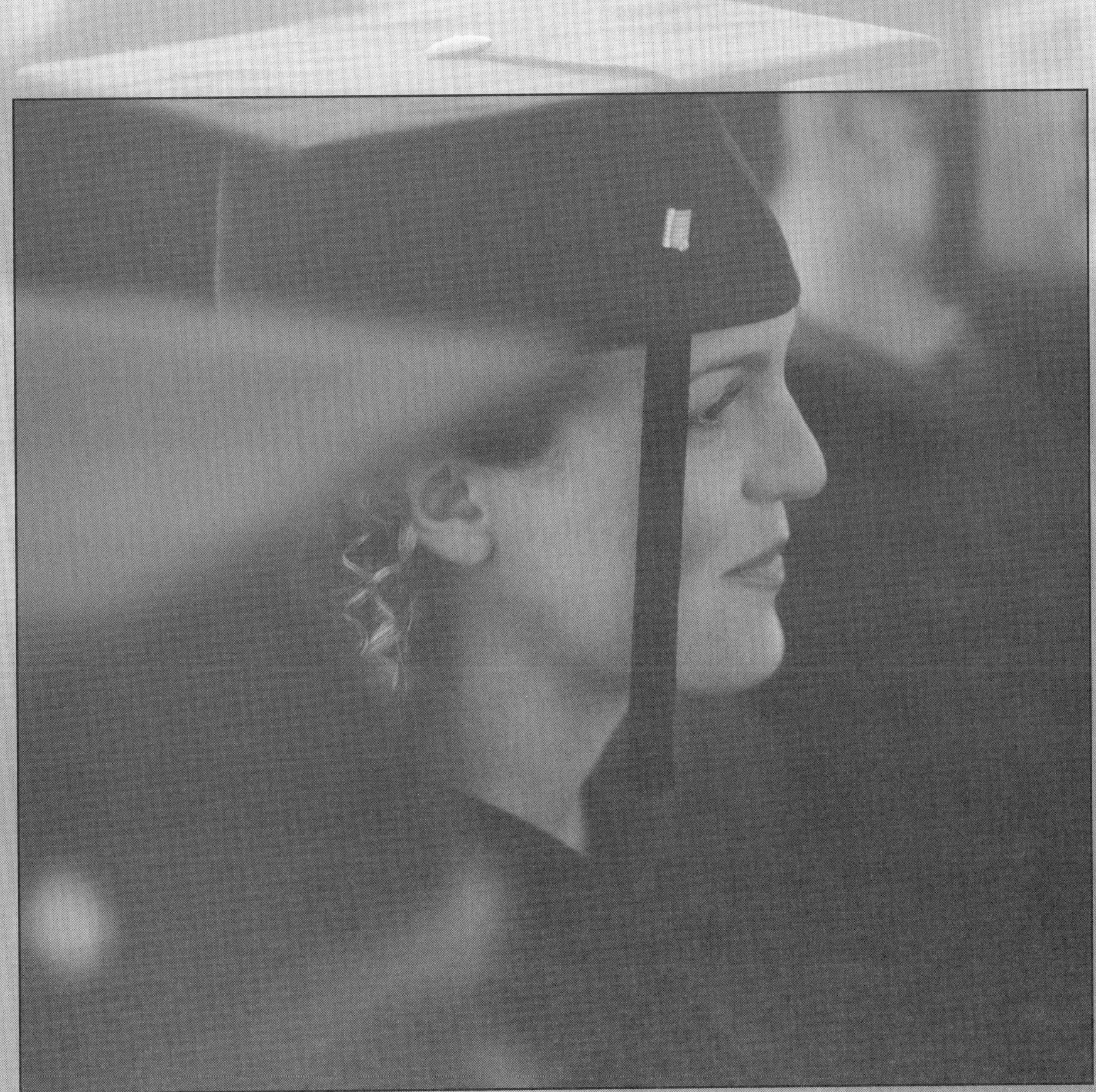

www.tomorrowsdoctors.org

MSAR AAMC

MEDICAL SCHOOL ADMISSION REQUIREMENTS

The Nature of Medical Education

1

Programs of medical education that award the degree of doctor of medicine in the United States and Canada are accredited by the Liaison Committee on Medical Education (LCME). This voluntary accrediting agency is sponsored by the Association of American Medical Colleges and the American Medical Association. All state medical practice laws recognize the accreditation status conferred by the LCME on the medical schools. Holders of the M.D. degree awarded by the LCME-accredited schools are provided the opportunity for licensure subject to certain examinations and other requirements imposed by each state. The LCME has traditionally avoided narrowly dictating curriculum content and has encouraged institutions, while meeting national minimal standards of quality, to approach the education of physicians in a variety of ways. This philosophy has led to a significant diversity of educational approaches. The extent of this diversity may be observed in the annual *AAMC Curriculum Directory,* which provides details about the curriculum of each U.S. and Canadian medical school.

THE MEDICAL SCHOOL CURRICULUM

Medical school curricula, although quite varied, have as their goal the preparation of students to enter a three- to seven-year period of graduate medical education. Many curricula are problem based as contrasted to topical and discipline focused. The teaching methodologies include lecture, small-group discussion, self-instruction, and laboratory experience.

• The First Two Years

Instruction is provided in anatomy, biochemistry, physiology, microbiology, pharmacology, pathology, and behavioral sciences during the first several academic periods after matriculation. These basic sciences may be taught independently by departmental faculties or by interdisciplinary groups of faculty. The interdisciplinary approach often focuses on organ systems. In this approach, instruction in anatomy, biochemistry, physiology, pharmacology, and pathology of an organ system, such as the heart and blood vessels, is integrated with normal and abnormal functions of the system. Whether the basic sciences are taught by discipline or in an interdisciplinary fashion, there is a major emphasis in almost all medical schools on introducing contact with clinical problems early in the curriculum. In some schools students begin to learn in their first year how to interview and examine patients; in other schools the first clinical contact may be demonstrations of patients by faculty. In all schools, however, by the middle of their second year, students have begun to learn how to obtain historical data from patients and conduct physical and selected basic laboratory examinations. The teaching of bioethics, legal medicine, disease prevention, medical sociology, and characteristics of the health care delivery system occurs parallel to or interspersed within the basic and clinical sciences.

• The Clinical Years

The last two years of medical school are usually devoted to education in the clinical setting. The immediate and specific aims of clinical education are to enable the student to establish desirable physician-patient relationships, to take a medical history, to conduct a physical examination, and to recognize the more familiar disease patterns. The overall aim, however, is to develop in the student both an understanding of the patient as a total human being and the sense of professional maturity that medicine demands.

• Clinical Clerkships

The length and number of required clinical educational periods (clinical clerkships) vary from school to school. Clinical clerkships are usually required in family medicine, internal medicine, obstetrics-gynecology, pediatrics, psychiatry, and surgery. These required clerkships vary in length from 6 to 12 weeks. During clerkships, students are usually assigned to a hospital clinical service where they assume responsibility for "working-up," that is, collecting data and presenting to the faculty a specified number of patient studies each week. Students also participate with post-M.D. trainees (residents) and faculty in caring for patients admitted to the clinical service to which they are assigned. When feasible, students are provided the opportunity to follow their patients before and after discharge from the hospital in ambulatory care settings. During clinical science education, basic science knowledge and fundamental clinical skills are applied to the solution of diagnostic and treatment problems. Lectures and seminars augment the bedside learning provided during patient visits, so-called "rounds," with teaching physicians.

• Clinical Elective Courses

As students progress through these clinical experiences, the range of opportunity for career development becomes apparent.

Elective courses in the basic, behavioral, and clinical sciences permit students to explore career options. In many institutions, courses taken in other colleges of the university may be applied for credit toward the M.D. degree. Depending upon individual interests and talent, students are provided the opportunity to arrange part of their program. In the fourth year, many schools permit students to arrange their entire program on an elective basis. Clinical electives include clerkships in the primary specialties and in their many subspecialties. Elective opportunities in clinical settings are often provided in other academic centers or in nonacademic settings. These may vary from a preceptorship with a practicing physician to a period of time spent in a research laboratory. Such settings allow students to become acquainted with the career possibilities of the medical specialties of their interest, while enriching their education.

At present a major emphasis is placed on encouraging students to develop careers in the primary care specialties of family medicine, general internal medicine, and general pediatrics. This emphasis should not, however, deter students interested in other specialties, research, and/or teaching from seeking the M.D. degree. There is also a need for well-prepared physicians and physician-scientists to translate the rapid advances in biomedical knowledge into clinical applications.

EVALUATION, PROMOTION, GRADUATION

Each medical school's faculty is responsible for establishing the criteria for evaluating student performance, promotion, and graduation. Many faculties have written learning objectives for the overall medical education program and for each course or segment of the curriculum. Determining whether students have met these objectives is accomplished by a combination of direct observation and written and/or oral assessments. The frequency and pattern of evaluation vary from institution to institution. Some form of year-end comprehensive exam is often required. Ninety-five schools report that they currently require students to pass Step 1 of the United States Medical Licensing Examination (USMLE) at the end of their basic science sequence or in order to graduate. Sixty-eight schools report that they currently require students to pass Step 2 of the USMLE to graduate.

• What is the USMLE?

The USMLE is a single, three-step examination for medical licensure in the United States. The Federation of State Medical Boards (FSMB) and the National Board of Medical Examiners (NBME) sponsor the USMLE. The USMLE provides a common evaluation system for all applicants for medical licensure. It consists of three steps and is designed to assess a physician's ability to apply knowledge, concepts and principles that are important in health and disease and that constitute the basis of safe and effective patient care.

Step 1 assesses the knowledge acquired in the basic medical sciences and also the scientific principles required for maintenance of competence through lifelong learning. Step 2 assesses the examinee's ability to apply the medical knowledge and understanding of clinical science including emphasis on health promotion and disease prevention. Step 3 assesses the examinee's ability to apply the medical knowledge and understanding of biomedical and clinical science considered essential for the unsupervised practice of medicine.

The USMLE is a computer-based test. Step 1 is to be completed in an eight hour testing day and Step 2 encompasses a nine-hour testing day. Step 3 is taken over one and one-half days and includes computer-based case simulations.

• How Am I Graded?

Grading in less than half of the schools is pass/fail or honors/pass/fail. Regardless of the pattern or frequency of evaluation used, individual students' abilities are carefully scrutinized. This is particularly true in the clinical clerkships where one-to-one relationships between faculty and students permit close observation. Although student evaluation is rigorous, the rate of attrition in U.S. medical schools is low—slightly over three percent. Students with detected deficiencies in knowledge or skills are provided counseling and assistance. Students who are having difficulty may be offered the opportunity to repeat course work. However, all faculties reserve the right to drop students whose academic or personal characteristics are found to be incompatible with the professional responsibilities of a physician in this society.

GRADUATE MEDICAL EDUCATION

• Residency Training

Exposure to the various branches and aspects of medicine helps students to determine the course their education will take during the training period following medical school (residency). For students who have made a career decision to practice in a medical or surgical specialty, the requirements of the certifying board in that particular specialty will mold the choice of the first-postgraduate-year program. Specialties such as family medicine, internal medicine, pediatrics, and surgery encourage students to enter directly into first-postgraduate-year programs in that specialty and to continue in these programs until they have completed specialty board requirements. Satisfactory completion of three years of training in family medicine, internal medicine, or pediatrics generally qualifies an individual to take the examination(s) administered by the certifying boards of these specialties. General surgery requires five years of training while other surgical specialties require additional training.

Students seeking careers in other specialties will find they are encouraged or required to spend their first postgraduate year in a program offering a broad clinical experience. Examples of these specialties are anesthesiology, dermatology, psychiatry, and radiology. Usually these students will apply for a single year of internal medicine or for a diversified, transitional first-postgraduate year with the expectation they will enter a program in the specialty of their choice in their second-postgraduate year. In some cases a year of broad clinical experience may be located in the same institution where subsequent subspecialty training occurs. In other instances, specialty training must be completed elsewhere.

By the end of the third year of medical school, almost all students have made a career decision regarding the area of medicine in which they will specialize. Nearly all will eventually seek certification by one of the 24 specialty boards. Some will take one to two years of additional training in a subspecialty and will seek recognition through additional certification in that subspecialty. Descriptions of recognized specialties and subspecialties can be found in *Which Medical Specialist for You,* a brochure published by the American Board of Medical Specialties (ABMS). The ABMS also publishes a brochure entitled *Medical Specialty Certification and Related Matters* that provides information about the medical profession and specialty certification for the medical student, the resident, and others, and lists sources of additional information. For more information, contact the ABMS at 1007 Church Street, Suite 404, Evanston, Illinois 60201-5913, or E-mail: smiller@abms.org.

SPECIAL PROGRAMS

Individual medical schools offer a number of special programs. Many of these are listed in the *AAMC Curriculum Directory.* Specific details of the characteristics of a school's special programs may be obtained from that school. Several of the more common special programs are described below.

• B.A.- or B.S.-M.D. Degree Programs

In 1999–2000 a small number of U.S. medical schools provided programs beginning after high school that combined undergraduate college study and medical education. (These schools are listed in Table 2 in Chapter 2 and are fully described in Chapter 10.) Students are admitted provisionally to these programs based upon their high school credentials and, if their performance is satisfactory, are permitted to progress to the M.D. degree. This generally requires six to eight years. Students interested in this type of program should request information from the prospective medical school as early as possible.

• Accelerated Programs

There are options for accelerating the standard four-year medical education curriculum. Since these options vary among schools, interested students should investigate the possibilities by consulting the dean of admissions' office at the institutions to which they intend to apply.

Several schools now offer programs that combine the medical school (M.D.) program and the first year of graduate medical education. These programs are especially designed to encourage careers in primary care through family practice or internal medicine. Students interested in these programs should inquire about their availability at the schools to which they apply.

• Research Training

There is a continuing need for physicians who have the ability both to conduct research and to interpret research findings. Students interested in research will find that most faculties are highly receptive to allowing them to engage in research projects. Depending upon the availability of resources and the student's willingness to invest time in research, programs ranging from a few months to a year or more can be arranged. These opportunities can be used by students to explore their creative talents for biomedical research. Such exploration can help students decide whether to pursue preparation for a career in academic medicine during graduate medical education.

• Medical Scientist Training Program (MSTP)

Within the biomedical science community, the need for clinical investigators who have been well trained in basic research has long been recognized. To help meet this need, the National Institute of General Medical Sciences (NIGMS) established the Medical Scientist Training Program (MSTP) to encourage and to support the training of students with outstanding credentials and potential who, through an integrated program of scientific and medical study leading to the combined M.D.-Ph.D. degree, are motivated to undertake a career in biomedical research and academic medicine. The program's goal is to prepare its graduates to function independently in both basic research and clinical investigation. The majority of MSTP graduates go on to careers in basic biomedical or clinical research.

The MSTP was established in 1964. It currently has 33 participating programs involving 37 degree-granting institutions with a total of 828 trainees. (There are approximately 75 medical schools that do not have NIGMS MSTP training grants but offer opportunities for M.D.-Ph.D. studies.)

MSTP participants may choose from a wide range of research training programs in the biological, chemical, or physical sciences. Other disciplines in which MSTP participants can pursue graduate study are the computer sciences, social and behavioral sciences, economics, epidemiology, public health, bioengineering, biostatistics, and bioethics.

MSTP grants are made to universities and their medical schools, which are responsible for program operation and trainee selection. About 170 positions for new students are available nationwide each year. (Many institutions also support additional students using funds from other sources.) Selection for admission is highly competitive. For those selected, the program provides a maximum of six years of support, although an individual's course of study for the combined degree may take somewhat longer. All institutions identify other sources of support for a trainee's additional years of study. Trainee support provided by an MSTP grant includes the following:

- stipend of $11,748 a year;
- tuition allowance; and
- modest sums for travel, equipment, and supplies.

Many institutions supplement the basic stipend provided by the MSTP grant.

Continued support for an individual student is subject to annual renewal based on the trainee's satisfactory performance in the program and the institution's successful competition for funds at the time of grant renewal every three to five years. Since MSTP grants are a type of National Research Service Award (NRSA), trainees must be citizens or noncitizen nationals of the United States or have been lawfully admitted for permanent residence (i.e., possess an alien registration receipt card I-151 or I-551). Trainees incur no payback obligation.

The 34 schools offering the MSTP are listed in Table 1-A. Other information about the MSTP may be obtained by contacting:

Program Director
Medical Scientist Training Program
National Institute of General Medicine Sciences
45 Center Drive MSC 6200
Bethesda, MD 20892-6200
(301) 594-3830

• M.D.-Ph.D. Degree Programs

In 1999–2000, 113 schools provided students the opportunity to earn both the M.D. and the Ph.D. in an area pertinent to medicine. Although Table 1-A lists only 34 Medical Scientist Training Programs that are supported by NIH, other medical schools have similar programs. Since these options vary among schools, students should investigate the funding packages that are offered and the number of funded positions available for other M.D.-Ph.D. programs. These schools and some of the disciplines in which the Ph.D. is offered are listed in Table 1-B. This table does not include all disciplines and should be used only as a guide. A list of the names of the contact persons at each school precedes this table. For a list of M.D.-Ph.D. programs and their related Web sites, visit www.aamc.org/research/dbr/mdphd/programs.htm.

• Independent Study

Several schools provide an option for students to pursue selected required courses of study at their own pace, using learning techniques of their own choosing. Characteristically, students engaged in independent study must meet periodically with faculty tutors to demonstrate their progress and must pass the comprehensive exams required of all students for promotion and graduation.

• Other Combined-Degree Programs

Table 1-C provides information about other medical school combined-degree programs.

TABLE 1-A

U.S. Medical Schools Offering Medical Scientist Training Programs Supported by National Institutes of Health, 1999–2000

Alabama	New York University
Albert Einstein	Northwestern
Baylor	Pennsylvania State University
California, Los Angeles (UCLA)	Pennsylvania, University of
California, San Diego	Rochester
California, San Francisco	Stanford
Case Western Reserve	SUNY-Stony Brook
Chicago	Texas, Dallas (Southwestern)
Colorado	Tufts
Columbia	Vanderbilt
Duke	Virginia, University of
Emory	Washington University (St. Louis)
Harvard†	Washington, University of
Iowa	Weill* (Cornell)
Johns Hopkins	Wisconsin, University of
Michigan, University of	Yale
Minnesota, University of	
Mount Sinai	

*Conducted in cooperation with Rockefeller University—Sloan Kettering Institute
†Conducted in cooperation with the Massachusetts Institute of Technology

Contact Persons for M.D.-Ph.D. Programs at U.S. Medical Schools

ALABAMA

University of Alabama School of Medicine
Dr. Jeffrey E. Kudlow
Director, Medical Scientist Training Program
Web Site: http://w3.lhl.uab.edu/mdphd/

University of South Alabama College of Medicine
Dr. Mark Gillespie
Director, Basic Medical Sciences Graduate Program

ARIZONA

University of Arizona College of Medicine
Nancy Suttle
M.D.-Ph.D. Program Coordinator

ARKANSAS

University of Arkansas for Medical Sciences College of Medicine
Dr. Lee Soderberg
Professor of Microbiology and Immunology
Web Site: http://www.uams.edu

CALIFORNIA

University of California, Davis School of Medicine
Edward D. Dagang
Director of Admissions
Web Site: www.ucdavis.edu

University of California, Irvine College of Medicine
Christine Varrone
Program Administrator
Web Site: www/med.uci.edu/~md-phd

University of California, Los Angeles UCLA School of Medicine
Alice del Rosario
Program Administrator
Web Site: www.medstudents.ucla.edu/admissions

University of California, San Diego School of Medicine
Christine Moran
Program Director
Professor of Pharmacology
Web Site: http://medschool.ucsd.edu/students/MSTP/newbroc.html

University of California, San Francisco, School of Medicine
Jana M. Toutolmin
Program Administrator, Recruitment and Admissions
Web Site: http://www.som.ucsf.edu

Loma Linda University School of Medicine
Dr. Anthony J. Zuccarelli
Director, Medical Scientist Program
Web Site: http://www.llu/grad/bulletin/medsci.html

Keck School of Medicine of University of Southern California
Sandra M. Mosteller
Administrative Director

Stanford University School of Medicine
Marjorie Weesner
Administrator for Medical Scientist Training Program
Web Site: http://www-med.stanford.edu/MSTP/

COLORADO

University of Colorado School of Medicine
Terri B. Wood
Administrator
Web Site: http://www.uchsc.edu/sm/mstp/

CONNECTICUT

University of Connecticut School of Medicine
Dr. Dominick L. Cinti
Director, Combined Degree Program
Professor of Pharmacology
Web Site: www.uchc.edu

Yale University School of Medicine
Marybeth Brandi
Program Coordinator
Web Site: http://info.med.yale.edu/mdphd/

DISTRICT OF COLUMBIA

George Washington University School of Medicine and Health Sciences
Diane P. McQuail
Director of Admissions
E-mail: medadmit@gwu.edu

Georgetown University School of Medicine
W. Taylor Johnson
Coordinator, Graduate Biomedical Education
Web Site: http://macpost.odr.georgetown.edu/aboutgraded.html

Howard University College of Medicine
Dr. Verle Headings
Director, M.D.-Ph.D. Program

FLORIDA

University of Florida College of Medicine
Robyn Sheppard
Admissions Coordinator
Web Site: www.ufl.edu.oea/admiss/

University of Miami School of Medicine
Jeff Coulter
Coordinator, M.D.-Ph.D. Program
Web Site: http://spider.med.miami.edu/mdphd

GEORGIA

Emory University School of Medicine
Mary E. Kollmer Horton
Administrative Director, M.D.-Ph.D. Program
Web Site: http://omesa.medadm.emory.edu/mdphd

Medical College of Georgia School of Medicine
Dr. James R. Goldenring
Director, M.D.-Ph.D. Program
Web Site: http://www.mcg.edu/som/mdphd/index.html

Morehouse School of Medicine
Karen A. Lewis
Assistant Director of Admissions
Web Site: www.msm.edu

HAWAII

University of Hawai'i at Mānoa John A. Burns School of Medicine
Marilyn M. Nishiki
Admissions Officer/Registrar
Web Site: http://medworld.biomed.hawaii.edu

ILLINOIS

University of Chicago Pritzker School of Medicine
Jackie McKissack
MSTP/M.D.-Ph.D. Coordinator
Web Site: http://pritzker.bsd.uchicago.edu

Finch University of Health Sciences Chicago Medical School
Dr. Yoon Berm Kim
Chair, M.D.-Ph.D. Program
Web Site: www.finchcms.edu

University of Illinois College of Medicine (Chicago)
Susan M. Stuecheli
Recruitment and Admissions Counselor
Web Site: www/uic.edu

University of Illinois College of Medicine at Urbana-Champaign
Jennifer Bloom
Coordinator, Medical Scholars Program
Web Site: http://soma.npa.uiuc.edu/msp/

Loyola University Chicago Stritch School of Medicine
Paula Griffin-Arnold
Coordinator
Web Site: www.lumen.luc.edu/ssom/studres/mdphd/index.htm

Northwestern University Medical School
Dr. David Engman
Director, Northwestern MSTP
Web Site: www.mstp.nwu.edu

Rush Medical College of Rush University
Jan L. Schmidt
Director of Admissions
Web Site: www.rush.edu

INDIANA

Indiana University School of Medicine
Dr. William F. Bosron
Assistant Dean for Graduate Studies
Web Site: www.iupui.edu/it/medschl/

IOWA

University of Iowa College of Medicine
Pamela Geyer
Director, MSTP
Web Site: http://www.uiowa.edu/~mstp

KANSAS

University of Kansas Medical Center School of Medicine
Dr. Joseph D. Bast
Dean of Graduate Studies
Web Site: http://www2.kumc.edu/gsr/

KENTUCKY

University of Kentucky College of Medicine
Dr. Charles Snow
Director of Graduate Studies, M.D.-Ph.D. Program
Web Site: http://www.uky.edu/

LOUISIANA

Louisiana State University School of Medicine in New Orleans
Dr. Adele Spence
Assistant Dean, School of Graduate Studies
Web Site: www.medschool.lsuhsc.edu

Louisiana State University School of Medicine in Shreveport
Dr. Leonard L. Seelig
Assistant Dean, Graduate Studies
Web Site: http://gradsch.shreveport.lsumc.edu/

Tulane University School of Medicine
Dr. Joseph C. Pisano
Associate Dean
Web Site: http://www.mcl.tulane.edu

MARYLAND

Johns Hopkins University School of Medicine
Thomasine Williams
Program Administrator
Web Site: www.med.jhu.edu/mdphd.html

University of Maryland School of Medicine
Dr. Terry B. Rogers
Director, M.D.–Ph.D. Program
Web Site: http://mdphd.umaryland.edu

Uniformed Services University of the Health Sciences F. Edward Hébert School of Medicine
Dr. Richard M. MacDonald
Associate Dean for Student Affairs

MASSACHUSETTS

Boston University School of Medicine
Sheila Welch
M.D.–Ph.D. Admissions Coordinator
Web Site: http://www.bumc.bu.edu

Harvard Medical School
Linda Burnley
Deputy Director
Web Site: www.hms.harvard.edu/md_phd/

University of Massachusetts Medical School
Judith Mondor
Administrative Coordinator
Web Site: http://www.ummed.edu/dept/med_school_admissions/admissions.html

Tufts University School of Medicine
Carolyn F. Locke
Associate Dean
E-mail: sschool@infonet.tufts.edu

MICHIGAN

Michigan State University
College of Human Medicine
Dr. Lynda J. Farquhar
Director, Medical Scientist Program
Web Site: http://www.chm.msu.edu/

University of Michigan Medical School
Penelope C. Morris
Assistant Director, MSTP
Web Site: www.med.umich.edu/medschool/mstp/

MINNESOTA

Mayo Medical School
Dr. Richard McGee
M.D.-Ph.D. Admissions Director
Web Site: http://www.mayo.edu/mgs/md_phd.htm

University of Minnesota Medical School–Minneapolis
Dana Rechtzigel
Associate Administrator

MISSISSIPPI

University of Mississippi
School of Medicine
Dr. Steven T. Case
Chairman, Medical School Admissions Committee
Web Site: http://umc.edu/medicine

MISSOURI

University of Missouri–Columbia
School of Medicine
Dr. Michael Misfeldt
Interim Associate Dean for Research and Academic Affairs
Web Site: www.hsc.missouri.edu/cares

Saint Louis University
Health Sciences Center
Dr. Andrew J. Lechner
Chairman, M.D.-Ph.D. Program
Professor and Director of Medical Physiology

Washington University
School of Medicine
Brian P. Sullivan
Assistant Director, MSTP
Web Site: http://dbbs.wustl.edu/mstp

NEBRASKA

Creighton University
School of Medicine
Dr. William L. Pancoe
Associate Dean for Student Affairs

University of Nebraska
College of Medicine
Dr. C. Kirk Phares
Associate Dean for Research and Development
Web Site: http://www.unmc.edu

NEVADA

University of Nevada
School of Medicine
Dr. Gale Starich
Assistant Professor

NEW HAMPSHIRE

Dartmouth Medical School
Ann M. Coady
Assistant Director M.D.–Ph.D. Program
Web Site: www.Dartmouth.edu/dms/mdphd/

NEW JERSEY

University of Medicine and Dentistry of New Jersey
New Jersey Medical School
Dr. Jeffrey Wilusz
Associate Professor of Microbiology
Director, M.D.–Ph.D. Program
Web Site: www.umdnj.edu/njmsweb/md_phd_program/

University of Medicine and Dentistry of New Jersey
Robert Wood Johnson Medical School
Dr. Michael J. Leibowitz
Associate Dean
Web Site: www2.umdnj.edu/~gsbspisc

NEW YORK

Albany Medical School
Dr. John Kaplan
Associate Dean for Graduate Studies
Web Site: www.AMC.EDU

Albert Einstein College of Medicine of Yeshiva University
Cecile A. Brown
Assistant Director, Graduate Education

Columbia University
College of Physicians and Surgeons
Dr. Michael Shelanski
Chairman, Department of Pathology

Weill Medical College of Cornell University
Ruth Gotián
Program Coordinator
Web Site: www.med.cornell.edu/mdphd

Mount Sinai School of Medicine of New York University
C. Gita Bosch
Assistant Dean
Web Site: http://www.mssm.edu

New York Medical College
Dr. Mario A. Inchiosa, Jr.
Director, M.D.-Ph.D. Program

New York University
School of Medicine
Arlene Kohler
Program Administrator
Web Site: http://www.med.nyu.edu/HomePage.html

University of Rochester
School of Medicine and Dentistry
Catherine Senecal-Rice
Coordinator, M.D.-Ph.D. Program
Web Site: http://www.urmc.rochester.edu/smd/mdphd/homepage.htm

State University of New York at Buffalo
School of Medicine and Biomedical Sciences
Dr. Jerome A. Roth
Director, MSTP
Web Site: www.smbs.buffalo.edu/mdphd/

State University of New York
Downstate Medical Center
College of Medicine
Dr. Stanley Friedman
Director, MSTP; Professor
Web Site: www.hscbklyn.edu

SUNY Stony Brook
School of Medicine
Toni Daraio
Program Administrator
Web Site: www.informatics.sunysb.edu/mstp

State University of New York Upstate Medical University College of Medicine
Terri Brown
Coordinator of Graduate Programs
Web Site: www.hscy.edu/home/medicine'

NORTH CAROLINA

The Brody School of Medicine at East Carolina University
Dr. Sam D. Pennington
Associate Dean, Research and Graduate Studies
Web Site: http://www.research.ecu.edu/grad/prg_info/menu.html

Duke University School of Medicine
Pat Burks
Program Coordinator
Web Site: http://www2.mc.duke.edu/som/

University of North Carolina at Chapel Hill School of Medicine
Kelly Collier
Administrative Coordinator

Wake Forest University School of Medicine
Dr. David A. Bass
Director, M.D.-Ph.D. Program
Web Site: www.wfubmc.edu/graduate/mdphd.html

NORTH DAKOTA

University of North Dakota School of Medicine
Dr. Robert F. Rubeck
Associate Dean, Academic Affairs and Information Services
Web Site: http://www.medicine.nodak.edu/

OHIO

Case Western Reserve University School of Medicine
Felicité Katz
MSTP Coordinator

University of Cincinnati College of Medicine
Dr. Leslie Myatt
Director, Physician Scientist Training Program
Web Site: www.med.uc.edu/pstp/index.htm

Medical College of Ohio
Dr. James C. Willey
Associate Professor of Medicine
Chairperson, M.D.-Ph.D. Committee
Web Site: www.mco.edu/grad/addegree.html

Northeastern Ohio Universities College of Medicine
Dr. Gary B. Schneider
Director, Division of Basic Medical Sciences
Associate Dean for Research
Web Site: http://www.neoucom.edu

Ohio State University College of Medicine
Catherine M. Kelly
Program Coordinator

Wright State University School of Medicine
Stephen Peterson
Assistant Dean for Admissions

OKLAHOMA

University of Oklahoma College of Medicine
Dr. O. Ray Kling
Dean, Graduate College
Web Site: www.ouhsc.edu

OREGON

Oregon Health Sciences University School of Medicine
Vicki Fields
Director of Admissions
Web Site: http://www.OHSU.edu

PENNSYLVANIA

Jefferson Medical College of Thomas Jefferson University
Dr. Benjamin Bacharach
Associate Dean for Admissions
Web Site: www.tju.edu

MCP Hahnemann School of Medicine
Dr. Daniel Rukstalis
Associate Professor of Surgery
Web Site: www.mcphu.edu

Pennsylvania State University College of Medicine
Barbara J. Noll
Staff Assistant
Web Site: http://www.collmed.psu.edu/mdphd/

University of Pennsylvania School of Medicine
Maggie Krall
Associate Director, Combined Degree Programs

University of Pittsburgh School of Medicine
Dr. Manjit K. Singh
Program Administrator
E-mail: mdphd@fsl.dean-med.pitt.edu

Temple University School of Medicine
Dr. Peter N. Walsh
Director, M.D.-Ph.D. Program
E-mail: mdphd@blue.temple.edu

RHODE ISLAND

Brown University Program in Medicine
Dr. Kim Boekelheide
Director, M.D.-Ph.D. Program
Web Site: www.brown.edu

SOUTH CAROLINA

Medical University of South Carolina
Dr. Perry V. Halushka
Director, Medical Scientist Training Program
Web Site: www2.musc.edu/MSTP/MSTP.html

University of South Carolina School of Medicine
Dr. James Buggy
Assistant Dean for Graduate Studies
Web Site: www.med.sc.edu

TENNESSEE

Meharry Medical College
Dr. Fred Jones
Acting Dean, School of Graduate Studies
Vice President for Research

University of Tennessee, Memphis College of Medicine
Dr. Edward G. Schneider
Associate Dean, College of Graduate Health Sciences
Web Site: http://www.utmem.edu

Vanderbilt University School of Medicine
Kimberly Ainsworth
MSTP Coordinator
Web Site: http://bret.mc.vanderbilt.edu/mstp

TEXAS

Baylor College of Medicine
Suzie Barnes
Program Administrator
Web Site: www.bcm.tmc.edu/mstp

Texas A&M University Health Science Center College of Medicine
Dr. George E. Davis
Director, M.D.–Ph.D. Program Associate Professor
Web Site: http://tamushsc.tamu.edu/COM/COMmain.html

Texas Tech University Health Sciences Center School of Medicine
Pamela Johnson
Director of Graduate Programs
Web Site: http://www.ttuhsc.edu/pages/grad/default.htm

University of Texas Southwestern Medical Center at Dallas Southwestern Medical School
Dr. Rodney Ulane
Associate Dean, MSTP
Web Site: www.swmed.edu

University of Texas Medical School at Galveston
Jessica E. Thorp
Program Coordinator
Web Site: www.utmb.edu/

University of Texas—Houston Medical School
Dr. Dianna M. Milewicz
Associate Professor
Director, M.D.–Ph.D. Program
Web Site: www.uth.tmc.edu

University of Texas Medical School at San Antonio
Dr. Terry Mikiten
Associate Dean, Graduate School

UTAH

University of Utah School of Medicine
Dr. Jerry Kaplan
Department of Ph.D. Programs
Web Site: www-medlib.med.utah.edu/som/education/mstp/mstp2.html

VERMONT

University of Vermont College of Medicine
Dr. Paula B. Tracy
Chair, Graduate Recruitment and Admissions Committee
Web Site: www.med.uvm.edu

VIRGINIA

Virginia Commonwealth University School of Medicine
Dr. Earl F. Ellis
M.D.-Ph.D. Program Director
Web Site: http://views.vcu.edu/mdphd

University of Virginia School of Medicine
Jane Cornelius
M.D.-Ph.D. Program Coordinator
Web Site: www.med.virginia.edu/mstp/

WASHINGTON

University of Washington School of Medicine
Maureen Levell
Program Administrator
Web Site: www.pathology.washington.edu/MSTP.html

WEST VIRGINIA

Marshall University School of Medicine
Marlene P. Gruetter
Senior Administrative Assistant
Web Site: http://meb.marshall.edu/graduate

West Virginia University School of Medicine
Dr. Charles R. Craig
Professor of Pharmacology, Director, M.D.-Ph.D. Training Program

WISCONSIN

Medical College of Wisconsin
Sharon Carpenter
Director of Admissions—Medical School
Web Site: www.mcw.edu/acad/

University of Wisconsin Medical School
Paul Cook
Program Administrator
Web Site: www.medsch.wisc.edu/education/mdphd

TABLE 1-B

Combined M.D.-Ph.D. Programs at U.S. Medical Schools, 1999–2000

Medical School	Anatomy	Biochemistry	Biomedical Engineering	Biophysics	Cell Biology	Genetics	Immunology	Microbiology	Molecular Biology	Neurosciences	Pathology	Pharmacology	Physiology	Other Disciplines
Alabama														
Alabama	•	•		•	•	•	•	•	•	•	•	•	•	
South Alabama	•	•			•	•	•	•	•	•		•	•	•
Arizona														
Arizona	•	•	•		•	•	•	•	•	•		•	•	•
Arkansas														
Arkansas	•	•		•			•	•	•			•	•	•
California														
University of California														
Davis		•	•		•	•	•	•	•	•	•	•	•	•
Irvine	•	•		•				•	•			•	•	•
Los Angeles	•	•	•	•	•	•	•	•	•	•	•	•	•	•
San Diego		•	•	•	•	•	•		•	•	•	•	•	•
San Francisco	•	•		•	•	•	•	•	•	•	•	•	•	
Loma Linda	•	•			•		•	•	•			•	•	
Keck (Southern California)	•	•	•	•	•	•	•	•	•	•	•	•	•	•
Stanford		•	•	•	•	•	•	•		•		•	•	•
Colorado														
Colorado		•		•	•	•	•	•	•	•	•	•	•	
Connecticut														
Connecticut		•			•	•	•		•	•		•		
Yale		•		•	•	•	•	•	•	•	•	•	•	•
District of Columbia														
George Washington	•	•	•		•	•	•	•	•	•	•	•	•	
Georgetown		•		•	•		•	•	•	•	•	•	•	•
Howard	•	•				•		•				•	•	•
Florida														
Florida	•					•	•		•	•		•	•	
Miami	•	•		•	•		•	•	•	•		•	•	•
Georgia														
Emory	•	•	•	•	•	•	•	•	•	•	•	•	•	•
Medical College of Georgia	•	•			•	•	•		•			•	•	
Morehouse														•
Hawai'i														
Hawai'i	•	•		•		•		•	•			•	•	
Illinois														
Finch University/Chicago Medical	•	•		•	•		•	•	•	•	•	•	•	
Chicago-Pritzker	•	•			•	•	•		•	•	•	•	•	•
Illinois, Chicago	•	•	•	•	•	•	•	•	•	•	•	•	•	
Illinois, Urbana-Champaign		•		•	•		•	•	•	•			•	•
Loyola-Stritch	•	•			•		•	•	•	•	•	•	•	

TABLE 1-B (continued)

Combined M.D.-Ph.D. Programs at U.S. Medical Schools, 1999–2000

Medical School	Anatomy	Biochemistry	Biomedical Engineering	Biophysics	Cell Biology	Genetics	Immunology	Microbiology	Molecular Biology	Neurosciences	Pathology	Pharmacology	Physiology	Other Disciplines
Illinois (Continued)														
Northwestern	•	•	•	•	•	•	•	•	•	•	•	•	•	
Rush	•	•					•	•		•		•	•	•
Indiana														
Indiana	•	•		•		•	•	•	•	•	•	•	•	
Iowa														
Iowa	•	•	•	•	•	•	•	•	•	•		•	•	•
Kansas														
Kansas	•	•			•	•	•	•	•	•	•	•	•	•
Kentucky														
Kentucky	•	•	•	•	•	•	•	•	•	•		•	•	•
Louisiana														
Louisiana State-New Orleans	•	•			•	•		•	•	•	•	•	•	
Louisiana State-Shreveport	•	•			•		•		•	•		•	•	
Tulane	•	•	•		•	•	•	•	•	•		•	•	
Maryland														
Johns Hopkins	•	•	•	•	•	•	•		•	•	•	•	•	•
Maryland	•	•	•		•	•	•	•	•	•	•	•	•	•
Uniformed Services	•	•			•			•	•	•	•		•	
Massachusetts														
Boston	•	•	•	•	•	•	•	•	•	•	•	•	•	•
Harvard		•	•	•	•	•	•	•	•	•	•	•		•
Massachusetts	•	•	•	•	•	•	•	•	•	•	•	•	•	•
Tufts	•	•			•	•	•	•	•	•	•	•	•	
Michigan														
Michigan State		•			•	•		•		•		•	•	
University of Michigan	•	•	•	•	•	•	•	•	•	•	•	•	•	
Minnesota														
Mayo		•	•	•			•		•	•		•	•	•
Minnesota—Minneapolis		•	•	•	•	•	•	•	•	•		•	•	•
Mississippi														
Mississippi	•	•						•			•	•	•	
Missouri														
Missouri—Columbia		•	•			•	•	•			•	•	•	
Saint Louis	•	•			•	•	•	•	•	•	•	•	•	
Washington University (Saint Louis)		•	•	•	•	•	•	•	•	•				•
Nebraska														
Creighton	•	•						•				•	•	
Nebraska	•	•			•	•	•	•	•	•	•	•	•	
Nevada														
Nevada		•	•		•							•	•	

TABLE 1-B (continued)

Combined M.D.-Ph.D. Programs at U.S. Medical Schools, 1999–2000

Medical School	Anatomy	Biochemistry	Biomedical Engineering	Biophysics	Cell Biology	Genetics	Immunology	Microbiology	Molecular Biology	Neurosciences	Pathology	Pharmacology	Physiology	Other Disciplines
New Hampshire														
Dartmouth		•	•		•		•	•	•			•	•	•
New Jersey														
New Jersey Medical	•	•			•	•	•	•	•	•	•	•	•	
Robert Wood Johnson		•	•		•			•				•	•	•
New York														
Albany		•			•	•	•	•	•	•	•	•	•	
Albert Einstein	•	•		•	•	•	•	•	•	•	•	•	•	
Columbia	•	•		•	•	•	•	•	•	•	•	•	•	•
Mount Sinai	•	•	•	•	•	•	•	•	•	•	•	•	•	•
New York Medical	•	•			•		•	•			•	•	•	
New York University		•		•	•	•		•	•	•	•	•	•	•
Rochester	•	•	•	•	•	•	•	•	•	•	•	•	•	•
SUNY-Buffalo	•	•		•	•	•	•	•	•	•	•	•	•	•
SUNY-Downstate									•	•				
SUNY-Stony Brook	•	•	•	•	•	•		•	•	•	•	•	•	
SUNY-Upstate	•	•			•			•		•		•	•	
Weill (Cornell)	•	•		•	•	•	•	•	•	•	•	•	•	
North Carolina														
Brody (East Carolina)	•	•			•		•	•			•	•	•	
Duke		•	•		•	•	•	•	•	•	•	•		
North Carolina	•	•	•	•	•	•	•	•	•	•	•	•	•	•
Wake Forest		•	•			•	•	•	•	•		•	•	•
North Dakota														
North Dakota	•	•			•		•	•	•			•	•	
Ohio														
Case Western Reserve		•	•	•	•	•	•	•	•	•	•	•	•	
Cincinnati	•	•		•	•	•	•	•	•	•	•	•	•	•
Medical College of Ohio					•				•	•				•
Northeastern Ohio Universities	•	•			•		•	•	•	•		•	•	•
Ohio State	•	•	•	•	•	•	•	•	•	•	•	•	•	•
Wright State														•
Oklahoma														
Oklahoma		•			•		•	•	•	•	•	•	•	
Oregon														
Oregon	•	•		•	•	•	•	•	•	•		•	•	•
Pennsylvania														
Jefferson	•	•	•		•	•	•	•	•		•	•	•	•
MCP Hahnemann					•	•	•	•	•	•	•	•	•	•
Pennsylvania State		•	•		•		•	•	•	•		•	•	•
University of Pennsylvania		•	•	•	•	•	•	•	•	•		•		•

TABLE 1-B (continued)

Combined M.D.-Ph.D. Programs at U.S. Medical Schools, 1999–2000

Medical School	Anatomy	Biochemistry	Biomedical Engineering	Biophysics	Cell Biology	Genetics	Immunology	Microbiology	Molecular Biology	Neurosciences	Pathology	Pharmacology	Physiology	Other Disciplines
Pennsylvania (continued)														
Pittsburgh	•	•	•	•	•	•	•	•	•	•	•	•	•	•
Temple	•	•			•	•	•	•	•		•	•	•	
Rhode Island														
Brown		•			•				•	•			•	•
South Carolina														
Medical University of South Carolina	•	•			•	•	•	•	•	•	•	•	•	
University of South Carolina	•				•		•	•		•	•	•	•	
Tennessee														
Meharry		•			•			•	•	•		•	•	
Tennessee-Memphis	•	•	•		•		•	•	•	•	•	•	•	
Vanderbilt		•	•	•		•	•	•	•	•	•	•	•	
Texas														
Baylor	•	•	•	•	•	•	•	•	•	•		•	•	
Texas A&M	•	•				•	•	•		•	•	•	•	
Texas Tech	•	•						•				•	•	
University of Texas														
Southwestern, Dallas		•		•	•	•	•	•	•	•				•
Galveston	•	•		•	•	•	•	•	•	•	•	•	•	•
Houston														•
San Antonio		•			•	•	•	•	•	•		•	•	•
Utah														
Utah		•			•	•	•		•					•
Vermont														
Vermont	•	•		•	•	•		•	•	•	•	•	•	•
Virginia														
University of Virginia		•	•	•	•		•	•	•	•		•	•	•
Virginia Commonwealth	•	•				•	•	•	•	•	•	•	•	•
Washington														
University of Washington		•	•	•	•	•	•	•	•	•	•	•	•	•
West Virginia														
Marshall	•	•			•	•	•	•	•	•		•	•	•
West Virginia	•	•	•		•		•	•		•	•	•	•	
Wisconsin														
Medical College of Wisconsin	•	•		•	•			•	•	•	•	•	•	
University of Wisconsin	•	•		•	•	•	•	•	•	•	•	•	•	•

TABLE 1-C

Other Combined Degree Programs at U.S. Medical Schools, 1998–99

Medical School	B.A.-M.D.	B.S.-M.D.	M.A.-M.D.	M.S.-M.D.	M.D.-J.D.	M.D.-M.B.A.	M.D.-M.P.A.	M.D.-M.P.H	Other
Alabama									
Alabama								•	
South Alabama		•							
Arizona									
Arizona								•	
California									
University of California									
Davis			•	•		•		•	
Irvine				•		•			
Loma Linda			•						
Los Angeles		•				•		•	
San Diego	•	•						•	
San Francisco				•					
Keck (Southern California)									
Stanford			•						
Colorado									
Colorado						•			
Connecticut									
Connecticut						•		•	
Yale	•				•	•		•	
District of Columbia									
George Washington	•	•							
Georgetown						•			
Howard		•							
Florida									
Florida		•			•	•			
Miami		•							
South Florida								•	M.D.-M.M.
Georgia									
Emory								•	
Illinois									
Finch University/Chicago Medical		•		•					
Illinois, Chicago	•	•			•			•	
Southern Illinois					•				
Northwestern		•				•		•	
Kentucky									
Kentucky						•		•	
Louisville			•	•		•			
Louisiana									
Louisiana State-New Orleans								•	
Tulane				•				•	

TABLE 1-C (continued)

Other Combined Degree Programs at U.S. Medical Schools, 1998–99

Medical School	B.A.-M.D.	B.S.-M.D.	M.A.-M.D.	M.S.-M.D.	M.D.-J.D.	M.D.-M.B.A.	M.D.-M.P.A.	M.D.-M.P.H.	Other
Maryland									
Johns Hopkins								•	
Maryland				•					
Massachusetts									
Boston	•		•					•	
Tufts						•		•	
Michigan									
Michigan State	•	•	•	•					
University of Michigan								•	
Minnesota									
Mayo									M.D.-O.M.S.
Missouri									
Missouri—Columbia				•					
Missouri—Kansas City	•								
Saint Louis								•	
New Hampshire									
Dartmouth						•			
New Jersey									
New Jersey Medical	•	•	•	•	•			•	
Robert Wood Johnson	•			•	•	•		•	
New York									
Albany	•	•				•			B.S.-M.S.-M.D.
Columbia				•	•			•	
Mount Sinai				•					
New York Medical								•	
New York University			•						
Rochester	•	•		•				•	
SUNY-Buffalo						•			
SUNY-Downstate	•								
SUNY-Stony Brook	•								
SUNY-Upstate	•								
North Carolina									
Brody (East Carolina)								•	
Duke					•			•	
Wake Forest			•			•			
North Dakota									
North Dakota									
Ohio									
Case Western Reserve	•	•		•	•	•		•	
Cincinnati						•			
Medical College of Ohio				•				•	

TABLE 1-C (continued)

Other Combined Degree Programs at U.S. Medical Schools, 1998–99

Medical School	B.A.-M.D.	B.S.-M.D.	M.A.-M.D.	M.S.-M.D.	M.D.-J.D.	M.D.-M.B.A.	M.D.-M.P.A.	M.D.-M.P.H.	Other
Ohio (Continued)									
Northeastern Ohio Universities		•							
Ohio State		•		•		•		•	
Oklahoma									
Oklahoma								•	
Oregon									
Oregon								•	
Pennsylvania									
Jefferson		•				•			M.D.-M.H.A.
MCP Hahnemann	•	•				•		•	
University of Pennsylvania			•	•	•				
Pittsburgh									
Temple	•	•						•	
Puerto Rico									
Ponce						•			Binary partnership with Catholic Univ. of Puerto Rico
Tennessee									
Meharry	•			•				•	
Vanderbilt					•			•	
Texas									
Baylor	•	•				•			
Texas A&M	•	•							
University of Texas Houston								•	
Utah									
Utah								•	M.D.-M.S.P.H.
Virginia									
Eastern Virginia		•						•	
University of Virginia			•	•					
Virginia Commonwealth		•						•	
Washington									
University of Washington			•						
West Virginia									
Marshall				•					
West Virginia								•	
Wisconsin									
Medical College of Wisconsin			•	•					

Options for Individuals Considering a Career in Medicine

2

The wide range of practice options and specialty choices, and the availability of locations provide substantial diversity to individuals choosing a career in medicine. Benefits include the reward of caring for others, the intellectual challenge of medicine, and the social and economic rewards of providing services that are highly valued by society. The demands of a medical career are great in terms of the time, energy, and responsibility for other people's lives, and a commitment to continuing service and education is essential.

CAREERS IN MEDICINE

• In General

Medicine offers multiple opportunities. New career options emerge with each advance in medical knowledge and with each development in the organization of medical services. The physician's responsibilities cover a wide range of functions in health maintenance, including both acute care, preventive care involving substantial patient education, and palliative care at the end of life. These responsibilities include diagnosing disease, supervising the care of patients, prescribing treatment, and participating in improved delivery of health care. Although most physicians provide direct patient care, some concentrate on basic or applied research, some become teachers or administrators, and others combine various elements of these activities. Students begin to consider these career decisions during medical school and finalize decisions near completion of medical school as they apply for residency.

• Specialties

Graduating students select an area of medicine for further training and eventual practice. Some physicians practice in one of the generalist specialties (general internal medicine, general pediatrics, or family practice). Others choose from among the following specialties: allergy and immunology, anesthesiology, dermatology, emergency medicine, obstetrics and gynecology, pathology, psychiatry, radiology, physical medicine (rehabilitation), nuclear medicine, opthalmology, and surgery (general, colon, neuro, orthopedic, plastic, thoracic, urology, vascular).

• Practice Modes

New patterns of practice are emerging. Physicians may be salaried, in partnership, or self-employed. A physician may choose from such varied settings as a Health Maintenance Organization (HMO), a managed care group practice that participates in a regional Preferred Provider Organization (PPO), private practice, clinic, hospital, laboratory, industry, military, university, government, or various combinations of these. The United States has a shortage of doctors in rural and center-city areas. Outstanding career opportunities are found in these locations.

New scientific breakthroughs have extended the limits of treatment to the young and old, and to individuals with serious, complex diseases. More and more medical care can be provided in the office, the clinic, and at home. Physicians are becoming more attuned to the promotion of health and the prevention of disease by risk screening and influencing healthier behaviors as well as to the need for palliative care at the end of life.

• AMA-FREIDA

Another valuable source to both applicants and advisors is the American Medical Association Fellowship and Residency Electronic Interactive Database Access (AMA-FREIDA) Online. The FREIDA Online is available at <http://www.ama-assn.org/freida>. FREIDA users can search all ACGME-accredited graduate medical education programs and board-approved combined specialty programs by specialty/subspecialty, state/region, program size, and educational requirements, among other variables. For AMA student and resident members, FREIDA Online provides a mailing label service. After making a search selection and viewing and saving the program listings, a student can request mailing labels at no charge for 30 or fewer programs. FREIDA Online also includes physician workforce information reported by residents and practicing physicians about their employment seeking experiences, professional job status, and work environment. For additional information, E-mail: freida@ama-assn.org.

EDUCATIONAL PREPARATION

What does it take to be a physician? Briefly, it takes physical, emotional, and intellectual stamina; the desire to work with and for people; and, particularly, the ability to use critical thinking to solve problems. The educational pipeline involves four (occasionally three) years of college, four years of medical school, and three or more years of residency.

While it has been a tradition for students to begin medical school immediately after graduation from college, several other options are now common. Some students enter a combined

TABLE 2

U.S. Medical Schools Offering Combined College-M.D. Programs Provisionally Admitting Students After Senior Year in High School, 1999–2000

Schools offering programs of instruction combined with their undergraduate division:	Schools offering programs in collaboration with other undergraduate institutions:
South Alabama	Albany
Boston	Baylor
Brown	California, Los Angeles (UCLA)
California, San Diego*	Chicago Medical
Southern California	Cincinnati
Case Western Reserve	Jefferson
Cincinnati	Medical College of Pennsylvania, Hahnemann
Florida	Meharry Medical College
George Washington	Miami*
Howard	UMDNJ—New Jersey Medical
Illinois, Chicago*†	UMDNJ—Robert Wood Johnson†
Michigan State	SUNY Brooklyn
Michigan, University of	SUNY Syracuse*
Missouri—Kansas City	Ohio, Northeastern
New York University	Pennsylvania State
Rochester	Virginia, Eastern
Northwestern	
SUNY Stony Book	
East Tennessee State	
Texas A&M*	
Wisconsin, University of	
Virginia Commonwealth	

*Program acceptance limited to state residents.

†Students are selected at the end of their sophomore year in college.

college/medical school program, delay medical school for a number of years, or choose to prepare for medical school after a successful experience in another career.

• Combined College/Medical School Programs

There are a number of programs beginning after high school graduation that combine the undergraduate college and medical school curricula. Approximately five percent of medical students begin their medical education in this path. Some of these programs result from special arrangements between a school of medicine and a particular undergraduate college and thus require enrollment in that respective undergraduate institution. For the 1999–2000 academic year, those medical schools offering combined programs accepting high school seniors into the M.D. program on a provisional basis are indicated in Table 2. Several programs are limited to residents of the state where the medical school is located. See Chapter 10 for further information about specific programs.

• Traditional Route

Most students apply to medical school during their senior year of undergraduate college. Admissions procedures are outlined in Chapter 7.

• Deferred Entry

An increasing number of medical schools consider requests from accepted applicants for a one-year deferral of their matriculation to undertakc a special opportunity or for specific personal reasons. Most schools require a specific request and review this request individually.

• Postbaccalaureate Programs

For those individuals who have completed college and perhaps embarked on another career before deciding to apply to medical school, a number of postbaccalaureate programs offer the opportunity to complete premedical courses and to participate in advising/counseling programs for premedical students. These programs are numerous and exist in every part of the country. Some provide a one- to two-year package of courses and health-related experiences for the individual who wishes to prepare on a half- or full-time schedule. Other programs are less structured and permit individuals to take premedical courses at their own pace while continuing their employment. Any U.S. medical school can provide the names of colleges and universities in the area that offer postbaccalaureate programs.

DECIDING WHEN TO APPLY

• Advice for High School Students

Choosing a medical career is a big decision, and the application process for a combined program should not be entered into lightly. High school students considering medicine need to weigh the relative advantages of combined undergraduate/medical school programs with those of the traditional route and consult carefully with high school advisors as well as appropriate college and medical school personnel in making a decision.

Medical schools accepting students in combined undergraduate college/medical school programs look for a high level of academic achievement, maturity, well-developed communication skills, intellectual abilities, and social adjustment as well as a carefully thought-through career decision. Normally students applying for combined programs will have had some health-related experience while in high school.

• Advice for College Students

By far, the majority of premedical students apply to medical school during the senior year of undergraduate college. College students are encouraged to make full use of their undergraduate experience to establish an early contact with the preprofessional advisor at their college. Chapter 3 provides more detailed information as well as links to the National Association of Advisors for the Health Professions.

Before applying, it is necessary to complete the premedical course requirements by taking or repeating the specific science and other course requirements that medical schools require of all applicants.

To complete premedical courses, postbaccalaureate students may choose between a structured program, which offers the opportunity to complete courses within one to two years, and a less structured approach, where courses are taken one at a time while the individual continues to work. Students are encouraged to investigate both types of programs, obtain information about the placement record of each, and weigh the pluses and minuses of each program with respect to their own personal needs. Prehealth advisors are available on most campuses, and postbaccalaureate students are encouraged to consult these individuals and to make use of the services provided by their offices (Chapter 3).

Postbaccalaureate students can expect their applications to be reviewed in competition with the entire applicant pool, with consideration given to both personal and academic qualifications, as discussed in Chapter 7. Admissions committees are interested in the process and experience that led to the applicant's choice of medicine as a career goal.

FINANCIAL PLANNING

In the United States, much attention is currently directed at the rising costs of acquiring a higher education and the need for more financial assistance for students. Significant amounts of aid are available, but the award of aid to medical students is generally based on financial need. Parents of students of any age seeking assistance in medical school will almost certainly be asked to file a confidential report about their income, financial assets, and liabilities.

It is important to start carefully estimating expenses for undergraduate college and medical school and analyzing the actual and potential income available from family resources, student earnings, and loans from a variety of national, regional, state, local, and institutional sources. Chapter 8 provides substantial detail regarding the types of financial aid (including loans and service commitment scholarships) available to medical students. In addition, readers are encouraged to consult the *Financial Planning and Management Manual*, available through the AAMC's Section for Publication Orders.

While substantial financial aid is available to medical students, much of this aid is in the form of loans. It is important to understand and plan for the accumulation of significant debt during medical school. In undergraduate college or during postbaccalaureate studies, it is wise to limit borrowing as much as possible. It is essential that an individual considering medicine maintain a clean credit record. The use of credit cards by undergraduates is discouraged. Good credit is required for federal loan programs. Undergraduate students may wish to work to defray expenses and reduce borrowing. Postbaccalaureate students who have accumulated financial assets during a prior career will find these assets invaluable in helping to finance both postbaccalaureate and medical studies.

Since a medical career can be financially rewarding, medical schools expect all students to fully use liquid assets to pay for medical school expenses.

OTHER HEALTH CAREERS

Applicants considering other careers are encouraged to consult the following professional associations and references.

1. American Association of Colleges of Osteopathic Medicine, Suite 310, 5500 Friendship Boulevard, Chevy Chase, Maryland 20815.
2. American Association of Colleges of Pharmacy, 1426 Prince Street, Alexandria, Virginia 22314-2841.
3. American Association of Colleges of Podiatric Medicine, Suite 322, 1350 Piccard Drive, Rockville, Maryland 20850-4307.
4. American Association of Dental Schools, 1625 Massachusetts Avenue, N.W., Suite 600, Washington, D.C. 20036-2212; <www.aads.jhu.edu>.
5. Association of American Veterinary Medical Colleges, Suite 710, 1101 Vermont Avenue, N.W., Washington, D.C. 20005-3521.
6. Association of Schools and Colleges of Optometry, Suite 510, 6110 Executive Boulevard, Rockville, Maryland 20852; <http://www.opted.org>.
7. Association of Schools of Public Health, Suite 204, 1660 L Street, N.W., Washington, D.C. 20036; <http://www.asph.org>.
8. *Health Professions Education Directory.* 27th edition. 1999–2000. $54.95, plus $8.95 for handling and shipping. Order No. OP-417599. (American Medical Association, P.O. Box 7046, Dover, Delaware 19903-7046; (800-621-8335); (312) 464-5600 (FAX); <http://www.ama-assn.org>.)
9. *270 Ways To Put Your Talent To Work in the Health Field.* Single copy, $15.00. (National Health Council, 1730 M Street, N.W., Suite 500, Washington, D.C. 20036)

INFORMATION SOURCES

For further information on educational and financial planning, the following may be of interest.

1. Cass-Liepmann, J., ed., *Cass & Birnbaum Guide to American Colleges,* 17th edition. $19.95 paperback. (Harper/Collins, Inc., Publications Department, Keystone Industrial Park, Scranton, Pennsylvania 18512.)
2. *The College Board Guide to 150 Popular Majors.* $16.00. Item #004000. Sales tax is applicable for the following states and Canada: CA, VA, PA, MA, GA, DC, WV, FL, IL, TX. Add $4.00 for postage and handling. (College Board Publications, Two College Way, Forrester Center, West Virginia 25438; Web Site: http://www.collegeboard.org.)
3. *The College Board College Costs and Financial Aid Handbook, 2000.* $21.95. Item #006283. Sales tax is applicable for the following states and Canada: CA, VA, PA, MA, GA, DC, WV, FL, IL, TX. Revised each September. Add $5.00 for postage and handling. (College Board Publications, Two College Way, Forrester Center, West Virginia 25438; Web Site: http://www.collegeboard.org.)
4. *The College Board College Handbook, 2000.* $25.95. Item #006259. Sales tax is applicable for the following states and Canada: CA, VA, PA, MA, GA, DC, WV, FL, IL, TX. Revised each September. Add $5.00 for postage and handling. (College Board Publications, Two College Way, Forrester Center, West Virginia 25438; Web Site: http://www.collegeboard.org.)
5. *Dollars for College: The Quick Guide to Scholarships, Fellowships, Loans, and Other Financial Aid Programs for Medicine, Dentistry, and Related Fields.* $7.95 prepaid. 1997. (Garrett Park Press, P.O. Box 190, Garrett Park, Maryland 20896; ISBN: 1-88077415-1.)
6. *Financial Planning and Management Manual for U.S. Medical Students, 1994.* $7.50 per copy. (Association of American Medical Colleges, 2450 N Street, N.W., Washington, D.C. 20037-1126.)
7. *The College Board Index of Majors and Graduate Degrees, 2000.* $21.95. Item #006291. Sales tax is applicable for the following states and Canada: CA, VA, PA, MA, GA, DC, WV, FL, IL, TX. Revised each September. Add $5.00 for postage and handling. (College Board Publications, Two College Way, Forrester Center, West Virginia 25438; Web Site: http://www.collegeboard.org.)
8. Keeslar, Santamaria/Santamaria *Financial Aids for Higher Education.* 1997. 17th edition. $43.00, subject to change. (Brown & Benchmark Publishers, 2460 Kerper Boulevard, Dubuque, Iowa 52004–0539; ISBN: 0-697-24151-3.)
9. *Need a Lift? College Financial Aid Handbook.* $3.00 prepaid. (The American Legion, P.O. Box 1050, Indianapolis, Indiana 46206; <http://www.legion.org>.)
10. *The Student Guide 1998–99.* U.S. Department of Education. Free. (Federal Student Aid Information Center, P.O. Box 84, Washington, D.C. 20044; 1-800-4-FED-AID, 1-800-433-3243.)

Premedical Advising

3

CHAPTER 3

Students looking into a career in medicine can get invaluable assistance from the prehealth advisor on their campus. Most U.S. colleges and universities designate an individual as the school's prehealth advisor. That person may be a faculty member, often in the sciences, who advises and teaches prehealth students and, perhaps, does scientific research; a member of the academic dean's office who oversees all academic advising at the institution; or a staff member of the school's career center, who specializes in advising on health careers. But, regardless of their specific location on campus, prehealth advisors are knowledgeable and supportive. Their role is to provide information and guidance to students preparing for a career in healthcare.

WITH WHICH STUDENTS DO PREHEALTH ADVISORS WORK?

- Anyone interested in medicine, regardless of age, or level of education, should consult with the prehealth advisor at their school or, if already graduated, their alma mater.
- Freshmen already certain that they want to pursue premedical studies should work with the prehealth advisor to get an overview of the medical school process, plan their specific courses, and develop a schedule for the upcoming years.
- All underclass students contemplating a health career can look to the advisor to learn about various professions, their requirements, and future career options.
- Students seeking to gain some health-related experience should consult the advisor to discuss possible volunteer opportunities in the local area.
- Students with academic difficulties can get help from the advisor, including referrals to other academic services on campus and a realistic assessment of the level of performance necessary for acceptance into medical school.
- Students who choose a medical career at a later point, during their college years, or after graduation, should ask the advisor about the available options for completing required course work and preparing to apply to medical school.
- Increasingly, advisors work with older or "nontraditional" students who have already graduated or have come to the school to do postbaccalaureate course work.

SPECIFICALLY, HOW CAN A PREHEALTH ADVISOR HELP YOU?

A prehealth advisor can help you:

- Determine which courses satisfy premedical requirements
- Determine the best sequence for individual courses
- Find tutoring or other academic support, if needed
- Figure out how to incorporate a study abroad program, a double major, or a senior honors thesis into the regular course of study, and still have sufficient preparation for medical school
- Seek experience in the health care field as a way of learning about the profession, as well as strengthening your medical school application
- Encourage and support students as they try to determine the best career paths for them, by taking stock of their individual strengths and weaknesses, values, and life goals.

WHAT SERVICES MIGHT A STUDENT EXPECT FROM THE PREHEALTH ADVISOR?

There are many different models of prehealth advising. Many advisors have other responsibilities on their campuses beyond advising prehealth students. Institutions vary, as well, in their organization and philosophy. Not every prehealth advisor at every college and university offers all of the services outlined below. Students are encouraged to meet with their advisor to learn which services are available to them.

Academics: All prehealth advisors can discuss course requirements and appropriate courses of study with their advisees.

- Often they know the instructors of premed courses quite well, and learn from them about key deadlines, programs, or trends in premedical and medical education.
- They may collaborate to target particular individuals or groups of students who need special attention.
- Some advisors work with academic support service staff at their college or university, to design study skills workshops or offer tutoring programs.

Volunteer/Internship Experiences: Prehealth advisors recognize the importance of health-related experience and encourage students to seek out opportunities for it.

- Some have listings of local volunteer opportunities and/or national internship programs in their offices.

- Coordinate a vacation-time "shadowing" program with alumni in medical practice.
- Design worthwhile volunteer programs with nearby health facilities, for which students receive academic credit.

Programming: Prehealth advisors frequently plan programs or sponsor speakers on campus, to help students understand the medical profession or the application process better.

- Physicians may visit as well as speak about their work.
- Admissions deans may give presentations about their schools and their admission's process.
- Financial aid officers may discuss the cost of medical school and explain how students can best position themselves before beginning their studies; and,
- Former students occasionally return to talk about their medical schools.

Personal Support: The prehealth advisor provides personal support to the many students whose goal is to become a physician, principally through individual conversations.

- An advisor's role is to encourage students to strive for their individual goals, and, at the same time, realistically convey what's necessary for success.
- Advisors may set up a peer advising program, with trained upperclassmen available to work with younger students; a mentoring program with medical students from a nearby medical school; and,
- Collaborative efforts with other professionals at their institutions who work with minority students.
- Medical schools are striving to diversify their classes and thereby reflect the U.S. population as a whole in the makeup of their classes.
- Prehealth advisors support that goal by encouraging medical school applications by minorities, providing information about special programs, and sharing accurate information regarding the current applicant pool.
- At times, minority affairs officers from nearby medical schools come to the undergraduate campus to speak with students.

Resources: All prehealth advisors have basic resources, such as the *Medical School Admission Requirements* book and CD-ROM available for their students, along with other helpful publications from the Association of American Medical Colleges (AAMC), the National Association of Advisors for the Health Professions (NAAHP), and other publishers. Key applicant and advisor information may be found on the AAMC Web site at <www.aamc.org/stuapps>.

- Listings of internships, mentors, and volunteer opportunities may be available as well.
- Many advisors distribute information on useful Internet sites that constitute a valuable resource to students interested in researching medicine, medical schools, and admissions.
- Some advisors have their own Web page as one section of their institution's Web site, available to both their own students and the general public.
- Increasingly, even high school students are accessing these sites in selecting the college or university they wish to attend.

WHAT HAPPENS WHEN YOU ARE READY TO APPLY?

When a student is ready to apply to medical school, the advisor becomes an indispensable resource. The application process for medical school is lengthy, complex, and often stressful. However, with good planning and the support of a knowledgeable advisor, these challenges can be minimized and chances of acceptance optimized. While there are no real secrets about the best way to gain acceptance into medical school, an experienced advisor will usually know more than most applicants can learn from their own research. In addition, the advisor will know about his/her own institution's experience with different medical schools.

- Prehealth advisors work with students throughout the application process to enhance each student's candidacy.
- Often, the process begins with a workshop, instruction booklet (or both), outlining the steps in the entire process. A time line aimed at preparing well and applying early, to take advantage of the rolling admissions schedule used by most medical schools, is often the first piece of advice conveyed. Advisors will discuss the Medical College Admissions Test (MCAT) with applicants, telling them when it's offered and providing the registration materials. Applicants may discuss which test date is best for them and how best to prepare for the exam.
- Although applicants can obtain the American Medical College Application Service (AMCAS) application directly from the AAMC, advisors will likely have copies available too. The advisor can explain any elements of AMCAS that are unclear to the applicant, provide any school-specific information needed to complete the application, and trouble shoot for the applicant, if necessary, by using a special advisor service that is provided by AMCAS. Also, prehealth advisors may offer suggestions for improving the personal statement that each student must write for the AMCAS application.
- Once an applicant has his/her grades and MCAT scores, the advisor can help assist students in the selection of medical school. Taking into account the student's state of residency and his/her experience with other students' applications, prehealth advisors offer some guidance about which schools are most likely to meet his/her needs.

WHAT IS THE PREHEALTH COMMITTEE LETTER OF RECOMMENDATION?

One important service prehealth advisors provide to current students, to medical schools, and to a significant number of alumni is the prehealth committee letter of recommendation. Medical schools generally prefer a composite letter written on behalf of an applicant by the college or university's prehealth committee, if there is one. The prehealth advisor may be a member of this committee; he/she may write all the letters, some of them, or none. In all cases, the advisor informs applicants about the importance of the composite letter and details what work needs to be done with the committee in order to get a letter generated by it.

Medical school admissions committees look for a concise, informative overview of a student's academic strengths; previous exposure to health care environments; contributions to campus and community; and personal qualities such as maturity, integrity, and humanitarianism. A prehealth advisor and/or committee is generally in the best position to provide that overview. The advisor can also:

- provide background on any extenuating circumstances;
- put problems or shortcomings in perspective; and,
- explain special courses, activities, and programs at the institution.

Some schools do not provide a composite letter of recommendation, but do offer advice on the appropriate letters the students need. Often, a recommendation file service is provided, whereby the office can collect individual letters of recommendation and officially mail them to the medical schools. This facilitates the process for both the student and the recommendation writer. Applicants should inquire about the specific services their prehealth advisor can provide.

HOW CAN YOU FIND A PREHEALTH ADVISOR?

If a student cannot identify a prehealth advisor on campus or at their alma mater, he/she can contact the National Association of Advisors for the Health Professions (NAAHP) or its regional affiliates. NAAHP, the principal professional association for prehealth advisors, provides students with a venue for identifying a prehealth advisor. By supporting and informing prehealth advisors, this association helps ensure that students receive accurate, up-to-date information and skilled counseling from their advisors. The association maintains close working relationships with health professions groups such as the AAMC, to keep advisors informed and to plan collaborative efforts on behalf of the students. In addition, NAAHP offers official publications to supplement the *Medical School Admission Requirements* to help students prepare for medical school.

You can visit the NAAHP Web site to learn more about this service at: <http://www.naahp.org>. There, students can search their current institution or alma mater to learn the name of the individual prehealth advisor at that college or university. For more information:

National Association of Advisors for the Health Professions (NAAHP)
P.O. Box 1518
Champaign, IL 61824-1518
Phone: (217) 355-0063
Fax: (217) 355-1287
E-mail: staff@naahp.org
Web site: http://www.naahp.org

Premedical Planning

4

CHAPTER 4

This chapter presents general recommendations for the individual who is seeking information about criteria for admission in order to plan a program that satisfies academic requirements as well as enhances the student's own intellectual, personal, and social development. Supplementary information for students from minority groups traditionally underrepresented in medicine (black Americans, Native Americans, Mexican Americans, mainland Puerto Ricans) is presented in Chapter 9.

Although the process of selecting medical school applicants necessarily involves a variety of considerations (Chapter 5), in general, medical schools are concerned with academic, nonacademic, and personal characteristics of applicants. As medical schools respond to national social issues and problems in medical care, they are making efforts to select individuals whose personal and career goals are compatible with the needs of society. Prospective applicants should give careful attention to the selection factors and school characteristics presented for each medical school listed in Part 2.

UNDERGRADUATE ACADEMIC PROGRAM

The medical profession needs individuals from diverse educational backgrounds who bring to the profession a variety of talents and interests. Educational philosophies and goals, systems of education, and specific undergraduate course requirements and other qualifications for admission vary among the nation's medical schools. All, however, recognize the importance of a strong foundation in the natural sciences (biology, chemistry, mathematics, and physics), highly developed communication skills, and a solid background in the social sciences and humanities. Although most medical schools require a minimum of three years of undergraduate work before entrance to their regular M.D. programs, the majority of entering medical students have four years of college and a baccalaureate degree.

• Science Preparation

An understanding of the principles of the sciences basic to medicine is required of entering medical students. A thorough understanding of modern concepts in biology, chemistry, and physics is necessary since the study and practice of medicine are based on these disciplines. In order to achieve the minimum level of understanding, medical schools generally require one year of biology, two years of chemistry (through organic chemistry), and one year of physics (Table 4-A). The courses should be rigorous and, in general, acceptable for students majoring in those areas. The courses should include adequate laboratory experience. The importance of these requirements is threefold: (1) to confirm interest in and capacity for proceeding further in these fields, (2) to enable medical schools to estimate an applicant's achievement and potential in these areas, and (3) to meet the requirements of state laws governing physician licensure.

Additional science courses are not required. Students may take upper-level science courses out of educational interest or to fulfill the requirements of their undergraduate major course of study. The practice of taking additional science courses that cover material taught within the medical school curriculum in the belief that they will be useful in gaining admission to medical school is not recommended.

Although only a small number of medical schools demand a specific course sequence in mathematics, all value mathematical competence, and many require or strongly recommend mathematics and computer science courses. Mathematics courses provide a good basis for the student's understanding of rigorous courses in chemistry, physics, and modern biology. Increasingly, medical schools utilize computer theory and statistics in the curriculum.

• Breadth of Education

Breadth of education is expected. The pursuit of some discipline in depth is encouraged. A successful medical student must effectively acquire, synthesize, apply, and communicate information. These are skills that can be developed through a great variety of academic disciplines. Studies in the humanities and in the social and behavioral sciences are strongly suggested.

• Advanced Work

Honors courses and independent study or research are encouraged, because they permit the student to explore, in depth, an area of knowledge and provide a scholarly experience that will facilitate a lifelong habit of self-education.

• Undergraduate Major

The selection of an undergraduate major area of study should be a carefully considered decision. Students should select a major area of study that is of interest and that will provide a foundation of knowledge necessary for the pursuit of several career alternatives. Students who select a major area of study solely or primarily because of the perception that it will enhance the chance of acceptance to a school of medicine are not making a decision in their best interest.

A science major is not a prerequisite for medical school, and students should not major in science simply because they believe this will increase their chances for acceptance. Medical schools are concerned with the overall quality and scope of undergraduate work. Students need to do well in the required premedical courses to ensure adequate preparation and favorable consideration by admission committees. For most physicians, however, the undergraduate years are the last available opportunity to pursue in depth a nonscience subject of interest, and all who hope to practice medicine should bear this in mind when selecting an undergraduate major.

Table 4-B indicates that, while there is some variation at the national level in the acceptance rates of applicants from different major fields of study in liberal arts programs, those majoring in certain areas of the humanities, for example, fared as well, or better, in gaining acceptance to the 1999–2000 entering class as applicants majoring in certain scientific disciplines. These data also show, however, that students who concentrated in such professional fields as medical technology, nursing, and pharmacy were less successful in gaining admission to medical school that year.

TABLE 4-A

Subjects Required by 10 or More U.S. Medical Schools, 2000–2001 Entering Class

Required Subject	No. of Schools (n=114)
Physics	110
Inorganic (general) chemistry	110
Organic chemistry	110
English	57
Biology	67
Biology or zoology	50
Calculus	21
Humanities	16
College mathematics	19
Social sciences	15
Behavioral sciences	13

NOTE: Figures based on data provided fall 1999. Eleven of the 125 medical schools (Florida, Northwestern, Southern Illinois, Weill, SUNY Syracuse, Northeastern Ohio, University of Pennsylvania, Medical University of South Carolina, Texas Tech, and University of Washington) did not indicate specific course requirements and are not included in the tabulations.

• Selection Factors

Decisions about the undergraduate academic program can be made more realistically if the student is aware of the medical school selection process. Medical schools review candidate qualifications in four areas: personal qualifications, academic qualifications, communication skills, and motivation. Chapter 5 discusses specific considerations for an applicant in choosing to which medical schools to apply.

• Personal Qualities

Medicine demands superior personal attributes of its students and practitioners. Integrity and responsibility assume major importance in the classroom and research laboratory as well as in relationships with patients and colleagues. Diversity within an entering class is highly desirable. Medical schools also look for evidence of other traits such as leadership, social maturity, purpose, motivation, initiative, curiosity, common sense, perseverance, and breadth of interests.

• Academic Qualifications

Medical schools seek candidates with high levels of scholastic achievement and intellectual potential, as well as the motivation and humanistic concern necessary for success as a physician. These qualities are measured by college grades, particularly science grades; recommendations from undergraduate faculty, including premedical advisors; Medical College Admission Test (MCAT) scores; interview assessments; an applicant's personal statement and application; and occasionally the use of psychological tests of educational development, mental aptitude, and nonintellectual qualities.

College grades are perhaps the most important single predictor of medical school performance in the first two years. Medical schools recognize that grading policies may differ from one college to another or even within departments of the same institution. Most first-year medical students have achieved undergraduate averages of A or B. In 1999–2000, only .3 percent of the applicants accepted to the first-year class had grade-point averages (GPAs) of equal to or less than 2.5. The mean undergraduate GPA of first-year entrants for the 1999–2000 entering class was 3.59. In recent years those individuals admitted with less than a 3.00 GPA have either achieved strikingly improved performances in their later years of college or demonstrated other characteristics deemed desirable for medicine by the various medical school admission committees.

It is also important for students to demonstrate an understanding of course content in ways other than by grades achieved. For example, the student who undertakes special projects or independent study may provide evidence of ability that is not reflected by grades alone.

• Communication Skills

Anyone considering a career as a physician must be able to relate to people effectively. The increasing emphasis on a team approach to medical care adds another dimension to the need for this skill.

• Motivation

Because of the demanding nature of both the training for and the practice of medicine, motivation is perhaps the most salient nonintellectual trait sought by most admission committees. It is assumed that a qualified applicant to medical school will have not only a general understanding of the profession but also a demonstrated interest in and knowledge of what the field of medicine encompasses. This could be accomplished, in part, by having experiences in health care settings (especially in a clinical setting), talking with health professionals, reading appropriate literature, and experiencing an exposure to research at the undergraduate level.

In all aspects of premedical planning, the prospective medical student is encouraged to consider not only the information and advice contained in this publication but also the resources and counseling available from undergraduate prehealth advisors. The prehealth advisor is an important source of information and guidance in the undergraduate institution on matters related to the application to medical school (Chapter 3).

TABLE 4-B

Acceptance to Medical School by Undergraduate Major, 1999–2000 Entering Class

Undergraduate Major	Total Applicants No.	Total Applicants % of Total	Accepted Applicants No.	Accepted Applicants % of Major
Biological Sciences				
Biology	14,249	37.0	6,137	43.1
Microbiology	1,041	2.7	431	41.4
Physiology	558	1.4	212	38.0
Science (other biology)	1,061	2.8	510	48.1
Zoology	735	1.9	327	44.5
Subtotal	17,644	45.8	7,617	43.2
Physical Sciences				
Biochemistry	2,389	6.2	1,172	49.1
Biomedical Engineering	368	1.01	212	57.6
Chemical Engineering	321	.8	173	53.9
Chemistry	2,110	5.5	1,020	48.3
Chemistry and Biology	314	.8	128	40.8
Electrical Engineering	173	.4	81	46.8
Mathematics	225	.6	99	44.0
Natural Sciences	204	.5	91	44.6
Physics	188	.5	88	46.8
Science (General)	176	.5	70	39.8
Subtotal	6,468	16.8	3,134	48.5
Nonscience Subjects				
Anthropology	329	.9	182	55.3
Economics	340	.9	193	56.8
English	463	1.2	244	52.7
Foreign Language	279	.7	142	50.9
History	414	1.1	244	58.9
Philosophy	184	.5	95	51.6
Political Science	254	.7	131	51.6
Psychobiology	304	.8	168	55.3
Psychology	1,802	4.7	769	42.7
Sociology	195	.5	85	43.6
Subtotal	4,564	11.8	2,253	49.4
Other Health Professions				
Medical Technology	170	.4	31	18.2
Nursing	267	.7	72	27.0
Pharmacy	193	.5	48	24.9
Subtotal	630	1.6	151	24.0
Mixed Disciplines				
Double Major Science	869	2.3	433	49.8
Double Major Science/Nonscience	1,487	3.9	834	56.1
Interdisciplinary Studies	221	.6	130	58.8
Premedical	563	1.5	204	36.2
Preprofessional	139	.4	66	47.5
Subtotal	3,279	8.5	1,667	50.8
Other*				
Other	5,944	15.4	2,623	44.1
Subtotal	5,944	15.4	2,623	44.1
Grand Total	38,529	100.0	17,445	45.3

*Those applicants not reporting an undergraduate major are included in "Other."
Source: AAMC Data Warehouse: Applicant Matriculant File. As of November 15, 1999.

Deciding Whether and Where to Apply to Medical School

5

CHAPTER 5

The practice of medicine has never been more challenging and rewarding, offered more opportunities for accomplishing good, or provided more selection in styles of practice and practice patterns than it does today. Deciding whether to apply to medical school must be the outcome of serious personal reflection about one's motivations and aspirations as these relate to the realities of medical practice. In this process of self-exploration, candid discussions with premedical advisors, knowledgeable faculty, and one's personal physician about the reasons for wanting to be a physician can be very helpful. Consulting books about medical education can provide an added perspective.

Medical schools have broadened the scientific foundation of medical training to include education in nutrition, geriatrics, epidemiology, environmental health and preventive medicine, medical humanities and bioethics, clinical decision making, medical socioeconomics, and the systems and cost-effective application of health care.

The more complex therapies and the special opportunities for care present complicated ethical and social questions that demand the unique guidance of the entire health care team and new interrelationships among the several health care professions. The trends named here are by no means all of the important changes that are occurring in the medical profession. Prospective medical students will want to seek more information by reading nationally distributed newspapers as well as medical periodicals, such as *The New England Journal of Medicine*.

If convinced that they genuinely want to study and practice medicine, students must decide whether they have a moderately good chance of being accepted to medical school and, if so, where to apply.

CHANCES FOR ACCEPTANCE

• Total Applications/Percent Matriculated

Admission to medical school has always been highly competitive. However, it is important for each applicant to assess his or her competitiveness relative to the applicant pool at the time of application. Over the period 1988–96, the applicant pool increased, making it more competitive for applicants to gain admission to medical school, but this increase has leveled off. For the 1988 entering class, 59.8 percent of the 26,721 candidates who applied matriculated; whereas, for the 1996 entering class 34.5 percent of the 46,968 candidates who applied matriculated. For the 1999 entering class, 42.1 percent of 38,529 applicants matriculated.

• Grades/MCAT Scores

Although many factors other than college grades and test scores enter into the admission decision, these two factors receive considerable attention in the preliminary review of each application. In 1999, 82.9 percent of matriculants had undergraduate grade-point averages (GPAs) of 3.26 or above. The majority of accepted applicants with GPAs below 3.26 achieved relatively high scores on the nationally standardized preadmission examination for medical school applicants, the Medical College Admission Test (MCAT). Only 4.6 percent of 1999 accepted applicants had GPAs lower than 3.0.

• Other Admissions Considerations

It is important to recognize that medical schools consider not only grades and test scores but also such factors as personality, character, place of residence, career plans, motivation and interest in medicine, communication and interpersonal skills, leadership, critical thinking skills, maturity, integrity, empathy, level of difficulty of course work, and whether the applicant is from a minority and/or disadvantaged background.

Again, students are encouraged to consult their premedical advisors, who ordinarily have access to pertinent data regarding the success of applicants from their institutions.

Admission committees understand that grades may not always measure a student's true ability; extenuating circumstances, such as prolonged illness, unsettled family circumstances, or the need to work while in school, can affect academic performance.

The relationship between MCAT performance and performance in specific undergraduate courses can be evaluated through the examination of individual test scores. A low score in the physical sciences may reflect the fact that a student has not completed introductory college-level physics prior to taking the test. Admission committees take such circumstances into consideration when evaluating an application. Although schools encourage students to schedule the MCAT, where possible, for a time when the premedical prerequisites are complete.

MEDICAL SCHOOL CHARACTERISTICS

• Medical School Accreditation

All medical schools listed in this resource maintain the high standards necessary for accreditation by the Liaison Committee on Medical Education (LCME). Most have similar basic undergraduate course requirements, and all seek to admit students with demonstrated learning, critical thinking, and communication skills and with the qualities of integrity, maturity, and caring.

The Association of American Medical Colleges (AAMC) and all its member schools strongly endorse the principle of equal opportunity for education and practice in the health professions without regard to sex, age, race, creed, national origin, disability, or sexual orientation. (See AAMC Position on Equal Opportunity.)

Medical schools differ, however, with respect to other factors, for example, policies and requirements regarding state or regional residence. They also vary considerably in such characteristics as size of student body, size of faculty, number and type of patients with whom medical students will have contact, general philosophy of education, geographic location, student services, sources of financial support, and opportunities for special activities such as research. Moreover, opportunities for postgraduate study and the aspects of medicine generally chosen as career paths by graduates differ among medical schools as well.

It is important to review the individual school entries in Part II of this book to identify the specific medical schools that meet an individual's needs, and appear to be competitive choices, given the individual's qualifications.

STATE AND REGIONAL RESIDENCE POLICIES

The residence restrictions noted in the individual entries in Chapters 10 and 11 are generally not subject to change. State-supported medical schools are required to give preference to state residents; some state-supported schools consider nonresidents only under the Early Decision Program discussed in Chapter 7. Some schools have requirements with respect to counties or regions of the state. State residents pay a substantially lower tuition in publicly supported schools. Some private schools give preference to residents of the state in which the school is located, because the school receives its financial support from its state government. Some states without medical schools within their boundaries participate in special interstate and regional agreements. These and similar arrangements are described later in this section.

• Residency Data

Table 5-A shows the number of applicants, new entrants, and total enrollment for each medical school. Within each of these categories, percentages of in-state residents and women are also provided. For applicants and new entrants the in-state figure represents the percentage of individuals in that category who claim as their legal residence the state in which the medical school is located. (For example, of the 1,548 applicants to the University of Alabama, 30.5 percent were Alabama residents; and of the 160 new entrants, 88.1 percent were Alabama residents.) Overall, 67.8 percent of 1999–2000 first-year students entered schools within their own states; 86.7 percent of public school entrants and 39.5 percent of private school entrants were in-state residents. Selection by a public school in

AAMC Position on Equal Opportunity

The Association strongly reaffirms the principle of equal opportunity for individuals who are qualified for education and training in, and the practice of, the health professions, without regard to sex, race, creed, color, national origin, age, or handicap. In pursuit of this principle and policy, the AAMC:

1. Requests member institutions to continue to monitor their admission policies and practices to ensure equal opportunity of admission to their educational and training programs.
2. Requests member institutions to continue to undertake and to reinforce programs of affirmative action to increase the numbers and proportions of students in the health professions from groups that are presently underrepresented in those professions.

Further, recognizing that the underrepresentation of some groups in health professions educational and training programs is but a symptom of broad social and economic problems, the AAMC:

1. Actively supports the organized study of the basic causes of underrepresentation and possible cures.
2. Actively supports the initiation of new programs, and the broadening of existing programs, which are designed to overcome these problems. These programs include, but are not limited to, those designed to permit women to fulfill their educational-professional goals and their cultural roles without sacrifice to either, programs designed to eliminate economic barriers to education in the health professions, and programs designed to develop increased interest in careers in the health professions on the part of members of underrepresented groups at the secondary school and college levels.

another state is highly improbable unless the nonresident candidate has exceptionally strong credentials.

An applicant may be a resident of only one state at any given time. In view of the relationship between geographic residence and chances for admission, applicants are strongly urged to clarify their official residency status, if it is uncertain, with the schools of their choice prior to making formal application. In most instances, the committee on admission will be responsible for official residency rulings regarding medical school applicants or will know what university office is responsible. University definitions of residency status may not always be identical with definitions of "legal residency" used for other purposes (for example, to determine liability for payment of state income taxes or voting registration).

The individual school entries in Chapters 11 and 12 present nonresident statistics and note preference given to applicants on the basis of residence.

• Special Opportunities for Residents of Some States

Three interstate agreements that provide special opportunities for residents of some states are:

WICHE. All accredited western medical schools except the University of Washington participate in the Western Interstate Commission for Higher Education (WICHE) Professional Student Exchange Program. After certification by their states, students from Montana and Wyoming can attend a participating school and pay the in-state tuition at a public institution or a reduced tuition at a private school. The student's home state then pays a support fee to the receiving school. In order to qualify for WICHE certification, a student must be a legal resident of the sending state and meet its eligibility requirements. Receiving WICHE certification does not guarantee admission to a participating school, however. Students must also apply directly to the participating schools of their choice, where they are considered on the basis of each school's admission criteria. Because funds available to the sending states for payment of support fees are limited, it is also possible that some students cannot be supported by their home states as exchange students, even though they are otherwise qualified for the exchange program. Further information is available from:

Professional Student Exchange Program
Western Interstate Commission for
Higher Education
P.O. Box 9752
Boulder, Colorado 80301-9752

WWAMI. The University of Washington School of Medicine serves as the medical school for the five states of Washington, Wyoming, Alaska, Montana, and Idaho (WWAMI). The WWAMI program of decentralized regional medical education began in 1971. Through this program, students from Alaska, Idaho, Montana, and Wyoming are admitted to the University of Washington School of Medicine and pay in-state tuition and fees. Under the supervision of the University of Washington School of Medicine, students from these states take their first year of medical school at participating universities in their home states. All students spend their second year at the University of Washington in Seattle. Clerkship opportunities are available for third- and fourth-year students throughout the WWAMI region. This decentralized medical education program serves the health care needs of states without medical schools by offering an opportunity for a larger number of individuals from these states to obtain a medical education. Additional information about the WWAMI program is available from:

Admissions Office
School of Medicine, Box 356340
University of Washington
Seattle, Washington 98195-6340
E-mail: askuwsom@u.washington.edu

Southern Regional Education Board Program. Certain students from the states of Alabama, Georgia, North Carolina, and Tennessee who are accepted at Meharry Medical College pay a reduced tuition under a program administered by the Southern Regional Education Board. Similar arrangements exist for a certain number of students from Georgia who are accepted at Morehouse School of Medicine. Georgia residents also have this opportunity at Emory University and Mercer University School of Medicine. Further information is available from:

Southern Regional Education Board
592 Tenth Street, N.W.
Atlanta, Georgia 30318-5790

• Citizenship

In 1999–2000, 155 foreign students entered the first-year class.

Prospective applicants from other countries should study carefully the application considerations and admission criteria discussed in this resource, since they apply equally to both U.S. and non-U.S. citizens. Successful applicants from other countries will ordinarily have completed several years of their undergraduate college work in the United States. Proficiency in the English language is required, and medical schools may require proficiency certification either from the appropriate official agency in the applicant's own country or from the American undergraduate college the applicant has attended.

A majority of U.S. schools are required to give preference to applicants from their own states or regions.

Most of the financial aid available for use at U.S. medical schools comes from federal sources, which require U.S. citizenship or permanent residency. Since some countries impose severe restrictions on the exportation of currency, applicants should investigate the accessibility of financial resources before applying. In no case should foreign applicants assume that financial aid will be available in the United States. Foreign applicants should be prepared to present detailed plans for financing their medical education.

(Text continued on page 38)

TABLE 5-A

U.S. Medical School Applicants and New Entrants by Residence and Sex, 1999–2000

	Applicants			New Entrants		
Medical School[1]	Total	Percent In-State	Percent Women	Total	Percent In-State	Percent Women
Alabama	1,548	30.5	43.2	160	88.1	40.0
Alabama, South	1,008	42.7	41.6	64	89.1	60.9
Albany	7,110	24.0	43.2	124	34.7	50.8
Albert Einstein	7,096	23.8	43.6	180	44.4	53.9
Arizona	1,089	49.9	41.5	100	100.0	45.0
Arkansas	675	46.5	38.1	144	97.2	32.6
Baylor	2,041	51.5	46.5	167	77.2	48.5
Boston	9,941	6.8	45.2	150	25.3	35.3
Brody (East Carolina)	1,459	51.7	43.9	72	100.0	45.8
Brown	129	8.5	56.6	65	13.8	55.4
California, University of						
Davis	4,255	81.3	44.1	93	100.0	54.8
Irvine	3,812	89.6	43.2	92	100.0	45.7
Los Angeles (UCLA) (and Drew program)	7,358	65.3	44.6	170	84.7	55.3
San Diego	4,625	71.3	43.9	122	96.7	39.3
San Francisco (and Berkeley program)	5,152	51.5	44.8	153	75.8	54.2
Caribe	923	35.9	44.9	60	80.0	53.3
Case Western Reserve	6,570	14.7	43.2	145	54.5	40.0
Chicago Medical	9,081	12.7	41.7	165	36.4	38.2
Chicago-Pritzker	7,485	13.7	43.4	104	38.5	50.0
Cincinnati	3,716	32.5	43.2	159	84.9	37.7
Colorado	2,347	27.7	42.5	122	87.7	50.8
Columbia	3,186	24.0	47.5	152	27.0	41.4
Connecticut	2,167	15.5	48.4	77	77.9	55.8
Creighton	4,672	5.0	37.6	115	11.3	50.4
Dartmouth	6,271	1.1	42.4	72	11.1	51.4
Duke	5,728	6.6	40.5	100	17.0	45.0
Emory	6,948	8.5	45.4	111	38.7	46.8
Florida (and FSU/FAMU/UWF program)	3,122	63.2	43.3	115	93.9	47.0
Florida, South	1,619	76.0	43.5	96	100.0	46.9
George Washington	9,693	0.5	46.0	151	2.0	47.0
Georgetown	8,373	0.5	43.7	171	5.3	46.2
Georgia, Medical College of	1,519	52.8	44.0	180	98.9	34.4
Harvard	6,097	7.3	41.3	165	12.7	44.8

TABLE 5-A (continued)

U.S. Medical School Applicants and New Entrants by Residence and Sex, 1999–2000

Medical School[1]	Applicants Total	Applicants Percent In-State	Applicants Percent Women	New Entrants Total	New Entrants Percent In-State	New Entrants Percent Women
Hawai'i	1,099	15.7	40.9	62	83.9	43.5
Howard	5,341	0.7	49.7	110	3.6	49.1
Illinois, Southern	1,492	70.3	42.6	72	100.0	45.8
Illinois, University of	4,193	40.3	43.5	300	94.0	38.7
Indiana	2,171	28.9	42.7	280	92.9	39.6
Iowa	2,512	13.2	42.2	157	72.0	41.4
Jefferson	8,204	12.7	43.3	223	39.9	46.2
Johns Hopkins	2,775	9.2	48.2	119	12.6	40.3
Kansas	1,424	29.3	41.8	175	87.4	42.3
Keck (Southern Cal.)	5,712	57.2	42.9	174	83.9	36.2
Kentucky	1,380	33.5	40.0	95	91.6	43.2
Loma Linda	3,788	47.3	40.9	159	50.9	43.4
Louisiana State—New Orleans	1,236	64.4	42.7	165	100.0	42.4
Louisiana State—Shreveport	947	73.8	43.4	100	100.0	44.0
Louisville	1,472	30.6	43.5	141	87.9	48.2
Loyola-Stritch	7,910	17.5	43.9	130	50.0	46.2
Marshall	953	30.8	41.3	48	97.9	50.0
Maryland	3,328	24.8	49.1	138	83.3	59.4
Massachusetts	1,329	62.7	48.8	100	100.0	55.0
Mayo	3,346	10.0	40.6	42	35.7	59.5
MCP Hahnemann	7,568	12.9	47.5	235	45.1	60.9
Meharry	4,361	5.1	48.5	80	22.5	63.8
Mercer	1,042	53.2	43.0	54	100.0	42.6
Miami	2,148	56.2	44.4	143	99.3	55.2
Michigan State	3,232	32.6	46.0	105	81.9	54.3
Michigan, University of	5,095	18.2	40.6	171	55.0	44.4
Minnesota—Duluth[2]	842	56.3	43.5	52	92.3	55.8
Minnesota—Minneapolis	1,885	38.8	44.6	166	88.0	45.2
Mississippi	592	51.0	43.6	100	100.0	42.0
Missouri—Columbia	933	51.0	42.0	96	100.0	47.9
Missouri—Kansas City	71	74.6	57.7	71	74.6	57.7
Morehouse	2,872	10.7	52.2	40	65.0	67.5
Mount Sinai	7,978	23.3	45.4	105	54.3	48.6
Nebraska	927	35.3	41.1	120	91.7	43.3
Nevada	848	20.5	40.6	55	87.3	36.4

TABLE 5-A (continued)

U.S. Medical School Applicants and New Entrants by Residence and Sex, 1999–2000

Medical School[1]	Applicants			New Entrants		
	Total	Percent In-State	Percent Women	Total	Percent In-State	Percent Women
New Jersey:						
UMDNJ—New Jersey Medical	2,756	37.2	50.4	170	93.5	46.5
UMDNJ—Robert Wood Johnson	2,483	42.4	49.2	155	87.7	47.7
New Mexico	1,090	30.2	47.3	73	97.3	53.4
New York Medical	9,372	19.5	43.0	184	34.3	47.3
New York University	3,647	27.8	47.9	160	50.0	46.3
New York:						
SUNY—Brooklyn	3,110	68.3	49.2	189	96.3	48.1
SUNY—Buffalo	2,198	82.2	45.2	142	99.3	54.2
SUNY—Stony Brook	3,310	66.1	47.4	100	100.0	49.0
SUNY—Syracuse	2,758	72.4	47.1	153	95.4	38.6
North Carolina	2,970	27.5	44.7	160	87.5	50.0
North Dakota	289	26.6	45.3	57	71.9	52.6
Northwestern	8,748	12.6	43.7	170	26.5	45.9
Ohio, Medical College of	3,136	35.7	40.2	140	90.7	35.7
Ohio, Northeastern	1,109	72.7	40.8	105	95.2	47.6
Ohio State	3,334	36.3	40.2	210	82.[illegible]	39.5
Oklahoma	1,050	30.5	40.5	150	92.[illegible]	38.7
Oregon	2,499	11.4	44.1	96	78.[illegible]	41.7
Pennsylvania State	6,414	16.0	43.5	106	49.1	48.1
Pennsylvania, University of	6,633	11.7	43.4	144	19.[illegible]	45.8
Pittsburgh	4,629	19.5	43.9	145	49.[illegible]	52.4
Ponce	999	36.5	44.2	59	76.[illegible]	42.4
Puerto Rico	899	38.2	45.6	110	93.[illegible]	50.0
Rochester	5,941	24.1	44.2	100	43.[illegible]	48.0
Rush	4,573	31.6	45.2	119	79.[illegible]	48.7
Saint Louis	5,492	7.3	38.8	151	33.[illegible]	47.7
South Carolina, Medical University of	2,063	24.3	44.9	139	95.[illegible]	46.0
South Carolina, University of	1,314	33.3	44.2	74	94.[illegible]	37.8
South Dakota	654	19.3	42.0	50	88.[illegible]	42.0
Stanford	6,476	36.1	42.7	86	44.[illegible]	53.5
Temple	7,500	13.9	44.2	206	63.[illegible]	35.0
Tennessee State, East	1,470	38.5	40.3	60	83.3	53.3
Tennessee, University of	1,652	37.4	43.9	162	88.9	37.0
Texas A&M	2,306	65.2	44.9	78	94.9	56.4
Texas Tech	1,484	95.8	42.0	123	91.9	36.6

TABLE 5-A (continued)

U.S. Medical School Applicants and New Entrants by Residence and Sex, 1999–2000

	Applicants			New Entrants		
Medical School[1]	Total	Percent In-State	Percent Women	Total	Percent In-State	Percent Women
Texas, University of						
Dallas (Southwestern)	2,543	80.8	44.0	203	84.2	37.9
Galveston	2,600	84.9	44.3	200	97.0	40.5
Houston	2,652	83.1	44.6	202	96.5	39.6
San Antonio	2,643	83.6	43.9	204	93.6	52.5
Tufts	9,369	7.7	45.4	168	29.8	43.5
Tulane	8,285	6.3	42.2	152	16.4	42.1
Uniformed Services University	2,473	7.1	32.7	165	9.7	26.1
Utah	1,336	31.2	31.6	102	73.5	39.2
Vanderbilt	4,459	6.2	40.0	103	9.7	41.7
VCU/MCV	4,152	21.4	43.4	172	70.3	43.0
Vermont	5,836	1.6	43.2	95	33.7	56.8
Virginia, Eastern	3,958	20.4	47.0	102	67.6	45.1
Virginia, University of	4,181	19.2	45.2	139	66.9	48.9
Wake Forest	5,439	12.4	41.7	108	62.0	41.7
Washington University (St. Louis)	5,086	4.5	41.8	121	8.3	51.2
Washington, University of[3]	3,056	31.0	44.6	175	87.4	57.7
Wayne State	3,171	37.9	43.6	252	89.7	45.2
Weill *(Cornell)*	6,845	20.7	44.3	101	44.6	54.5
West Virginia	1,012	29.7	43.0	88	94.3	43.2
Wisconsin, Medical College of	5,368	9.9	40.3	204	46.1	36.8
Wisconsin, University of	2,230	24.9	45.2	146	89.0	57.5
Wright State	3,068	35.6	46.1	90	88.9	55.6
Yale	2,439	4.5	47.0	104	7.7	45.2
Total[4]	38,529	n/a	45.2	16,221	n/a	45.7

Source: AAMC Data Warehouse: Applicant Matriculant File. As of November 15, 1999.

Notes:
[1] Italics indicate privately supported schools.
[2] Two-year school of basic medical sciences.
[3] In-state residents include residents of Alaska, Idaho, Montana, and Wyoming.
[4] These applicants submitted a total of 454,380 applications.

• Age

Medical schools review applications without regard to the candidate's age.

The proportion of older applicants has decreased slightly since 1996. For the 1999–2000 entering class, 27.3 percent of the 2,355 applicants who were 32 years or older were accepted; this represents about 3.7 percent of the total number of accepted applicants. Additional information will be found in Chapter 2.

• Disabled Applicants

Medical school graduates must have the knowledge and skills to function in a broad variety of clinical situations and to render a wide spectrum of patient care. Schools may ask applicants to respond to a statement of technical standards, describing the standards expected of students who will be candidates for the M.D. degree. Applicants may be questioned on their ability to meet these standards and may be asked to provide documentation to support their statement.

The LCME standards for accreditation of medical schools state: "While physical disability should not preclude a student from consideration for admission, each school should develop and publish technical standards for the admission of handicapped applicants, in accordance with legal requirements." The AAMC has distributed information regarding the development of technical standards by institutions to ensure that admission policies of medical schools are in compliance with the Americans with Disabilities Act (ADA).

• Special Information for Women

The AAMC continues to assist medical schools in creating an educational environment as conducive to the professional development of women as it is to that of men. Currently, about 20 percent of U.S. physicians are women, up from less than 8 percent in 1970. The proportion of women in the applicant pool has increased to 45.2 percent (Table 5-C). In 1970–71, 2,734 women and 22,253 men applied to medical school. The corresponding figures for 1999–2000 were 17,433 and 21,096 (Table 5-D). In 1999–2000 the acceptance rates of both men and women were virtually the same, 44.9 percent and 45.8 percent, respectively. Data for 1994–95 were essentially the same as well. Many of these individuals have acquired experience in another health career or in community service.

Table 5-A shows the proportion of new entrants into each U.S. medical school who are women. Large school-to-school variations are apparent, from a low of 26.1 percent to a high of 67.5 percent. At 40 schools, women make up at least 50 percent of new entrants. In recent years the proportion of minorities who are women has been increasing; in 1999–2000, 59.2 percent of those minorities accepted were women.

Women considering medicine as a career often have questions about the medical school environment, future career options, and combining a medical career with parenting responsibilities. Changes in the health care system are creating opportunities in primary care and team building that women physicians are particularly well positioned to lead. Likewise, with increasing attention being focused on women's health needs, there has never been a more exciting time for women to enter the medical field.

Overall, women currently in practice report a high level of satisfaction with both their professional and personal lives. Approximately two-thirds of practicing physicians have children, and medical students are increasingly likely to meet female residents and faculty members who are also mothers. For applicants with questions along these lines, student chapters of the American Medical Women's Association (AMWA), present at many of the medical schools, can be good resources. Some of the local AMWA chapters offer housing arrangements for women applicants interviewing at their institution. At schools without such chapters, the admission office may be able to provide names of local women physicians who could talk with applicants about their experiences in the practice of medicine.

Women students are finding more women faculty members at medical schools each year. Since 1968 the percentage of women faculty in U.S. medical schools has grown from 13.3 percent to 26 percent. However, women are far from being proportionately represented in leadership positions in academic medicine. Only 10 percent of women faculty are full professors, compared to 31 percent of men faculty. The low number of women reaching this rank partially explains the low number of women who chair academic departments; there are currently about 183 women chairs.

• Women in Medicine Program

The AAMC's Women in Medicine Program, steered by its Women in Medicine Coordinating Committee, works on programs and avenues to address this paucity of women leaders. This includes annual Women in Medicine professional development seminars for junior and senior faculty desiring to increase their leadership skills. All U.S. medical schools and many teaching hospitals have designated an individual to serve as the Women Liaison Officer (WLO) to the AAMC and with others outside their medical centers on matters of special interest and concern to women in academic medicine. WLOs are periodically surveyed regarding the activities they have initiated to improve the environment for women students and faculty at their institutions. Their responses are compiled into a handbook and distributed among the WLOs. The name and address of the WLO at any institution and data about women in medical education are available from:

Staff, Women in Medicine Program
Division of Institutional Planning
and Development
Association of American Medical Colleges
2450 N Street, N.W.
Washington, D.C. 20037-1126
<http://www.aamc.org>

RESOURCES FOR AND REFERENCES ABOUT WOMEN IN MEDICINE

Women with questions that pertain more to the practice of medicine than to medical education are encouraged to contact the AMA Department of Women in Medicine (515 N. State St., Chicago, Illinois 60610; (312) 464-4392), or AMWA (801 North Fairfax Street, Alexandria, Virginia 22314; (703) 838-0500); <http://www.amwa–doc.org>. The American Medical Students Association (1890 Preston White Drive, Reston, Virginia 22091; (703) 620-6600) has a Standing Committee on Women in Medicine that can connect female students to sources of support and information. As noted above, many medical schools have student AMWA chapters. Moreover, AMWA publishes the *Journal of the American Medical Women's Association,* which includes diverse articles of interest to women physicians and medical students.

• References About Women in Medicine

The books and articles included in the following bibliography are also valuable resources. Familiarity with information included in any of the following may be of great advantage in responding to interviewers' questions, especially inquiries related to combining family and career, and to gender-related issues in medicine.

1. Association of Women Surgeons. *Pocket Mentor: A Manual for Surgical Residents.* Westmont, Illinois: AWS, 1996 (708/655-0394).
2. Bickel, J., Croft, K. *Women in Medicine: Getting in, Surviving and Advancing.* Sage Publishers. March 2000.
3. Bickel, J. Scenarios for Success—Enhancing Women Physicians' Professional Advancement. *Western Journal of Medicine,*162:165–9, 1995.
4. Bickel, J., Croft, K., and Marshall, R., *Enhancing the Environment for Women in Academic Medicine: Resources and Pathways.* Washington, DC: AAMC, 1996.
5. Bickel, J., Povar, G. Women as Health Professionals: Contemporary Issues. *Encyclopedia of Bioethics,* ed. W. Reich, New York: Simon and Schuster, 1995.
6. Bickel, J., Ruffin, A. Gender-associated Differences in Matriculating and Graduating Medical Students. *Academic Medicine,* 70:552-559, June 1994.
7. Bongiovi, M., et al. Maternity Leave Experiences of Resident Physicians. *Journal of the American Medical Women's Association,* 48 (6): 185–93, 1993.
8. Carr, P., et. al., Comparing the Status of Women and Men in Academic Medicine. *Annals of Internal Medicine,* 119:908–13, 1993.
9. Crandall, S.J., et al., Medical Students' Attitudes Toward Providing Care for the Underserved: Are We Training Socially Responsible Physicians? *Journal of the American Medical Association,* 269: 2519–23, 1993.
10. Elgin, S.H., *Genderspeak: Men, Women, and the Gentle Art of Verbal Self-Defense.* New York, NY: John Wiley & Sons, 1993.
11. Fried, L., et al., Career Development for Women in Academic Medicine: Multiple Interventions in One Department of Medicine, *Journal of the American Medical Association,*176:898–905, 1996.
12. Hostler, S. and Gressard, R., Perceptions of Gender Fairness of the Medical Education Environment, *Journal of the American Medical Women's Association,* 48:51–57, 1993.
13. Jeruchim, J. and Shapiro, P. *Women, Mentors, and Success.* New York: Ballantine Books, 1992.
14. Klebanoff, M.A., et. al. Outcomes of Pregnancy in a National Sample of Resident Physicians. *New England Journal of Medicine,* 323:1040–45, 1990.
15. Komaromy, J., et al., Sexual Harassment in Medical Training, *New England Journal of Medicine,* 328:322–326, 1993.
16. Lenhart, S., Evans C. Sexual harassment of gender discrimination: A primer for women physicians. *Journal of American Medical Womens' Association,* 46:77–82, May/June 1991.
17. Levinson, W., Tolle, S. W., and Lewis, C. Women in Academic Medicine: Combining Career and Family. *New England Journal of Medicine,* 321:1511–7, 1989.
18. Lillemoe, K., et. al. Surgery—Still an "Old Boys" Club? *Surgery,* 116:255–61, 1994.
19. Mendelsohn, K., et. al. Sex and Gender Bias in Anatomy and Physical Diagnosis Text Illustrations. *Journal of the American Medical Association,* 272:1267–70, 1994.
20. Morantz-Sanchez, R. *Sympathy & Science: Women Physicians in American Medicine.* 1987. $12.95. ISBN: 0195049853. (Oxford University Press, (800) 451-7556).
21. Sandrick, J. The Residency Experience: The Woman's Perspective. *American College of Surgeons Bulletin,* 77:10–17, August 1992.
22. Sonnert, G. and Holton, G., *Who Succeeds in Science? The Gender Dimension,* Camden, NJ: Rutgers University Press, 1995.
23. Tannen, D. *Talking from 9 to 5: Language, Sex and Power.* New York: Ballantine Books, 1990.
24. Tesch, B., et. al. Promotion of Women Physicians: Glass Ceiling or Sticky Floor? *Journal of the American Medical Association,* 273:1022-5, 1995.
25. Wear, D. (ed.), *Women in Medical Education: An Anthology of Experience,* Albany, NY: SUNY Press, 1996.
26. Wear, D. and Nixon, L.L. *Literary Anatomies: Women's Bodies and Health in Literature.* Ithaca: SUNY Press, 1994. $15.00 (607/277-2211).

INFORMATION ABOUT FINANCIAL AID AND SPECIAL PROGRAMS

Because of the strong national movement encouraging women to pursue professional careers, a number of informational resources have been designed specifically for women.

The following list of published resources was developed from a publication prepared by the Project on the Status and Education of Women (Association of American Colleges, 1818 R Street, N.W., Washington, D.C. 20009).

1. American Fellowships and Selected Professions Fellowships, American Association of University Women (AAUW) Educational Foundation, 2201 N. Dodge Street, Department 67, Iowa City, Iowa 52243–4030; (319) 337-1716, ext. 67. Awarded to American women to conduct research or study in the final year at the following levels: dissertation and post-doctoral in any field of study and selected professions (including medicine and osteopathic medicine underrepresented for minorities). Request announcement flier and applications from August through November only. Applications must be postmarked for dissertation/post-doctoral by November 15 and for selected professions by December 15.

2. American Medical Women's Association (AMWA), Medical Education Loan Program, 801 North Fairfax Street, Suite 400, Alexandria, Virginia 22314. Women in their first, second, or third year of medical school are eligible to apply. Loans of $2,000 to $2,500 at 10 percent interest are granted. Applicants must be U.S. citizens or permanent residents attending a U.S. institution full time and be student members of AMWA. No interest until after graduation.

   American Medical Women's Association Wilhelm-Frankowski Medical Education Scholarship of $4,000 to women in their first, second, or third year of medical school. Applicants must be U.S. citizens or permanent residents attending a U.S. institution full time and be student members of AMWA. Criteria include community service, AMWA activities, and women's health. Web Site: http://www.amwa-doc.org; or contact Marie Glanz at <mglanz@amwa-doc.org>.

3. Business and Professional Women's Foundation Scholarship Program, 2012 Massachusetts Avenue, N.W., Washington, D.C. 20036–1070. This program awards scholarships to nontraditional female students with critical financial need who are seeking the education necessary for entry into, re-entry into, or advancement within the work force. Applicants must be 25 years of age or older, have U.S. citizenship, and be within 24 months of completing an accredited program at a U.S. institution. Applicants may be full- or part-time students in the fields of computer science, teacher education, paralegal studies, engineering, science, or professional (J.D., M.D., D.D.S.) degrees. Applications are available only between October 1 and April 1. The deadline is April 15. To receive additional information, submit a business-size, self-addressed, double-stamped envelope to the above address for each request.

4. *Financial Aid for Minorities in Health Fields.* 1996. $5.95. ISBN 0-912048-96-4. (Garrett Park Press, P.O. Box 190, Garrett Park, Maryland 20896)

5. Schlachter, G. A. *Directory of Financial Aids for Women.* 1999–2001 Published since 1977. $45, plus $5 shipping. (Reference Service Press, 5000 Windplay Drive, Suite 4, El Dorado Hills, CA 95762.) ISBN 0-918276-80-2. A list of over 1,700 scholarships, fellowships, loans, grants, internships, awards, and prizes is available to women. Also included are a list of state sources of educational benefits and a bibliography of financial aid directories.

Information about other sources of medical student financing is presented in Chapter 8.

• Marital Status

Medical school admission decisions are made without regard to marital status.

• Minority Status

Efforts continue to be made to encourage better representation in medical schools of students from racial/ethnic groups underrepresented in medicine and students from nontraditional or economically disadvantaged backgrounds. Medical schools focus their affirmative action recruitment on ethnic minority groups that have been traditionally underrepresented among the physician work force in the United States. These groups are black Americans, mainland Puerto Ricans, Mexican Americans, and Native Americans (including American Indians, Alaskan Natives, and Native Hawaiians).

Many schools have programs directed at the preparation of the prospective minority medical school applicant; recruitment and retention programs; programs that offer funds for scholarships to minority undergraduate and medical students; establishment of more direct relationships between the medical schools and the predominantly minority colleges; and special projects, such as summer study programs, for minority undergraduate students.

Table 5-F shows first-year new entrants and total enrollments, by racial/ethnic categories, for 1999–2000. Chapter 9 provides more detailed information and a list of information sources for minority group students.

TABLE 5-B

Acceptance Rates of Applicants by Sex and by Age at Anticipated Enrollment, 1997 Through 1999 First-Year Classes

1997	All Applicants				By Gender							
					Men				Women			
	Applicants		Acceptees		Applicants		Acceptees		Applicants		Acceptees	
	No.	%	No.	%	No.	%	No.	%	No.	%	No.	%
Age												
20 and Under	719	1.7	500	2.9	378	1.5	266	2.7	341	1.9	234	3.1
21–23	22,682	52.7	10,832	62.6	12,498	50.5	5,987	60.9	10,184	55.7	4,845	64.7
24–27	12,667	29.4	4,069	23.5	7,751	31.3	2,482	25.3	4,916	26.9	1,587	21.2
28–31	3,921	9.1	1,175	6.8	2,423	9.8	699	7.1	1,498	8.2	476	6.4
32–34	1,353	3.1	373	2.2	777	3.1	205	2.1	576	3.2	168	2.2
35–37	707	1.6	163	0.9	400	1.6	90	0.9	307	1.7	73	1
38 and Over	971	2.3	201	1.2	520	2.1	99	1	451	2.5	102	1.4
Total	43,020	100	17,313	100	24,747	100	9,828	100	18,273	100	7,485	100

1998	All Applicants				By Gender							
					Men				Women			
	Applicants		Acceptees		Applicants		Acceptees		Applicants		Acceptees	
	No.	%	No.	%	No.	%	No.	%	No.	%	No.	%
Age												
20 and Under	671	1.6	473	2.7	305	1.3	226	2.3	366	2.1	247	3.2
21–23	21,807	53.2	10,887	62.6	11,781	50.7	5,881	60.7	10,026	56.4	5,006	65.1
24–27	12,094	29.5	4,114	23.7	7,290	31.4	2,449	25.3	4,804	27	1,665	21.7
28–31	3,773	9.2	1,224	7	2,360	10.2	757	7.8	1,413	7.9	467	6.1
32–34	1,132	2.8	333	1.9	649	2.8	185	1.9	483	2.7	148	1.9
35–37	700	1.7	182	1	396	1.7	108	1.1	304	1.7	74	1
38 and Over	826	2	166	1	435	1.9	87	0.9	391	2.2	79	1
Total	41,003	100	17,379	100	23,216	100	9,693	100	17,787	100	7,686	100

1999	All Applicants				By Gender							
					Men				Women			
	Applicants		Acceptees		Applicants		Acceptees		Applicants		Acceptees	
	No.	%	No.	%	No.	%	No.	%	No.	%	No.	%
Age*												
20 and Under	620	1.6	412	2.4	295	1.4	198	2.1	325	1.9	214	2.7
21–23	20,770	53.9	10,912	62.6	10,776	51.1	5,720	60.4	9,994	57.3	5,192	65.1
24–27	11,336	29.4	4,309	24.7	6,709	31.8	2,538	26.8	4,627	26.5	1,771	22.2
28–31	3,448	8.9	1,169	6.7	2,022	9.6	661	7	1,426	8.2	508	6.4
32–34	1,007	2.6	299	1.7	584	2.8	178	1.9	423	2.4	121	1.5
35–37	585	1.5	166	1	336	1.6	90	1	249	1.4	76	1
38 and Over	763	2	178	1	374	1.8	80	0.8	389	2.2	98	1.2
Total	38,529	100	17,445	100	21,096	100	9,465	100	17,433	100	7,980	100

Source: AAMC Data Warehouse: Applicant Matriculant File. As of November 15, 1999.

*In 1999 the mean ages for these applicant groups were as follows: 24 (all applicants), 24 (applicants accepted), 25 (men applicants), 24 (men accepted), 24 (women applicants), 24 (women accepted).

TABLE 5-C

Women Applicants and First-Year Women New Entrants to U.S. Medical Schools, 1995–96 Through 1999–2000

First-Year Class	Total Applicants	Women Applicants	% of Total Applicants	Total First-Year New Entrants*	Women First-Year New Entrants*	% of Total First-Year New Entrants*
1995–96	46,591	19,779	42.5	16,253	6,941	42.7
1996–97	46,968	20,031	42.6	16,201	6,918	42.7
1997–98	43,020	18,273	42.5	16,165	6,995	43.3
1998–99	41,003	17,787	43.4	16,170	7,162	44.3
1999–00	38,529	17,433	45.2	16,221	7,412	45.7

Source: AAMC Data Warehouse: Applicant Matriculant File. As of November 15, 1999.

*New entrants are those students entering medical school for the first time.

TABLE 5-D

Comparative Acceptance Data for Men and Women Applicants, 1995–96 Through 1999–2000

First-Year Class	No. of Applicants		No. Accepted		% Accepted	
	Men	Women	Men	Women	Men	Women
1995–96	26,812	19,779	9,920	7,437	37.0	37.6
1996–97	26,937	20,031	9,946	7,439	36.9	37.1
1997–98	24,747	18,273	9,828	7,485	39.7	41.0
1998–99	23,216	17,787	9,693	7,686	41.8	43.2
1999–00	21,096	17,433	9,465	7,980	44.9	45.8

Source: AAMC Data Warehouse: Applicant Matriculant File. As of November 15, 1999.

TABLE 5-E*

Application and Acceptance Rate of Selected Minority Group Applicants to First-Year Classes in U.S. Medical Schools, 1995–96 Through 1999–2000

First-Year Class	Black American				American Indian			
	Applicants		Acceptees		Applicants		Acceptees	
	No.	% of All Applicants	No.	% Accepted	No.	% of All Applicants	No.	% Accepted
1995–96	3,487	7.5	1,365	39.1	358	0.8	152	42.7
1996–97	3,524	7.5	1,266	35.9	383	0.8	154	40.2
1997–98	3,168	7.4	1,202	37.9	330	0.8	137	41.5
1998–99	3,151	7.7	1,269	40.3	294	0.7	155	52.7
1999–00	2,940	7.6	1,199	40.8	247	0.6	117	47.4

First-Year Class	Mexican American/Chicano				Mainland Puerto Rican			
	Applicants		Acceptees		Applicants		Acceptees	
	No.	% of All Applicants	No.	% Accepted	No.	% of All Applicants	No.	% Accepted
1995–96	933	2.0	504	54.0	267	0.6	116	43.4
1996–97	975	2.1	470	48.2	272	0.6	146	53.7
1997–98	838	1.9	418	49.9	214	0.5	116	54.2
1998–99	822	2.0	435	52.9	220	0.5	111	50.5
1999–00	777	2.0	415	53.4	217	0.6	119	54.8

Source: AAMC Data Warehouse: Applicant Matriculant File. As of November 15, 1999.

*Data on applicants are based upon the newly developed AAMC Data Warehouse. The Data Warehouse provides more complete data on racial/ethnic self-description and consistent definitions across all years reported. As a result, the data published this year from the Data Warehouse may not match previously published numbers.

TABLE 5-F

U.S. Medical School New Entrants, 1999–2000

Racial/Ethnic Category	New Entrants* Total	New Entrants* % of Grand Total
Underrepresented Minorities		
Black	1,122	6.9
Native American†	109	0.7
Mexican American/Chicano	389	2.4
Puerto Rican (Mainland)	112	0.7
Subtotal	**1,732**	**10.7**
Other Minorities		
Asian or Pacific Islander	3,225	19.9
Puerto Rican (Commonwealth)	199	1.2
Other Hispanic	349	2.2
Subtotal	**3,773**	**23.3**
Non Minorities		
White	10,276	63.3
Other Race/Ethnicity		
Unidentified Race/Ethnicity	385	1.8
Foreign	155	1.0
Grand Total	**16,221**	**100.0**

Source: AAMC Data Warehouse: Applicant Matriculant and Student Enrollment Files.

*New entrants are students entering medical school for the first time. As of November 15, 1999.
†Native American includes American Indians, Alaskan Natives, and Native Hawaiians.

MCAT and AMCAS

6

This chapter provides information on the Medical College Admission Test (MCAT) and the American Medical College Application Service (AMCAS). Details concerning application and selection procedures are presented in Chapter 7.

MEDICAL COLLEGE ADMISSION TEST (MCAT)

The MCAT is a standardized examination comprised of multiple-choice questions and a writing assessment, designed to help admission committees predict which of their applicants will perform adequately in the medical school curriculum. It provides these committees with a standardized measure of academic performance for all examinees under equivalent conditions. The test battery was developed by medical school admission officers, premedical instructors, medical educators, practicing physicians, the Association of American Medical Colleges (AAMC), and a group of testing experts under contract to the AAMC.

The MCAT is designed to encourage students interested in medicine to pursue broad undergraduate study in the natural and social sciences and in the humanities. The MCAT assesses facility with scientific problem solving, critical thinking, and writing skills, as well as understanding of science concepts and principles identified as prerequisite to the study of medicine. The four parts of the MCAT are Verbal Reasoning, Physical Sciences, Writing Sample, and Biological Sciences.

• Verbal Reasoning

Verbal Reasoning is designed to assess students' abilities to comprehend, reason, and think critically. It draws upon materials from the humanities, social sciences, and natural sciences. Subject matter knowledge is not tested; content information necessary to answer test questions is presented in each passage. In preparation for this section of the MCAT, examinees are encouraged to familiarize themselves with the practice of critical thinking and the use of reasoning skills in these disciplines.

• Biological Sciences and Physical Sciences

The Biological Sciences and Physical Sciences sections are constructed to test material covered in first-year or introductory undergraduate courses in biology; chemistry, including inorganic chemistry, organic chemistry; and general, noncalculus physics. Both sections consist entirely of science problems and may include data presented in graphs, tables, and charts. Each section is designed to assess knowledge of basic concepts and facility with scientific problem solving as well as the ability to interpret data presented in a tabular or graphic format.

• Writing Sample

The essay topics that constitute the Writing Sample section are designed to provide examinees with an opportunity to demonstrate their writing and analytical skills. The Writing Sample section begins after a lunch break. Examinees are allowed 30 minutes to write an essay on the first assigned topic. A second topic statement is then issued, and they have a 30-minute period to complete an essay on the second topic. Each essay question provides a specific topic that requires an expository response. Essay topics do not pertain to the technical content of biology, chemistry, physics, or mathematics; the medical school application process or reasons for the choice of medicine as a career; social or cultural issues not in the general experience of MCAT examinees; or religious or other emotionally charged issues.

The test-day schedule is as follows:

Section	Number of Questions	Time in Minutes
Verbal Reasoning	65	85
Physical Sciences	77	100
Writing Sample	2	60
Biological Sciences	77	100

Total testing time: 5-3/4 hours

Four scores are reported, one for each section. Verbal Reasoning, Physical Sciences, and Biological Sciences are presented on a scale ranging from 1 (lowest) to 15 (highest). The Writing Sample is presented on a scale ranging from J (lowest) to T (highest).

Information about the specific content of the examination, its organization, and scoring scheme appears in the MCAT Student Manual available from the AAMC and at some college and university bookstores. The manual includes detailed descriptions of the content and cognitive skills assessed and a full-length practice test with a scoring key.

• Test Dates and Registration

The MCAT is administered twice a year—on a Saturday in April and August. It is recommended that students take it about 18 months before they expect to enter medical school. Testing dates for the MCAT in 2000 are April 15 and August 19. All students, especially those taking the test in August, should bear in mind that there is no provision for makeup examinations. Where possible, special Sunday testings are arranged for applicants presenting, in advance, satisfactory evidence that (1) their religious convictions prevent them from taking the examination on Saturday or (2) unavoidable conflicts prevent them from taking the examination on one of the regularly scheduled dates. An additional $10 fee is charged for these special testing arrangements. Only those persons who plan to apply to a school of allopathic, osteopathic, podiatric, and/or veterinary medicine will be permitted to take the MCAT without special permission.

Most medical schools prefer that the test be taken in April because of the short period of time between the availability of the August test scores and application deadlines. Taking the April test decreases the possibility that procedural problems will prevent the completion of an applicant's file and its timely review. Furthermore, in most cases, very little content that would be helpful to a student for the test is covered between the April and the August administrations, except institutions in which the introductory science courses are taken during the intervening summer months. For these students, the August testing date may be preferable.

The MCAT is administered and scored by the MCAT Program Office at the direction of the AAMC. The examination fee is $165 for the 2000 administrations. A registration packet that contains an announcement, registration card, and all up-to-date information about the MCAT (including test dates, testing locations, distribution of scores, and deadlines) is available in February through premedical advisory offices and at major university testing centers. It may also be obtained by writing directly to:

MCAT Program Office
P.O. Box 4056
Iowa City, Iowa 52243
Telephone: (319) 337-1357

It is essential that students apprise themselves of the information provided in this packet.

• Fee Reduction

The Fee Reduction Program makes the MCAT accessible to financially disadvantaged individuals by lowering the MCAT testing fee for eligible individuals to $60. The MCAT Fee Reduction Program is operated according to eligibility policies and processing procedures established by the Association of American Medical Colleges. Instructions and deadline information are published in the MCAT Fee Reduction Request Form. Fee Reduction Request Forms are contained in the MCAT registration packet, or the form may be downloaded and printed from the AAMC's Web Site <http://www.aamc.org/stuapps/admiss/mcat/forms.htm>. You may also request that materials be sent to you by calling the Section for Student Services, AAMC, at (202) 828-0600.

• Score Reporting

Payment of the examination fee will entitle the candidate to have test scores sent to six medical schools, **provided the scores are released by the examinee at the time of the examination.** Students need to direct these six free reports only to medical schools not participating in AMCAS, since AMCAS automatically provides official reports of MCAT scores released by the candidate to the participating schools to which the candidate applies. MCAT examinees are encouraged to request at the time of registration that their scores be sent, at no added cost, directly to their current premedical advisors. MCAT examinees may not cancel or delete their scores.

An MCAT Additional Score Report request form should be used for (1) additional non-AMCAS score reports beyond the six included in the MCAT examination fee; (2) score reports from previous MCAT administrations to non-AMCAS destinations; or (3) reports of pre-1991 MCAT scores to any institution. Completed MCAT Additional Score Report forms along with the appropriate fees should be submitted to the address below. Further information is provided in the *1999 MCAT Announcement*. The form is available from the AAMC Web Site <http://www.aamc.org/stuapps/admiss/mcat/forms.htm>, and from:

Additional Score Reports
Section for Student Services
Association of American Medical Colleges
2501 M Street, N.W., Suite 1
Washington, D.C. 20037-1300

AAMC policy does not permit the waiver of fees for additional score reports. This policy applies to all examinees.

• Publications

To help students prepare for the MCAT, the AAMC publishes a variety of materials, including four Practice Tests. The first includes the *MCAT Student Manual* and the full-length *MCAT Practice Test I*. The *MCAT Student Manual* describes the four sections of the test and the content and reasoning skills covered by each of the sections; it also offers suggestions for preparing to take the test.

A second set of publications includes *MCAT Practice Items: Verbal Reasoning and Writing Sample, MCAT Practice Items: Physical Science* and *Biological Science*, and *MCAT Practice Test II*. *MCAT Practice Test II* is a released operational test form. Items in the *Practice Item* booklets are similar to test materials used in an actual MCAT. They have not, however, received the same level of review and testing as the materials that appear on the MCAT examination; they are intended to provide examinees with additional practice with MCAT item formats and do not constitute a sample test.

The *MCAT Practice Test III* and *Practice Test IV* are also released operational test forms. Included with these publications is a set of tables that allows individuals to conduct an in-depth analysis of their strengths and weaknesses. Extensive information on the Writing Sample is included with Practice Test III and a solutions booklet accompanies Practice Test III and Practice Test IV.

The AAMC also produces a videocassette, *Preparing for the MCAT.* Designed to be used in conjunction with the *MCAT Student Manual,* this tape provides information about the knowledge and skills tested by the MCAT and discusses preparation strategies for each of the four sections of the test. Other information about the MCAT, including an annotated bibliography of MCAT research, is available on the AAMC Web Site, http://www.aamc.org/stuapps/admiss/mcat/start.htm.

For information about purchasing publications from the AAMC, call the AAMC's Section for Membership and Publication Orders at (202) 828-0416, <http://www.aamc.org>, or write to them at the following address:

Membership and Publication Orders
Association of American Medical Colleges
2450 N Street, N.W.
Washington, D.C. 20037-1129

The MCAT pages on the AAMC Web Site also contain data on the latest score distributions and on Writing Sample topics that may be used on future tests.

• Retaking the Test

If an applicant's MCAT scores are low, the advisability of retaking the test may be discussed with a premedical advisor. Legitimate reasons for retaking the test include: unusual discrepancy between college grades and MCAT scores; having taken the MCAT prematurely, that is, before completing the introductory science courses that provide the necessary background for the science areas of the test; serious illness at the time of the test; and recommendation by a member of a medical school admission committee that the test be retaken. Application procedures for retaking the test are identical to those for initial testing.

THE AMERICAN MEDICAL COLLEGE APPLICATION SERVICE (AMCAS)

• General Information

- AMCAS is a nonprofit, centralized application service developed by medical school admission officers to facilitate the process of applying to participating U.S. medical schools.
- AMCAS does not render any admission decisions or advise applicants where to submit applications. Each participating school is completely autonomous in its admission decisions. AMCAS provides only the processing service.
- AMCAS benefits both the applicant and the participating medical schools by efficiently collecting, coordinating, and processing data, which frequently reduces the time and expense of application. The total operation neither alters nor depersonalizes the principles of traditional application procedures.
- AMCAS further assists admissions committees by providing rosters and statistical reports relative to the individual medical school and the national applicant pools. For example, a list of accepted applicants is forwarded to all medical schools beginning in April and continuing through October of the matriculation year. This list identifies each applicant holding an acceptance and the schools where those acceptances are being held.
- AMCAS also enables the AAMC to initiate research projects focusing on the medical school admission process.

For the 1999–2000 entering class 96.5 percent of all applicants applied to at least one AMCAS-participating school. One hundred and thirteen medical schools and two programs are participating in AMCAS for the 2000 entering class. AMCAS participation is indicated in individual school entries in Chapter 11.

• The AMCAS Application

All individuals applying to medical schools participating in the AMCAS for the first-year entering class must apply through AMCAS.

Applicants can complete their AMCAS application using a personal computer and software developed by the Association of American Medical Colleges.

- The software, **AMCAS-E,** significantly reduces the time needed to supply data required by AMCAS, while preserving the final product forwarded by AMCAS to designated medical schools—the standard verified AMCAS application.
- The process is simple.
- Applicants using AMCAS-E software supply required information in response to prompts, making use of pull-down tables for common data elements such as colleges attended, state and county of legal residence, etc.
- In addition, the process of standardizing course-work grades and credit hours is automated. These prompts, supporting data tables, automation of grade/credit-hour conversion, and an audit of all required data fields ensure that all required information is provided to AMCAS, speeding the processing of the application.
- In addition, AMCAS-E software includes the AMCAS Fee Waiver Request Form, the Additional Designation Form used by applicants to apply to other medical schools after their initial application has been submitted, and the Post Submission Change Forms, which applicants may use to change information after they have submitted their initial application.
- Applicants will also be able to print a "replica" copy of the AMCAS application and text-only copies of other forms for their personal records.

Applicants without access to a personal computer are able to complete the traditional AMCAS paper application.

• How to Get the AMCAS Application

The AMCAS application is available in April, and can be obtained from a variety of sources.

- Applicants can download AMCAS-E software from the AAMC's Web site at http://www.aamc.org.
- Both AMCAS-E and the paper materials are available either from preprofessional health advisors, participating medical schools, or by contacting AMCAS at the following address:

AMCAS
Section for Student Services
Association of American Medical Colleges
2501 M Street, N.W., Lobby–26
Washington, DC 20037-1300
(202) 828-0600

- In addition to written and telephone requests, applicants may also order materials from the AAMC's Web Site or by sending an E-mail message to amcas@aamc.org.

• Transcript Requirements and Deadlines

Before submitting application materials, the applicant should request that one set of official transcripts be forwarded directly to AMCAS by the registrar of every school at which he or she has registered. Official transcripts are required from each junior college, community college, college, university, graduate school, U.S. medical school, trade school, or professional school within the United States, Canada, or U.S. Territories, regardless of whether credit was earned. The applicant is also encouraged to simultaneously request a personal copy of each transcript in order to properly complete his or her AMCAS application materials.

Transcripts submitted to AMCAS in prior years cannot be reactivated and will not be used.

The Early Decision Program application materials and official transcripts must be received by August 1; all official transcripts must be received no later than two weeks following the deadline for application materials. Refer to the AMCAS instructions for detailed information on official transcript requirements and deadlines. **AMCAS begins accepting official transcripts on March 15.**

• Application Processing

Applicants submit only one set of application materials **(paper or data diskette)** and have one set of official transcripts forwarded to AMCAS regardless of the number of AMCAS participating medical schools to which they are applying. The service fee is based on the number of schools an applicant designates and can be paid by check, money order, or credit card.

• AMCAS Fee Waiver Program

The AMCAS Fee Waiver Program is provided by the AAMC for applicants whose inability to pay the AMCAS service fee would absolutely prohibit them from applying to medical school. Applicants must complete and forward to AMCAS the Fee Waiver Request Form found in both the paper AMCAS application packet and in the AMCAS-E software to determine eligibility prior to submitting their application materials.

AMCAS will not accept completed applications (paper or diskette) until June 1, 2000. Materials received prior to June 1 will be returned to the applicant. The deadline for submitting applications to AMCAS for each medical school is listed in Chapter 11.

The processing of an application is contingent upon receipt by AMCAS of both the completed application and all required official transcripts by the published deadlines.

Upon receiving the completed application, AMCAS verifies the applicant's academic record against the required transcripts to ensure accuracy. After verification, grade point averages and credit-hour totals are computed, these data, as well as other information extracted from the application (paper or diskette), are forwarded to the applicant's designated medical schools with a copy of the application form.

After receiving application materials from AMCAS, medical schools will notify the applicant directly of any supplemental items that may be required, such as additional fees, letters of recommendation, or updated transcripts. These items should be forwarded by the applicant directly to the medical schools upon request.

The fee listed in Chapter 11 under each school entry is the supplemental fee to be paid directly to that school upon request; not the AMCAS service fee. Applicants should contact individual schools regarding the waiver of supplemental fees.

FIGURE 6

Sample AMCAS Application (Paper Format)

1. SSN	AMCAS® APPLICATION FOR THE 1998 ENTERING CLASS	AMCAS USE ONLY
028-26-2288		

2A. Last Name	2B. First Name	2C. Middle Name	2D. Suffix
ZYLER	Richard	Ross	III

3A. Permanent Address - Street	3B. City (and Province)	3C. St	3D. Zip/Postal Code
434 Columbus Avenue, Apt. 2	New Haven	CT	06519 - 1234

3E. County (if in U.S.A.)	3F. Country (if not U.S.A.)	4. Telephone
New Haven		(203) 555-5125

5. PARENTS OR GUARDIAN

	Name	Living? Yes	Living? No	Occupation	Legal Residence	Education/College (Highest Level)
Father	Ralph E. Zyler	x		Teacher	Mass.	M.A., Boston Univ.
Mother	Edwina Alexander	x		Economist	Calif.	Ph.D., Harvard
Guardian						

6A. Ages of your Brothers	6B. Ages of your Sisters	7A. Secondary School – Name	7B. Location	7C. Grad Yr.
9		William Penn H. S.	Davis, CA	1988

8. ALL COLLEGES, GRADUATE AND PROFESSIONAL SCHOOLS ATTENDED (list in chronological order)

Name	Location	Dates of Attendance MM/YY to MM/YY	Check if summer only	Check if Jr/Comm College	Major	Degree Granted or Expected (with date)
Sorbonne	Paris, France	6/88 to 8/88	x		French	None
Bennett College	Millbrook, NY	9/88 to 8/89		x	Science	None
Nassau Cmty. Col.	Garden City, NY	9/89 to 6/90		x	Biology	None
Michigan State U.	East Lansing, MI	9/90 to 8/91			Biology	None
EFGH College	Washington, DC	9/91 to 6/92			Biology	B.S. 6/92
St. Mercy Hospital	Duncannon, PA	1/92 to 6/92			Med Tech	None
XY State Univ.	Washington, DC	9/92 to 6/96			Psych	M.A. 6/96
Abcd University	Washington, DC	9/96 to 6/97			Microbiol	None
		to to				

9. POST-SECONDARY HONORS/AWARDS:

Phi Beta Kappa; Dean's List for three semesters; National Biology Honor Society; National Psychology Honor Society; Biology Student of the Year (EFGH College); Varsity Lacrosse Player (Michigan State); Outstanding Volunteer Award from St. Mercy Hospital (continued)

10. EXTRACURRICULAR, COMMUNITY, AND AVOCATIONAL ACTIVITIES:

Community activities: Sickle Cell Anemia screening, XY State Univ.

11. CHRONOLOGICAL POST-SECONDARY HISTORY, INCLUDING VOLUNTEER, PART-TIME AND FULL-TIME EMPLOYMENT

Summer 1990 - Lab Technician, Allstate Labs.

1990-91 - Junior Year - Waiter/Cook, Pizza Restaurant - 20 hrs/wk

1996-97 Academic Year - Lab Assistant, Hematology - 15 hrs/wk

See AMCAS instructions before completing this form.

PERSONAL COMMENTS (Your comments must not exceed the space provided. Use a font at least 10 points in size.)	NAME (LAST NAME FIRST)

This is your opportunity to provide personal information that is otherwise not included on the application. Consider and construct your comments carefully; many admissions committees place significant weight on this section.

SSN	ACADEMIC RECORD	AMCAS USE ONLY
028-26-2288		

Last Name	First Name	Middle Name	Suffix
ZYLER	Richard	Ross	III

College Name / Location	Academic Status	BCPM/A	Academic Year	Term	Course Name	Number	Type	Transcript Grade	Semester Hours Attempted	AMCAS Grade	AMCAS Use
Bennett College,	FR	A	88	SS	Credit (French)		PF	S	6	P	
Transfer Credit		A			Adv. French Convers			B+			
(Sorbonne/Paris)		A			French Civiliz.(Art)			A			
Bennett College		A		S1	Elementary French		AP		6	G	
Millbrook, N.Y.		A			Intermed French I		AP	B	3	B	
		A			American History		CL		6	L	
		C			Gen Chemistry I+Lab	115		A-	4	A-	
		A			Volleyball	118		A+	1	A	
		A			Philosophy	101		A+	3	A	
		A			Fresh. English Comp	180	H	A-	3	A-	
		P			General Physics I	125		B	4	B	
		M		SM	Calculus I	125		B-	4	B-	
		A		S2	English Literature	109		A	3	A	
		C			Gen Chemistry II+Lab	116		B	4	B	
		A			First Aid & Safety	116		B	2	B	
		A			European History	104		B	3	B	
		M			Calculus II	126		B	4	B	
	SO	P	89	SS	Electromagnetism	103		B	4.5	B	
		A			Literature	131		A-	3	A-	
Nassau Cmty. Col		A		S1	French Literature	001	EX				
Garden City, NY		B			General Biology	201		B+	4	AB	
		C			Organic Chemistry	223		B	3	B	
		A			Medical Ethics	225	AU	NG			
		C			Organic Chem Lab	223		C	1	C	
		B		S2	General Biology	202		B	4	B	
		C			Organic Chemistry	224	PF	S	3	P	
		C			Organic Chem Lab	224	PF	U	1	N	
		A			Social Psychology	227		A	3	A	
		P			General Physics II	222		C+	3	BC	
Michigan State U.	JR	A	90	Q1	Political Science	241		3.5	2.7	AB	
E. Lansing, MI		A			Revolution and War	243	H/I	2.0	2.7	C	
[Narrative		C			Basic Biochemistry	401		3.5	3.3	AB	
Evaluations		B			Comp Vertebrate Anat	314	R	1.0	3.3	D	
Enclosed]		A			Military Drill	259		4.0	0.7	A	
		B		Q2	Comp Vertebrate Anat	314	R	4.0	3.3	A	
		A			Mythology	250		2.0	2.7	C	
		M			Statistics I	201		2.5	2.7	BC	
		A			Modern Ideologies	242		1.5	2.7	CD	
		A		Q3	Anthropology	171		2.0	2.7	C	
		B			Zoology	331		3.0	2.0	B	
		A			Humanities	251		0.0	2.7	F	
Michigan State U.		M	91	QS	Linear Functions	302		3.0	2.7	B	
Study Abroad Prog		A			History of England I	307		4.0	2.7	A	
(Oxfrd/Londn,Eng)		A			Hist of England II	308		2.0	2.7	C	
EFGH College,	SR	M		Q1	Statistics II	91		P	3	C	
Washington, DC		B			Cell & Molec Biol	122		HP	3	B	
		B			Physiology	163		HH	4	A	
		M			Scientific Analysis	22		HH	4	A	
		A			Economics (micro)	2		P	4	C	

-3-

Be sure to complete and sign page 4. >>

College Name / Location	Academic Status	BCPM/A	Academic Year	Term	Course Name	Number	Type	Transcript Grade	Semester Hours Attempted	AMCAS Grade	AMCAS Use
EFGH College,	SR	B	91	Q2	Med Tech Internship:		PF	CR	16	P	
Washington, DC		B			Hematology	101		86			
Transfer Credit		B			Serology	107		91			
(St. Mercy Hsp, PA)		B			Lab Techniques	111		96			
		B			Virology	113		92			
Penn State Univ.	PB	A	92	T1	Occult Literature	120	W	WF			
Univ. Park, PA		A			Tolstoy	220		A	3	A	
		A			Modern Novel	224		A	3	A	
		A	93	T1	Physio. Psychology	301		A	3	A	
		A			Psych. of Learning	304	W	WN			
		A		T2	Research Psychology	340		A	2	A	
		A		T3	Semantics	307	NR	NG	3		
	GR	A	94	T1	Child Psychology	435		A	4	A	
		A			Educ. Psychology	441		B	4	B	
		A		T2	Social Psychology	415		A	4	A	
		A			Abnormal Psychology	460		A	4	A	
		A			Psych. Field Work	490	I	INC	4		
		A	95	T1	Advanced Research	477	PF	PS	4	P	
		A		T2	Death and Dying	503	DG	DF	4		
		A			Advanced Research	477	PF	PS	4	P	
		A		T3	Death and Dying	503		A	4	A	
Abcd University,	GR	M	96	S1	Quantitative Data	668		H	3	A	
Washington, DC		B			Epidemiology	635		HP	4	A-	
		B		S2	Microbiology	665		P	3	B	
		B	97	S1	Biology of Tumors	230	CC		2		
		B			Microbiology	665	CC		3		
		B		S2	Virus Infections	668	CC		1		

14. MCAT Testing Status

Number of MCATs taken since April 1991: 3

Have you taken, or do you plan to take, the August 1997 MCAT?

YES [X] NO [ ]

15. Medical School

You must answer this Question

Have you ever matriculated at or attended any medical school as a candidate for the M.D. degree?

YES [ ] NO [X]

16. Institutional Action

You must answer this Question

[Refer to AMCAS instructions before answering.] Were you ever the recipient of any action (e.g., dismissal, disqualification, suspension, etc.) by any college or medical school for: (1) unacceptable academic performance or (2) conduct violations? If "YES," explain fully in the "Personal Comments" section (page 2).

YES [ ] NO [X]

Certification Statement

I have read and understand the AMCAS instructions. I certify that the information submitted in this application and associated materials is current, complete, and accurate to the best of my knowledge.

Signature (Black Ink Only)	Date
	June 15, 1997

No. E-6 Rev. 1/97 DCIC No. 97-XXX -4-

The Medical School Application and Selection Process

7

Each medical school faculty has the responsibility and authority to select the individuals who will be admitted to the school. This faculty responsibility is handled by the Medical School Admissions Committee, a standing committee of the faculty of medicine. Responsibility for the administrative process is delegated to an admission officer who, with the assistance of an office staff, organizes and conducts the procedures for the receipt and processing of applications. Through this process, candidates' credentials are reviewed, and decisions to admit or reject a candidate are made by a faculty admission committee. The composition of admission committees and the selection process vary from school to school, but each school follows the general principles discussed below.

• Composition of Committees

Admission committees are composed principally of faculty members from both basic science and clinical departments. Frequently one or more medical student members are included. At a few schools, committees include faculty members from other colleges in the university and/or individuals from the community.

• Processing of Applications

Applications are screened and placed in priority categories according to policies established by the faculty. Supplementary application materials may be requested from all applicants or from only those in specified categories. A general discussion of the criteria and approach used by admissions committees in the evaluation of applicants is found in Chapters 4 and 5.

Applicants in the highest priority are contacted by the admission office to arrange an interview appointment. As the process continues, applicants in successively lower categories are contacted.

The admission committee schedules interviews regularly throughout the fall, winter, and spring. Applicants are interviewed by one or more committee members, either sequentially or by several committee members together. Subsequently, the full committee reviews the complete file of all interviewed candidates.

Interviewed applicants are informed of the committee's decision sometime after the interview. The exact schedule will vary from school to school.

The decision will be to offer an acceptance, reject the applicant, or place the applicant on an alternate list.

Investigation Policies and Procedures

One significant responsibility of the Association of American Medical Colleges (AAMC) is to promote integrity and high ethical standards in the processes associated with admission to and enrollment in medical school. Applicants are expected to provide complete, current, and accurate information at the time application materials are submitted and during all phases of this process. Registrants for the MCAT are also obligated to present accurate and current information at the time registration materials are submitted and to adhere to all Test Center Regulations and Procedures as outlined in the *MCAT Announcement*.

Any falsification, omission, or discrepancy in application materials, including incomplete or invalid financial transactions, as well as any irregular behavior exhibited during the administration of the MCAT will prompt an inquiry by the AAMC. An investigation is conducted in accordance with procedures established by the AAMC's Executive Council as outlined in *AAMC Policies and Procedures for Investigating Reported Violations of Admission and Enrollment Standards,* which is available upon request.

If the investigation confirms that such an action has occurred, a report thereof will be issued to all current and future medical schools to which the individual has applied or matriculated and all MCAT score recipients. In addition, it is the position of the AAMC to cooperate with report requests from duly constituted agencies, because reports may contain information relevant to academic or disciplinary proceedings, criminal investigations, graduate medical education, and/or professional licensure.

As the process continues through the admission cycle, acceptances are offered until the requisite number of acceptees is achieved to fill all the positions in the entering class for that year.

• Number in Entering Classes

Each medical school predetermines the number of students to be matriculated each year. (An estimate of the expected size of the entering class is provided in each school entry in

TABLE 7

Trends Related to Medical School Applications for First-Year Entering Classes, 1995–96 Through 1999–2000

Entering Year	Individuals Filing Applications	Applications Filed	Number of New Entrants*
1995–96	46,591	595,975	16,253
1996–97	46,968	566,122	16,201
1997–98	43,020	512,878	16,165
1998–99	41,003	481,335	16,170
1999–00	38,529	454,380	16,221

Source: AAMC Data Warehouse: Applicant Matriculant File. As of November 15, 1999.
*New entrants are those students entering medical school for the very first time.

Chapter 11.) Budgetary and other policies may modify this number in any given year, so it is wise to check directly with the school. There were 16,221 new entrants in 1999 (Table 7).

• Number of Applicants

Nationwide, 38,529 individuals applied for the 1999 entering class, a 6.0 percent decrease from the number of applicants for the entering class of 1998. The ratio of applicants to entering students was 2.4:1 in 1999, indicating a slight decrease from the previous year.

• Proportion of Applicants Accepted

Overall, 45.3 percent of the candidates applying in 1999 were accepted. This is a slight increase from 1998. Among first-time applicants, who numbered 26,200, the acceptance rate was 47.8 percent. Those 5,687 candidates who had applied for the second time after not being admitted in 1998 had a 39.9 percent acceptance rate.

• Timing of Applications

Applicants are encouraged to submit their application as early as feasible in the admission cycle. For schools participating in the American Medical College Application Service (AMCAS), applications received beginning June 1 will be processed and forwarded to the schools designated by each applicant. (Any application received prior to June 1 will be returned to the applicant.) The 12 schools not participating in AMCAS have varying dates for the earliest receipt of applications (see school entries in Chapter 11).

All schools (whether using or not using AMCAS) determine the closing date for applications. For AMCAS-participating schools, the deadline date shown in the school's Chapter 11 entry is the date when the application must be received at AMCAS.

• Early Decision Program (EDP)

The Early Decision Program (EDP) provides the well-qualified applicant who has a strong preference for a particular school with the opportunity to secure an acceptance by October 1. By applying as an EDP candidate, the individual agrees not to apply to any other U.S. medical school (AMCAS or non-AMCAS) until any of the following occurs: (1) receipt of an EDP rejection; (2) receipt of a formal release from the EDP commitment, or (3) the October 1 notification deadline has passed. In addition, the applicant agrees to attend the school if offered an EDP acceptance. Any violation of these conditions will be investigated and, if confirmed, reported to legitimately interested parties.

For the 1999 entering class, 91 medical schools offered admission through EDP. The EDP deadline for the receipt of application materials and official transcripts for AMCAS-participating schools is August 1. The EDP deadlines for non-AMCAS schools are listed in Chapter 11. If an EDP applicant is not accepted by the school, the applicant still has sufficient time to apply to other schools.

• Number of Applications

Early Decision Program applicants initially file only one application. In 1999, there were 2,049 EDP candidates, and 1,202 (58.7 percent) were offered acceptances under the EDP. For the 1999 entering class, AMCAS applicants applied to an average of 11.5 AMCAS-participating schools. AMCAS applicants who applied to from 7 to 19 AMCAS-participating schools for the 1999 entering class had an average acceptance rate of 46.0 percent at these institutions. AMCAS applicants who applied to 20 or more AMCAS-participating schools for the 1999 entering class had an average acceptance rate of 50.1 percent at these institutions.

The number of applications an applicant should file depends upon the qualifications of the individual relative to the overall level of competition of the schools to which the individual is applying. The decision of how many schools and to which schools to apply is important and should be made only after careful consultation with the premedical advisor. The considerations detailed in Chapter 5 should be used as a guideline.

• Admissions Selection Factors

Decisions to admit candidates are based upon multiple criteria developed by each individual school and related to the mission and objectives of the school. In general, however, all schools are looking for (1) evidence of an ability to accomplish the academic work necessary to progress through the school's curriculum, (2) evidence of possession of the personal qualities and attributes of physicians, and (3) potential to exemplify the goals of the school.

• Academic Ability

An admission committee seeks students who have acquired the knowledge and study skills needed to progress through the medical curriculum and to be active learners throughout their medical careers. To evaluate this, committees rely on candidates' college records and on the scores achieved on the MCAT. College transcripts are carefully reviewed from the standpoint of the grades earned, the credit hours carried during successive academic periods, and the distribution of courses among the biological, physical, and social sciences and the humanities. Although each school sets its own scale of preferences, schools prefer candidates who have accomplished their college work on a normal schedule, who have a balanced distribution of credits among the sciences and humanities, and who have consistently earned grades in the 3.0 to 4.0 range.

In analyzing candidates' transcripts, the characteristics of the colleges they have attended are also considered. Thus, work accomplished and grades earned at colleges known by admission committees to have rigorous standards will be accorded greater weight than those from colleges considered to have lesser standards. The acceptability of advanced placement (AP) credits earned in high school varies from school to school. The individual school entries in Chapter 11 should be reviewed regarding their policies. If a school's policies for AP are unclear, the school's admission office should be consulted.

Scores on the MCAT provide ancillary information on candidates' academic ability. Each school establishes the method by which the scores achieved on the MCAT are factored into determining whether candidates can reasonably be expected to accomplish the academic work necessary to progress through a school's curriculum. The range of acceptable MCAT scores varies among schools. MCAT scores are given greater attention when evaluating the academic records of candidates from colleges that are unfamiliar to an admission committee. Comparing MCAT scores with grades earned provides an estimation of such candidates' academic accomplishments in relation to candidates from colleges that are familiar to the committee.

In summary, academic ability is an important selection factor, but judgments of academic ability vary among schools. Assessments of the academic ability of older candidates will include their achievement in postbaccalaureate courses as well as their overall college record. The academic abilities of socioeconomically disadvantaged and minority candidates require special assessments (see Chapter 9 and the AAMC publication, *Minority Student Opportunities in United States Medical Schools)*.

• Personal Qualities and Attributes

Candidates' personal qualities are important factors in selection decisions. Evidence of maturity, character and integrity, self-discipline, concern with helping others, and leadership is sought through information obtained from the personal statement on the application, evaluations by premedical advisors and college faculty members, and interviews.

In writing a personal statement, the applicant should discuss not only the reasons for desiring a career in medicine but also extracurricular and work accomplishments. Particularly significant activities should be described clearly and succinctly.

All medical schools ask the applicant to designate the persons from whom letters of evaluation will come. Generally, a letter from the premedical committee at the applicant's undergraduate college or university where premedical courses are taken is required. Evaluations from premedical advisors and college faculty members who know the applicant as a student are given much greater weight by admission committees than letters of recommendation from friends, family members, or political figures. If the applicant has worked extensively during college or is applying several years after college, letters from employers and supervisors are helpful.

Character, integrity, and maturity are important factors to medical schools. Applicants who have experienced disciplinary action in college for infractions of citizenship codes of conduct are expected to disclose this information in their application and to discuss the incident on their personal growth in a personal statement. Failure to disclose such official college action will prompt an investigation.

• Interviews

Policies regarding scheduling of interviews vary from school to school. Some will grant interviews to all candidates requesting one. Others invite candidates for an interview only after initial screening and priority categorization. In almost all cases, acceptances are offered only after candidates have been interviewed. Usually, the applicant will be asked to come to the school for the interview. Some schools have designated interviewers in various regions of the country to reduce the financial and time expenditures for candidates. However, the interview trip is a good opportunity for the applicant to see the medical school and meet students.

Information about a school's interview policies and procedures is generally provided to candidates in the initial stage of the school's selection process. If this information is not clear, applicants should ask for clarification from the admission office. At the interview, applicants should be prepared to discuss their personal histories and motivation for medicine.

• Notification of Acceptance

Since 1961, the constituent medical schools of the AAMC have agreed to observe a set of recommendations concerning medical school acceptance procedures for first-year entering students, commonly referred to as the "traffic rules." The purpose of these recommendations is to complete the admissions cycle in as timely a fashion as possible so that both students and schools will know who is entering the first year prior to the summer months.

The earliest and latest dates for notification and the time allowed for the applicant's response to an acceptance are shown in each school's entry in Chapter 11. Some schools permit accepted students to defer their entrance for one or more years. Applicants desiring to defer entrance to medical school should request deferment no later than when responding to a school's offer of acceptance.

The AAMC recommends that deposits required of accepted students not exceed $100 and that they be refundable until May 15. The amount of the deposit and the refund policy for each school are shown in the school entries in Chapter 11.

• Applicant Responsibilities

In order for medical school admission committees to fully consider an application, the applicant must assume certain responsibilities in the application process. The observance of the responsibilities in the box below will ensure both applicants and admission committees of an orderly and timely process of student selection.

• Applicants Offered Multiple Acceptances

In 1999, 6,670 applicants were accepted by two or more medical schools. To provide an orderly and fair admission process, applicants are obligated to hold no more than one acceptance at a time. An applicant receiving acceptances from two or more schools simultaneously is expected to accept the offer of the most preferred school and notify the others that their offers are not accepted. If subsequent offers are received from other schools, the applicant may withdraw from the school originally accepted and accept the offer of a more preferred school. The schools are expected not to offer acceptances to students who have already arrived at another medical school for orientation and matriculation.

Responsibilities of Medical School Applicants

1. Applicants are expected to become familiar with and observe the application procedures at each school to which they apply. All application documents, including primary and secondary application forms, transcript(s), letters of evaluation, fees, etc., must be submitted in a timely manner.
2. Applicants must promptly notify AMCAS and medical schools not participating in AMCAS of any change of address.
3. Applicants must respond promptly to all invitations for a medical school interview. In those instances when an applicant cannot appear for a previously scheduled interview, the applicant is responsible for promptly notifying the school of the cancellation of the appointment. The cancellation should be undertaken by telephone, followed by a letter.
4. Applicants in need of financial aid must initiate the steps necessary to determine their eligibility as early as possible. This includes filing the appropriate need analysis forms in January or February and encouraging their parents (if required) to file their income tax forms early.
5. Applicants who remain under consideration for admission should keep the medical schools informed of the address and telephone number where they can be reached. Applicants who are unavailable (e.g. foreign travel) should instruct and grant authority to a parent or other individual to act on their behalf.
6. Applicants who have made a final decision on the medical school they plan to attend have the obligation to promptly withdraw their applications from all other schools.

AAMC Recommendations Concerning Medical School Acceptance Procedures for First-Year Entering Students

For the information of prospective medical students and their advisors, the recommended procedures for offering acceptance to medical school and for student responses to those offers are as follows:

1. Each school of medicine should prepare and distribute to applicants and college advisors a detailed schedule of its application and acceptance procedures and should adhere to this schedule unless it is publicly amended.

2. Each school of medicine should agree not to notify its applicants (except for those applying via Early Decision Program [EDP]) of acceptance prior to October 15 of each admission cycle.

3. By March 15 of the year of matriculation, each school of medicine should have issued a number of acceptances at least equal to the size of its first-year entering class.

4. Only after May 15 are schools free to apply appropriate rules for dealing with accepted applicants who, without adequate explanation, hold one or more places in other schools. These rules should recognize the problems of the applicant who has multiple offers and also of those applicants who have not yet been accepted. Only schools whose first official day of classes begins prior to August 1 may start to request decisions from accepted applicants prior to May 15 but not earlier than April 15. This rule applies to all accepted applicants for the entering medical school class, including those individuals entering M.D./Ph.D. programs and individuals to whom merit scholarships or other special scholarships have been awarded.

5. By May 15 of the year of matriculation, an applicant who has received offers of admission from more than one school should choose the one school that he or she prefers and withdraw from all other schools to which he or she has been accepted.

*6. Prior to May 15 of the year of matriculation, an applicant should be given at least two weeks to reply to an offer of admission. After May 15, schools may require applicants to respond to acceptance offers in less than two weeks. An applicant may be required to file a statement of intent, a deposit, or both. The statement of intent should provide freedom to withdraw if the applicant is later accepted by a school that he or she prefers. Under no circumstances should an applicant be asked to withdraw from waiting lists as a condition of accepting a place.

*7. It is recommended that the acceptance deposit not exceed $100 and be refundable until May 15. After that date, a school may retain the deposit as a late withdrawal fee. If the applicant matriculates at the school, the school is encouraged to credit the deposit toward tuition.

8. Subsequent to June 1, a school of medicine seeking to admit an applicant already known to be accepted by another school for that entering class should advise that school of its intent. Because of the administrative problems involved in filling a place vacated just prior to the commencement of the academic year, schools should communicate fully with each other with respect to anticipated late roster changes in order to keep misunderstandings at a minimum.

9. After an applicant has enrolled in a U.S. school of medicine or begun a brief orientation program contiguous to enrollment, no further acceptances should be offered to that individual. Once enrolled in a school, students have an obligation to withdraw their applications promptly from all other schools. Enrollment is defined as being officially registered as a member of the first-year entering class at a school.

10. All letters of recommendation submitted in support of an applicant to a medical school are confidential. No portion of the letter should be read to an applicant during an interview. This requirement is subject to any Sunshine Laws within specific states.

*Most of what is stated in these two procedures does not pertain to students accepted through the Early Decision Program (EDP), because such students agree in advance to attend a given medical school if offered a place during the "early decision" segment of the application year.

Financial Information for Medical Students

8

This chapter, which is designed for individuals seeking to finance their medical education, includes general information on financial planning and debt management, financial aid application procedures, distribution of aid, and common sources of student funding. Medical school applicants who need to supplement their resources to pay for the cost of a medical education need not feel intimidated by the profusion of financial aid programs, the amount of paperwork involved, or the variety of requirements. However, the following points should be kept in mind:

1. The primary responsibility for financing a medical education rests with the student and/or the student's family.
2. Borrowing is the most common form of assistance.
3. Applicants who are in default on federal educational loans or who owe refunds to federal grant programs are prohibited from obtaining additional support from a number of federal programs.
4. The amount of assistance available and how it is awarded to students differs from one medical school to another.
5. Funding and eligibility requirements for federal programs may change at any time.
6. The financial aid officer is responsible for coordinating all sources of financial assistance for each enrolled student.
7. **Students with outstanding credit card and other consumer debts will find it difficult to finance medical school, as these obligations cannot be covered with student financial aid. In addition, students with adverse credit will likely have difficulty securing private loans that may be needed to supplement other student financial aid.**

FINANCIAL PLANNING

The cost of attaining a medical education has increased markedly in the last decade. Individual school entries in Chapter 11 provide information on the cost of attendance for the 1999–2000 academic year. Table 8-A provides tuition and student fees for 1999–2000 first-year medical students at U.S. medical schools. The average debt for indebted medical school graduates in the class of 1999 was $90,745, inclusive of premed debt. The primary source of financial aid is in the form of loans. For students who must depend extensively on loans to pay for medical school, two fundamental concepts are critical.

First, borrowing is defined as obligating future income. It is income yet to be earned that is obligated today for some benefit such as buying a car or paying for tuition to acquire an M.D. degree. When that income is finally earned, the amount that has been obligated cannot be used for any purpose other than the repayment of the past debt.

The second concept is a corollary to the first—an individual who decides to borrow to obtain an M.D. degree has also decided implicitly that the degree is equal in value to the amount of future income that has been obligated in order to attend medical school. Borrowing, therefore, has a direct effect on future professional and personal lifestyle; it is also an investment in one's own future. In deciding whether to pursue a medical education, the individual assesses whether the return is worth the investment.

Even if a student must borrow, it is possible to acquire a sense of fiscal awareness and responsibility that will permit significant control over the amount of future income obligated. Following the guidelines described below—and these are guidelines that will serve a lifetime—has the two-fold benefit of setting limits on the level of indebtedness while the student is in school and of successfully dealing with repayments after graduation.

DEBT MANAGEMENT

Formulating a budget and living within its limits are essential. It requires delaying gratification in terms of purchases and lifestyle decisions while the individual is enrolled in school. Doing so can mean borrowing less and having more money in the future. To assist students, each medical school prepares a standard student budget, which can serve as a guideline for creating an individual budget. It is possible to live on less than the amount budgeted—by having roommates, sharing transportation, and preparing meals at home, for example. Participating in seemingly small economies can free literally thousands of dollars of future income for purposes other than repaying educational debts. Formulating budgeting skills during medical school will also help during residency, when many loans enter repayment and when many residents attempt to accelerate payment on their loans.

The AAMC-sponsored MEDLOANS Program has a Debt Management Program available on the Web at www.aamc.org/medloans. Simply click on MEDLOANS Debt Management Program to begin the PowerPoint slide presentation.

TABLE 8-A

Tuition and Student Fees for 1999–2000 First-Year Students in U.S. Medical Schools (In Dollars)

	Private Schools			Public Schools		
Categories of Students	Range	Median	Average	Range	Median	Average
Resident	7,513–35,975	28,224	26,991	3,286–22,139	10,941	11,375
Nonresident	17,898–35,975	28,852	28,733	11,401–56,750	24,245	25,195

Figures based on data provided summer 1999. Uniformed Services University of the Health Sciences, a public institution, does not charge tuition or student fees; books and equipment are also furnished without charge.

• Meeting Deadlines

Meeting deadlines for assistance is fundamental to receiving both sufficient and the least expensive funding while in school. Students are urged to maintain personal calendars in which due dates for applications, other documents, and tuition payments can be recorded. Meeting all deadlines will prevent late fees on tuition bills and, later on, defaults on educational loans while enhancing a good credit rating.

• Debt Reduction Methods

Limiting undergraduate borrowing, working (as long as academic standing is not jeopardized), and aggressively seeking private sources of assistance are very effective methods for reducing debt and increasing future disposable earnings. For more information on private organizations and agencies—medical societies, state programs, brotherhoods, sisterhoods, and church groups—applicants are urged to explore their college libraries, contact their state departments of education, and review the material offered by their medical school's financial aid office. Although the search for private assistance requires considerable effort, the prospect of meeting the cost of education and decreasing the level of indebtedness makes the effort worthwhile. Students who borrow unsubsidized loans (loans that accrue interest during school, grace, and deferment periods) might ask their family to consider paying the interest on these loans during school. Although this will not reduce the initial principal amount a student borrows, it will help reduce the overall amount the student owes in repayment and is another way to help reduce overall borrowing costs.

• Keeping Good Records

Maintaining good records is the responsibility of the borrower and is indispensable to the financial health of that borrower. Students should not expect others to maintain their records. The maintenance of precise records, including copies of application forms and signed promissory notes, enables the borrower to verify any errors and potentially save money that may be inappropriately assigned. Further, lenders often sell their loans to other lenders. A borrower with poor records may inadvertently default because deferment forms or payments are forwarded to the wrong financial institution. Some loan programs provide students access to information on their loan portfolios, including current balances, on their Web sites as a means of helping borrowers keep track of their loans.

• Borrower Responsibility

Students are responsible for keeping in touch with the lender or servicer of their student loans. This means always letting them know when you change your name, address, telephone number, or in-school status. Students who fail to keep in touch with their lender or servicer, especially when filling out deferment or other loan forms, run the risk of becoming either delinquent or in default on their student loans, BOTH of which have a long term adverse impact on the borrower's credit rating.

SOURCES OF ASSISTANCE AND APPLICATION PROCEDURES

This chapter describes the rudiments of financial aid; each medical school has its own policies and procedures for distributing funds to students. Applicants must, therefore, maintain close contact with the financial aid offices at the schools to which they have been accepted.

Despite the variations of policies, procedures, application forms, and deadlines among institutions, a calendar showing general deadlines and dates of procedures is included here to help applicants with their plans for financing a medical education (Table 8-C); individual schools may deviate somewhat from the schedule in the table.

In addition to understanding the financial aid award cycle and the need to meet program deadlines, applicants should be

(Text continued on page 61)

TABLE 8-B

Federal Loan Programs for Students

Characteristic	Primary Care Loan	Federal Perkins	Federal Subsidized Stafford	Federal Unsubsidized Stafford
Lender	Medical school financial aid office on behalf of the Department of Health and Human Services	Medical school financial aid office on behalf of the Federal Government	Bank or other lending institution, the Federal Government or an eligible institution	Bank or other lending institution, the Federal Government or an eligible institution
Based on need	Note[1]	Yes	Yes	No
Citizenship Requirement	U.S. citizen, U.S. National, or U.S. permanent resident	U.S. citizen, U.S. National, or U.S. permanent resident	U.S. citizen, U.S. National, or U.S. permanent resident	U.S. citizen, U.S. National, or U.S. permanent resident
Borrowing limits	Up to cost of attendance (Third- and fourth-year students may receive additional funds to repay previous educational loans received while attending the medical school)	$5,000/year $30,000 aggregate undergraduate and graduate	$8,500 annual maximum; $65,500 cumulative maximum including premed and medical borrowing[2]	$38,500 less Subsidized Stafford annual maximum; $138,500 less Subsidized Stafford cumulative maximum premed and medical borrowing[2]
Interest rate	Note[3]	5%	In school, grace, and deferment: 91-Day Treasury Bill rate plus 1.7%, not to exceed 8.25%. In repayment: 91-Day Treasury Bill rate plus 2.3%, not to exceed 8.25%.	In school, grace, and deferment: 91-Day Treasury Bill rate plus 1.7%, not to exceed 8.25%. In repayment: 91-Day Treasury Bill rate plus 2.3%, not to exceed 8.25%.
Borrower is responsible for interest during:				
School	No	No	No	Yes
Deferments	No	No	No	Yes
Grace Period	No	No	No	Yes

[1]Yes; in addition, borrower must agree upon signing loan agreement to enter and complete primary care residency and practice in a primary care field until the loan is repaid in full. Family resource information is required for consideration.

[2]Both annual and cumulative maximums are subject to change pending Congressional action.

[3]Five percent; however, rate is recomputed at 18% from the date of noncompliance should borrower fail to meet primary care requirements.

CHAPTER 8

TABLE 8-B (continued)

Federal Loan Programs for Students

Characteristic	Primary Care Loan	Federal Perkins	Federal Subsidized Stafford	Federal Unsubsidized Stafford
Grace Period	1 year after graduation	9 months after graduation	6 months after graduation	6 months after graduation
Deferments	During school, grace, and throughout residency; check your promissory note	During school and applicable grace periods; few deferments available other than economic hardship; check your promissory note and ask your financial aid officer	During school and applicable grace periods; few deferments available other than economic hardship; check your promissory note and ask your financial aid officer	During school and applicable grace periods; few deferments available other than economic hardship; check your promissory note and ask your financial aid officer
Repayment requirements	Minimum: $40/month minimum paymeht; 10 to 25 years to repay; not eligible for loan consolidation	Minimum: $40/month including interest; maximum 10 years to repay; eligible for loan consolidation	Minimum: $50/month; level, graduated, income-based, and extended repayment options available; eligible for loan consolidation	Minimum: $50/month; level, graduated, income-based, and extended repayment options available; eligible for loan consolidation
Prepayment penalties	None	None	None	None
Allowable cancellations	Death, total, and permanent disability	Death, total, and permanent disability	Death, total, and permanent disability	Death, total, and permanent disability

TABLE 8-C

Calendar of Deadlines and Procedures for Financial Aid for Incoming Students

Event	*Dates*
Free Application for Federal Student Assistance (FAFSA) available for students	November–March
Financial aid information available for students	January–March
School-based aid application available for students	January–March
Deadline for submission of state scholarship applications by students	February–March
Deadline for submission of need analysis forms by students	March–May
Processing of applications to Federal loan programs begins	March–August
Deadline for submission of institutional aid forms by students	March–June
Notification to students of estimated award of school-based aid	April–August
Notification to students of complete award package	April–August

NOTE: This schedule is approximate. Contact individual schools for specific dates.

aware that there are some general eligibility requirements and some specific requirements based on particular programs.

• General Eligibility Criteria

Most programs—federal and private, need- and cost-based—will normally require that the applicant be a U.S. citizen or permanent resident of the United States, make satisfactory academic progress, and comply with Selective Service registration requirements. Further, the student may not be in default on other loans. Applicants who have defaulted on prior educational debts will be unable to obtain loans from most federal programs. An individual in this circumstance may be prevented from attending medical school because of being barred from a substantial source of aid—the federal government. It is critical, therefore, to remain in good standing with all loan and scholarship programs. Some programs also may require a commitment of service as a condition for receiving financial assistance.

• Need-Based Funds

Financial need is determined by subtracting the student's family resources from the school's standard student budget. The family contribution is calculated using a national need analysis service. Supporting materials such as tax returns are often required. Most medical schools expect full disclosure of parents' financial information—even for independent, older, or married students—to be considered for grants, scholarships, and low interest loans administered by the institution. It is important for applicants to ask their parents to file their income tax forms as early in the year as possible. Applicants should submit the required need analysis form(s) in March, April, or May of the year they expect to be accepted to medical school. Medical school financial aid officers can assist accepted students in determining their financial assistance requirements in a timely manner *only if applicants submit the necessary forms early.*

Table 8-B lists the various Federal loan programs available to medical students. School-administered programs and a number of private sources are also need-based. Individual medical schools, state departments of education, and college libraries are the best sources of information for these programs.

• Cost-Based Funds

Some programs are cost based, which means a formal need analysis of family contribution is not required. The student's resources must still be taken into account and subtracted from the budget established by the school in order to determine the amount that may be obtained. The Federal Unsubsidized Stafford Loan is not based on financial need. In addition, private loans such as the MEDLOANS' Alternative Loan Program (ALP) Loan are not need based, but rather based on a student's annual cost of attendance or financial aid budget. Information on the ALP is provided in the section on MEDLOANS.

• Credit

Many students require assistance beyond that provided by their family, the Federal government, and their medical school. This assistance often comes in the form of private loans such as the ALP. Students must not only have a cost of attendance, which supports their borrowing from these private loans, they must also be "credit ready." Credit ready means a student has either a) no credit history, or b) no adverse credit history. Students who have a history of late payments on consumer obligations will find it extremely difficult to borrow from private loans and are well advised to clean up their credit history as soon as possible. Some medical school financial aid offices require a copy of a student's credit history as part of their financial aid application.

It is also important to note that students with no adverse credit history (i.e., a solid record of on-time consumer payments), but who still have outstanding obligations, will find it very difficult to finance medical school. Even though they may be able to secure private loans, they will not be able to secure financial aid to cover their monthly consumer obligations.

Applicants to medical school are strongly encouraged to contact their medical school financial aid officer as soon as possible regarding the impact of credit on medical school financing.

AAMC MEDLOANS℠ PROGRAM

Designed exclusively with the unique needs of medical students in mind, the MEDLOANS Program is the smart choice for financing your medical education. The MEDLOANS Program has provided more than $2 billion to medical students over the last 15 years, and is the only student loan program in the country that is sponsored, endorsed and managed by the Association of American Medical Colleges. MEDLOANS provides medical students with a comprehensive package of student loans including the Federal Stafford Loan, the private Alternative Loan Program (ALP), and MEDEX for fourth-year students needing funds for residency interview and travel expenses. MEDLOANS remains the leader in medical school loan programs by offering:

- *Competitive Cost and More Money Up Front.* Besides being affordable, the MEDLOANS Program saves you money. In addition to no guarantee fee on Federal Stafford Loans and no up-front insurance premiums on the private Alternative Loan Program (ALP), the MEDLOANS Program rewards borrowers for prompt repayment. You will receive interest rate reductions and account credits for making scheduled payments on time! See the accompanying chart for more details on MEDLOANS' 2000–2001 terms and conditions.
- *One Easy Source of Funding and Life of Loan Servicing.* MEDLOANS borrowers get responsive customer service from start to finish, giving you peace of mind when calling with questions or concerns regarding your student loan portfolio. The MEDLOANS Program combines low-cost federal and private loans into one package, and can fund up to the total cost of your medical school education. And the MEDLOANS Program guarantees you one servicer throughout the life of your loans; such servicing is an essential element in avoiding unnecessary paperwork and confusion during your residency and repayment years. The MEDLOANS Program lets you select the repayment plan that works best for you, whether you need standard, graduated or income-sensitive plans—or even if you'd like to consolidate your loans.
- *Debt Management Assistance.* No other loan program offers you more debt management assistance than the MEDLOANS Program. As a MEDLOANS borrower you get the MEDLOANS Electronic Loan Portfolio (ELP), debt management software created specifically for medical students. You also get the MEDLOANS Borrower Notebooks, which feature loan terms and conditions, budgeting materials and a convenient centralized place to keep your loan promissory notes and records. You also get web-access to your student loan portfolio for up-to-the-minute information on your loan disbursements and balances.

MEDLOANS wants to help should you need financial assistance for medical school. However, your first call regarding financial aid of any kind should be to your medical school's financial aid office; your financial aid officer is the professional who will be working with you on financing matters throughout medical school.

For complete, up-to-date information (including current terms and conditions) on the MEDLOANS Program, please call MEDLOANS Customer Assistance at 1-800-858-5050, or visit our Web site at:

www.aamc.org/MEDLOANS

SERVICE COMMITMENT PROGRAMS

The commitment service scholarship programs—military awards available through the Army, Navy, and Air Force are not need-based or cost-based, nor are they, strictly speaking, financial aid.

The Armed Forces Health Professions Scholarship Program essentially offers full support to the medical student while in school in exchange for service in the funding organization once the scholarship recipient has received the M.D. degree. Participation in a postgraduate training program conducted at a military facility does not count toward the service commitment. Applications are very competitive and are handled by military recruiters. Addresses and further information are outlined in Table 8-D.

Medical students have the opportunity to enlist in the National Health Service Corps (NHSC) Scholarship Program upon matriculation to medical school. The NHSC is administered by the Bureau of Health Care Delivery and Assistance in the Health Resources and Services Administration, an agency

MEDLOANS 2000–2001 Terms and Conditions

	Federal Stafford Loans Subsidized and Unsubsidized	Alternative Loan Program (ALP)
Eligibility	Be enrolled in an eligible school at least ½ time. Meet other eligibility criteria in the Federal Stafford Loan Promissory Note.	Meet established credit criteria. Be currently enrolled at an approved school. All outstanting student loans in good standing.
Loan Limits	Annual $38,500 Aggregate Limits $189,125 *Unsubsidized loan limit is less any subsidized loan amount. (Subsidized limit: $8,500).	Minimum: $500 Annual Maximum: Cost of education minus other financial aid. Aggregate Maximum: $200,000 (total educational indebtedness from all sources)
Interest Rates	*In–school, grace and deferment:* Bond-equivalent rate for 91-day T-bills plus 1.7%, not to exceed 8.25%. *In Repayment:* Bond-equivalent rate for 91-day T-bills plus 2.3%, not to exceed 8.25%.	*Prior to repayment:* Variable, adjusted quarterly to the Prime Rate +0% *In repayment:* Variable, adjusted quarterly to the Prime Rate +0.25%. See Borrower Benefits for further details.
Subsidy & Capitalization	No interest on the subsidized Stafford while in school, grace and deferment. For Unsubsidized Stafford loans, interest is deferred and capitalized immediately before the commencement of repayment.	Interest is deferred and capitalized immediately before the commencement of repayment.
Fees	Guarantee fee: 0% Origination fee: 3% (subtracted from loan proceeds)	0% at loan origination. *At repayment:* Between 0% and 6%, based on a borrower's credit analysis at repayment and voluntary payments made during residency. Repayment insurance premium will be lower if minimum $50 payments are made in residency.
Repayment	Begins following six month grace period after leaving school or dropping to less than half time status. Deferment and forbearance options for residency. Borrowers have a maximum of 10 years to repay. Standard Repayment Graduated Repayment Income Sensitive Repayment	Begins three years after graduation, or nine months after enrollment status drops to less than half time. Borrowers have a maximum of 20 years to repay. Standard Repayment Alternative Repayment Terms
Borrower Benefits	***MEDLOANS Direct Repay Plan*** Pay electronically and receive a 0.25 percentage point interest rate reduction. ***MEDLOANS Healthy Returns Program*** Make your first 12 scheduled monthly payments on time and receive an account credit of 1% of your original Stafford loan balance, make 24 on time payments and receive a credit of another 1% of your original Stafford loan balance, and make 36 on time payments and receive a final credit of 1% of your original Stafford loan balance. ***MEDLOANS Great Rewards® Program*** Make your first 48 scheduled monthly payments on time and receive a 2.0 percentage point interest rate reduction for the remaining term of your Stafford loans.	The ALP Repayment Rate of Prime Rate +0.25% is available to those borrowers participating in the MEDLOANS Direct Repay Plan and the MEDLOANS Great Rewards® Program; otherwise the rate is Prime Rate +1.0%. ***MEDLOANS Direct Repay Plan*** Pay electronically and receive a 0.25 percentage point interest rate reduction. ***MEDLOANS Great Rewards® Program*** Maintain a schedule of on time monthly payments and receive a 0.50 percentage point interest rate reduction.

of the U.S. Public Health Service. Among the goals of the NHSC is the improvement of the delivery of primary care health services in health professional shortage areas (HPSA). The NHSC offers two major types of financial support in exchange for professional services: competitive scholarships and loan repayment. Awards are made in various amounts and service obligations range from two to four years.

Students applying for service scholarship programs should ask their financial aid officer about the treatment of these scholarships for tax purposes by the IRS.

Information on both scholarship and loan repayment programs can be found in the *State and Other Loan Repayment/Forgiveness and Scholarship Programs*, reference book, also available at www.aamc.org/about/gsa/stloan/start.htm.

• The Federal Scholarship Program

This program awards tuition and fees; payment towards books, supplies, and equipment; and a monthly stipend. In return, awardees commit to service in a federally designated HPSA one year for each year the scholarship is awarded with a minimum two-year obligation.

• The Federal Loan Repayment Program

This program provides payment towards both government and commercial education loans—up to $25,000 per year for the first two years and up to $35,000 for every year thereafter with a minimum two-year commitment. The program also provides funds for increased income taxes resulting from loan repayment. This is in addition to full salary and benefits.

The NHSC also provides a State Loan Repayment Program and Community Scholarship Program in selected states. For more information contact:

National Health Service Corps
Scholarship Program
U.S. Public Health Recruitment
2070 Chain Bridge Road, Suite 450
Vienna, Virginia 22182
1-800-221-9393

Students may also want to inquire about whether the state in which they intend to eventually practice has a loan forgiveness or repayment program in return for a commitment to serve in that state's areas of need. These programs are often aimed at residents and practicing physicians, though some are available to medical students who are still in school. Financial aid officers in the medical schools are a good source of information in this area. Inquire about the reference handbook, *State and Other Loan Repayment/Forgiveness and Scholarship Programs* (www.aamc.org/about/gsa/stloan/start.htm), when you are gathering other information from the medical school financial aid office.

• Loan Consolidation

Loan consolidation simply means paying off existing student loans with one new loan. In this regard, loan consolidation may be an attractive option for students who have multiple loans through multiple lenders, which sometimes results in the borrower working with different loan servicers during repayment, and who want the convenience of working with just one organization during repayment. Students who borrow their entire loan portfolio from one organization may already have the convenience of working with just one organization on repayment issues.

There are both advantages and disadvantages to consolidating your student loans. Students are well advised to check with their financial aid officer or loan servicer before consolidating.

INFORMATION SOURCES

The following books, articles, brochures, and newsletters should be readily available in libraries, university counseling offices, and medical school student affairs and financial aid offices, or they may be ordered directly from the publishers. Study of these materials may help students in their financial planning and lead them to further sources of financial aid.

1. *The Student Guide, 1998–99.* U.S. Department of Education. Free. (Federal Student Aid Information Center, P.O. Box 84, Washington, D.C. 20044; 1-800-4-FED AID (1-800-433-3243).
2. *Dollars for College: The Quick Guide to Scholarships, Fellowships, Loans, and Other Financial Aid Programs for Medicine, Dentistry, and Related Fields.* $7.95 prepaid. 1997. (Garrett Park Press, P.O. Box 190, Garrett Park, Maryland 20896; ISBN: 1-880774-15-1.)
3. *Financial Planning and Management Manual for U.S. Medical Students, 1994.* Association of American Medical Colleges. $7.50 plus shipping and handling. (Association of American Medical Colleges, Department 66, Washington, D.C. 20055; (202) 828-0416.)
4. *Informed Decision-Making: Part I, Financial Planning and Management for Medical Students; Part II, Sources of Financial Assistance for Medical School.* National Medical Fellowships, Inc. 1993. $15.00 per set. (Scholarship Department, National Medical Fellowships, Inc., 110 West 32nd Street, 8th Floor, New York, New York 10001).

FINANCIAL AID APPLICATION REQUIREMENTS FOR AMERICAN MEDICAL COLLEGES: A REFERENCE GUIDE FOR APPLICANTS AND PREMEDICAL ADVISORS

• What is the purpose of this guide?

The purpose of this guide is to provide medical school applicants and premedical advisors with a single directory of basic information about the process of applying for financial aid at medical schools across the United States. Each medical school entry includes information about how to contact its financial aid office; the school's U.S. Department of Education School ID Code (see Financial Aid Glossary); applications

TABLE 8-D

Federal Programs for Students

	Source of Grant		
Characteristic	Air Force	Army	Navy
Provider	Medical Recruiting Division HQ USAFRS/RSOC 550 D Street West, Suite 1 Randolph AFB, TX 78150-4527	U.S. Army Recruiting Command Attn: RCRO-HS-MC 1307 Third Avenue Fort Knox, KY 40121-2726 1-800-USA-ARMY; (502) 626-0368; 626-0376 http://www.goarmy.com	Commander, Navy Recruiting Command (Code 32B) 5722 Integrity Drive Millington, TN 38054-5057
Based on need	No	No	No
Citizenship requirement	U.S. citizen only	U.S. citizen only	U.S. citizen only
Service commitment	Yes	Yes	Yes
Nature of commitment	One year of service for each year of support	One year of service for each year of support	One year of service for each year of support (minimum three year obligation)
Level of support	Full tuition, monthly living stipend, book and supply allowance	Full tuition, monthly living stipend, book and supply allowance	Full tuition, monthly living stipend, book and supply allowance

that must be completed to be considered for financial assistance; filing deadlines for these applications; and, an indication as to whether the institution requires parental financial data to determine students' eligibility for its own financial aid funds. Table 8-E lists the necessary financial aid forms required by each medical school.

- **When was the data collected, and is it still accurate?**

The data in this publication were solicited directly from financial aid officials within the last year, although contact information or policies and procedures may have changed since that time. You are advised to contact all institutions in which you are interested, to verify the current accuracy of the information and to ask additional questions.

- **Is there anything I should know that is NOT contained in this guide?**

You should in no way perceive this guide to be a complete statement of institutional requirements for financial aid eligibility. Medical schools manage funds from various sources, all of which have unique requirements. You should request a complete list of all application requirements and procedures, as well as a copy of the institution's financial aid handbook, before initiating the financial aid application process.

- **When is parental financial information required?**

Please note that any medical student who wishes to borrow *only* a Federal Stafford Loan or Federal Direct Stafford Loan need only complete the Free Application for Federal Student Aid (FAFSA) and is not required to include parental financial data on that form. *However, if you wish to be considered for financial assistance programs offered by the U.S. Department of Health and Human Services (exclusive to health professions students) you must provide parental financial data on all forms the school requires, which may include the FAFSA.* The requirements of various schools will only differ with respect to whether any forms other than the FAFSA must be filed, and whether parental financial data is required for the school's own (non-federal) financial aid.

• Where may I find definitions of the terms used in this guide?

All of the terminology and abbreviations used are defined in the Financial Aid Glossary. If you have additional questions, you should contact the financial aid office(s) of the school(s) you are interested in attending.

This resource was created and compiled by the Group on Student Affairs' Committee on Student Financial Aid (COSFA) of the Association of American Medical Colleges (AAMC).

• Financial Aid Glossary

FAFSA (Free Application for Federal Student Aid)— This form serves as the application for all federal aid administered by the U.S. Department of Education. Information on the FAFSA may also be used by schools to determine eligibility for other financial assistance. To be considered for *all* sources of financial assistance for which you may be eligible (including low-interest loan and scholarship funds regulated by the U.S. Department of Health and Human Services), you may be requested to include parental financial data on the FAFSA.

Federal Direct Stafford Loan—A federally guaranteed loan made to students directly by the U.S. Department of Education to finance the costs of their attendance at postsecondary schools.

Federal School ID Code—An identification number assigned by the U.S. Department of Education to schools that participate in its financial aid programs. In order for a school to receive the data reported on the FAFSA, you must identify the school by using this number in Section H of the FAFSA.

Federal Stafford Loan—A federally guaranteed loan made to students by private lenders to finance the costs of their attendance at postsecondary schools.

U.S. Department of Education—The government agency that regulates all federal financial aid programs, with the exception of programs available only to health professions students.

U.S. Department of Health and Human Services (HHS)—The government agency that regulates federal loan and scholarship programs exclusive to health professions students.

Parent and Student Supplemental Application—This form serves as the application for aid administered by many schools. It may be used to determine your eligibility for aid administered by HHS, such as the exceptional need scholarships and Primary Care Loan program. Names of these applications include: Need Access, CSS Financial Aid PROFILE, and others. Check this guide to determine which forms you may need to complete.

FINANCIAL AID CONTACTS

University of Alabama School of Medicine
Office of Financial Aid
P-100 Volker Hall
1530 3rd Avenue, South
Birmingham, AL 35294-0019
Contact: Mark H. Martin
E-mail: mmartin@uab.edu
Web Site: http://main.uab.edu/show.asp?durki=2160
(205) 934-8707; 934-8724 (FAX)
Direct Lending: Yes
Federal School ID Code: 001052
Supplemental Application School Code: N/A

University of South Alabama College of Medicine
Office of Financial Aid
307 University Boulevard, Room 1005
Mobile, AL 36688-0002
Contact: Sharon Hera
Web Site: www.usouthal.edu
(334) 460-7918; 460-6761 (FAX)
Direct Lending: No
Federal School ID Code: 001057
Supplemental Application School Code: N/A

University of Arizona College of Medicine
Office of Financial Aid
P.O. Box 245026
Tucson, AZ 85724-5026
Contact: Maggie Gumble
Web Site: www.medicine.arizona.edu/financial_aid/
(520) 626-7145; 626-6300 (FAX)
Direct Lending: No
Federal School ID Code: 001083
Supplemental Application School Code: N/A

University of Arkansas College of Medicine
Student and Academic Affairs
4301 W. Markham Street
Financial Aid Slot 709
Little Rock, AR 72205-7199
Contact: Tom South
E-mail: SouthTomG@exchange.uams.edu
(501) 686-5813; 686-5873 (FAX)
Direct Lending: No
Federal School ID Code: 001109-01
Supplemental Application School Code: E00600

University of California, Davis, School of Medicine
Student Affairs Office
One Shields Avenue
Davis, CA 95616
Contact: Jay A. Conner
E-mail: medfinancialaid@ucdavis.edu
Web Site: www.ucdavis.edu/
(530) 752-6618; 752-2376 (FAX)
Direct Lending: Yes
Federal School ID: 001313
Supplemental Application School Code: N/A

University of California, Irvine, College of Medicine
Financial Aid Office
Medical Education Building 802, Room 106
Irvine, CA 92697-4089
Contact: James Miles
Web Site: www.fao.uci.edu/med
(949) 824-6476; 824-2485 (FAX)
Direct Lending: Yes
Federal School ID Code: 001314
Supplemental Application School Code: N/A

University of California, Los Angeles, UCLA School of Medicine
Financial Aid Office
12-109 CHS
Los Angeles, CA 90095
Contact: Teddie J. Milner
E-mail: Teddie@deans.medsch.ucla.edu
(310) 825-4181; 794-1629 (FAX)
Direct Lending: No
Federal School ID Code: 001315
Supplemental Application School Code: N/A

University of California, San Diego, School of Medicine
Student Financial Services Office
9500 Gilman Drive, Department 0621
La Jolla, CA 92093-0621
Contact: Carol Hartupee
Web Site: http://cybermed.ucsd.edu/catalog/
(858) 534-4664; 534-1513 (FAX)
Direct Lending: No
Federal School ID Code: 001317-03
Supplemental Application School Code: N/A

University of California, San Francisco, School of Medicine
Office of Financial Aid
500 Parnassus Avenue, MU201W
San Francisco, CA 94143-0246
E-mail: finaid_at_saa@ccmail.ucsf.edu
(415) 476-4181; 476-6652 (FAX)
Direct Lending: No
Federal School ID Code: 001319
Supplemental Application School Code: N/A

Loma Linda University School of Medicine
Office of Financial Aid
11139 Anderson Street
Loma Linda, CA 92350
Contact: Verdell Schaefer
Web Site: www.llu.edu
(909) 558-4509 or (800) 422-4558;
(909) 558-4879 (FAX)
Direct Lending: No
Federal School ID Code: 001218
Supplemental Application School Code: N/A

Keck School of Medicine
(University of Southern California)
Office of Financial Aid
1975 Zonal Avenue, KAM-420
Los Angeles, CA 90033
Contact: Linda Lewis
Web Site: www.usc.edu/schools/medicine
(323) 442-1016; 442-2943 (FAX)
Direct Lending: No
Federal School ID Code: 001328
Supplemental Application School Code: N/A

Stanford University School of Medicine
Office of Financial Aid
SUMC, Room M105
Stanford, CA 94305-5301
Contact: Edward Caron
Web Site: www.med.stanford.edu/school
(650) 723-6958; 725-6106 (FAX)
Direct Lending: No
Federal School ID: 001305-01
Supplemental Application School Code: N/A

University of Colorado School of Medicine
Office of Financial Aid
4200 East 9th Avenue, #A088
Denver, CO 80262
Contact: Veronica Van Gulick
Web Site: www.uchsc.edu/csa/finaid/
favahomg.htm
(303) 315-8364; 315-3350 (FAX)
Direct Lending: Yes
Federal School ID Code: 004508
Supplemental Application School Code: N/A

University of Connecticut School of Medicine
Student Financial Services
263 Farmington Avenue, MC1827
Farmington, CT 06030-1827
Contact: Patricia Lawson
E-mail: lawson@nso.uchc.edu
Web Site: www.uchc.edu
(860) 679-3574; 679-1877 (FAX)
Direct Lending: No
Federal School ID Code: G09867; 009867
Supplemental Application School Code: N/A

Yale University School of Medicine
Office of Financial Aid
367 Cedar Street
New Haven, CT 06510
(203) 785-2645; 785-3234
Direct Lending: No
Federal School ID Code: E00450
Supplemental Application School Code: N/A

George Washington University School of Medicine and Health Sciences
Office of Financial Aid
2300 Eye Street, N.W.
Washington, DC 20037
Contact: Charles Carpenter
E-mail: medfinan@gwis2.circ.gwu.edu
Web Site: www.gwumc.edu
(202) 994-2960; 728-0765 (FAX)
Direct Lending: No
Federal School ID Code: E00197
Supplemental Application School Code: N/A

Georgetown University School of Medicine
Office of Financial Aid
3900 Reservoir Road, N.W.
Butler Annex, Room #6
Washington, DC 20007
Contact: David Pollock
Web Site: www.dml.georgetown.edu/schmed/finaid/
(202) 687-1693; 687-2201 (FAX)
Direct Lending: No
Federal School ID Code: 001445-01
Supplemental Application School Code: N/A

Howard University College of Medicine
Office of Financial Aid
520 W Street, N.W.
Washington, DC 20059
Contact: Antoinette Christian-Rodgers
Web Site: www.med.howard.edu
(202) 806-6270; 806-7934 (FAX)
Direct Lending: Yes
Federal School ID Code: 001448
Supplemental Application School Code: N/A

University of Florida College of Medicine
Office of Financial Aid
P.O. Box 100216 HSC
Gainesville, FL 32610-0216
Contact: Eileen Parris

Web Site: www.med.ufl.edu/oea/finaid/
(352) 392-7800; 846-0812 (FAX)
Direct Lending: Yes
Federal School ID Code: 001535
Supplemental Application School Code: N/A

University of Miami School of Medicine
Office of Financial Aid
1600 N.W. 10 Avenue Room 2097
Miami, FL 33136
Contact: Laura L. Horsley
Web Site: www.med.miami.edu/
(305) 243-6211; 243-6748 (FAX)
Direct Lending: No
Federal School ID Code: E00533
Supplemental Application School Code: N/A

University of South Florida College of Medicine
Office of Financial Aid
12901 Bruce B. Downs Boulevard
MDC Box 4
Tampa, FL 33612-4799
Contact: Michelle Williamson
E-mail: MiWillia@com1.med.usf.edu
Web Site: www.med.usf.edu/
(813) 974-2068; 974-8181 (FAX)
Direct Lending: No
Federal School ID Code: E00568
Supplemental Application School Code: N/A

Emory University School of Medicine
Office of Financial Aid
300 B. Jones Center
Atlanta, GA 30322
Contact: Douglas Futch
E-mail: finaid@emory.edu
Web Site: www.emory.edu
(404) 727-6039; 727-6709 (FAX)
Direct Lending: No
Federal School ID Code: 001564
Supplemental Application School Code: 5187

Medical College of Georgia School of Medicine
Office of Student Financial Aid
1120 - 15th Street (AA2013)
Augusta, GA 30912-7320
Contact: Sandra D. Fowler
E-mail: osfa@mail.mcg.edu
Web Site: www.mcg.edu
(706) 721-4901
Direct Lending: No
Federal School ID Code: 001579
Supplemental Application School Code: N/A

Mercer University School of Medicine
Office of Financial Aid
1550 College Street
Macon, GA 31207
Contact: Youvette Hudson
Web Site: www.mercer.edu
(912) 301-2853; 301-5617 (FAX)
Direct Lending: Yes
Federal School ID Code: E00560
Supplemental Application School Code: N/A

Morehouse School of Medicine
Student Fiscal Affairs Office
720 Westview Drive, S.W.
Atlanta, GA 30310-1495
Contact: Cynthia H. Handy
Web Site: www.msm.edu
(404) 752-1655; 752-1053 (FAX)
Direct Lending: No
Federal School ID Code: G24821
Supplemental Application School Code: N/A

University of Hawai‘i at Mānoa
John A. Burns School of Medicine
Financial Aid Services
2600 Campus Road
Honolulu, HI 96822
Contact: Gail Koki
Web Site: www2.hawaii.edu/osa/Financial_Aid_Services.html
(808) 956-7251; 956-3985 (FAX)
Direct Lending: No
Federal School ID Code: 001610
Supplemental Application School Code: N/A

University of Chicago Division of the Biological Sciences Pritzker School of Medicine
Office of Financial Aid
924 East 57th Street, Suite 104
Chicago, IL 60637-5416
Contact: Mary Murray
Web Site: http://pritzker.bsd.uchicago.edu/
(773) 702-1938; 702-2598 (FAX)
Direct Lending: No
Federal School ID Code: G10141
Supplemental Application School Code: N/A

Finch University of Health Sciences/Chicago Medical School
Office of Financial Aid
3333 Green Bay Road
North Chicago, IL 60064
Contact: Jennifer Johnson
E-mail: johnsonj@finchcms.edu

Web Site: www.finchcms.edu
(847) 578-3217; 578-3284 (FAX)
Direct Lending: No
Federal School ID Code: 001659
Supplemental Application School Code: N/A

University of Illinois at Chicago College of Medicine
Office of Student Financial Aid
808 South Wood Street, Room 163 (M/C 782)
Chicago, IL 60612-7301
Contact: James Mendez
E-mail: jmendez@uic.edu
Web Site: www.uic.edu/depts/mcam/
(312) 413-0127; 996-2467 (FAX)
Direct Lending: Yes
Federal School ID Code: 001776
Supplemental Application School Code: N/A

Loyola University of Chicago Stritch School of Medicine
Office of Financial Aid
2160 South First Avenue, Room 210
Maywood, IL 60153
Contact: Donna J. Sobie
Web Site: www.lumen.edu/
(708) 216-3227; 216-0480 (FAX)
Direct Lending: No
Federal School ID Code: 001710-02
Supplemental Application School Code: G09188

Northwestern University Medical School
Office of Financial Aid
710 North Lake Shore Drive, #629 (C315)
Chicago, IL 60611-3078
Contact: Financial Aid Officer
(312) 503-8722; 503-8700 (FAX)
Direct Lending: No
Federal School ID Code: 00173901
Supplemental Application School Code: N/A

Rush Medical College of Rush University
Office of Financial Aid
600 South Paulina Street
Chicago, IL 60612
Contact: Robert Dame
Web Site: www.rush.edu/
(312) 942-6256; 942-2219 (FAX)
Direct Lending: No
Federal School ID Code: 009800
Supplemental Application School Code: N/A

Southern Illinois University School of Medicine
Office of Financial Aid
P.O. Box 19624
Springfield, IL 62794-9624
Contact: Nancy Calvert
E-mail: ncalvert@slumed.edu
Web Site: www.siumed.edu
(217) 785-2224; 785-5538 (FAX)
Direct Lending: Yes
Federal School ID Code: E00569
Supplemental Application School Code: N/A

Indiana University School of Medicine
635 Barnhill Drive, MS119
Indianapolis, IN 46202-5120
Contact: Jose R. Espada
Web Site: www.medicine.iupui.edu
(317) 274-1967; 274-4309 (FAX)
Direct Lending: No
Federal School ID Code: 001813
Supplemental Application School Code: N/A

University of Iowa College of Medicine
Office of Financial Aid
112 Medicine Administration Building
Iowa City, IA 52242-1101
Contact: Linda G. Bissell
E-mail: linda-bissell@uiowa.edu
Web Site: www.medicine.uiowa.edu/osac/finaid99
(319) 335-8059; 335-8049 (FAX)
Direct Lending: Yes
Federal School ID Code: 001892
Supplemental Application School Code: N/A

University of Kansas School of Medicine
Office of Financial Aid
3901 Rainbow Boulevard
4008 Student Center Building
Kansas City, KS 66160-7192
Contact: Financial Aid Officer
(913) 588-5170; 588-2597 (FAX)
Direct Lending: No
Federal School ID Code: 004605
Supplemental Application School Code: N/A

University of Kentucky College of Medicine
Office of Financial Aid
MN109A-Medical Center
800 Rose Street
Lexington, KY 40536-0084
Contact: Linda A. Gilbert
E-mail: lagilbo1@pop.uky.edu
Web Site: www.comed.uky.edu
(606) 323-6271; 323-2076 (FAX)
Direct Lending: Yes
Federal School ID Code: 001989-02
Supplemental Application School Code: N/A

University of Louisville School of Medicine
Office of Financial Aid
Abell Administration Center, Suite 402
323 East Chestnut Street
Louisville, KY 40202-3866

Contact: Leslie R. Kaelin
Web Site: www.louisville.edu
(502) 852-5187; 852-0302 (FAX)
Direct Lending: No
Federal School ID Code: 001999
Supplemental Application School Code: N/A

Louisiana State University School of Medicine in New Orleans
Office of Financial Aid
433 Bolivar Street, Suite 215
New Orleans, LA 70112
Contact: Daisy Engram
E-mail: pgorma@lsumc.edu
Web Site: www.lsumc.edu
(504) 568-4820; 599-1390 (FAX)
Direct Lending: No
Federal School ID Code: 002014
Supplemental Application School Code: N/A

Louisiana State University School of Medicine in Shreveport
Office of Financial Aid
1501 Kings Highway
P.O. Box 33932
Shreveport, LA 71130-3932
Contact: Sherry Gladney
E-mail: shufinaid@lsumc.edu
(318) 675-5561; 675-7893 (FAX)
Direct Lending: No
Federal School ID Code: 008067
Supplemental Application School Code: N/A

Tulane University School of Medicine
Office of Financial Aid
1430 Tulane Avenue, TB1
New Orleans, LA 70112-2699
Contact: Michael T. Goodman
Web Site: www1.omi.tulane.edu/
(504) 585-6135; 585-6136 (FAX)
Direct Lending: No
Federal School ID Code: 002029-01
Supplemental Application School Code: N/A

Johns Hopkins University School of Medicine
Office of Financial Aid
720 Rutland Avenue
Administration Building, Room 128
Baltimore, MD 21205-2196
Contact: Paula Abernethy
(410) 955-1324; 955-0544 (FAX)
Direct Lending: Yes
Federal School ID Code: E00235
Supplemental Application School Code: N/A

University of Maryland School of Medicine
Student Financial Aid
621 West Lombard Street, Room 334
Baltimore, MD 21201-1575
Contact: Melissa Fritz
Web Site: www.umaryland.edu/fin/
(410) 706-7347; 706-0824 (FAX)
Direct Lending: No
Federal School ID Code: 002104
Supplemental Application School Code: N/A

Boston University School of Medicine
Office of Student Financial Management
715 Albany Street, A401
Boston, MA 02118
Contact: Sonji Justice
Web Site: www.bumc.bu.edu/osfm
(617) 638-5130; 638-5116 (FAX)
Direct Lending: Yes
Federal School ID Code: 002130
Supplemental Application School Code: Profile: 3116

Harvard Medical School
Financial Aid Office
25 Shattuck Street, Room 150
Boston, MA 02115-6092
Contact: Sharon P. Clayborne
E-mail: hmsfao@warren.med.harvard.edu
Web Site: www.hms.harvard.edu/finaid/
(617) 432-1575; 432-4308 (FAX)
Direct Lending: Yes
Federal School ID Code: E00472
Supplemental Application School Code: 3445

University of Massachusetts Medical School
Financial Aid Office, UMMS
55 Lake Avenue North
Worcester, MA 01655
(508) 856-2265; 856-1899 (FAX)
Direct Lending: No
Federal School ID Code: N/A
Supplemental Application School Code: N/A

Tufts University School of Medicine
Office of Financial Aid
136 Harrison Avenue
Boston, MA 02111
Contact: Ellen C. Cost
Web Site: www.tufts.edu/med
(617) 636-6574; 636-3447 (FAX)
Direct Lending: No
Federal School ID Code: E00520
Supplemental Application School Code: N/A

Michigan State University College of Human Medicine
Financial Aid Office
252 Student Services Building
East Lansing, MI 48824-1113
Contact: Diane Batten
E-mail: Batten@pilot.msu.edu
Web Site: www.esp.msu.edu/
(517) 353 5188; 432 1155 (FAX)
Direct Lending: Yes
Federal School ID Code: 002290
Supplemental Application School Code: N/A

University of Michigan Medical School
Office of Financial Aid
C4130 MED SCI 1
1301 Catherine
Ann Arbor, MI 48109-0611
Contact: Carmen Colby
Web Site: www.med.umich.edu/
(734) 763-4147; 763-0453 (FAX)
Direct Lending: Yes
Federal School ID Code: E00398
Supplemental Application School Code: N/A

Wayne State University School of Medicine
Office of Financial Aid
540 East Canfield, 1374 Scott Hall
Detroit, MI 48201
Contact: Laurinda Osterbur
E-mail: losterb@wayne.edu
Web Site: www.med.wayne.edu
(313) 577-1039; 544-3434 (FAX)
Direct Lending: No
Federal School ID Code: E00570
Supplemental Application School Code: N/A

Mayo Medical School
Office of Financial Aid
200 First Street, S.W.
Rochester, MN 55905
Contact: Glenda Tucker
Web Site: www.mayo.edu/mms
(507) 284-4839; 266-5298 (FAX)
Direct Lending: No
Federal School ID Code: 011732; G11732
Supplemental Application School Code: N/A

University of Minnesota Medical School—Minneapolis
Office of Financial Aid
Box 293, 420 Delaware Street
Minneapolis, MN 55455
Contact: B.J. Gibson
E-mail: b-gibs@tc.umn.edu
(612) 624-7675; 626-4794 (FAX)
Direct Lending: Yes
Federal School ID Code: 003969
Supplemental Application School Code: N/A

University of Mississippi School of Medicine
Office of Financial Aid
2500 North State Street
Jackson, MS 39216
Contact: Steve Greenough
E-mail: Sgreenough@registrar.umsmed.edu
Web Site: umc.edu/medicine/
(601) 984-1117; 984-6984 (FAX)
Direct Lending: No
Federal School ID Code: 004688
Supplemental Application School Code: N/A

University of Missouri—Columbia School of Medicine
Financial Aid Office
MA202 Medical Sciences Building
Columbia, MO 65212
Contact: Conway A. Jones
E-mail: JonesCA@health.missouri.edu
Web Site: www.hscmissouri.edu/~medicine/
(573) 882-2923; 884-4808 (FAX)
Direct Lending: Yes
Federal School ID Code: 002516
Supplemental Application School Code: N/A

University of Missouri—Kansas City School of Medicine
Financial Aid and Scholarships Office
5100 Rockhill Road, Administrative Center 101
Kansas City, MO 64110
Contact: Nate Shatto
Web Site: www.umkc.edu/finaid
(816) 235-1154; 235-5511 (FAX)
Direct Lending: Yes
Federal School ID Code: 002518
Supplemental Application School Code: N/A

Saint Louis University School of Medicine
Office of Financial Aid
1402 South Grand Boulevard, MS229
St. Louis, MO 63104
Contact: Mary B.W. Fenton
Web Site: www.slu.edu/colleges/med/sfp
(314) 577-8617; 268-5489 (FAX)
Direct Lending: No
Federal School ID Code: E00318
Supplemental Application School Code: N/A

Washington University School of Medicine
Committee on Student Financial Aid
660 South Euclid Avenue, #8059
St. Louis, MO 63110
Contact: John F. Walters
E-mail: money@msnotes.wustl.edu

Web Site: http://medschool.wustl.edu/
(314) 362-6845; 362-3045 (FAX)
Direct Lending: No
Federal School ID Code: G24620
Supplemental Application School Code: N/A

Creighton University School of Medicine
Office of Financial Aid
2500 California Street
Criss II Room 106
Omaha, NE 68178
Contact: Tanya T. Avant
E-mail: tavant@creighton.edu
Web Site: www.creighton.edu
(402) 280-2666; 280-2599 (FAX)
Direct Lending: No
Federal School ID Code: 002542
Supplemental Application School Code: N/A

University of Nebraska College of Medicine
Office of Financial Aid
984265 Nebraska Medical Center
Omaha, NE 68198-4265
Contact: Judi Walker
E-mail: jdwalker@unmcvm.unmc.edu
Web Site: www.unmc.edu/
(402) 559-4199; 559-6796 (FAX)
Direct Lending: No
Federal School ID Code: 006895
Supplemental Application School Code: N/A

University of Nevada School of Medicine
Office of Admissions and Student Affairs
Manville Medical Building, Mail Stop 357
Reno, NV 89557
Contact: Barbara Hall-Bellows
E-mail: asa@unr.edu
Web Site: www.unr.edu/med/
(702) 784-6063; 784-6194 (FAX)
Direct Lending: No
Federal School ID Code: 002568
Supplemental Application School Code: N/A

Dartmouth Medical School
Office of Financial Aid
7021 Remsen Building, 305A
Hanover, NH 03755-3833
Contact: Nanci G. Cirone
E-mail: dms.financial.aid@dartmouth.edu
Web Site: www.dartmouth.edu/dms/dms_finaid/
(603) 650-1919; 650-1614 (FAX)
Direct Lending: No
Federal School ID Code: 002573
Supplemental Application School Code: N/A

UMDNJ—New Jersey Medical School
Office of Financial Aid
ADMC 1208, 30 Bergen Street
Newark, NJ 07107-3000
Contact: Cheryl White
Web Site: www.umdnj.edu
(973) 972-4376; 972-7436 (FAX)
Direct Lending: No
Federal School ID Code: 010394
Supplemental Application School Code: 013645

University of Medicine and Dentistry of New Jersey-Robert Wood Johnson Medical School
Office of Financial Aid
675 Hoes Lane, C-103
Piscataway, NJ 08854
Contact: Paul D. Koch
Web Site: www.umdnj.edu
(732) 235-4689; 235-3264 (FAX)
Direct Lending: No
Federal School ID Code: 013645
Supplemental Application School Code: N/A

University of New Mexico School of Medicine
Office of Admissions and Student Affairs
BMSB, Room B83
Albuquerque, NM 87131-5166
Contact: Ed Wyckoff
E-mail: ewyck@unm.deu
Web Site: www.unm.edu
(505) 272-8008; 272-8239 (FAX)
Direct Lending: Yes
Federal School ID Code: 002663
Supplemental Application School Code: N/A

Albany Medical College
Financial Aid Office
47 New Scotland Avenue
Administration R214, Mailcode 1
Albany, NY 12208-3479
Contact: Tor Shekerjian
Web Site: www.amc.edu/
(518) 262-5435; 262-5914 (FAX)
Direct Lending: No
Federal School ID Code: G02887
Supplemental Application School Code: N/A

Albert Einstein College of Medicine of Yeshiva University
Office of Financial Aid
1300 Morris Park Avenue, Room B208A
Bronx, NY 10461
Contact: Lloyd Greenberg
Web Site: www.aecom.yu.edu/
(718) 430-2336; 430-8825 (FAX)

Direct Lending: No
Federal School ID Code: G09895
Supplemental Application School Code: 2995

Columbia University College of Physicians and Surgeons
Office of Student Financial Planning
630 West 168th Street
New York, NY 10032
Contact: Sanora Garcia
Web Site: www.columbia.edu
(212) 305-4100; 305-0221 (FAX)
Direct Lending: No
Federal School ID Code: 002707/16
Supplemental Application School Code: N/A

Weill Medical College of Cornell University
Office of Financial Aid
445 E. 69th Street
New York, NY 10021
Contact: Gladys Laden
Web Site: www.med.cornell.edu/
(212) 746-1066; 746-8211 (FAX)
Direct Lending: Yes
Federal School ID Code: G04762
Supplemental Application School Code: N/A

Mount Sinai School of Medicine of New York University
Student Financial Services
One Gustave L. Levy Place, Box 1002
New York, NY 10029
Contact: Dale Fuller
Web Site: www.mssm.edu
(212) 241-5245; 876-4658 (FAX)
Direct Lending: No
Federal School ID Code: 007026-00
Supplemental Application School Code: N/A

New York Medical College
Office of Student Financial Planning
Administration Building, Room 125B
Valhalla, NY 10595
Contact: Beverly Bello
Web Site: www.NYMC.EDU
(914) 594-4491; 594-4613 (FAX)
Direct Lending: No
Federal School ID Code: G02784
Supplemental Application School Code: N/A

New York University School of Medicine
Office of Financial Aid
550 First Avenue
New York, NY 10016
Contact: Joanne M. Horan
Web Site: www.med.nyu.edu/som/
(212) 263-5286
Direct Lending: No
Federal School ID Code: G24543
Supplemental Application School Code: N/A

University of Rochester School of Medicine and Dentistry
Office of Financial Aid
601 Elmwood Avenue, Box 601
Rochester, NY 14642
Contact: Nancy Janson
E-mail: finaid@URMC.Rochester.edu
WebSite: www.urmc.rochester.edu/smd/finaid/
(716) 275-7245; 273-1016 (FAX)
Direct Lending: Yes
Federal School ID Code: G24601
Supplemental Application School Code: N/A

State University of New York Downstate Medical Center College of Medicine
Student Financial Aid Services
450 Clarkson Avenue, Box 110
Brooklyn, New York 11203-2098
Contact: Julia B. Clayton
E-mail: jclayton@netmail.hscbklyn.edu
Web Site: www.hscbklyn.edu
(718) 270-2488: 270-7592 (FAX)
Direct Lending: No
Federal School ID Code: 002839
Supplemental Application School Code: N/A

State University of New York at Buffalo School of Medicine and Biomedical Sciences
Financial Aid Office
Hayes Annex C
3435 Main Street
Buffalo, NY 14214
Contact: Any financial aid advisor
Web Site: http://wings.buffalo.edu/
(716) 829-3724; 829-2022 (FAX)
Direct Lending: Yes
Federal School ID Code: 002837
Supplemental Application School Code: N/A

State University of New York at Stony Brook Health Sciences Center School of Medicine
Office of Student Affairs
HSC Level 4, Room 147
Stony Brook, NY 11794-8436
Contact: Mary Jean Allen
Web Site: www.uhmc.sunysb.edu/som/
(516) 444-2341; 444-8921 (FAX)
Direct Lending: No

Federal School ID Code: 002838
Supplemental Application School Code: N/A

State University of New York Upstate Medical University College of Medicine
Financial Aid Office
155 Elizabeth Blackwell Street
Syracuse, NY 13210
E-mail: finaid@vax.cs.hscsyr.edu
Web Site: www.hscsyr.edu
(315) 464-4329; 464-8857 (FAX)
Direct Lending: No
Federal School ID Code: 002840
Supplemental Application School Code: N/A

The Brody School of Medicine at East Carolina University
Office of Financial Aid
2S-20 Brody
Greenville, NC 27858-4354
Contact: Vickie Ogden
Web Site: www.med.ecu.edu/
(252) 816-2278; 816-3250 (FAX)
Direct Lending: No
Federal School ID Code: 002923
Supplemental Application School Code: N/A

Duke University School of Medicine
Office of Financial Aid
DUMC Box 3067
Durham, NC 27710
Contact: Karen Robinette or Karen Woedlief
E-mail: financial_aid@mc.duke.edu
Web Site: www2.mc.duke.edu/som/
(919) 684-6649; 684-2593 (FAX)
Direct Lending: No
Federal School ID Code: 002920-01
Supplemental Application School Code: N/A

University of North Carolina at Chapel Hill School of Medicine
Office of Student Affairs, Student Aid Section
CB# 7000, 121 MacNider Building
Chapel Hill, NC 27599-7000
Contact: Sheila M. Graham
Web Site: www.med.unc.edu
(919) 962-6117; 966-9153 (FAX)
Direct Lending: No
Federal School ID Code: 002974-01
Supplemental Application School Code: N/A

Wake Forest University School of Medicine
Office of Financial Aid
Medical Center Boulevard
Winston-Salem, NC 27157-1090
Contact: Melissa Stevens
Web Site: www.wfubmc.edu
(336) 716-2889; 716-5807 (FAX)
Direct Lending: No
Federal School ID Code: E00524
Supplemental Application School Code: 5084

University of North Dakota School of Medicine and Health Sciences
Office of Financial Aid
P.O. Box 9037
501 North Columbia Road
Grand Forks, ND 58202
Contact: Sandra K. Elshaug
Web Site: www.med.und.nodak.edu
(701) 777-2849; 777-4942 (FAX)
Direct Lending: No
Federal School ID Code: 003005
Supplemental Application School Code: N/A

Case Western Reserve University School of Medicine
Office of Financial Aid
10900 Euclid Avenue, T-303
Cleveland, OH 44106-4920
Contact: Wanda L. Rollins or Shelley Spera
E-mail: medfa@po.cwru.edu
Web Site: http://mediwww.meds.cwru.edu
(216) 368-3666; 368-6011 (FAX)
Direct Lending: No
Federal School ID Code: E00079
Supplemental Application School Code: N/A

University of Cincinnati College of Medicine
Financial Aid Office
P.O. Box 670552
Cincinnati, OH 45267-0552
Contact: Daniel A. Burr
E-mail: burrda@uc.edu
Web Site: www.med.uc.edu
(513) 558-6797; 558-1165 (FAX)
Direct Lending: No
Federal School ID Code: E00385
Supplemental Application School Code: N/A

Medical College of Ohio
Office of Financial Aid
3045 Arlington Avenue
Toledo, OH 43614-5805
Contact: Deb Heineman
E-mail: bpettaway@mco.edu
Web Site: www.mco.edu
(419) 383-3444; 383-4005 (FAX)
Direct Lending: No
Federal School ID Code: 007737
Supplemental Application School Code: N/A

Northeastern Ohio Universities College of Medicine
Office of Financial Aid
4209 State Route 44
P.O. Box 95
Rootstown, OH 44272-0095
Contact: Michelle L. Cassetty
Web Site: www.neoucom.edu
(330) 325-6481; 325-5905 (FAX)
Direct Lending: No
Federal School ID Code: 024544
Supplemental Application School Code: N/A

Ohio State University College of Medicine and Public Health
Office of Financial Aid
370 West 9th Avenue
Columbus, OH 43210
Contact: Donna Cavell
Web Site: www.osu.edu
(614) 292-4838; 292-1544 (FAX)
Direct Lending: Yes
Federal School ID Code: 003090
Supplemental Application School Code: N/A

Wright State University School of Medicine
Student Affairs/Admissions
P.O. Box 1751
Dayton, OH 45401-1751
Contact: Gwen Sloas
E-mail: gwen.sloas@wright.edu
Web Site: www.med.wright.edu/
(937) 775-2934; 775-3322 (FAX)
Direct Lending: No
Federal School ID Code: 003078
Supplemental Application School Code: N/A

University of Oklahoma College of Medicine
Financial Aid Office
P. O. Box 26901
Oklahoma City, Ok 73190
Contact: Martha Starling
Web Site: www.ouhsc.edu/sfs
(405) 271-2118; 271-5446 (FAX)
Direct Lending: No
Federal School ID Code: 005889
Supplemental Application School Code: N/A

Oregon Health Sciences University School of Medicine
3181 S.W. Sam Jackson Park Road, L109
Portland, OR 97201
Contact: Rebecca Cady
E-mail: finaid@ohsu.edu
Web Site: www.ohsu.edu/
(503) 494-7800; 494-4629 (FAX)
Direct Lending: Yes
Federal School ID Code: 004883
Supplemental Application School Code: N/A

Jefferson Medical College of Thomas Jefferson University
Office of Financial Aid
1025 Walnut Street, Room G-1
Philadelphia, PA 19107
Contact: Raelynn Cooter
E-mail: financial.aid@jefferson.edu
Web Site: www.tju.edu
(215) 955-2867
Direct Lending: No
Federal School ID Code: 010021
Supplemental Application School Code: N/A

MCP Hahnemann School of Medicine
Office of Financial Aid
2900 Queen Lane
Philadelphia, PA 19129
Contact: Cindy DeLone
E-mail: Iannuzzij@wpo.auhs.edu
Web Site: www.auhs.edu
(215) 991-8210; 843-5243 (FAX)
Direct Lending: No
Federal School ID Code: 003271
Supplemental Application School Code: N/A

Pennsylvania State University College of Medicine
Office of Student Affairs H060
Attn: Financial Aid
500 University Drive
Hershey, PA 17033
Contact: Kathy Greider
Web Site: www.collmed.psu.edu/
(717) 531-4103; 531-6225 (FAX)
Direct Lending: No
Federal School ID Code: G06813
Supplemental Application School Code: N/A

University of Pennsylvania School of Medicine
Office of Financial Aid
Suite 100, Stemmler Hall
3450 Hamilton Walk
Philadelphia, PA 19104-6056
Contact: Ann Marie Hunt
Web Site: www.med.upenn.edu
(215) 573-3423: 573-6645 (FAX)
Direct Lending: No
Federal School ID Code: 003378
Supplemental Application School Code: N/A

University of Pittsburgh School of Medicine
Office of Financial Aid
M219 Scaife Hall
Pittsburgh, PA 15261
Contact: Judy Manjerovic

E-mail: financial_aid@fs1.dean-med.pitt.edu
Web Site: www.dean-med.pitt.edu
(412) 648-8936; 648-1236 (FAX)
Direct Lending: No
Federal School ID Code: E00516
Supplemental Application School Code: N/A

Temple University School of Medicine
Office of Financial Aid
SFC, Building LB-41
Broad and Ontario Streets
Philadelphia, PA 19140
Contact: Thomas K. Malloy
Web Site: www.temple.edu/medschool
(215) 707-2667; 707-2917 (FAX)
Direct Lending: No
Federal School ID Code: E00352
Supplemental Application School Code: N/A

Universidad Central del Caribe School of Medicine
Office of Financial Aid
P.O. Box 60327
Bayamon, PR 00960
Contact: Vivian Cintron-Diaz
E-mail: vcintron@uccaribe.edu
Web Site: www.uccaribe.edu
(787) 740-1611; 269-7550 (FAX)
Direct Lending: No
Federal School ID Code: 021633-00
Supplemental Application School Code: N/A

Ponce School of Medicine
Office of Financial Aid
P.O. Box 7004
Ponce, PR 00732
Contact: Rosalia Martinez
E-mail: psmfinstu@hotmail.com
(787) 840-2575 ext. 260; 842-1563 (FAX)
Direct Lending: No
Federal School ID Code: 024824
Supplemental Application School Code: N/A

University of Puerto Rico School of Medicine
Office of Financial Aid
P.O. Box 365067
San Juan, PR 00936-5067
Contact: Lourdes Pont
(787) 758-2525; 282-7117 (FAX)
E-mail: 1_pont@rcmaxp.upr.clu.edu
Web Site: wwwrcm.upr.clu.edu
Direct Lending: No
Federal School ID Code: 003945
Supplemental Application School Code: N/A

Brown University School of Medicine
Office of Admissions and Financial Aid
97 Waterman Street, Box G-A212
Providence, RI 02912-9706
Contact: Kathleen Massone Baer
Web Site: www.brown.edu
(401) 863-1142; 863-3801 (FAX)
Direct Lending: Yes
Federal School ID Code: E00059
Supplemental Application School Code: N/A

Medical University of South Carolina College of Medicine
Financial Aid Services
45 Courtenay Drive
P.O. Box 250176
Charleston, SC 29425
Contact: Pearl M. Givens
Web Site: www.musc.edu
(843) 792-2536; 792-2535 (FAX)
Direct Lending: No
Federal School ID Code: 003438
Supplemental Application School Code: N/A

University of South Carolina School of Medicine
Office of Financial Aid
Basic Science Building #1
Columbia, SC 29208
Contact: Peggy J. Lynch
E-mail: plynch@med.sc.edu
Web Site: www.med.sc.edu/
(803) 733-3135; 733-1585 (FAX)
Direct Lending: No
Federal School ID Code: 003448
Supplemental Application School Code: N/A

University of South Dakota School of Medicine
Medical Student Affairs
414 East Clark Street
Vermillion, SD 57069
Contact: Carol Hemmingson
E-mail: chemming@usd.edu
Web Site: www.usd.edu/med/md/saserv.htm
(605) 677-5112; 677-5109 (FAX)
Direct Lending: No
Federal School ID Code: 003474
Supplemental Application School Code: N/A

East Tennessee State University James H. Quillen College of Medicine
Office of Financial Aid
Box 70580
Johnson City, TN 37614-0580
Contact: Ruth Angle
Web Site: http://qcom.etsu.edu

(423) 439-4751; 439-4760 (FAX)
Direct Lending: No
Federal School ID Code: 003487-01
Supplemental Application School Code: N/A

Meharry Medical College School of Medicine
Office of Student Financial Aid
1005 D.B. Todd Jr. Boulevard
LRC Building, Suite 606
Nashville, TN 37208
Contact: Vickie L. Johnson
Web Site: www.mmc.edu/
(615) 327-6826; 327-6951 (FAX)
Direct Lending: No
Federal School ID Code: 003506-00
Supplemental Application School Code: N/A

University of Tennessee, Memphis, College of Medicine
Office of Financial Aid
800 Madison, SAC 311
Memphis, TN 38163
Contact: Lori A. Hartman
E-mail: osfa@utmem.edu
Web Site: www.utmem.edu
(901) 448-5568; 448-1570 (FAX)
Direct Lending: No
Federal School ID Code: 006725
Supplemental Application School Code: N/A

Vanderbilt University School of Medicine
Office of Student Financial Services
404 Light Hall
Nashville, TN 37232-0740
Contact: Vicky L. Cagle
E-mail: vicky.cagle@mcmail.vanderbilt.edu
Web Site: www.mc.vanderbilt.edu/medschool/finaid.html
(615) 343-6310; 343-8397 (FAX)
Direct Lending: No
Federal School ID Code: E00459
Supplemental Application School Code: N/A

Baylor College of Medicine
Office of Financial Aid
One Baylor Plaza, Suite N104
Houston, TX 77030
E-mail: finaid@bcm.tmc.edu
Web Site: www.bcm.tmc.edu/osa/osa- financial.html
(713) 798-4603; 798-5563 (FAX)
Direct Lending: No
Federal School ID Code: 015170
Supplemental Application School Code: N/A

Texas A&M University Health Science Center College of Medicine
Office of Financial Aid
159 Reynolds Medical Building
College Station, TX 77843-1114
Contact: Jack Falks
E-mail: med-stu-aff@tamu.edu
Web Site: www.tamu.edu/
(409) 845-7743; 845-5533 (FAX)
Direct Lending: No
Federal School ID Code: 003632
Supplemental Application School Code: NA

Texas Tech University Health Sciences Center School of Medicine
Office of Financial Aid
3601 4th Street, 3B 310
Lubbock, TX 79430
Contact: Sherri Henry
E-mail: financial.aid@ttuhsc.edu
Web Site: www.ttuhsc.edu
(806) 743-3025; 743-3027 (FAX)
Direct Lending: No
Federal School ID Code: 010674
Supplemental Application School Code: N/A

University of Texas Southwestern Medical Center at Dallas Southwestern Medical School
Office of Student Financial Aid
5323 Harry Hines Boulevard
Dallas, TX 75235-9064
Contact: Karen Mangum
E-mail: admissions@email.swmed.edu
Web Site: www.swmed.edu
(214) 648-3611; 648-3289 (FAX)
Direct Lending: No
Federal School ID Code: 010019
Supplemental Application School Code: N/A

University of Texas Medical Branch University of Texas Medical School at Galveston
Office of Financial Aid
301 University Boulevard
Galveston, TX 77555-1312
Contact: Betty Hazelbaker
Web Site: www2.utmb.edu/finaid
(409) 772-4955; 772-4466 (FAX)
Direct Lending: Yes
Federal School ID Code: 004952
Supplemental Application School Code: N/A

University of Texas—Houston Medical School
Office of Financial Aid
P.O. Box 20036
Houston, TX 77225
Contact: Financial officer
Web Site: www.uth.tmc.edu/
(713) 500-3860; 500-3863 (FAX)
Direct Lending: No
Federal School ID Code: 013956
Supplemental Application School Code: 004951

University of Texas Medical School at San Antonio
Financial Aid Office
7703 Floyd Curl Drive
San Antonio, TX 78284-7708
Contact: Lynn A. McConnell
E-mail: mcconnell@uthscsa.edu
Web Site: www.uthscsa.edu
(210) 567-2635; 567-6643 (FAX)
Direct Lending: No
Federal School ID Code: 003659
Supplemental Application School Code: N/A

University of Utah School of Medicine
Office of Financial Aid
1C102 Medical Center
50 North Medical Drive
Salt Lake City, UT 84132
Contact: Rita Litsas
Web Site: www.saff.utah.edu/finance/
(801) 581-6474; 585-3300 (FAX)
Direct Lending: No
Federal School ID Code: 003675
Supplemental Application School Code: N/A

University of Vermont College of Medicine
Financial Aid Office
105 A Rowell
Burlington, VT 05405
Contact: Sean P. McGivney
E-mail: medfao@zoo.uvm.edu
Web Site: www.uvm.edu/medfao
(802) 656-8293
Direct Lending: No
Federal School ID Code: 003696
Supplemental Application School Code: N/A

Eastern Virginia Medical School of the Medical College of Hampton Roads
Office of Financial Aid
700 Olney Road, Room 1147
Norfolk, VA 23507
Contact: Patricia Ashkenazi
Web Site: www.evms.edu
(757) 446-5813; 446-5817 (FAX)
Direct Lending: No
Federal School ID Code: 010338
Supplemental Application School Code: N/A

Virginia Commonwealth University School of Medicine
Office of Financial Aid
1101 East Marshall Street
P.O. Box 980565
Richmond, VA 23298-0565
Contact: Sean L. Bates
E-mail: SLBates@VCU.edu
(804) 828-4006; 828-5115 (FAX)
Direct Lending: Yes
Federal School ID Code: 003735
Supplemental Application School Code: N/A

University of Virginia School of Medicine
Financial Aid Office
416 HSC
Charlottesville, VA 22908
Contact: Catharine Anas
Web Site: www.med.virginia.edu
(804) 924-0033; 924-2279
Direct Lending: Yes
Federal School ID Code: 003745
Supplemental Application School Code: N/A

University of Washington School of Medicine
Office of Financial Aid
Box 357430
Seattle, WA 98195-7430
Contact: Diane Noecker
E-mail: dnoecker@u.washington.edu
Web Site: www.washington.edu
(206) 685-2520: 543-9063 (FAX)
Direct Lending: Yes
Federal School ID Code: 003798
Supplemental Application School Code: N/A

Marshall University School of Medicine
Office of Financial Aid
400 Hal Greer Boulevard
Huntington, WV 25755
Contact: Nadine A. Hamrick
Web Site: www.marshall.edu/sfa/
(304) 696-3162 or 1 (800) 438-5390; 696-3242 (FAX)
Direct Lending: Yes

Federal School ID Code: 003815
Supplemental Application School Code: N/A

West Virginia University School of Medicine
Financial Aid Office-WVU
Health and Sciences Center
P.O. Box 9810
Morgantown, WV 26506-9810
Contact: Candance Hostutler
E-mail: hscfao@wvnvm.wvnet.edu
Web Site: www.hsu.wvu.edu/fin/
(304) 293-3706; 293-6861 (FAX)
Direct Lending: Yes
Federal School ID Code: 003827
Supplemental Application School Code: N/A

Medical College of Wisconsin
Office of Financial Aid
8701 Watertown Plank Road
Milwaukee, WI 53226
Contact: Linda L. Paschal
E-mail: finaid@mcw.edu
Web Site: www.mcw.edu/
(414) 456-8208; 456-6506 (FAX)
Direct Lending: No
Federal School ID Code: 015611
Supplemental Application School Code: N/A

University of Wisconsin Medical School
Office of Financial Aid
432 North Murray Street
Madison, WI 53706
Contact: John Selbo
E-mail: financialaid.uw-madison@
mail.admin.wisc.edu
Web Site: www.wisc.edu
(608) 262-3060; 262-9068 (FAX)
Direct Lending: No
Federal School ID Code: 003895
Supplemental Application School Code: N/A

FINANCIAL AID CONTACTS—CANADIAN MEDICAL SCHOOLS

University of Calgary Faculty of Medicine
Student Awards and Financial Aid
2500 University Drive, N.W.
Calgary, Alberta
Canada T2N 1N4
Contact: Sharon Westlund
E-mail: ucawards@ucalgary.ca
Web Site: www.ucalgary.ca/uofc/students/awards
(403) 220-6925; 282-2999 (FAX)
Direct Lending: No
Federal School ID Code: 007874
Supplemental Application School Code: N/A

University of British Columbia Faculty of Medicine
Awards and Financial Aid-UBC
Awards and Financial Aid
Room 1036, 1874 East Mall
Vancouver, British Columbia
Canada V6T 1Z1
Contact: Daniel R. Worsley
E-mail: worsley@regi.ubc.ca
Web Site: www.awards.ubc.ca
(604) 822-6279; 822-6929 (FAX)
Direct Lending: No
Federal School ID Code: 008369
Supplemental Application School Code: N/A

University of Manitoba Faculty of Medicine
753 McDermot Avenue
Winnipeg, Manitoba
Canada R3E 0W3
Contact: Charles K. Paragg
E-mail: parragg@ms.umanitoba.ca
Web Site: www.umanitoba.ca/
(204) 789-3569; 789-3929 (FAX)
Direct Lending: Yes
Federal School ID Code: N/A
Supplemental Application School Code: N/A

Memorial University of Newfoundland
Faculty of Medicine
Health Sciences Center
300 Prince Phillip Drive
St. John's, Newfoundland
Canada AIB 3V6
Contact: Mary Dray
E-mail: mdray@morgan.ucs.mun.ca
Web Site: www.mun.ca
(709) 737-6029; 737-5029 (FAX)
Direct Lending: No
Federal School ID Code: 009500
Supplemental Application School Code: 009500

Dalhousie University Faculty of Medicine
Office of Financial Aid
Room C-132 CRC
5849 University Avenue
Halifax, Nova Scotia
Canada B3H 4H7
Contact: Carl Stevens
Web Site: www.mcms.dal.ca

(902) 494-1874; 494-8884 (FAX)
Direct Lending: N/A
Federal School ID Code: N/A
Supplemental Application School Code: N/A

Queen's University Faculty of Health Sciences
Student Awards Office
110 Alfred Street
Kingston, Ontario
Canada K7L 3N6
Contact: Patricia A. Bogstad
Web Site: www.queensu.ca/registrar/awards/index.html
(613) 545-2216; 545-6409 (FAX)
Direct Lending: No
Federal School ID Code: G06679
Supplemental Application School Code: N/A

University of Western Ontario Faculty of Medicine & Dentistry
Financial Aid Services, Office of the Registrar
Room 180, Stevenson-Lawson Building
1151 Richmond Street North
London, Ontario
Canada N6A 5B8
Contact: Carol West
E-mail: cwest@julian.uwo.ca
Web Site: www.med.uwo.ca/
(519) 661-3775; 661-3388 (FAX)
Direct Lending: No
Federal School ID Code: 008446-00
Supplemental Application School Code: N/A

McGill University Faculty of Medicine
Student Aid Office
3637 Peel Street, Room 200
Montreal, Quebec
Canada H3A 1X1
Web Site: www.mcgill.ca/
(514) 398-6015; 398-7352 (FAX)
Direct Lending: No
Federal School ID Code: 006677
Supplemental Application School Code: N/A

Université de Montréal Faculty of Medicine
Bureau des Affaires Etudiantes
C.P. 6128, Succ. Centre-ville
Montreal, Quebec
Canada H3C 3J7
Contact: Marc Girard
Web Site: www.umontreal.ca/
(514) 343-6603; 343-6629 (FAX)
Direct Lending: Yes
Federal School ID Code: N/A
Supplemental Application School Code: N/A

TABLE 8-E

Which School? Which Form?

Medical School	FAFSA				Institutional Financial Aid Application (IFAA)				Parent and Student Supplemental Application				
	Is parent information required for non-federal institutional funds?	For all applications?	For first-time applicants?	Deadline	Is parent information required for non-federal institutional funds?	For all applications?	For first-time applicants?	Deadline	Does school use parent and student supplemental application?	Name of supplemental application?	For all applications?	For first-time applicants?	Deadline
Alabama													
Alabama	Yes	—	—	April	Yes	—	—	April	No	—	—	—	—
South Alabama	Yes	Yes	—	—	Yes	Yes	—	—	No	—	—	—	—
Arizona													
Arizona	No	—	—	March	No	—	—	March	Yes	Health Professions Program Parental Information Form	Yes	—	March
Arkansas													
Arkansas	No	—	—	March	Yes	Yes	—	March	No	—	—	—	—
California													
UC, Davis	Yes	Yes	—	March	—	—	—	—	Yes	School-based application	Yes	—	—
UC, Irvine	No	—	—	March	—	—	—	—	No	—	—	—	—
UCLA	No	No	No	—	Yes	Yes	Yes	—	Yes	Access	Yes	Yes	—
UC, San Diego	Yes	Yes	—	Varies	Yes	Yes	—	Varies	No	—	—	—	—
UC, San Francisco	Yes	Yes	Yes	March	Yes	Yes	—	February	Yes	Parents' Information	No	Yes	February
Loma Linda	Yes	Yes	Yes	April	Yes	Yes	Yes	April	No	—	—	—	—
Keck (Southern California)	Yes	No	No	March	Yes	Yes	Yes	March	Yes	Supplemental Form for Grad. & Prof. Students	Yes	Yes	March
Stanford	No	—	—	June	Yes	Yes	Yes	June	Yes	Need Access	Yes	Yes	June
Colorado													
Colorado	No	No	No	March	Yes	Yes	Yes	—	No	—	No	No	—
Connecticut													
Connecticut	Yes	Yes	Yes	March	Yes	Yes	Yes	March	No	—	—	—	—
Yale	No	Yes	Yes	April	Yes	Yes	Yes	April	Yes	Need Access	Yes	Yes	April
District of Columbia													
George Washington	Yes	Yes	Yes	—	Yes	Yes	Yes	—	No	—	—	—	—
Georgetown	Yes	Yes	—	March	Yes	Yes	—	April	No	—	—	—	—
Howard	Yes	Yes	Yes	April	Yes	Yes	Yes	April	No	—	—	—	—

TABLE 8-E (continued)

Which School? Which Form?

Medical School	FAFSA: Is parent information required for non-federal institutional funds?	FAFSA: For all applications?	FAFSA: For first-time applicants?	FAFSA: Deadline	IFAA: Is parent information required for non-federal institutional funds?	IFAA: For all applications?	IFAA: For first-time applicants?	IFAA: Deadline	Parent and Student Supplemental Application: Does school use parent and student supplemental applications?	Name of supplemental application?	For all applications?	For first-time applicants?	Deadline
Florida													
Florida	Yes	Yes	—	April	Yes	Yes	—	April	No	—	—	—	—
Miami	Yes	Yes	—	—	No	—	—	—	No	—	—	—	—
South Florida	Yes	Yes	—	April	Yes	Yes	—	April	No	—	—	—	—
Georgia													
Emory	No	No	No	April	—	—	—	—	Yes	CSS Profile	Yes	Yes	April
Medical College of Georgia	Yes	Yes	—	March	Yes	Yes	—	March	No	—	—	—	—
Mercer	Yes	Yes	Yes	April	Yes	Yes	Yes	April	No	—	—	—	—
Morehouse	Yes	Yes	—	April	Yes	Yes	—	April	No	—	—	—	—
Hawaii													
Hawai'i at Mānoa	No	No	No	March	No	No	No	March	No	—	—	—	—
Illinois													
Chicago-Pritzker	Yes	Yes	Yes	April	Yes	Yes	Yes	April	Yes	Need Access	Yes	Yes	April
Finch Univ./Chicago Medical	No	—	—	—	—	—	—	—	Yes	—	Yes	Yes	—
Univ. Illinois	No	No	No	—	—	—	—	—	No	—	—	—	—
Loyola-Stritch	Yes	Yes	Yes	March	Yes	Yes	Yes	March	Yes	Parent Supplemental	Yes	Yes	March
Northwestern	Yes	Yes	Yes	April	Yes	—	—	April	Yes	Parents' Financial Supplement	Yes	Yes	April
Rush	Yes	Yes	Yes	May	Yes	Yes	Yes	May	No	—	—	—	—
Southern Illinois	No	—	—	—	Yes	—	Yes	March	No	—	—	—	—
Indiana													
Indiana	Yes	Yes	Yes	March	Yes	Yes	Yes	May	No	—	—	—	—
Iowa													
Iowa	Yes	Yes	Yes	—	No	—	—	—	Yes	U. of Iowa Verification Form	Yes	Yes	—
Kansas													
Kansas	No	No	No	April	—	—	—	—	Yes	Univ. of KS Medical Center Student Data Sheet	Yes	Yes	April
Kentucky													
Kentucky	No	—	—	—	—	—	—	—	No	—	—	—	—

CHAPTER 8

TABLE 8-E (continued)

Which School? Which Form?

Medical School	FAFSA				Institutional Financial Aid Application (IFAA)				Parent and Student Supplemental Application				
	Is parent information required for non-federal institutional funds?	For all applications?	For first-time applicants?	Deadline	Is parent information required for non-federal institutional funds?	For all applications?	For first-time applicants?	Deadline	Does school use parent and student supplemental application?	Name of supplemental application?	For all applications?	For first-time applicants?	Deadline
Louisville	No	—	—	—	—	—	—	—	No	—	—	—	—
Louisiana													
LSU-New Orleans	Yes	No	Yes	April	—	—	—	—	No	—	—	—	—
LSU-Shreveport	No	—	—	—	No	—	—	—	No		—	—	—
Tulane	Yes	Yes	—	April	Yes	Yes		April	No	—	—	—	—
Maryland													
Johns Hopkins	Yes	Yes	Yes	April	Yes	Yes	Yes	April	Yes	Need Access	Yes	Yes	April
Maryland	No	—	—	March	No	—	—	—	No	N/A	No	No	N/A
Massachusetts													
Boston	Yes	Yes	Yes	April	Yes	Yes	Yes	April	Yes	Divorced/ Separated Parents; Business/Form Supplement	Yes	Yes	April
Harvard	Yes	Yes	Yes	March	Yes	Yes	Yes	March	Yes	CSS Profile	Yes	Yes	March
Massachusetts	Yes	No	Yes	March	Yes	Yes	—	March	Yes	Need Access CSS Profile	—	—	March
Tufts	Yes	Yes	—	March	Yes	Yes	—	March	Yes	Tufts Parents' Information Form	Yes	—	March
Michigan													
Michigan State	Yes	Yes	—	—	No	—	—	—	No	—	—	—	—
Univ. Michigan	Yes	Yes	—	March	Yes	Yes	Yes	March	No	—	—	—	—
Wayne State	Yes	No	Optional	March	Yes	Yes	Yes	May	No	—	—	—	—
Minnesota													
Mayo	No	No	No	—	No	No	No	—	No	—	No	No	—
Minnesota-Minneapolis	Yes	Yes	Yes	March	No	—	—	—	No	—	—	—	—
Mississippi													
Mississippi	No	—	—	—	No	—	—	—	No	—	—	—	—
Missouri													
Missouri-Columbia	Yes	Yes	Yes	August	Yes	Yes	Yes	August	No	—	—	—	—
Missouri-Kansas City	No	—	—	—	No	—	—	—	No	—	—	—	—
Saint Louis	Yes	Yes	Yes	—	Yes	Yes	Yes	April	Yes	Need Access	Yes	Yes	April
Washington Univ. (Saint Louis)	Yes	Yes	Yes	April	Yes	Yes	Yes	April	No	—	—	—	—

TABLE 8-E (continued)

Which School? Which Form?

Medical School	FAFSA				Institutional Financial Aid Application (IFAA)				Parent and Student Supplemental Application				
	Is parent information required for non-federal institutional funds?	For all applications?	For first-time applicants?	Deadline	Is parent information required for non-federal institutional funds?	For all applications?	For first-time applicants?	Deadline	Does school use parent and student supplemental application?	Name of supplemental application?	For all applications?	For first-time applicants?	Deadline
Nebraska													
Creighton	Yes	No	Yes	March	Yes	Yes	Yes	—	Yes	Creighton U. Aid Application	Yes	Yes	—
Nebraska	No	—	—	—	Yes	Yes	Yes	February	No	—	—	—	—
Nevada													
Nevada	Yes	Yes	Yes	March	No	No	No	—	Yes	School of Medicine Scholarship Application	Yes	Yes	—
New Hampshire													
Dartmouth	Yes	No	Yes	May	Yes	Yes	Yes	May	Yes	Need Access	Yes	Yes	May
New Jersey													
UMDNJ-New Jersey Medical	No	Yes	—	May	No	—	—	May	No	—	—	—	—
UMDNJ-Robert Wood Johnson	No	—	—	—	No	—	—	—	No	—	—	—	—
New Mexico													
New Mexico	No	—	—	March	No	—	—	April	No	—	—	—	—
New York													
Albany	No	No	No	February	Yes	Yes	—	February	Yes	Need Access	Yes	—	February
Albert Einstein	No	No	No	—	Yes	Yes	Yes	—	No	—	—	—	—
Columbia	Yes	Yes	Yes	—	Yes	Yes	Yes	—	Yes	Institutional Application	—	—	—
Mount Sinai	No	Yes	—	May	Yes	—	—	May	Yes	Need Access	Yes	Yes	May
New York Medical	Yes	Yes	—	April	Yes	Yes	—	April	No	—	—	—	—
New York University	Yes	Yes	Yes	May	No	—	—	—	No	—	—	—	—
Rochester	No	—	—	—	No	Yes	—	August	Yes	Need Access	Yes	—	August
SUNY-Buffalo	No	—	—	—	No	—	—	—	No	—	—	—	—
SUNY-Downstate	Yes	Yes	—	March	Yes	Yes	—	March	No	—	—	—	—
SUNY-Stony Brook	No	No	No	—	Yes	Yes	—	N/A	No	—	—	—	—
SUNY-Upstate	Yes	Yes	—	March	—	—	—	—	No	—	—	—	—
Weill (Cornell)	No	—	—	—	Yes	Yes	Yes	May	Yes	Need Access	Yes	Yes	May

TABLE 8-E (continued)

Which School? Which Form?

Medical School	FAFSA				Institutional Financial Aid Application (IFAA)				Parent and Student Supplemental Application				
	Is parent information required for non-federal institutional funds?	For all applications?	For first-time applicants?	Deadline	Is parent information required for non-federal institutional funds?	For all applications?	For first-time applicants?	Deadline	Does school use parent and student supplemental application?	Name of supplemental application?	For all applications?	For first-time applicants?	Deadline
North Carolina													
Brody (East Carolina)	No	—	—	—	N/A	—	—	—	No	N/A	—	—	—
Duke	No	No	No	May	Yes	Yes	Yes	May	No	—	—	—	—
North Carolina	No	—	—	—	—	—	—	—	No	—	—	—	—
Wake Forest	No	Yes	Yes	May	Yes	Yes	Yes	May	Yes	Profile	Yes	Yes	May
North Dakota													
North Dakota	No	—	—	—	—	—	—	—	No	—	—	—	—
Ohio													
Case Western	No	No	No	March	Yes	Yes	Yes	April	Yes	Need Access	Yes	Yes	March
Cincinnati	No	—	—	May	No	—	—	May	Yes	Need Access	Yes	Yes	May
Medical College of Ohio	Yes	Yes	—	May	No	—	—	—	No	—	—	—	—
Northeastern Ohio	Yes	Yes	Yes	April	Yes	Yes	Yes	April	No	—	—	—	—
Ohio State	Yes	Yes	—	N/A	No	—	—	—	No	—	—	—	—
Wright State	Yes	Yes	Yes	March	Yes	Yes	Yes	March	No	—	—	—	—
Oklahoma													
Oklahoma	No	—	—	—	No	—	—	—	Yes	Questionnaire	Yes	—	April
Oregon													
Oregon	No	—	—	March	No	—	—	March	Yes	DHHS Scholarship and Loan Program Application	Yes	—	June
Pennsylvania													
Jefferson	Yes	Yes	Yes	March	No	—	—	—	No	—	—	—	—
MCP Hahnemann	Yes	Yes	Yes	May	Yes	Yes	Yes	May	No	—	—	—	—
Penn State	Yes	Yes	Yes	February	No	—	—	—	No	—	—	—	—
Pennsylvania	Yes	Yes	—	—	Yes	Yes	—	—	Yes	Penn Institutional Application	—	—	—
Pittsburgh	Yes	Yes	Yes	February/ March	Yes	Yes	Yes	April	Yes	Application for Institutional Aid	Yes	Yes	March/ April
Temple	Yes	Yes	Yes	March	No	No	No	—	No	—	—	—	—

TABLE 8-E (continued)

Which School? Which Form?

Medical School	FAFSA				Institutional Financial Aid Application (IFAA)				Parent and Student Supplemental Application				
	Is parent information required for non-federal institutional funds?	For all applications?	For first-time applicants?	Deadline	Is parent information required for non-federal institutional funds?	For all applications?	For first-time applicants?	Deadline	Does school use parent and student supplemental application?	Name of supplemental application?	For all applications?	For first-time applicants?	Deadline
Puerto Rico													
Caribe	Yes	Yes	Yes	September	No	—	—	—	No	—	—	—	—
Ponce	Yes	Yes	Yes	May	Yes	Yes	Yes	May	No	—	—	—	—
Puerto Rico	Yes	No	—	June	No	—	—	—	No	—	—	—	—
Rhode Island													
Brown	Yes	Yes	Yes	May	Yes	Yes	Yes	May	Yes	Need Access Report	Yes	Yes	May
South Carolina													
Medical Univ. South Carolina	No	Yes	Yes	April	Yes	—	—	—	No	—	—	—	—
South Carolina	No	—	—	—	No	—	—	—	No	—	—	—	—
South Dakota													
South Dakota	Yes	Yes	Yes	June	Yes	Yes	Yes	July	No	—	—	—	—
Tennessee													
East Tennessee	No	—	—	—	No	—	—	—	No	—	—	—	—
Meharry	No	No	No	—	No	—	—	—	No	—	—	—	—
Tennessee-Memphis	No	No	No	—	Yes	Yes	Yes	April	No	—	—	—	—
Vanderbilt	Yes	Yes	Yes	—	Yes	Yes	Yes	—	No	—	—	—	—
Texas													
Baylor	Yes	Yes	—	May	Yes	Yes	—	May	Yes	Parents' Verification Worksheet	Yes	—	May
Texas A&M	Yes	Yes	Yes	April	No	No	No	—	No	—	—	—	—
Texas Tech	No	—	—	—	No	—	—	—	No	—	—	—	—
Southwestern, Dallas	Yes	Yes	—	April	N/A	—	—	—	No	—	—	—	—
Galveston	No	—	—	—	No	—	—	—	No	—	—	—	—
Houston	No	—	—	—	No	—	—	—	No	—	—	—	—
San Antonio	Yes	Yes	Yes	—	Yes	Yes	Yes	—	No	—	—	—	—
Utah													
Utah	No	—	—	—	No	—	—	—	No	—	—	—	—
Vermont													
Vermont	Yes	Yes	Yes	March	No	—	—	—	No	—	—	—	—
Virginia													
Eastern Virginia	Yes	Yes	Yes	May	No	—	—	—	No	—	—	—	—
Univ. Virginia	Yes	Yes	—	March	Yes	Yes	—	March	No	—	—	—	—
Virginia Commonwealth	No	—	—	—	No	—	—	—	No	—	—	—	—

CHAPTER 8

TABLE 8-E (continued)

Which School? Which Form?

Medical School	FAFSA				Institutional Financial Aid Application (IFAA)				Parent and Student Supplemental Application				
	Is parent information required for non-federal institutional funds?	For all applications?	For first-time applicants?	Deadline	Is parent information required for non-federal institutional funds?	For all applications?	For first-time applicants?	Deadline	Does school use parent and student supplemental application?	Name of supplemental application?	For all applications?	For first-time applicants?	Deadline
Washington													
Washington Univ.	Yes	Yes	Yes	February	No	—	—	—	No	—	—	—	—
West Virginia													
Marshall	Yes	No	Yes	None	Yes	No	Yes	None	No	—	—	—	—
West Virginia	No	—	—	—	No	—	—	—	No	—	—	—	—
Wisconsin													
Medical College Wisconsin	No	Yes	Yes	April	Yes	Yes	Yes	April	No	—	—	—	—
Univ. Wisconsin	Yes	Yes	Yes	(rolling)	Yes	Yes	Yes	(rolling)	Yes	Student & Parent Tax Form Requirements	Yes	Yes	(rolling)
Canada													
Calgary (Alberta)	Yes	Yes	—	—	Yes	Yes	—	August	No	—	—	—	—
British-Columbia	Yes	Yes	Yes	June	Yes	Yes	Yes	October	No	—	—	—	—
Manitoba	No	—	—	—	Yes	Yes	Yes	—	No	—	—	—	—
Newfoundland	Yes	Yes	Yes	—	No	—	—	—	No	—	—	—	—
Dalhousie (Nova Scotia)	No	—	—	—	—	—	—	—	No	—	—	—	—
Queen's (Ontario)	Yes	Yes	Yes	—	Yes	Yes	Yes	December	Yes	Plus Loan Application	No	—	—
Western Ontario (Ontario)	Yes	Yes	Yes	October	Yes	Yes	Yes	October	Yes	Bursary Application and Scholarship Application	Yes	Yes	October
McGill (Quebec)	N/A	—	—	—	N/A	—	—	—	No	—	—	—	—
Montreal (Quebec)	No	—	—	—	No	—	—	—	No	—	—	—	—

Information for Minority Group Students

9

This chapter provides information on applying to medical school for students from minority groups underrepresented in medicine—blacks, Native Americans (American Indian, Alaskan Native or Native Hawaiian), Mexican Americans, and mainland Puerto Ricans. These four groups were designated as underrepresented in medicine more than 20 years ago by the Association of American Medical Colleges (AAMC). They continue to be underrepresented in medical school enrollment—underrepresented minorities constitute 19.4 percent of the U.S. population (1990 U.S. Census) but only 10.7 percent of the 1999 medical school matriculants. In 1998, they were 11.6 percent. Designation as underrepresented not only reflects these groups' numerical score underrepresentation but also a history of discrimination and exclusion in the United States.

Increasing the number of physicians from racial and ethnic groups underrepresented in medicine has been a priority of medical schools for many years. The Executive Council of the AAMC issued a policy statement in 1970 on the medical education of minority group students. The AAMC reaffirmed this commitment in 1987 by issuing the "AAMC Statement on Medical Education of Minority Group Students" (page 89). In 1991 AAMC officially launched *Project 3000 by 2000*. The goal of this project is to increase the number of underrepresented minority students entering medical school each year to 3,000 by the Year 2000. The project emphasizes the development of partnerships linking medical school systems with undergraduate colleges and local school systems.

Most medical schools have programs and resources specifically designed to assist in the recruitment and enrollment of minority students. Premedical advisors at undergraduate colleges can also provide pertinent information on medical school admissions or refer students to appropriate contact persons or offices.

The applicant pool for U.S. medical schools declined for the third straight year to 38,529, a drop of 6 percent (total applicants in 1998 was 41,003). In 1996, the number of applicants to medical school reached an all-time high of 46,968. With regard to underrepresented minority applicants, in 1999, the percentage of underrepresented minority applicants fell 6 percent to 4,181 (total underrepresented minority applicants in 1998 was 4,487). The number of total applicants and applicants from underrepresented minority groups represent the lowest figures since 1992.

Despite the fluctuations in the number of applicants, the number of matriculating (new entrants) medical students has remained roughly the same over the past 20 years. In 1999, 16,221 individuals entered medical school (the number of matriculants in 1998 was 16,170). The number of underrepresented minority matriculants to the 1999 entering class was 1,732, comprising 10.68 percent of new entrants. In 1998, underrepresented minority new entrants was 11.57 percent of new entrants. Therefore the number of underrepresented minority new entrants in 1999 dropped approximately 7 percent to 1,732 from 1,871 in 1998. The peak enrollment occurred in 1994 and 1995 when 2,022 underrepresented minorities matriculated to medical school.

Overall, the number of males applying to medical school dropped 9 percent from 23,216 in 1998 to 21,096 in 1999. The number of underrepresented minority male applicants dropped 14 percent from 1,896 in 1998 to 1,629 in 1999. The highest number of underrepresented male applicants was 2,236 in 1996. The number of underrepresented minority male new entrants was 706—15 percent less than in 1998 (831).

The number of females applying to medical school in 1999 was 17,433, only 2 percent less than in 1998 (17,787). The number of underrepresented minority females applying to medical school was 2,552, only 1 percent less than in 1998 (2,591). The number of underrepresented minority female new entrants was 1,026, approximately 1 percent less than in 1998 (1,040).

The number of underrepresented minority male new entrants (706) continues to be lower than the number of underrepresented minority female new entrants (1,026).

Table 9A shows the trend in underrepresented minority new entrants/matriculants to U.S. medical schools.

Once enrolled in medical school, academic and personal support programs are available to students. These support systems promote the successful completion of medical studies by minority students to help achieve the ultimate goal: increasing the numbers of minority physicians entering careers in patient care, teaching, and research.

Table 9-B identifies the individual primarily responsible for minority affairs at each U.S. medical school. This individual can provide more detailed information on their school's programs and admissions procedures. Enrollment data on underrepresented minority new entrants for each medical school is also included in the table.

Additional information concerning programs at medical schools for minority students can be obtained from the medical school contact persons or offices listed in Table 9-B, from premedical advisors at the undergraduate colleges, and in the AAMC Division of Community and Minority Programs' publication, *Minority Student Opportunities in the United States Medical Schools, 2000.*

MEDICAL MINORITY APPLICANT REGISTRY (MED-MAR)

The Medical Minority Applicant Registry (Med-MAR) is one of the services initiated by the AAMC for students from minority groups. This program provides the opportunity for any medical school applicant belonging to a minority group traditionally underrepresented in medicine—black; Mexican American; Native American (American Indian, Alaskan Native, or Native Hawaiian); mainland Puerto Rican; and/or disadvantaged students—to have basic biographical information and the Medical College Admission Test (MCAT) scores circulated automatically, at no cost, to minority affairs and admission offices of all U.S. medical schools as well as to other health-related services organizations and institutions that request the Med-MAR lists. Students elect to participate in Med-MAR by indicating their interest on a questionnaire completed at the time they take the MCAT. The Med-MAR lists are circulated twice a year (usually in July and November) following the administration of the MCAT. Medical schools correspond directly with students and may request from them more detailed information.

Inclusion of an applicant's name on a Med-MAR list does not automatically waive the application fees. Waiver of medical school application fees is determined by each school on an individual basis. Similarly, fees for the American Medical College Application Service (AMCAS) are waived on an individual basis. MCAT fees are not waived, but a fee reduction program is in place (see Chapter 6).

For information about matters related to minority students, the applicant should write to:

Minority Student Information Clearinghouse
Division of Community and Minority Programs
Association of American Medical Colleges
2450 N Street, N.W.
Washington, D.C. 20037-1126

SUMMER AND ENRICHMENT PROGRAMS

To encourage and prepare minority students for a career in medicine, a variety of academic enrichment programs are available. There are programs designed for almost every stage in the educational continuum—middle school and high school programs, college programs, and postbaccalaureate programs, as well as research opportunities. There are also laboratory research internships available for high school and college students.

Information can be obtained from the minority affairs contact person at each medical school, from premedical advisors at the undergraduate colleges, from guidance counselors at high schools, from the AAMC publication *Minority Student Opportunities in United States Medical Schools, 2000,* from *Getting into Medical School: A Planning Guide for Minority Students*, from computer searches, and from libraries.

FINANCIAL AID

Because of the variety and scope of financial assistance plans, applicants to both public and private medical schools should not think that they are unqualified for admission solely because of financial status. Generally, medical schools have been successful in providing adequate funding to meet the needs of their students, regardless of financial means. However, it is the responsibility of applicants to devote careful and thorough attention to all aspects of their educational financing. Before enrolling, applicants should obtain specific information from the medical schools about possibilities of financial assistance. (See Chapter 8.)

Financial assistance is often made available to medical students in the form of loans or a combination of grants, scholarships, and loans. Eligibility is most often determined on the basis of a student's demonstrated financial need, as well as the total cost of attendance, as opposed to the student's academic performance. As referenced in Chapter 8, it is important to remember that some cost-based loan programs are based, in part, on a student being "credit ready," so a sound credit history may play a critical part in helping a student secure enough financial aid for medical school.

Although you should always check with your financial aid officer on the availability of funds, the following is a list of various sources of financial aid most often available to medical students:

1. Institutional support directly from the medical school, which usually comes in the form of grants, scholarships, and low-interest subsidized loans.
2. Federal Subsidized and Federal Unsubsidized Stafford loans, which are low-interest loan funds made available from either a private lender or the Federal Government. Check with your financial aid officer for a list of potential lenders for the Federal Stafford Loan.
3. Federal Perkins Loans, which are low-interest loan funds made available through the school.

Hints for Applicants

- Submit **completed** applications early. Many medical schools have rolling admissions.
- **Incomplete applications** *will not* be processed
- For accurate information on medical school admissions procedures, application requirements, and deadline dates, review each medical school entry in the *Medical School Admission Requirements*. When in doubt, contact the school directly.
- AMCAS *does not* grant deadline extensions for any reason; you must contact the individual medical school directly.
- Financial aid/Credit ready—having a good credit rating is necessary for obtaining financial aid.

AAMC Statement on Medical Education of Minority Group Students

The findings and recommendations of the 1970 AAMC Task Force on Minority Student Opportunities in Medical Education, combined with federal and private philanthropy support, provided the first impetus for the academic medical community to address the issue of access to the profession of medicine for individuals of underrepresented minority groups in our society.

The following decade witnessed significant progress as total enrollment of underrepresented minorities surged from 3.12 percent in 1969 to 8.0 percent in 1979. Whereas in 1969 Howard and Meharry accounted for 75 percent of all black medical students, by 1979 they accounted for only 20 percent.

Minority enrollments in U.S. medical schools reached their peak in 1975, when minorities represented 8.1 percent of the total student body. Since then, however, a leveling-off effect has dominated, and no significant increase in the number of underrepresented minorities entering medical school has occurred.

This long-term plateau indicates that if the progress achieved in providing access for more minorities to pursue careers in medicine is to continue, educational institutions, the federal government, and philanthropic organizations must reaffirm their commitment to the education of underrepresented minorities for careers in medicine as a national goal.

The AAMC and its constituent members are directing an earnest effort toward the goal of increasing opportunities for underrepresented minorities who wish to pursue careers in medical service, teaching, and research. These goals are described in detail in the 1970 "Report of the AAMC Task Force to the Inter-Association Committee on Expanding Educational Opportunities in Medicine for Blacks and Other Minority Students." These goals were also reaffirmed in the 1978 "Report of the AAMC Task Force on Minority Student Opportunities in Medicine."

Medical schools, working with cooperating undergraduate institutions, the AAMC, other agencies, and interested entities, are urged to help increase minority student awareness of the opportunities for professional education and specific preparation necessary for medical school. Minority students, thus motivated, prepared, and recruited, should be provided with the necessary encouragement and support to ensure their retention in and graduation from medical schools. To strengthen these efforts, medical schools are encouraged to continue to identify a faculty member or administrator who can be specifically charged with responsibility for minority student affairs. The person designated for this role should be a member of a minority group and should work closely with the AAMC Group on Student Affairs to represent the medical school in the activities of the Group on Student Affairs' Minority Affairs Section.

Medical schools are encouraged to pursue actively the expansion of minority student support funds from local, state, and federal levels. The AAMC is making known to the American public and to the federal government these needs to increase financial aid for minority students and for all students.

The AAMC-AMA Liaison Committee on Medical Education (LCME) is strongly encouraged to review critically the degree of individual opportunity provided to minority students. The LCME should continue to include in its membership and accreditation teams representatives from minority group members who have experience and knowledge in the education of minority group students.

The AAMC and its constituent members reaffirm their commitment to these efforts. Many current trends point to the urgency and timeliness of this affirmation: a perceived physician surplus in the face of an underrepresentation of minority physicians, the continuing physician maldistribution vis-a-vis minority and other underserved areas, the lack of opportunity for minorities in graduate medical programs, the underrepresentation of both minority medical students and faculty members in medical education, and the increasing cost of medical education to minorities and other low-income individuals. The AAMC and its member schools urge that, in any deliberations regarding physician manpower, the recruitment and graduation of individuals from underrepresented minorities in medical education be considered with particular care.

Approved by the AAMC Executive Council
June 1987

4. Loan and scholarship funds targeted to students in primary care, which include the Scholarships for Disadvantaged Students (SDS) and the Primary Care Loan (PCL).
5. National Medical Fellowships, Inc., which provide grants to help minority students finance their medical school education.
6. State-supported loan and scholarship programs, for which the availability and amount will vary widely by state.
7. Service scholarship programs, such as the National Health Service Corps (NHSC) and the Armed Forces Health Professions Scholarship Program (the military) that are programs that most often provide tuition, a living stipend, and other financial support in exchange for a service commitment. These programs, especially the NHSC, tend to be very competitive, so students should apply early.
8. Loans, grants, and scholarships made available through various philanthropic organizations are also available.

The federal financial assistance programs described in the preceding list are subject to change due to congressional and executive review. Students should obtain up-to-date information on each of these programs from the school's financial aid office either when interviewed or when accepted.

Further information about these sources and about financial aid programs in general is provided in Chapter 8. Information on admission procedures for individual medical schools is given in Chapter 11.

INFORMATION SOURCES

Students may find the following articles, books, and brochures helpful in planning the\ir medical careers.

1. *Choosing a Health Professional Career: A Reference Guide.* National Medical Fellowships, Inc. 1993. $15.00 per set. (National Medical Fellowships, Inc., 110 West 32nd Street, Eighth Floor, New York, New York 10001; (212) 714-1007)

2. *Dollars for College: The Quick Guide to Scholarships, Fellowships, Loans, and Other Financial Aid Programs for Medicine, Dentistry, and Related Fields 1997.* $7.95 prepaid. (Garrett Park Press, P.O. Box 190, Garrett Park, Maryland 20896) ISBN: 1-880774-15-1

3. *Educational Survival Skills Study Guide.* Free. (Office of Statewide Health Planning and Development, Health Professions Career Opportunity Program, 1600 Ninth Street, Room 441, Sacramento, California 95814)

4. Epps, A. C., and Pisano, J. C. *MEDREP at Tulane: Effectiveness of a Medical Education Reinforcement and Enrichment Program for Minorities in the Health Professions.* 1985. $12.00. (Futura Publishing Company, Inc., 2 Bedford Ridge Road, Mount Kisco, New York 10549)

5. *Financial Advice and Health Careers Resources Directory for Minority Students.* Free. (Office of Statewide Health Planning and Development, Health Professions Career Opportunity Program, 1600 Ninth Street, Room 441, Sacramento, California 95814)

6. *Financial Aid for Minorities in Health Fields.* 1996. $5.95. ISBN 0-912048-96-4. (Garrett Park Press, P.O. Box 190, Garrett Park, Maryland 20896)

7. *Financing Medical Education, 1997–1998.* $7.00 (includes shipping and handling) Checks made payable to NAMME (Charles Terrell, Associate Dean for Student Affairs, Boston University School of Medicine, 80 East Concord Street, Boston, Massachusetts 02118); (617) 638-5130; 638-5116 (FAX).

8. *Financing Your Health Professions Education and Financial Planning and Debt Management for Health Professions Students.* National Medical Fellowships, Inc. 1993. $15.00 per set. (National Medical Fellowships, Inc., 110 West 32nd Street, Eighth Floor, New York, New York 10001; (212) 714-1007)

9. Haller, E. H., and Myers, R. A. (Eds.). *Searching, Teaching, Healing: American Indians and Alaskan Natives in Biomedical Research Careers.* 1986. $9.95. (Futura Publishing Company, Inc., 2 Bedford Ridge Road, Mount Kisco, New York 10549)

10. *Health Pathways Quarterly Newsletter.* Free. (Office of Statewide Health Planning and Development, Health Professions Career Opportunity Program, 1600 Ninth Street, Room 441, Sacramento, California 95814)

11. *Informed Decision-Making: Part I, Financial Planning and Management for Medical Students; Part II, Sources of Financial Assistance for Medical School.* National Medical Fellowships, Inc. 1993. $15.00 per set. (National Medical Fellowships, Inc., 110 West 32nd Street, New York, New York 10001; (212) 714-1007)

12. James, E.J., and Hamilton, K.E. (Eds.). *Getting into Medical School: A Planning Guide for Minority Students.* 1996. A book by doctors for prospective doctors. $12.50 includes shipping and handling. (Betz Publishing Company, a division of Williams and Wilkins, 351 West Camden Street, Baltimore, Maryland 21201–2436; (610) 892-6637)

13. *The Journal for Minority Medical Students.* Published quarterly by Spectrum Unlimited. $10.00 annually. (Spectrum Unlimited, 4203 Canal Street, New Orleans, Louisiana 70119; 1 (800) 661-3319 or (504) 488-5100; 488-7072 (FAX); E-mail: JMMSmag@aol.com)

14. *Minorities in Medicine: A Guide for Premedical Students.* Free. (Office of Statewide Health Planning

FIGURE 9

URM Applicants, 1990-1999

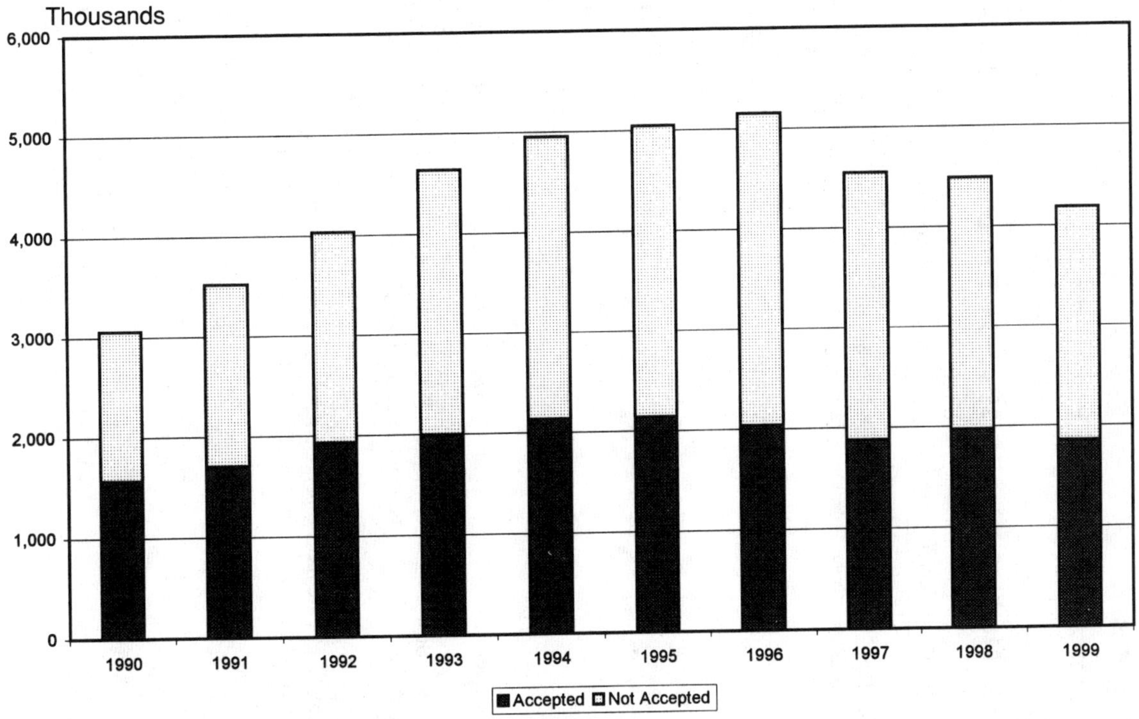

Source: AAMC Data Warehouse: Applicant Matriculant File. As of November 15, 1999.

and Development, Health Professions Career Opportunity Program, 1600 Ninth Street, Room 441, Sacramento, California 95814)

15. *Minority Student Opportunities in United States Medical Schools, 2000*. 15th edition. Association of American Medical Colleges. (Association of American Medical Colleges, Department 66, Washington, D.C. 20055; (202) 828-0416)

16. *Time Management for Students*. Free. (Office of Statewide Health Planning and Development, Health Professions Career Opportunity Program, 1600 Ninth Street, Room 441, Sacramento, California 95814)

CHAPTER 9

TABLE 9-A

Selected Minority Group Enrollment in First-Year Classes in U.S. Medical Schools, 1990–91 Through 1999–2000

Year	Black American: Number New Entrants*	Black American: % of Total First-Year New Entrants	Native American†: Number New Entrants	Native American†: % of Total First-Year New Entrants	Mexican American/Chicano: Number New Entrants	Mexican American/Chicano: % of Total First-Year New Entrants	Mainland Puerto Rican: Number New Entrants	Mainland Puerto Rican: % of Total First-Year New Entrants	Total New Entrants‡
1990–91	1,046	6.5	68	0.4	272	1.7	99	0.6	15,993
1991–92	1,063	6.6	94	0.6	313	1.9	110	0.7	16,211
1992–93	1,196	7.3	118	0.7	409	2.5	108	0.7	16,289
1993–94	1,275	7.8	129	0.8	382	2.3	96	0.6	16,307
1994–95	1,309	8.0	128	0.8	458	2.8	129	0.8	16,287
1995–96	1,289	7.9	145	0.9	480	3.0	109	0.7	16,253
1996–97	1,190	7.3	142	0.9	453	2.8	141	0.9	16,200
1997–98	1,134	7.0	123	0.8	397	2.5	108	0.7	16,165
1998–99	1,201	7.4	147	0.9	418	2.6	106	0.7	16,170
1999–00**	1,122	6.9	109	0.7	389	2.4	112	0.7	16,221

Source: AAMC Data Warehouse: Applicant Matriculant File

* These figures include Black Americans who were new entrants at predominantly black schools. In 1999, a total of 166 were new entrants at Howard, Meharry, and Morehouse medical schools.

** Data from Brown, Florida, and Missouri-Kansas City are not included. These data are as follows: Brown—Black American: 5; Native American: 0; Meximan-American: 3; Mainland Puerto Rican: 0. Florida—Black American: 10; Native American: 1; Mexican-American: 1; Mainland Puerto Rican: 2. Missouri-Kansas City—Black American: 5; Native American: 0; Mexican-American: 2; Mainland Puerto Rican: 0.

† Includes Native Americans, Alaskan Natives, and Native Hawaiians.

‡ New entrants are those students entering medical school for the very first time. Data on applicants are based upon the newly developed AAMC Data Warehouse. The Data Warehouse provides more complete data on racial/ethnic self-description and consistent definitions across all years reported. As a result, the data published this year from the Data Warehouse may not match previously published numbers.

As of November 15, 1999

TABLE 9-B

Minority Student Matriculants by Individual Medical School

Medical School	Contact Person or Office	Minority Enrollment, Fall 1999 (New Entrant)*			
		Black	Native† American	Mexican-American	Mainland Puerto Rican
Alabama	Dr. John Scott Assistant Dean (205) 934-7975	11	0	1	0
Alabama, South	Dr Hattie M. Myles Assistant Dean, Office of Special Programs and Student Affairs (334) 460-7313	7	2	0	0
Albany‡	Dr. Assie Bishop Director of Minority Affairs (518) 262-5824	3	0	2	0
Albert Einstein†	Dr. Milton Gumbs Assistant Dean (718) 430-3091 Nilda I. Soto Director, Minority Student Affairs (718) 430-3091	5	0	0	3
Arizona	Linda K. Don Director, Office of Minority Affairs (520) 621-5531	3	1	9	0
Arkansas	Dr. Billy R. Thomas Office of Minority Affairs (501) 686-7299	5	2	1	0
Baylor‡	Dr. James L. Phillips Senior Associate Dean/ Professor of Pediatrics (713) 798-6598	10	2	17	1
Boston‡	Dr. Kenneth Edelin Associate Dean for Students and Minority Affairs (617) 638-4163	9	1	8	3
Brody (East Carolina)	Dr. Julius J. Mallette Assistant Dean for Minority Affairs (252) 816-2278	15	1	0	1

CHAPTER 9

TABLE 9-B (continued)

Minority Student Matriculants by Individual Medical School

Medical School	Contact Person or Office	Minority Enrollment, Fall 1999 (New Entrant)*			
		Black	Native† American	Mexican-American	Mainland Puerto Rican
Brown‡	Dr. Alicia D. Monroe Assistant Dean for Minority Affairs (401) 863-3335	5**	0**	3**	0**
California, University of Davis	Dr. Lindy Kumagai Assistant Dean for Minority Affairs (916) 752-8119	1	0	5	0
Irvine	Dr. Ralph Purdy Associate Dean, Admissions and Outreach (714) 824-8358	2	0	4	1
Los Angeles (Drew and Riverside)	Dr. Patricia Pratt (UCLA) Director, Student Support Services (310) 825-3575 Dr. Theodore Miller (Drew) Associate Dean for Student Affairs (323) 563-4881	16	1	27	1
San Diego	Dr. Sandra Daley Assistant Dean for Student Development Community Affairs (619) 534-0764	3	0	2	0
San Francisco (and Berkeley)	Dr. Michael V. Drake Associate Dean, Admissions and External Programs (415) 476-8088	9	1	8	1
Caribe‡	Dr. Nereida Diaz Dean of Admission and Student Affairs (787) 740-1611	0	0	0	2
Case Western Reserve‡	Dr. Rubens Pamies Associate Dean, Student Affairs (216) 368-2212	16	1	1	2

TABLE 9-B (continued)

Minority Student Matriculants by Individual Medical School

Medical School	Contact Person or Office	Minority Enrollment, Fall 1999 (New Entrant)* Black	Native† American	Mexican-American	Mainland Puerto Rican
Finch UHS Chicago Medical‡	Dr. Timothy Hansen Associate Dean, Educational Affairs (847) 578-3314	10	1	1	1
Chicago-Pritzker‡	Rosita Ragin Director of Student Programs (773) 702-1939	10	0	4	0
Cincinnati	Clarice Fooks Assistant Dean for Admissions and Student Affairs (513) 558-7314	4	2	0	1
Colorado	J. Raul Armendariz Assistant Vice Chancellor, Diversity (303) 315-2559	3	1	6	0
Columbia‡	Dr. Gerald E. Thomson Senior Associate Dean and Assistant Vice President for Health Sciences (212) 305-4158	11	0	4	2
Connecticut	Dr. Marja Hurley Associate Dean for Health (860) 679-3483	8	0	1	3
Creighton	Darlene Brown Director, Minority Affairs for Health Sciences (402) 280-2981	1	2	3	0
Dartmouth‡	Dr. Lori Arviso Alvord Associate Dean, Student and Minority Affairs (603) 650-1509	3	0	2	2
Duke‡	Dr. Delbert R. Wigfall Associate Professor of Pediatrics (919) 684-4246	21	2	0	0

CHAPTER 9

TABLE 9-B (continued)

Minority Student Matriculants by Individual Medical School

Medical School	Contact Person or Office	Minority Enrollment, Fall 1999 (New Entrant)* Black	Native† American	Mexican-American	Mainland Puerto Rican
Emory‡	Dr. Robert Lee Associate Dean/Director, Office of Minority Affairs (404) 727-0016	8	0	1	0
Florida (and FSU/FAMU program)	Dr. Beverly V. Wright Assistant Dean (352) 392-3015 Dr. Donna M. Parker Assistant Dean, Office of Minority Affairs (352) 392-3015	10**	1**	1**	2**
Florida, South	Dr. Marvin T. Williams Professor and Associate Dean for Diversity Initiative (813) 974-3609	4	2	2	1
George Washington‡	Dr. John F. Williams, Jr. Interim Vice President for Medical Affairs George Washington University Medical Center (202) 994-3727	18	0	3	0
Georgetown‡	Joy P. Williams Assistant Dean for Students and Special Programs (202) 687-1645	7	1	4	0
Georgia, Medical College of	Dr. Rosie Allen-Noble Associate Dean, Special Academic Programs (706) 721-2522	10	1	0	0
Harvard	Dr. Alvin F. Poussaint Associate Dean for Student Affairs (617) 432-1572	18	2	6	2
Hawaii	Dr. Benjamin Young Associate Dean for Minority Affairs (808) 956-5826	0	4	0	0

TABLE 9-B (continued)

Minority Student Matriculants by Individual Medical School

Medical School	Contact Person or Office	Minority Enrollment, Fall 1999 (New Entrant)*			
		Black	Native† American	Mexican-American	Mainland Puerto Rican
Howard‡	Dr. Dawn L. Cannon Assistant Dean for Student Affairs (202) 806-6270	78	1	0	0
Illinois	Dr. Jorge A. Girotti Associate Dean and Director of Urban Health Program (312) 996-4493	24	4	16	2
Illinois, Southern	Dr. Harold R. Bardo Assistant Dean, Minority Affairs (618) 453-1650	4	1	2	0
Indiana	Dr. William Agbor-Baiyee Director of Special Programs (317) 278-1724	9	1	0	1
Iowa	Barbara Barlow Program Associate for Equal Opportunity Programs (319) 335-8056	4	0	4	1
Jefferson‡	Dr. Edward Christian Assistant Dean for Student Affairs and Special Projects (215) 503-6763	4	1	2	3
Johns Hopkins‡	Dr. Roland T. Smoot Assistant Dean for Student Affairs (410) 955-3416	11	0	0	0
Kansas	Dr. Patricia A. Thomas Director of Cytopathology (913) 588-7070	9	2	6	0
California, Southern‡ (Keck)	Althea Alexander Assistant Dean for Minority Affairs (323) 342-1050	9	0	15	0
Kentucky	Dr. Carol Elam Assistant Dean for Admissions (606) 323-6161	4	0	0	0

CHAPTER 9

TABLE 9-B (continued)

Minority Student Matriculants by Individual Medical School

Medical School	Contact Person or Office	Minority Enrollment, Fall 1999 (New Entrant)* Black	Native† American	Mexican-American	Mainland Puerto Rican
Loma Linda‡	Dr. Daisy DeLeon Assistant to the Dean for Diversity (909) 824-2757	8	1	1	1
Louisiana State—New Orleans	Dr. Edward Helm Associate Dean, Community and Minority Health (504) 568-8501	18	0	0	1
Louisiana State—Shreveport	Shirley Roberson Director, Multicultural Affairs (318) 675-5049	2	0	1	1
Louisville	Michael Byrne Director, Health Sciences Center, Special Programs (502) 852-7159	12	2	0	0
Loyola-Stritch‡	Teresa J. Wronski Associate Dean for Student Affairs (708) 216-8140	3	0	1	1
Marshall	Dr. Patrick I. Brown Associate Dean, Student Affairs and Academic Affairs (304) 691-1730	1	0	1	0
Maryland	Dr. Willarda Edwards Assistant Dean of Student and Minority Affairs (410) 706-7689	18	0	0	0
Massachusetts	Dr. Danna B. Peterson Assistant Dean of Student Affairs and Minority Support (508) 856-3866	2	0	1	2
Mayo‡	Dr. Richard McGee, Jr. Associate Dean for Student Affairs (507) 284-0339	1	0	2	0

TABLE 9-B (continued)

Minority Student Matriculants by Individual Medical School

		Minority Enrollment, Fall 1999 (New Entrant)*			
Medical School	**Contact Person or Office**	Black	Native† American	Mexican-American	Mainland Puerto Rican
MCP Hahnemann	Dr. Emily Pollard Associate Dean for Minority Affairs (215) 991-8216	32	1	10	0
Meharry‡	Dr. Pamela C. Williams Associate Dean for Student/Academic Affairs (615) 327-6413	53	0	1	0
Mercer‡	Dr. Roger Comeau Associate Dean for Admissions/ Student Affairs (912) 752-2542	1	0	0	0
Miami‡	Dr. Astrid Mack Associate Dean for Minority Affairs (305) 243-5998	13	0	0	2
Michigan State	Dr. Wanda Lipscomb Assistant Dean for Student Affairs and Services (517) 353-7140	10	1	6	3
Michigan, University of	Dr. Joyce M. Mitchell Assistant Dean for Student and Minority Affairs (313) 764-8185	14	2	7	0
Minnesota—Duluth§	Dr. Gerald L. Hill Director, CAIMH (218) 726-7235	0	5	2	0
Minnesota—Minneapolis	Mary Tate Director of Minority Affairs (612) 625-1494	4	4	0	0
Mississippi	Dr. Leon Anderson, Jr. Director of Minority Affairs (601) 984-1340	3	0	0	0
Missouri—Columbia	Dr. Michael Hosokawa Assistant Dean for Curriculum and Minority Affairs (573) 882-9219	3	0	0	0

CHAPTER 9

TABLE 9-B (continued)

Minority Student Matriculants by Individual Medical School

Medical School	Contact Person or Office	Minority Enrollment, Fall 1999 (New Entrant)* Black	Native† American	Mexican-American	Mainland Puerto Rican
Missouri—Kansas City	Dr. Reaner Shannon Director, Office of Minority Affairs (816) 235-1780	5**	0**	2**	0**
Morehouse‡	Dr. Angela Franklin Associate Dean for Student Affairs and Curriculum (404) 752-1651	35	0	0	0
Mount Sinai‡	Dr. Gary C. Butts Associate Dean, Student Affairs (212) 241-8276	7	3	4	1
Nebraska	Dr. Jeffrey W. Hill Associate Dean, Office of Academic and Student Affairs (402) 559-2258	2	0	0	0
Nevada—Reno	Ann Diggins Director of Recruitment (775) 784-1317	0	0	1	0
UMDNJ—New Jersey Medical	Dr. Maria Soto-Greene Acting Associate Dean for Student Programs (973) 972-3762	22	0	0	6
UMDNJ—Robert Wood Johnson	Dr. Geoffrey Young Assistant Dean, Multicultural and Student Affairs (732) 235-4060	15	0	1	8
New Mexico	Dr. Roberto Gomez Associate Dean (505) 272-2728	1	3	14	0
New York Medical College‡	Dr. Gladys Ayala Associate Dean for Student and Minority Affairs (914) 594-3013	5	0	1	2
New York University‡	Dr. Margaret Haynes Associate Dean, Office of Minority Affairs Dean, Student Services (212) 263-8948	6	0	0	1

TABLE 9-B (continued)

Minority Student Matriculants by Individual Medical School

Medical School	Contact Person or Office	Minority Enrollment, Fall 1999 (New Entrant)* Black	Native† American	Mexican-American	Mainland Puerto Rican
SUNY—Downstate	Dr. Constance Hill Associate Dean for Minority Affairs (718) 270-3765	21	0	0	0
SUNY—Buffalo	Dr. Carolyn Hamilton Assistant Dean, Minority Affairs (716) 829-2802	8	1	1	2
SUNY—Stony Brook	Dr. Aldustus E. Jordan Associate Dean for Student and Minority Affairs (516) 444-2341	5	0	0	1
SUNY—Upstate	Barbara Hamilton Assistant Dean, Multicultural Resources (315) 464-5433	8	0	0	2
(Binghamton Campus)	Dr. Gina Lynch Assistant Dean for Student Affairs (607) 770-8616				
North Carolina	Larry D. Keith Director, Medical Education (919) 966-3641	17	0	1	0
North Dakota	Eugene DeLorne Director, INMED (701) 777-3037	0	6	0	0
Northwestern‡	Dr. Tacoma A. McKnight Associate Dean for Minority Affairs (312) 503-0461	6	0	2	0
Ohio, Medical College of	Monica Smith-Scott Director of Multicultural Affairs (419) 383-3438	14	0	2	1

CHAPTER 9

TABLE 9-B (continued)

Minority Student Matriculants by Individual Medical School

Medical School	Contact Person or Office	Minority Enrollment, Fall 1999 (New Entrant)*			
		Black	Native† American	Mexican-American	Mainland Puerto Rican
Ohio, Northeastern	Dr. Kenneth B. Durgans Assistant to the President for Minority Affairs and Affirmative Action (330) 325-6223	5	0	3	3
Ohio State	Dr. Milton B. Armstrong Associate Dean for Minority Affairs (614) 293-8562	16	0	2	0
Oklahoma	Susan Massara Director of Student Services (405) 271-2316	6	10	0	0
Oregon	Jeff Butler Acting Director, Multicultural Affairs (503) 494-7574	0	1	0	2
Pennsylvania State‡	Dr. Alphonse E. Leure-duPree Associate Dean, Student Affairs (717) 531-6411	9	0	3	0
Pennsylvania,‡ University of	Dr. Karen Hamilton Assistant Dean for Student Affairs and Director, Minority Affairs (215) 898-4409	8	0	4	5
Pittsburgh‡	Paula K. Davis Assistant Dean, Office of Student and Minority Affairs (412) 648-8987	12	0	6	0
Ponce‡	Arvin Baez Assistant Dean, Student Affairs (787) 840-2575	0	0	0	4‖
Puerto Rico	Dr. America Facundo Director, Hispanic Center of Excellence (787) 756-6343	0	0	0	3‖

TABLE 9-B (continued)

Minority Student Matriculants by Individual Medical School

Medical School	Contact Person or Office	Minority Enrollment, Fall 1999 (New Entrant)* Black	Native† American	Mexican-American	Mainland Puerto Rican
Rochester‡	Dr. Nathaniel Holmes Director, Office of Ethnic and Multicultural Affairs (716) 275-2842	7	1	0	1
Rush‡	Dr. Cynthia E. Boyd Assistant Dean, Minority Affairs (312) 942-5496	7	0	1	1
Saint Louis	Dr. George Rausch Assistant Dean for Multicultural Affairs (314) 268-5398	18	1	2	0
South Carolina, Medical University of	Dr. Thaddeus J. Bell Director, University Diversity and Executive Assistant (843) 792-2146	15	0	0	0
South Carolina, University of	Dr. Carol L. McMahon Assistant Dean for Minority Affairs (803) 733-3319	3	0	0	0
South Dakota	Dr. Barbara E. Goodman Associate Professor Physiology/Pharmacology (605) 677-5158	0	1	0	0
Stanford‡	Dr. Fernando S. Mendoza Associate Dean for Student Affairs (650) 725-8314	4	0	8	0
Temple‡	Dr. Raul A. De La Cadena Assistant Dean, Director Recruitment, Admissions, and Retention Programs (215) 707-3595	23	1	7	4
Tennessee State, East	Dr. Dorothy Dobbins Associate Dean, Student Affairs (423) 439-6269	8	2	0	1

TABLE 9-B (continued)

Minority Student Matriculants by Individual Medical School

Medical School	Contact Person or Office	Minority Enrollment, Fall 1999 (New Entrant)*			
		Black	Native† American	Mexican-American	Mainland Puerto Rican
Tennessee, University of	Dr. Kenneth Robinson Assistant Dean, Admissions and Students (901) 448-7228	18	0	1	0
Texas A&M	Tommy Bosquez Special Assistant to VP for Health Affairs (409) 862-4065	2	0	4	0
Texas Tech	Dr. Eugene Trowers Associate Professor of Medicine (806) 743-3155	1	2	7	0
Texas—Dallas (Southwestern)	Dr. Byron Cryer Assistant Dean for Minority Student Affairs (214) 648-2168	11	1	10	0
Texas—Galveston	Dr. Billy R. Ballard Associate VP for Student Affairs Associate Dean for Student Affairs and Admissions (409) 772-1442	21	0	33	2
Texas—Houston	Dr. Patricia Butler Associate Dean for Educational Programs (713) 500-5140	4	1	8	0
Texas—San Antonio	Dr. Leonard E. Lawrence Medical Deans Office (210) 567-4429	2	0	27	1
Tufts‡	Colleen Romain Assistant Director of Student Affairs (617) 636-6576	5	2	4	2
Tulane‡	Dr. Dave Williams Assistant Dean of Student Affairs (504) 988-4555	5	1	1	0

TABLE 9-B (continued)

Minority Student Matriculants by Individual Medical School

Medical School	Contact Person or Office	Minority Enrollment, Fall 1999 (New Entrant)* Black	Native† American	Mexican-American	Mainland Puerto Rican
Uniformed Services University	Dr. Carolyn Miller Vice President, Minority Affairs (301) 295-9560	7	5	4	1
Utah	Kristi Ryujin Director, Diversity and Community Outreach (801) 585-2430	1	1	5	0
Vanderbilt‡	Dr. Michael Rodriguez Director, Minority Student Affairs (615) 343-0437	4	1	1	0
Vermont	Dr. Cathleen J. Gleeson Director of Admissions (802) 656-4170	0	0	0	0
Virginia Commonwealth	Aileen Edwards Director, Admissions and Minority Affairs (804) 828-0997	8	0	0	0
Virginia, Eastern‡	Gail C. Williams Assistant Dean for Student Affairs and Director of Minority Affairs (757) 446-5869	6	0	0	0
Virginia, University of	Dr. Maurice Apprey Associate Dean, Professor of Psychology (804) 924-1867	7	1	0	1
Wake Forest	Dr. Velma G. Watts Director of Minority Affairs (336) 716-4201	13	0	0	0
Washington University‡ (St. Louis)	Dr. Will Ross Associate Dean, Diversity Programs (314) 362-6854	5	0	8	0
Washington, University of	Charles Garcia Director, Multicultural Affairs (206) 685-2489	4	3	4	1

CHAPTER 9

TABLE 9-B (continued)

Minority Student Matriculants by Individual Medical School

Medical School	Contact Person or Office	Minority Enrollment, Fall 1999 (New Entrant)* Black	Native† American	Mexican-American	Mainland Puerto Rican
Wayne State	Dr. Jane Thomas Assistant Dean for Student Affairs (313) 577-1463	28	1	0	0
Weill‡	Dr. Bruce L. Ballard Associate Dean for Student Affairs and Equal Opportunity Programs (212) 746-1058	12	0	2	4
West Virginia	Dr. John W. Traubert Associate Dean for Student Affairs (304) 293-2408	2	0	0	0
Wisconsin,‡ Medical College of	Dr. Earnestine Willis Interim Associate Dean, Minority Student Affairs (414) 456-4131	4	2	0	0
Wisconsin, University of	Dr. Gloria V. Hawkins Assistant Dean for Minority Affairs (608) 263-3713	4	1	4	1
Wright State	Dr. Alonzo Patterson, III Assistant Dean for Minority Affairs (937) 775-2934	11	0	0	3
Yale‡	Dr. Forrester A. Lee Assistant Dean of Multicultural Affairs (203) 785-7545	10	0	2	1
Total New Entrants:		1,132	109	394	112

TABLE 9-B (continued)

Minority Student Information by Individual Medical School

* The first figure under each minority category is the number of those students who are new entrants for 1999. Data on applicants are based upon the newly developed AAMC Data Warehouse. The Data Warehouse provides more complete data on racial/ethnic self-description and consistent definitions across all years reported. As a result, the data published this year from the Data Warehouse may not match previously published numbers.

** Data self-reported from school.

† Includes Native Americans, Alaskan Natives, and Native Hawaiians.

‡ Privately supported medical schools.

§ Two-year school of basic medical sciences.

|| These figures represent students who are mainland Puerto Rican residents only and do not include residents of the Commonwealth of Puerto Rico.

Source: AAMC Data Warehouse: Applicant Matriculant Files. New entrants are students entering medical school for the first time.

CHAPTER 9

Information on Medical Schools Offering Combined College/M.D. Program for High School Students

10

Many of the medical schools providing programs of undergraduate college and medical education for high school students offer an accelerated course of study. These programs take a minimum of six to eight years to complete. The first two to four years of the curriculum consist of undergraduate courses and include the necessary premedical requirements. At various stages, a graduate receives a bachelor's degree from the university and then the M.D. degree from the medical school on completion of the program. There are several schools that offer an integrated curriculum and are primarily designed for students entering from high school.

Admission is open to highly qualified high school seniors with a strong desire to pursue medicine as a career. State-supported schools generally do not admit many out-of-state applicants into their programs. Prospective applicants seeking admission to state-supported schools will have a better chance of acceptance at institutions located in their own state of residence. Private schools are, for the most part, more flexible; enrollment is generally not limited to state residents.

Academic prerequisites for admission vary among the schools conducting these programs but usually include the following subjects: introductory calculus, biology, physics, chemistry, English, and social studies. Any high school student who has an early aspiration to become a physician should consult with a guidance counselor to be certain that the curriculum incorporates those specific courses required for the program(s) in which the student would like to enroll.

The following program descriptions were compiled from responses to a questionnaire sent to all medical schools with programs of interest to high school students. For medical school tuitions for the 1999–2000 entering class, refer to the school entries in Part 2. For further information, please contact the schools directly.

ABBREVIATIONS

Listed below are the abbreviations used in the school entries in this chapter.

ACT Assessment—American College Testing Program Assessment
CEEB—College Entrance Examination Board
FAFSA—Free Application for Federal Student Aid
GPA—Grade-point average
MCAT—Medical College Admission Test
SAT—Scholastic Aptitude Test
USMLE—United States Medical Licensing Examination

List of Medical Schools Offering Combined College/ M.D. Programs for High School Students

Alabama
University of South Alabama College of Medicine

California
University of California, Riverside and University of California, Los Angeles, UCLA School of Medicine
University of California, San Diego School of Medicine
University of Southern California College of Letters, Arts, and Sciences and School of Medicine

District of Columbia
George Washington University School of Medicine and Columbian School of Arts and Sciences
Howard University

Florida
University of Florida College of Medicine
University of Miami

Illinois
Finch University of Health Sciences/Chicago Medical School and Illinois Institute of Technology
Northwestern University
University of Illinois at Chicago

Massachusetts
Boston University

Michigan
Michigan State University College of Human Medicine
University of Michigan

Missouri
University of Missouri—Kansas City School of Medicine

New Jersey
UMDNJ—New Jersey Medical School
Rutgers University and University of Medicine and Dentistry of New Jersey Robert Wood Johnson Medical School

New York
Binghamton University and State University of New York Health Science Center at Syracuse College of Medicine
Brooklyn College and State University of New York Downstate Medical Center College of Medicine
New York University
Rensselaer Polytechnic Institute and Albany Medical College
Siena College and Albany Medical College
SUNY Stony Brook and SUNY Stony Brook School of Medicine
Union College and Albany Medical College
University of Rochester School of Medicine and Dentistry

Ohio
Case Western Reserve University
Northeastern Ohio Universities College of Medicine
University of Cincinnati College of Medicine

Pennsylvania
Lehigh University and MCP Hahnemann School of Medicine
Pennsylvania State University and Jefferson Medical College of Thomas Jefferson University

Rhode Island
Brown University

Tennessee
East Tennessee State University
Fisk University and Meharry Medical College

Texas
Rice University and Baylor College of Medicine
Texas A&M University Health Sciences Center College of Medicine

Virginia
Eastern Virginia Medical School
Virginia Commonwealth University

Wisconsin
University of Wisconsin Medical School

Number of Years Required by Undergraduate and U.S. Medical Schools to Complete the Combined College/M.D. Program

6 Years

University of Missouri—Kansas City School of Medicine
Rensselaer Polytechnic Institute and Albany Medical College
Pennsylvania State University and Jefferson Medical College of Thomas Jefferson University
Texas A&M University Health Science Center College of Medicine

6-7 Years

University of Miami
Lehigh University and MCP Hahnemann School of Medicine
Northeastern Ohio Universities College of Medicine

7 Years

University of California, Riverside and University of California, Los Angeles UCLA School of Medicine
George Washington University School of Medicine and Columbian School of Arts and Sciences
University of Florida College of Medicine
Northwestern University
Boston University*
UMDNJ—New Jersey Medical School
Sophie Davis School of Biomedical Education/City University of New York
Union College and Albany Medical College
Fisk University and Meharry Medical College
University of Wisconsin Medical School†

8 Years

University of South Alabama College of Medicine
University of California, San Diego School of Medicine
University of Southern California College of Letters, Arts, and Sciences School of Medicine
Howard University
Finch University of Health Sciences/Chicago Medical School and Illinois Institute of Technology
University of Illinois at Chicago
Michigan State University College of Human Medicine
University of Michigan
Rutgers University and University of Medicine and Dentistry of New Jersey Robert Wood Johnson Medical School
Binghamton University and State University of New York Health Sciences Center at Syracuse College of Medicine
Brooklyn College and State University of New York Downstate Medical Center College of Medicine
New York University
Siena College and Albany Medical College
SUNY Stony Brook School of Medicine
University of Rochester School of Medicine and Dentistry
Case Western Reserve University
University of Cincinnati College of Medicine
Brown University
East Tennessee State University
Rice University and Baylor College of Medicine
Eastern Virginia Medical College
Virginia Commonwealth University

9 Years

University of Cincinnati College of Medicine (College of Engineering—undergraduate)

*8-year option
†7- to 9-year program

University of South Alabama College of Medicine

Mobile, Alabama

ADDRESS INQUIRIES TO:

Office of Admissions
University of South Alabama
Administrative Building
Room 182
Mobile, Alabama 36688-0002
(334) 460-6141 or (800) 872-5247

PURPOSE

Candidates selected for the program will receive early acceptance from the University of South Alabama and College of Medicine. Students participating in the program are expected to enter the University of South Alabama College of Medicine following the fall after completion of the baccalaureate degree.

REQUIREMENTS FOR ENTRANCE

Students in the senior year of high school or recently graduated individuals who have not yet entered college will be eligible to apply for the program. Both residents and nonresidents of Alabama may apply.

SELECTION FACTORS

Candidates must have a minimum high school GPA of 3.5 as computed by the University of South Alabama and must present a minimum enhanced composite ACT score of 28 (or comparable SAT). Candidates must also have demonstrated leadership qualities and motivation toward the study of medicine.

CURRICULUM

The curriculum will include core requirements for the selected baccalaureate program and prerequisites for matriculation in medical school. Students in the program must maintain a minimum overall GPA of 3.5 and a minimum GPA of 3.4 in the sciences (biology, chemistry, physics) and mathematics. All required courses must be taken at the University of South Alabama unless otherwise approved in advance by their undergraduate program director and the associate dean of the College of Medicine.

Students will be required to participate in CP-200 (Career Planning; Clinical Observation) for a minimum of four quarters. Students will be given the opportunity to participate in a special summer premedical clerkship. The activities will be planned to give the participant a broad exposure to medical education.

Students will be required to take the MCAT for admission to the College of Medicine and will be required to score above the national average. A formal assessment, including an interview, will be conducted after the student has completed 96 quarter hours of work. At this time, the student's academic performance and continued interest in a medical career will be assessed.

EXPENSES

The 1999–2000 annual tuition for students at the University of South Alabama was $2,841 for residents; $5,481 for nonresidents. Medical school tuition for residents was $7,000; $14,000 for nonresidents.

FINANCIAL AID

Information can be obtained from the Office of Financial Aid, Administration Building, Room 260, University of South Alabama, Mobile, Alabama 36688-0002; or phone (334) 460-6231.

APPLICATION AND ACCEPTANCE POLICIES

Filing of application:
  Latest date: March
Application fee: $25
Acceptance notice:
  Earliest date: April
Applicant's response to acceptance offer:
  Maximum time: 2 weeks
Deposit to hold place in class: None
Starting date: Mid-August

INFORMATION ON 1999–2000 ENTERING CLASS

Number of	*In-State*	*Out-of-State*	*Total*
Applicants	90	65	155
Applicants Interviewed	30	10	40
New Entrants	10	5	15

University of California, Riverside, and University of California, Los Angeles UCLA School of Medicine

Riverside, California

ADDRESS INQUIRIES TO:

Student Affairs Officer
Division of Biomedical Sciences
University of California, Riverside
Riverside, California 92521-0121
(909) 787-4333
Web Site: http://www.biomed.ucr.edu

PURPOSE

This program offers an accelerated curriculum, which allows receipt of a B.S. degree after four years of college work and the M.D. degree seven years after matriculation as an undergraduate freshman.

REQUIREMENTS FOR ENTRANCE

Admission to this combined-degree program occurs in two phases: first, admission from high school to the University of California, Riverside, as a freshman; and second, admission to UCLA School of Medicine after completion of three undergraduate years at Riverside (UCR). Residents of California as well as out-of-state students are eligible to apply. For admission to Riverside, students are required to take the SAT I and three SAT II scholastic assessment tests. One test must be in writing, and one must be in mathematics. In addition, applicants are required to complete six semesters of laboratory science courses in chemistry, physics, or biology, plus eight semesters of mathematics and qualify for placement in calculus.

SELECTION FACTORS

To gain admission as a freshman in the combined-degree program at Riverside, an applicant must meet the selection criteria for the University of California, as mentioned above. Subsequent admission to UCLA School of Medicine depends on the student's undergraduate science GPA at Riverside, nonscience and overall GPA, results of the MCAT taken in the summer before the third year at Riverside, letters of recommendation, and three required interviews. In the 1999–2000 class entering UCLA School of Medicine from Riverside's combined-degree program, the 24 students had an average undergraduate GPA of 3.73, an average MCAT score of 9.8, and an average combined SAT score of 1327.

CURRICULUM

This program leads to a baccalaureate degree granted by the University of California, Riverside, and the M.D. degree awarded by the University of California, Los Angeles, UCLA School of Medicine.

The curriculum for both degrees takes seven years to complete. Students are expected to take Steps 1 and 2 of the USMLE examinations while at UCLA. In addition, passing these examinations is a graduation requirement.

EXPENSES

For California residents, there is no tuition for undergraduate work, but there are fees amounting to $3,747 per year. For out-of-state undergraduate students, tuition was $9,804 per year, plus fees. For years one and two of medical school, California residents pay fees of $10,128 annually; nonresidents pay an additional $9,804 annually.

FINANCIAL AID

Sources of aid are scholarships, grants, work-study, and student loans. Applicants can receive more information from the Financial Aid Office, University of California, Riverside, Riverside, California 92521.

APPLICATION AND ACCEPTANCE POLICIES FOR UNDERGRADUATE PORTION AT RIVERSIDE

Filing of application:
- Earliest date: Nov. 1
- Latest date: Nov. 30

Application fee: $40

Acceptance notice:
- Earliest date: March 1
- Latest date: Sept. 15

Applicant's response to acceptance offer:
- Maximum time: May 1

Deposit to hold place in class: $100; nonrefundable

Starting date: Sept. 28

INFORMATION ON 1999–2000 ENTERING CLASS UCLA SCHOOL OF MEDICINE FROM THE COMBINED-DEGREE PROGRAM AT RIVERSIDE

Number of	*In-State*	*Out-of-State*	*Total*
Applicants	42	2	44
Applicants Interviewed	42	2	44
New Entrants	24	1	25

University of California San Diego School of Medicine

La Jolla, California

ADDRESS INQUIRIES TO:

Linda Whitson
Director of Admissions
University of California, San Diego School of Medicine
Office of Admissions 0621
9500 Gilman Drive
La Jolla, California 92093
(858) 534-3880
Web Site: www.medicine.ucsd.edu

PURPOSE

The Medical Scholars Program has been established to encourage the recruitment of unusually talented high school students, who would then be attracted both to the University of California, San Diego (UCSD) undergraduate and medical schools, and to promote the goal of increasing diversity on both campuses.

REQUIREMENTS FOR ENTRANCE

Students are selected for this program during their senior year of high school. It is open to California residents only. Applicants must meet course requirements for UCSD undergraduate admission. They must take either the SAT or ACT and achieve a minimum score of 1450 on the SAT or 32 on the ACT.

SELECTION FACTORS

To be eligible for consideration, applicants must have a minimum high school GPA of 4.0 and 1450 on the SAT. The average high school grade-point average for the 1999–2000 entering class was 4.28. Applicants must also demonstrate strong extracurricular involvement, particularly in community service and leadership. Letters of recommendation and an essay are additional considerations. An interview is required. The MCAT is not required.

CURRICULUM

This program leads to a baccalaureate degree granted by the University of California, San Diego, and to an M.D. degree granted by the UCSD School of Medicine. It takes eight years to fulfill the requirements for both degrees. The specific course requirements for the baccalaureate degree include a minimum of 6 quarters in either Humanities or social sciences, and 15 quarters in the natural and physical sciences. Students must take Step 1 of the USMLE after the second year of medical school. The passage of Steps 1 and 2 of the USMLE is required in order to be promoted and graduate.

EXPENSES

In 1999–2000, tuition was $9,804. Undergraduate student fees were $3,847, and medical school fees were $10,324.

FINANCIAL AID

Sources of financial aid include scholarships, grants, loans, and work-study. Additional information is available through the undergraduate financial aid office: Building 201, University Center, La Jolla, California 92093-0013 or www.ucsd.edu/finaid.

APPLICATION AND ACCEPTANCE POLICIES

Filing of application:
- Earliest date: March 1
- Latest date: March 24

Application fee: None

Acceptance notice:
- Earliest date: April 1
- Latest date: May 1

Applicant's response to acceptance offer:
- Maximum time: 1 week

Deposit to hold place in class: None

Starting date: September

INFORMATION ON 1999–2000 ENTERING CLASS

Number of	*Total*
Applicants	180
Applicants Interviewed	19
New Entrants	3

CHAPTER 10

University of Southern California
College of Letters, Arts, and Sciences
School of Medicine

Los Angeles, California

ADDRESS INQUIRIES TO:

Office of Admission
College of Letters, Arts, and Sciences
University of Southern California
Los Angeles, California 90089-0152
(213) 740-5930
(213) 740-1338 (FAX)
Web Site: http://www.usc.edu/dept/las/md.html

PURPOSE

The goal of this program, initiated in 1993, is to encourage bright and highly motivated students to expand the breadth of their education through a diverse liberal arts education. Students accepted into this program have the opportunity to study a wide variety of disciplines beyond the course of the standard premedical curriculum. It is the hope of the University to graduate physicians who are educated in medical science, art, and the humanities.

REQUIREMENTS FOR ENTRANCE

Students are selected for this program in the senior year of high school. Both residents and nonresidents of California and international students are eligible to apply. There are no specific high school course requirements, but applicants are required to take either the SAT or ACT Assessment.

SELECTION FACTORS

Academic factors considered include grades and standardized test scores. Additionally, participation in extracurricular activities and demonstrated leadership and community service are highly valued. Students who enrolled in 1999 had a mean high school GPA of 4.22, and a mean SAT score of 1500 (recentered). An interview is required and is granted by invitation following careful evaluation of an applicant's file.

CURRICULUM

This program leads to a baccalaureate degree awarded by the University of Southern California, and the M.D. degree granted by the University of Southern California School of Medicine.

This is not an accelerated program; all students must complete four years of undergraduate education and four years of medical school.

Students must complete requirements for the bachelor's degree and may pursue any major offered in the university that is compatible with the requirements of the program. There are specific requirements for the bachelor's degree, which include the humanities, social, natural, and physical sciences.

Advancement to the medical school phase of the program is based on acceptable academic performance and MCAT scores as defined by the program. The MCAT is required and must be taken by the spring of junior year. Students must take steps 1 and 2, and pass Step 1 of the USMLE examinations in order to graduate.

EXPENSES

In 1999–2000, undergraduate tuition for residents and nonresidents was $22,200 plus annual fees of $477. The medical school tuition was $32,266 plus annual fees of $1,108.

FINANCIAL AID

Sources of aid include scholarships, grants, work-study programs, and loans. Contact the Office of Financial Aid, University of Southern California, Los Angeles, California 90089-0912; or call (213) 740-5466 for additional information.

APPLICATION AND ACCEPTANCE POLICIES

Filing of application:
  Earliest date: Aug. 1
  Latest date: Nov. 15
Application fee: None
Acceptance notice:
  Latest date: April 1
Applicant's response to acceptance offer:
  Maximum time: May 1
Deposit to hold place in class: $200; nonrefundable
Starting date: Aug. 2000

INFORMATION ON 1999–2000 ENTERING CLASS

Number of	*Total*
Applicants	520
Applicants Interviewed	102
New Entrants	21

George Washington University School of Medicine and Columbian College School of Arts and Sciences

Washington, D.C.

ADDRESS INQUIRIES TO:

Office of Admissions
George Washington University
2121 "I" Street, N.W.
Washington, D.C. 20052
(800) 447-3765
Web Site: http://www.gwu.edu/~go2gw

PURPOSE

The undergraduate program includes basic training in the premedical sciences with the opportunity to explore another field of interest. The baccalaureate degree is awarded after year four (first year of medical school).

REQUIREMENTS FOR ENTRANCE

Students are selected in their senior year of high school. There are no residency requirements. There are no specific high school course requirements. Applicants are required to take the SAT II Subject Tests in writing, mathematics, and science. Many students receive their undergraduate degrees before beginning medical school.

SELECTION FACTORS

Applicants should be in the top five percent of their class. The average GPA for the 1999–2000 entering class was 3.80. The average test score for the ACT was 32, and the average SAT score was 1450. In addition to academic factors, and extracurricular and health-related activities, letters of recommendation are reviewed. An interview is required.

CURRICULUM

This seven-year program leads to the baccalaureate degree granted by the George Washington University and the M.D. degree granted by the School of Medicine. The course requirements for the baccalaureate degree in the humanities and social sciences vary, but students must complete 32 semester hours in the natural and physical sciences. Passing the MCAT examination is not a factor in the admission or promotion phase to the medical school program. The medicine portion of the curriculum provides a course on the Practice of Medicine that involves primary care apprenticeship, group-mentor teams, and problem-based learning groups.

Students are required to take Step 1 of the USMLE at the end of Year 2 of medical school. Passing Step 1 is a requirement for promotion and graduation. Students must take Step 2 of the USMLE, but are not required to pass in order to graduate.

EXPENSES

In 1999–2000, tuition was $30,500 per year for seven years. This includes a $10,000-per-year scholarship.

FINANCIAL AID

Information may be obtained from the George Washington University, Office of Student Financial Assistance, 2121 "I" Street, N.W., Rice Hall, Washington, D.C. 20037.

APPLICATION AND ACCEPTANCE POLICIES

Filing of application:
- Earliest date: Sept.
- Latest date: Dec. 1 (Part I); Part II and Supplemental, Jan. 15

Application fee: $55
Acceptance notice:
- Earliest date: mid-March

Applicant's response to acceptance offer:
- Latest date: May 1

Deposit to hold place in class: $650; nonrefundable

INFORMATION ON 1999–2000 ENTERING CLASS

Number of	*Total*
Applicants	534
Applicants Interviewed	50
New Entrants	8

Howard University

Washington, D.C.

ADDRESS INQUIRIES TO:

Dr. G. Aboko-Cole, *Director*
Center for Preprofessional Education
College of Arts and Sciences
P.O. Box 473
Administration Building
Howard University
Washington, D.C. 20059
(202) 238-2363

PURPOSE

The goal of this combined-degree program is to encourage talented undergraduate students to choose medicine as a career and to retain these excellent students in the Howard University College of Medicine.

REQUIREMENTS FOR ENTRANCE

Students can be selected for this program during the senior year of high school or during the first year of college. There are no state residence requirements. Applicants are expected to have completed the following courses by the time they graduate from high school: at least two years of a foreign language; at least one year each of biology, chemistry, and physics; two years of mathematics; and four years of English, including literature. They must take either the SAT or the ACT Assessment.

SELECTION FACTORS

The academic factors considered in offering admission to an applicant are rank in high school class, GPA, and test scores. Applicants are expected to be in the top five percent of their high school class. In the 1999–2000 entering class, the average GPA was 3.7, and the average SAT combined score was 1300. ACT Assessment cumulative scores ranged from 25 to 29. Personal qualities considered include self-esteem, realistic self-appraisal, a realistic assessment of the medical profession, leadership, and superior writing skills. An interview is required.

CURRICULUM

This program leads to a bachelor's degree awarded by the College of Arts and Sciences at Howard University and the M.D. degree granted by the College of Medicine, also at Howard.

Students must complete work for a baccalaureate degree. They are expected to complete at least 40 semester hours of humanities and social sciences to fulfill general education requirements and at least 46 semester hours of natural and physical science. Students meet with the director (the advisor) of the Center for Preprofessional Education to design a curriculum tailored to individual needs. The specific course selection must have the advisor's approval. Students are encouraged to select a major of personal interest.

The curricula for both degrees are completed in six years. In the first two years the curriculum focuses on work toward the bachelor's degree and premedical requirements, and in the last four years the focus is on studies related to medicine. Students in this program must take the MCAT in April of the second year. The results of this test and the GPA are major factors in gaining admission to the medical school phase of the combined-degree program. Students are also expected to take Steps 1 and 2 of the USMLE examinations while at Howard University College of Medicine, and they must pass these examinations for graduation from that school.

EXPENSES

In 1999–2000 the annual tuition for students in the College of Arts and Sciences was $9,390. There are also student fees, which are subject to change.

FINANCIAL AID

Information can be obtained from the Office of Financial Aid, Howard University, Johnson Administration Building, 2400 – 6th Street, N.W., Washington, D.C. 20059.

APPLICATION AND ACCEPTANCE POLICIES

Filing of application:
  Latest date: Rolling admission
Application fee: $45
Deposit to hold place in class: $150; nonrefundable
Starting date: Late August

INFORMATION ON 1999–2000 ENTERING CLASS

Number of	*Total*
Applicants	40
Applicants Interviewed	20
New Entrants	10

University of Florida College of Medicine

Gainesville, Florida

ADDRESS INQUIRIES TO:

Medical Selection Committee
University of Florida College of Medicine
P.O. Box 100216
Gainesville, Florida 32610
(352) 392-4569; 846-0622 (FAX)
Web Site: http://www.med.ufl.edu

PURPOSE

The Junior Honors Medical Program is for undergraduate students who have chosen a career in the medical profession and who have demonstrated superior scholastic ability and personal development during their first two academic years.

REQUIREMENTS FOR ENTRANCE

Students are selected for our program during their sophomore year of college. Admission is open to all possible candidates. There are no specific high school course requirements; however, admissions tests such as SAT achievement tests are required.

SELECTION FACTORS

The academic factors considered in offering admission to an applicant are sophomore standing, GPA, and prerequisite courses. Applicants must take the MCAT in their fourth year. Although the MCAT is not a factor in admissions to the medical school phase of the program, it is a factor in promotion. Selected applicants are invited for a required interview.

CURRICULUM

The most frequent major for the baccalaureate degree is biomedical sciences, followed by neuroscience. Both are awarded at the University of Florida of Liberal Arts and Sciences. Requirements for that degree include four semesters each in the humanities, and five semesters in the natural and physical sciences. The Doctor of Medicine degree is awarded at the University of Florida College of Medicine. It takes seven years to complete requirements for both degrees.

The following chart shows the approximate percentage of liberal arts and medicine courses in the curriculum each year:

Year	*Percent Liberal Arts*	*Percent Medicine*
1	100	0
2	100	0
3	50	50
4	0	100
5	0	100
6	0	100
7	0	100

EXPENSES

Undergraduate tuition for residents in 1999–2000 was $1,480 and $8,136 for nonresidents. The medical school tuition in 1999–2000 was $9,684 for residents and $27,335 for nonresidents. Annual student fees were $662 for undergraduates and $1,343 for medical students.

FINANCIAL AID

There are several sources of financial aid available to students such as college scholarships and loans, Federal Stafford loans, possible state scholarships, National Merit and Robert Byrd, if eligible. For more information, contact Office of Financial Aid, P.O. Box 100216 HSC, Gainesville, Florida 32610, (352) 392-7800, E-mail: eparris@ufl.edu.

APPLICATION AND ACCEPTANCE POLICIES

Filing of application:
- Earliest date: Jan.13
- Latest date: Jan. 31

Application fee: None
Acceptance notice:
- Earliest date: May 15
- Latest date: August 20

Applicant's response to acceptance offer:
- Maximum time: 2 weeks

Deposit to hold place in class: None
Starting date: August 22

INFORMATION ON 1999–2000 ENTERING CLASS

Number of	*In-State*	*Out-of-State*	*Total*
Applicants	80	4	84
Applicants Interviewed	32	0	32
New Entrants	12	0	12

CHAPTER 10

University of Miami

Miami, Florida

ADDRESS INQUIRIES TO:

Office of Admissions
University of Miami
P.O. Box 248025
Coral Gables, FL 33124
(305) 284-4323
Web Sites: www.miami.edu
www.miami.edu/medical-admissions

PURPOSE

The Honors Program in Medicine (HPM) offers exceptionally motivated and talented students who have reached a mature and independent decision to study medicine, and an opportunity to earn the B.S. and M.D. degrees in either six or seven years.

REQUIREMENTS FOR ENTRANCE

Applicants must be residents of the state of Florida and in their last year of high school at the time of application. Applicants must have a minimum combined score of 1360 on the SAT or a composite score of 31 on the ACT, and take the SAT II Subject Tests in English, mathematics, and science (no minimum score required). All must have completed eight semesters of English and mathematics and two semesters each of biology and chemistry by the time they graduate from high school.

SELECTION FACTORS

Academic factors taken into account include scores on standardized tests, the quality of the high school curriculum including the number and nature of advanced placement courses, and the amount of university-level work already completed. Of equal importance to academic achievements are personal factors such as maturity of thought and action, common sense, empathy, interpersonal skills, appropriate freedom from parental influence, and social cognizance. Most importantly, the applicant must have made a practical decision to study medicine based on self-initiated patient-contact experiences. "Skipping" grades or graduating early from high school confers no advantage.

CURRICULUM

The first two years are spent on the Coral Gables campus taking required science and humanity courses and focusing almost exclusively on work related to the bachelor's degree. The undergraduate portion of the curriculum may be extended to three years if the student is in good academic standing and has established a clear plan of academic and personal growth. HPM students major in biology, most frequently followed by chemistry and microbiology. All HPM students must have a 3.2 science GPA and a 3.4 cumulative GPA, and take the MCAT before starting medical school. MCAT scores do not factor into subsequent promotion to medical school but are used as one indicator of the student's preparedness to study medicine. The medical curriculum is four years long. HPM students usually qualify for the B.S. degree after successfully completing the first year of medical school.

EXPENSES

In 1999–2000 tuition for the undergraduate portion of the HPM program was $21,350. Tuition at the School of Medicine was $25,670 and fees were $120.

FINANCIAL AID

Scholarships, work-study, loans and state tuition grants are sources of financial assistance. Information on undergraduate financial aid is available from the Office of Financial Assistance Services, (305) 284-5212.

APPLICATION AND ACCEPTANCE POLICIES

Filing of application:
Earliest date: October 15
Latest date for receipt of all materials: January 15
Application fee: $50
Acceptance notice:
All decisions are made on April 1
Applicant's response to acceptance offer:
No later than May 1
Deposit to hold place in class (applied to tuition):
$300; nonrefundable
Starting date: August

INFORMATION ON 1999–2000 ENTERING CLASS

Number of	*Total*
Applicants Interviewed	107
New Entrants	21

Finch University of Health Sciences/ Chicago Medical School and Illinois Institute of Technology

Chicago, Illinois

ADDRESS INQUIRIES TO:

Dean of Admission
Illinois Institute of Technology
B.S./M.D. Program
10 West 33rd Street
Chicago, Illinois 60616
(312) 567-3025; outside Chicago, 800-448-2329
Web Sites: http://www.iit.edu
http://www.finchcms.edu
On-line Application:
http://www.iit.edu/admission/undergrad/application

PURPOSE

The honors program allows superior students to earn both an Accreditation Board for Engineering and Technology (ABET) accredited Bachelor of Science degree in chemical, computer, electrical, mechanical engineering, molecular biochemistry and biophysics, computer science, and an M.D. degree in eight years. The goal is to produce graduates who understand the intricacies of technology applied to medicine who will be the future innovators in improving medical diagnoses and treatment for their patients.

REQUIREMENTS FOR ENTRANCE

Students are selected for this program during their senior year of high school. The program is open to U.S. citizens and permanent residents. Applicants are expected to have completed the following courses by the time they graduate from high school: four years of mathematics (through calculus) and three years of life sciences (chemistry, biology, and physics). Applicants must take either the SAT or the ACT Assessment.

Students must take the MCAT in their junior year, but scores are not a factor for admission to the medical school.

SELECTION FACTORS

Academic factors considered in offering admission to an applicant include high school class rank, GPA, curriculum, and essay and letters of recommendation. In the 1999–2000 entering class, the average score on the ACT was 31 and the SAT was 1350; the average high school grade-point average was 4.0. An interview is required. Students should also demonstrate an interest in engineering and medicine through medical-related research, hospital volunteer work, and participation in engineering and medical-related organizations.

CURRICULUM

This program leads to a baccalaureate degree granted by the Illinois Institute of Technology (IIT) and to an M.D. degree granted by the Finch University of Health Sciences/Chicago Medical School. The most frequent major for a baccalaureate degree is chemical engineering followed by computer science. The curriculum focuses on studies for the bachelor's degree in the first four years. Continuation on to medical school is contingent upon maintaining a 3.3 GPA, no course grade below a "C," and displaying ethical behavior appropriate for a future physician. Students enter medical school in the fifth year. Students are required to pass Step 1 and Step 2 of the USMLE before graduation.

EXPENSES

In 1999–2000, the undergraduate tuition was $17,500. The medical school tuition was $33,527, plus $100 in yearly fees. Tuition is subject to change at both institutions.

FINANCIAL AID

Sources of financial aid include university grants, work-study, loans, and merit scholarships. For more information, call the Illinois Institute of Technology Admissions Office at the numbers above.

APPLICATION AND ACCEPTANCE POLICIES

Filing of application:
Latest date: Jan. 15
Application fee: $30
Acceptance notice:
Latest date: April 1
Applicant's response to acceptance offer:
Maximum time: May 1
Deposit to hold place in class: $100; nonrefundable
Starting date: Aug. 28

INFORMATION ON 1999–2000 ENTERING CLASS

Number of	*In-State*	*Out-of-State*	*Total*
Applicants	45	222	267
Applicants Interviewed	8	35	43
New Entrants	2	12	14

Northwestern University

Evanston, Illinois

ADDRESS INQUIRIES TO:

Office of Admission and Financial Aid
Northwestern University
1801 Hinman Avenue
Evanston, Illinois 60204-3060
(847) 491-7271; 467-1317 (FAX)
E-mail: ug-admission.northwestern.edu

PURPOSE

The Honors Program in Medical Education (HPME), one of the oldest in the nation, provides highly motivated and gifted students an individualized undergraduate curriculum that shortens the premedical preparation and assures entry into medical school.

REQUIREMENTS FOR ENTRANCE

Students are selected for this program during the senior year of high school. Both residents and nonresidents of Illinois are eligible to apply. Applicants must meet the following high school course requirements: English, eight semesters; mathematics including differential and integral calculus, eight semesters; chemistry, two semesters; physics, two semesters; biology, two semesters; foreign language, four semesters. They must take either the SAT I or the ACT Assessment plus the SAT II Subject Tests in mathematics IIC, chemistry, and writing.

SELECTION FACTORS

Academic factors considered in selecting applicants include class rank, grades in high school, and scores on college entrance tests. Average test scores of students in the 1999–2000 entering class were: SAT Verbal, 749; SAT Mathematics, 768; CEEB Achievement Tests—Writing, 763; Mathematics II, 767; Chemistry, 750. Nonacademic factors considered are motivation, concern for others, maturity, and involvement in extracurricular activities. An interview is required.

CURRICULUM

The degrees offered in the Honors Program are a baccalaureate degree (B.S. in medicine, B.S. in biomedical engineering, B.S. in Speech, or B.A.) and the M.D., all from Northwestern University.

Students must complete requirements for a baccalaureate degree. Most students major in the biological sciences followed by psychology. Course requirements include the following: 11 quarters of natural and physical sciences and courses in the humanities and social sciences. The engineering curriculum also includes courses in basic and advanced engineering and mathematics. A third option is to study Communication Sciences and Disorders—Human Communication Sciences. It includes courses in that department in addition to the HPME requirements.

The curriculum normally takes seven years to complete. In years 1 through 3, the curriculum consists entirely of courses in the liberal arts and sciences, engineering, or speech. In years 4 through 7, the curriculum focuses on medicine. The MCAT is not required. Students must also take Step 1 of the USMLE, but passing that examination is not a requirement for graduation from the medical school.

EXPENSES

In 1999–2000 tuition for the B.S. degree was $23,496 per year. Medical school tuition was $30,417.

FINANCIAL AID

Sources of aid include Northwestern University and federal, state, and private programs. Undergraduate applicants can receive more information from the Office of Admission and Financial Aid, 1801 Hinman Avenue, Evanston, Illinois 60204–3060; or phone (847) 491-7271. Information about medical school financial aid can be obtained from Northwestern University, Financial Aid, 710 N. Lake Shore Drive, Chicago, Illinois 60611.

APPLICATION AND ACCEPTANCE POLICIES

Filing of application:
  Latest date: Jan. 1
    of applicant's senior year of high school
Application fee: $55
Acceptance notice:
  Earliest date: April 1
Applicant's response to acceptance offer:
  Maximum time: May 1
Deposit to hold place in class: $200; nonrefundable
Starting date: Sept. 13

INFORMATION ON 1999–2000 ENTERING CLASS

Number of	*Total*
Applicants	676
Applicants Interviewed	174
New Entrants	43

University of Illinois at Chicago

Chicago, Illinois

ADDRESS INQUIRIES TO:

Special Projects Unit
Office of Admissions and Records
University of Illinois at Chicago
P.O. Box 6020
Chicago, Illinois 60680-6020
(312) 996-8365; 413-7628 (FAX)
Web Site: http://www.uic.edu

PURPOSE

The purpose of this program is to encourage exceptionally motivated and talented students to choose medicine as a career and to enter the University of Illinois College of Medicine for their medical education.

REQUIREMENTS FOR ENTRANCE

Students are selected for this program during their senior year of high school. Admission is strictly for residents of Illinois. There are no specific high school course requirements; however, admissions tests such as the ACT or SAT achievement tests are required.

SELECTION FACTORS

The academic factors considered in offering admission to an applicant are rank in high school class, GPA, and test scores. Applicants must be in the top 15 percent of their high school class in order to be eligible to apply. Also, applicants must have an ACT composite of 28 or greater, or an SAT composite score of 1240 or greater in order to be eligible to apply. In the 1999–2000 entering class, the students had an ACT average of 32, and an average combined SAT score of 1410. In addition to academic factors, and extracurricular and health-related activities, letters of recommendation are required. Selected applicants are invited for a required interview.

CURRICULUM

Students in this program are required to complete a baccalaureate degree. The most frequent major for this degree is biological sciences awarded at the University of Illinois at Chicago. The Doctor of Medicine degree is awarded at the University of Illinois College of Medicine. It takes eight years to fulfill the requirements for both degrees.

EXPENSES

In 1999–2000, undergraduate tuition for residents was $3,138; for nonresidents, $9,414. Tuition for the medical school portion for residents was $16,294, for nonresidents, $39,826. Annual fees total $1,490 for undergraduates and medical students.

FINANCIAL AID

There are several sources of financial aid that can be obtained from the University of Illinois at Chicago, Office of Student Financial Aid, 1200 West Harrison Street, M/C 334, Chicago, Illinois 60607-7163; (312) 996-3126.

APPLICATION AND ACCEPTANCE POLICIES

Filing of application:
- Earliest date: Oct. 1
- Latest date: Jan. 15

Application fee: $40

Acceptance notice:
- Earliest date: March 15
- Latest date: March 15

Applicant's response to acceptance offer:
- Maximum time: 1½ months

Deposit to hold place in class: None

Starting date: August

INFORMATION ON 1999–2000 ENTERING CLASS

Number of	*Total*
Applicants	278
Applicants Interviewed	125
New Entrants	64

CHAPTER 10

Boston University

Boston, Massachusetts

ADDRESS INQUIRIES TO:

Office of Undergraduate Admissions
Boston University
121 Bay State Road
Boston, Massachusetts 02215
(617) 353-2300; 353-9695 (FAX)
Web Site: http://www.bu.edu/admissions/academics/esp/index.html

PURPOSE

This combined-degree program, one of the oldest in the nation, provides an undergraduate premedical preparation that also emphasizes the humanities and social sciences and affords a quality medical education even though the overall period of study is shortened.

REQUIREMENTS FOR ENTRANCE

Students are selected for the program at Boston University during the senior year of high school or after high school if they have not been enrolled in any other degree-granting program. There are no state residence requirements. Students who are completing their high school graduation requirements in three years in order to graduate early are not eligible for this program. Applicants are expected to have completed the following courses by the time they graduate from high school: four years each of English and mathematics (one year of calculus is required), three years of a foreign language, and one year each of biology, chemistry (AP chemistry is *strongly* recommended), and physics. They must take the SAT II Subject Exams in writing, mathematics Ic or IIc, and chemistry. The SAT II Subject Exam in a foreign language is recommended.

SELECTION FACTORS

The academic factors taken into account in offering admission to an applicant include the following: the high school GPA, the SAT I or ACT score, scores on the SAT II Subject Exams, rank in high school class, and the nature of the applicant's high school curriculum. In the 1999–2000 entering class, the average high school GPA was an unweighted 3.94 on a 4.0 scale, the average SAT Verbal was 744, SAT Mathematics was 769. SAT II Subject Exam scores averaged 750, and rank in class was in the top one percent. Personal characteristics sought in applicants are motivation, maturity, and understanding of a career in medicine. An interview with College of Arts and Sciences and School of Medicine faculty is required.

CURRICULUM

This program leads to a baccalaureate degree granted by the College of Arts and Sciences in Boston University and to the M.D. degree awarded by Boston University School of Medicine.

Students must complete work for the baccalaureate degree with a major in Medical Science. Requirements for this degree include four semester courses in the humanities, four courses in the social sciences, and nine courses in the natural and physical sciences. The program is seven years in length with an eight-year option.

Students must meet GPA and MCAT requirements of the program. They are also required to take Step 1 of the USMLE during the medical school portion of the program. Taking Step 2 of the USMLE is not a requirement for graduation, but is strongly recommended.

EXPENSES

In 1999–2000 undergraduate tuition was $23,770 per year for residents and nonresidents, plus $330 for student fees.

FINANCIAL AID

The usual sources of financial aid are available to students during the undergraduate portion of this program. Once into the medical school, students can qualify for need-based, low-interest, and government-sponsored loans. More information about aid can be obtained from the Office of Financial Assistance, Boston University, 881 Commonwealth Avenue, Boston, Massachusetts 02215; or phone (617) 353-2965.

APPLICATION AND ACCEPTANCE POLICIES

Filing of application:
- Earliest date: Sept. 1
- Latest date: Dec. 1

Application fee: $50

Acceptance notice:
- Earliest date: March 15
- Latest date: April 15

Applicant's response to acceptance offer:
- Maximum time: May 1

Deposit to hold place in class: $400; nonrefundable

INFORMATION ON 1999–2000 ENTERING CLASS

Number of	*In-State*	*Out-of-State*	*Total*
Applicants	23	557	580
Applicants Interviewed	3	97	100
New Entrants	1	19	20

Michigan State University College of Human Medicine

East Lansing, Michigan

ADDRESS INQUIRIES TO:

College of Human Medicine
Office of Admissions
A-239 Life Sciences
Michigan State University
East Lansing, Michigan 48824
(517) 353-9620
Web Site: http://www.chm.msu.edu/

PURPOSE

The goal of the program is to educate excellent primary care physicians who will establish caring relationships with patients, who will practice in Michigan, especially in underserved rural and inner-city areas, and who will commit to a lifetime of learning and ethical practices.

REQUIREMENTS FOR ENTRANCE

Students are selected for this program in the senior year of high school. Both residents and nonresidents of Michigan are eligible to apply. There are no specific high school course requirements, but applicants are required to have an ACT composite score in the range of 29 or higher, or an SAT composite score in the range of 1280 or higher.

SELECTION FACTORS

Academic factors considered in selecting applicants include consistently high grades or a strong upward trend, class rank in the top 10 percent, and a GPA of at least 3.6 or higher. College preparatory course work that includes at least three years each of basic science and mathematics, two years of foreign language, and one year of psychology/sociology or a communications-related course. An interview is required.

In the 1999–2000 entering class, the high school GPA averaged 3.89, and the average mean ACT score was 29.5; the SAT score averaged 1370.

CURRICULUM

This program leads to a baccalaureate degree awarded by the Michigan State University, and the M.D. degree granted by the Michigan State University College of Human Medicine. It is not an accelerated program; all students must complete requirements for a B.A. or B.S. degree, and four years of medical school.

The most frequent major for the baccalaureate degree is physiology followed by health studies (Interdisciplinary Social Science). Course requirements include eight semesters each of humanities, social sciences, and natural and physical sciences. These credit requirements are minimums and are dependent on the academic major.

Medical Scholars complete a component that may include a specialization in Health and Humanities. They participate in a research project under the direction of Michigan State University faculty. They complete a year of volunteer community service and at least a year of medical/clinical experience.

Students in this program are not required to take the MCAT for promotion or admission to the medical school. The student must pass Steps 1 and 2 of the USMLE in order to graduate. The USMLE Step 1 is administered at the completion of Year 2.

EXPENSES

In 1999–2000, undergraduate tuition was $4,670 for residents and $12,034 for nonresidents. Student fees averaged $626 for the year. Medical school tuition for residents was $15,420 (three semesters); nonresidents, $33,870 (three semesters). The average cost for student fees was $925.

FINANCIAL AID

A number of options are available for aid. These include college work-study, Pell Grants, student aid grants, Supplemental Educational Opportunities Grant, Subsidized and Unsubsidized Stafford loans, Parent Loans for Undergraduate Students, and private loans. Applicants can receive more information from Michigan State University, Office of Financial Aid, 252 Student Services, East Lansing, Michigan 48824; (517) 353-5940, 432-1155 (FAX), or E-mail: finaid@msu.edu.

APPLICATION AND ACCEPTANCE POLICIES

Filing of application:
  Earliest date: Aug. 15
  Latest date: Nov. 1
Application fee: $55
Acceptance notice: March 15
Applicant's response to acceptance offer:
  Maximum time: 2 weeks
Deposit to hold place in class: $55; nonrefundable
Starting date: Aug. 2001

INFORMATION ON 1999–2000 ENTERING CLASS

Number of	*In-State*	*Out-of-State*	*Total*
Applicants	155	82	257
Applicants Interviewed	29	16	45
New Entrants	8	2	10

CHAPTER 10

University of Michigan

Ann Arbor, Michigan

ADDRESS INQUIRIES TO:

Inteflex Program
1301 Catherine Street
3808 Medical Science Building II
University of Michigan
Ann Arbor, Michigan 48109-0608
(734) 763-3265; 936-1190 (FAX)
Web Site: http://www.umich.edu/

PURPOSE

The primary goal of the Integrated Premedical/Medical (Inteflex) Program is to educate physicians who are scientifically competent, compassionate, and socially conscious and who can apply the insights gained in the study of the humanities and social sciences in addressing the challenges of medicine in the twenty-first century.

REQUIREMENTS FOR ENTRANCE

Students are selected for this program during the senior year of high school. Both residents and nonresidents of Michigan are eligible to apply. Students must first apply to and be admitted to the College of Literature, Science, and Arts. In general, applicants are expected to have a solid background in mathematics and science. To be considered, they must take either the SAT or the ACT Assessment and achieve a minimum score of 1310 total on the SAT or 29 cumulative on the ACT Assessment.

SELECTION FACTORS

Academic factors considered in selecting applicants include the high school GPA, scores on college entrance tests, and type of high school courses completed. Personal factors such as extracurricular activities, honors and awards, letters of recommendation, and motivation to study medicine are evaluated. Students interested in a career as a generalist physician and students from minority groups are encouraged to apply. In 1998, the average SAT score for incoming Michigan resident students was 1412; the average for nonresidents was 1468. The average high school GPA for both groups was 3.94. An interview is required for admission.

CURRICULUM

Degrees offered in the Inteflex Program are a baccalaureate degree from the College of Literature, Science, and Arts at the University of Michigan and an M.D. degree from the University of Michigan Medical School.

Students may elect from a variety of liberal arts majors and must complete all requirements for the baccalaureate degree prior to advancement to the medical four years of the program. Most students major in the biomedical sciences. Some course requirements for the baccalaureate degree include three semesters of humanities, three semesters of social science, three semesters of natural and physical sciences, four semesters of a foreign language, and two semesters of writing.

The curriculum normally takes eight years to complete. The study of medicine is integrated with the study of liberal arts beginning with the first year of the program. Advancement to the medical school phase is based on the overall undergraduate record and a successful performance on the required MCAT examination. Students must complete all requirements of the standard four-year medical curriculum (including Steps 1 and 2 of the USMLE) to complete the program and receive the M.D. degree.

EXPENSES

Students are responsible for tuition and fees set by the university for four years of both undergraduate and medical school. For the 1998–99* entering class, the in-state annual tuition (including spring term) was $7,468; out-of-state tuition was $23,790. For reference, medical school annual tuition for 1999–2000 was $18,020 for in-state and $27,776 for out-of-state. University fees are approximately $185.38 per year. Costs for room and board are additional.

FINANCIAL AID

Sources of aid include grants, loans, and work-study, which are available through the Undergraduate Financial Aid Office (undergraduates in Inteflex), 2011 Student Activities Building, University of Michigan, Ann Arbor, Michigan 48109-1316.

*No entering class for the fall of 1999.

APPLICATION AND ACCEPTANCE POLICIES

Filing of application:
The future missions and curriculum of the Program are currently under review. No applications for admission will be accepted at this time.

INFORMATION ON 1998–99* ENTERING CLASS

Number of	*In-State*	*Out-of-State*	*Total*
Applicants	180	249	429
Applicants Interviewed	81	35	116
New Entrants	25	10	35

University of Missouri—Kansas City School of Medicine

Kansas City, Missouri

ADDRESS INQUIRIES TO:

Council on Selection
University of Missouri—Kansas City
School of Medicine
2411 Holmes
Kansas City, Missouri 64108–2792
(816) 235-1870; 235-5277 (FAX)
Web Site: http://www.med.umkc.edu

PURPOSE

This combined baccalaureate-M.D. degree program integrates the humanities, social sciences, basic sciences, and clinical medicine throughout the curriculum so graduates will have the background for lifelong learning in order to meet the needs of their patients, families, and communities. It is one of the few U.S. programs in which the vast majority of students are pursuing a combined degree.

REQUIREMENTS FOR ENTRANCE

The program is primarily designed for high school graduates who are entering college. Residents and nonresidents of Missouri are eligible to apply. An applicant's high school curriculum must include at a minimum the following: eight semesters of English; eight semesters of mathematics; six semesters of science, including two semesters of biology and two semesters of chemistry; six semesters of social studies; two semesters of fine arts; four semesters of a foreign language; and one semester of computer science is recommended, but not required. Applicants must meet a minimum academic screen based on the ACT composite score and rank in high school class.

SELECTION FACTORS

Applicants' academic potential is judged by the quality of high school courses, rank in high school class, and scores on the ACT. In the 1999–2000 entering class, the average ACT score was in the 90th percentile, and the average rank in class was in the 95th percentile. Personal qualities include maturity, leadership, stamina, reliability, motivation for medicine, range of interests, interpersonal skills, compassion, and job experience. Qualified applicants are invited for a required interview.

CURRICULUM

The six-year curriculum leads to a baccalaureate degree granted by the University of Missouri, Kansas City (UMKC) College of Arts and Sciences or the UMKC School of Biological Sciences and the doctor of medicine degree granted by the School of Medicine.

Students must complete requirements for the bachelor's degree. Students have a choice of majors, but most select liberal arts or psychology. Course requirements for the bachelor's degree in liberal arts include 21 semester hours of humanities, 21 semester hours of social sciences, and 50 semester hours of natural and physical sciences.

The curriculum normally takes six years to complete. During the first two years of the curriculum, students spend 75 percent of their time in course work related to the bachelor's degree. Conversely, in the last four years students spend 75 percent of their time in courses, clerkships, and electives related to the M.D. degree. Thus, the study of liberal arts, basic sciences, and clinical medicine is integrated throughout the entire curriculum. Students are assigned a faculty advisor (docent), and younger students are paired with older students. During the last four years of the curriculum students attend a general medicine outpatient clinic for a half-day each week.

Students in this program do not take the MCAT. They must pass Steps 1 and 2 of the USMLE for graduation.

An alternative path is available for extended study.

EXPENSES

In 1999–2000 estimated tuition for Years 1 and 2 of the six-year program was $19,948 in-state per year and $40,250 out-of-state, plus $601 for student fees. Estimated tuition for Years 3 through 6 of the six-year program was $22,918 in-state per year and $45,497 out-of-state, plus $791 for student fees.

FINANCIAL AID

Contact the UMKC Financial Aid Office at the Administrative Center, 5115 Oak, Kansas City, Missouri 64110.

APPLICATION AND ACCEPTANCE POLICIES

Filing of application:
  Earliest date: Aug. 1
  Latest date: Nov. 15
Application fee: $25 in-state; $50 out-of-state
Acceptance notice:
  Earliest date: April 1
Applicant's response to acceptance offer:
  Maximum time: No later than May 1
Deposit to hold place in class: $100; refundable before May 15
Starting date: Mid-August

INFORMATION ON 1999–2000 ENTERING CLASS

Number of	*In-State*	*Out-of-State*	*Total*
Applicants	330	314	644
Applicants Interviewed	204	78	282
New Entrants	104	16	120

CHAPTER 10

UMDNJ—New Jersey Medical School

Newark, New Jersey

ADDRESS INQUIRIES TO:

Office of Admissions
C653 MSB
UMDNJ—New Jersey Medical School
185 South Orange Avenue
Newark, New Jersey 07103-2714
(973) 972-4631

PURPOSE

New Jersey Medical School has established accelerated baccalaureate/M.D.-degree programs in collaboration with eight undergraduate institutions. The goal of these programs is to give highly qualified high school students an opportunity to broaden their premedical preparation without having to compete for admission to medical school.

REQUIREMENTS FOR ENTRANCE

The programs are open to all high school seniors who are either U.S. citizens or permanent residents. Application procedures vary slightly among the programs, but SATs are required.

SELECTION FACTORS

Applicants should be in the top 5 to 10 percent of their high school class and have a minimum combined SAT score of 1400. Applicants are screened on the basis of academic credentials, letters of recommendation, and an essay. Those who meet screening criteria are invited for an interview at the undergraduate school and at the medical school. The deadline for applications to the undergraduate college is January 7. However, early application is encouraged.

CURRICULUM

The course of study consists of three years at the undergraduate school, followed by the regular four-year medical program. Students must take the MCAT in their junior year, but scores are not a factor for promotion or admission to the medical school phase. Promotion to the medical school is contingent upon achieving grades of B or better in all premedical courses and maintaining an overall grade-point average of at least 3.4 each semester. The baccalaureate degree is awarded by the undergraduate institution upon completion of the first year of medical school. The M.D. degree is awarded by New Jersey Medical School.

Students are required to pass Step 1 of the USMLE for promotion to the fourth year. Passage of Step 2 is required for graduation.

Eight programs are currently available:

Boston University provides an undergraduate emphasis in liberal arts or humanities. This program is open only to residents of New Jersey. Mailing address: Office of Undergraduate Admissions, Boston University, Commonwealth Avenue, Boston, Massachusetts 02215; E-mail: admissions@bu.edu.

Drew University offers premedical preparation in all sciences and liberal arts subjects. Mailing address: College Admissions, Drew University, Madison, New Jersey 07940; (973) 408-3739; E-mail: cadm@drew. edu.

Montclair State University offers premedical preparation in biology, chemistry, biochemistry, molecular biology, computer science, mathematics, psychology, and anthropology. Mailing address: Dr. Judith Shillcock, Health Professions Committee, Department of Biology, Montclair State University, Upper Montclair, New Jersey 07043.

New Jersey Institute of Technology offers undergraduate study in the Honors Premedical Curriculum within the Engineering Science Program. Mailing address: Dr. Dennis Donahue, Director, Honors College, New Jersey Institute of Technology, University Heights, Newark, New Jersey 07102; (973) 596-3216; E-mail: honors@njit.edu.

Rutgers University–Newark Campus offers premedical preparation in the sciences. Mailing address: Michael Liloia, Admissions Officer, Office of Admissions, Rutgers University, 249 University Avenue, Newark, New Jersey; (973) 353-5205.

Stevens Institute of Technology offers premedical preparation in chemical biology. Mailing address: Edwina W. Fleming, Director of Honors Admissions Programs, Stevens Institute of Technology, Castle Point–on–the–Hudson, Hoboken, New Jersey 07030; (201) 216-5193; E-mail: efleming@stevens-tech.edu.

The College of New Jersey offers preparation in biology, chemistry, history, philosophy, and psychology. Mailing address: Dr. Dennis Shevlin, Chairman, Medical Careers Committee, The College of New Jersey, P.O. Box 7718, Ewing, NJ 08628-0718; (609) 771-2021.

The Richard Stockton College of New Jersey offers preparation in chemistry, biology, physics, and liberal arts. Mailing address: Dr. Mary Beth Krogh-Jespersen, Associate Vice President for Academic Affairs, Stockton State College, Pomona, New Jersey 08240-9988; (609) 652-4514; E-mail: admissions@stockton.edu.

Application is made through the undergraduate institutions listed above.

Rutgers University and University of Medicine and Dentistry of New Jersey Robert Wood Johnson Medical School

Piscataway, New Jersey

ADDRESS INQUIRIES TO:

Bachelor/Medical Degree Program
Health Professions Office
Nelson Biological Laboratory
Rutgers University
604 Allison Road
Piscataway, New Jersey 08854-8082
(732) 445-5667; 445-5870 (FAX)
Web Site: http://lifesci.rutgers.edu/~hpo
E-mail: hpo@nel-exchange.rutgers.edu

PURPOSE

The program permits the early identification and admission of high-quality medical students. It also integrates medical studies with liberal arts study.

REQUIREMENTS FOR ENTRANCE

Applicants must be students at Rutgers University and are selected for this program at the end of their sophomore year. Residents and nonresidents of New Jersey are considered.

SELECTION FACTORS

An applicant's high school and college transcripts plus faculty recommendations are taken into account in offering admission. In the 1999–2000 entering class, matriculants had achieved a 3.82 GPA at the end of two years of college. They had an average score of 645 on the SAT Verbal section and 692 on the Mathematics section. Maturity, motivation, and broad interests are personal characteristics sought in applicants. An interview is required. The MCAT is not used.

CURRICULUM

This program leads to the baccalaureate degree awarded by Rutgers University and to the M.D. degree granted by the University of Medicine and Dentistry of New Jersey Robert Wood Johnson Medical School. Students must complete requirements for a baccalaureate degree. The most frequent majors for that degree are biological sciences, followed by biochemistry.

The program is eight years in duration. As indicated in the curriculum chart below, the basic sciences and the liberal arts are studied together during a four-year period.

While in medical school, students must take and pass Steps 1 and 2 of the USMLE.

Year	*Percent Liberal Arts*	*Percent Basic Sciences*
1	100	0
2	100	0
3	50	50
4	50	50
5	20	80
6	0	100
7	0	100
8	0	100

EXPENSES

In 1999–2000 residents of New Jersey paid $4,762 per year in undergraduate tuition and $14,927 per year in medical school tuition. In the same year, nonresidents paid $9,692 per year in undergraduate tuition and $23,359 annually in medical school tuition. Fees averaged $1,182 for undergraduates each year and $285 for medical students per year.

FINANCIAL AID

Undergraduates should contact the Office of Financial Aid, 620 George Street, Rutgers University, New Brunswick, New Jersey 08901.

APPLICATION AND ACCEPTANCE POLICIES

Filing of application:
Latest date: June 1 of sophomore year at Rutgers University
Application fee: None
Acceptance notice:
Latest date: July 1
Applicant's response to acceptance offer:
Maximum time: 2 weeks
Deposit to hold place in class: None
Starting date: August

INFORMATION ON 1999–2000 ENTERING CLASS

Number of	*In-State*	*Out-of-State*	*Total*
Applicants	46	1	47
Applicants Interviewed	37	0	37
New Entrants	12	0	12

Binghamton University and State University of New York Health Science Center at Syracuse College of Medicine

This entry was not updated this year and is reprinted from the 1999–2000 edition of this publication.

Binghamton, New York

ADDRESS INQUIRIES TO:

The Early Acceptance Program for UMEDS
College of Medicine
State University of New York
Health Science Center at Syracuse
P.O. Box 1000
Binghamton, New York 13902
(607) 770-8515

PURPOSE

The UMEDS program will offer a unique pathway for underrepresented minorities in medicine who possess both academic and personal attributes that will lead to primary care practice in underserved areas.

REQUIREMENTS FOR ENTRANCE

Students are selected for this program during their senior year of high school. Only residents of New York are eligible to apply. Applicants must meet the entrance requirements of Binghamton University and take the SAT.

SELECTION FACTORS

To be considered for this program, applicants must have a grade-point average of 85 or above, a combined SAT of 900 or higher, and must be a U.S. citizen or permanent resident. An interview is required.

CURRICULUM

This eight-year program leads to a baccalaureate degree granted by Binghamton University, and to the M.D. degree awarded by the State University of New York Health Science Center at Syracuse.

Students are expected to complete work for the bachelor's degree. Requirements for that degree vary according to the major chosen, but all include course work in the humanities and two semesters each of social sciences, and natural and physical sciences. They are not required to take the MCAT to advance to the medical school.

Educational innovations include: (a) a primary care mentor in college; (b) health care-related classes; (c) participation in hospital and private practice settings; and (d) community-based clinical medical education in a primary care setting.

Students are required to take Step 1 of the USMLE, and passing this exam is required for promotion and graduation. Students also must take Step 2 of the USMLE.

EXPENSES

Annual tuition for undergraduates is $3,200, and $10,840 for the medical school.

FINANCIAL AID

For more information, applicants can contact the Early Acceptance Program for UMEDS, College of Medicine, State University of New York, Health Science Center at Syracuse, P.O. Box 1000, Binghamton University, New York 13902; or phone (607) 770-8515.

APPLICATION AND ACCEPTANCE POLICIES

Filing of application:
- Earliest date: Sept. 1
- Latest date: Jan. 1

Application fee: None

Applicant's response to acceptance offer:
- Maximum time: May 1

Starting date: Aug. 1999

INFORMATION ON 1997–98 ENTERING CLASS

Number of	*In-State*	*Out-of-State*	*Total*
Applicants	12	0	12
Applicants Interviewed	11	0	11
New Entrants	3	0	3

Brooklyn College and State University at New York Downstate Medical Center College of Medicine

Brooklyn, New York

ADDRESS INQUIRIES TO:

Jerrold Mirotznik, Ph.D., M.P.H.
Director, B.A./M.D. Honors Program
2231 Boylan Hall
Brooklyn College
2900 Bedford Avenue
Brooklyn, New York 11210
(718) 951-4706; 677-6185 (FAX)
E-mail: Jerrym@brooklyn.cuny.edu
Web Site: http://academic.brooklyn.cuny.edu/

PURPOSE

The aims of this program are to produce physicians who are humanists, concerned with the caring, as well as curing dimensions of medicine, and to offer an economically affordable baccalaureate and medical school education.

REQUIREMENTS FOR ENTRANCE

Students are selected in their senior year of high school. Preference is given to New York residents. Applicants are expected to have completed the following high school courses: a full year of biology, chemistry, and physics plus mathematics through trigonometry. Students must have at least a 90 percent CAA (College Admission Average, academic subjects only) and a combined score of at least 1200 on the new SAT scale.

SELECTION FACTORS

The academic factors taken into account in offering admission to an applicant include: the high school GPA, SAT scores, New York State Regents Examination scores, Advanced Placement courses, and CEEB Achievement Tests scores. In the 1999–2000 entering class, most students had a high school average of at least 95, and the median SAT combined score was 1400. Maturity and motivation are personal characteristics sought among applicants. An interview is required.

CURRICULUM

This program leads to a baccalaureate degree awarded by Brooklyn College and to the M.D. degree granted by the State University of New York Health Science Center at Brooklyn College of Medicine.

The baccalaureate program includes eight required semester courses in the natural and physical sciences, seven semester courses in humanities, and three semester courses in the social sciences. Several of these classes are honors sections specifically for students in the B.A.-M.D. program. The most frequent major is psychology. Students may major in any subject, but nonscience majors are encouraged. Students must maintain a 3.5 overall, and 3.5 science undergraduate GPA to progress to the medical school. Students must take the MCAT before the end of their senior year at Brooklyn College, achieving a score of at least 9 on each of the subtests in one exam administration.

The program is eight years in length. Students are encouraged to do an internship at the medical school during the summer after their second college year. The four-year medical school program focuses on the M.D. degree exclusively.

During medical school, students must take and pass Step 1 of the USMLE.

EXPENSES

In 1999–2000 the undergraduate tuition for state residents was $3,200 per year. The 1999–2000 medical school tuition was $10,840 for state residents. Student fees cost an additional $160 per year at Brooklyn College and $220 per year at the Medical College.

Brooklyn College has no dormitory facilities, so students must commute or find lodging in the community. Dormitory space is available during the medical school portion of the program.

FINANCIAL AID

Pell Grants, Stafford Student Loans, work-study, Hearst Scholarships for minority female students, and Brooklyn College Foundation scholarships are available. Applicants can receive more information from the Office of Admissions.

APPLICATION AND ACCEPTANCE POLICIES

Filing of application:
  Earliest date: Sept. 15
  Latest date: Dec. 31
Application fee: None
Acceptance notice: April 1
Applicant's response to acceptance offer:
  Maximum time: May 1
Deposit to hold place in class: None
Starting date: Aug. 29

INFORMATION ON 1999–2000 ENTERING CLASS

Number of	*In-State*	*Out-of-State*	*Total*
Applicants	350	30	380
Applicants Interviewed	60	0	60
New Entrants	15	0	15

CHAPTER 10

New York University

New York, New York

ADDRESS INQUIRIES TO:

Admissions Office
New York University
22 Washington Square North
New York, New York 10011
(212) 998-4500
Web Site: www.nyu.edu/ugadmissions/

PURPOSE

The goal of the B.A.-M.D. program is to train broadly educated doctors who are interested in people and their place in society and who are excited about the science of medicine.

REQUIREMENTS FOR ENTRANCE

Students are selected for this program only during the senior year of high school. There are no state residency requirements. No specific courses are required. Applicants must take the ACT Assessment or SAT I and either three CEEB Achievement Tests or three Advanced Placement Tests (one of which must be English in either case).

SELECTION FACTORS

Academic factors considered in offering admission include high school GPA, rank in high school class, and honors or advanced placement course work. The admissions committee looks very closely at each applicant's extracurricular and/or service activities, writing skills, knowledge of and enthusiasm for the medical profession, and general intellectual curiosity. Students with broad interests and backgrounds are sought. Minority applicants are encouraged to apply. Interviews at the College of Arts and Science and the School of Medicine are required.

CURRICULUM

The B.A.-M.D. program is not accelerated. All students must complete four years of undergraduate education and four years of medical school.

Students earn a bachelor's degree, which includes completion of a major and the Morse Academic Plan, the College's integrated general education curriculum in the liberal arts. Students in the combined-degree program are encouraged to pursue any liberal arts major they wish. Additionally, they are required to complete an independent interdisciplinary research project over a period of several semesters. Students are expected to maintain good progress and a satisfactory GPA while in college. They are not required to take the MCAT to advance to the medical school.

EXPENSES

The annual tuition and fees for the undergraduate portion of the combined-degree program totaled $23,456 in 1999–2000. The medical school portion was $27,605.

FINANCIAL AID

A full range of need-based and merit-based financial aid/scholarships are available to undergraduates. All applicants are automatically considered for merit scholarships, which may include participation in a scholars program. Candidates for financial aid are required to submit the Free Application for Federal Student Aid (FAFSA) by February 15. Applicants can receive more information from the Office of Financial Aid, 25 West 4th Street, New York, New York 10003; <www.nyu.edu/financialaid/>.

APPLICATION AND ACCEPTANCE POLICIES

Filing of application:
  Latest date: Jan. 15
Application fee: $50
Acceptance notice:
  Earliest date: April 1
Applicant's response to acceptance offer:
  Maximum time: May 1
Deposit to hold place in class: $200; nonrefundable
Starting date: September

INFORMATION ON 1999–2000 ENTERING CLASS

Number of	*Total*
Applicants	751
Applicants Interviewed	15
New Entrants	3

Rensselaer Polytechnic Institute and Albany Medical College

Troy, New York

ADDRESS INQUIRIES TO:

Dean of Undergraduate Admissions
Rensselaer Polytechnic Institute
110 Eighth Street
Troy, New York 12180-3590
(518) 276-6216
Western Regional Office: (800) 873-9369 or (760) 730-3132
E-mail: admissions@rpi.edu
Web Site: http://admissions.rpi.edu/

PURPOSE

The Accelerated Physician-Scientist Program offers qualified individuals the opportunity to become physicians who are intensively trained in medical research. This innovative approach provides a well-rounded perspective that prepares future practitioners and physician-scientists to perform with confidence and care in a technologically changing environment.

REQUIREMENTS FOR ENTRANCE

Students are selected for this program during the senior year of high school. Residents of New York as well as nonresidents of the state are eligible to apply. Applicants are expected to have completed the following courses by the time they graduate from high school: four years of English; one year each of biology, chemistry, and physics; and four years of mathematics (through pre-calculus). They must take the SAT I and the SAT II in mathematics (level IC or level IIC) and writing; and out of the sciences, physics, chemistry, or biology are required. In lieu of these tests, American College Testing (ACT) program scores may be submitted. All tests must be completed by the November testing date prior to the proposed September matriculation.

SELECTION FACTORS

Academic factors considered in offering admission to an applicant include the quality and nature of course work in high school, performance in those courses, rank in high school class, and test scores. The 1999–2000 entering class had an average score of 700 on the SAT Verbal and 730 on the SAT Math. Personal qualities sought in applicants are motivation, maturity, and intellectual capacity necessary to pursue the accelerated course of study. An interview is required.

CURRICULUM

The program leads to a B.S. degree awarded by Rensselaer Polytechnic Institute and the M.D. degree granted by Albany Medical College.

The curriculum for the B.S. and M.D. degrees normally requires seven years to complete. During the first three years of the program spent at Rensselaer, the curriculum involves 70 percent premedical science courses and 30 percent liberal arts courses. Students take 18 courses in the natural and physical sciences and 8 elective courses in the humanities and social sciences.

The medical college has replaced the traditional two years of basic science and two years of clinical science with an integrated four-year curriculum. Emphasis is placed on the pivotal role of primary care.

Students admitted to the program are not required to take the MCAT for admission to Albany Medical college. Students are expected to take Steps 1 and 2 of the USMLE while at Albany Medical College.

EXPENSES

The tuition and fees for 1999–2000 were $22,300 at Rensselaer, and $30,797 for residents at Albany Medical College.

FINANCIAL AID

Sources of financial aid are restricted and endowed scholarships based on need, merit scholarships, work-study, and student loans through federal and institutional programs. Applicants can receive more information by contacting the Financial Aid Office of Rensselaer Polytechnic Institute at (518) 276-6813 or Albany Medical College at (518) 262-5435.

APPLICATION AND ACCEPTANCE POLICIES

Filing of application:
- Earliest date: Sept. 1
- Latest date: Dec. 1

Application fee: $50 (RPI);
- $75 (Albany Medical College)

Acceptance notice:
- Earliest date: March
- Latest date: until class is filled

Applicant's response to acceptance offer:
- Maximum time: May 1

Deposit to hold place in class: $300; nonrefundable
Starting date: September

INFORMATION ON 1999–2000 ENTERING CLASS

Number of	*In-State*	*Out-of-State*	*Total*
Applicants	60	238	298
Applicants Interviewed	28	62	90
New Entrants	9	9	18

CHAPTER 10

Siena College and Albany Medical College

Loudonville, New York

ADDRESS INQUIRIES TO:

Siena College
Office of Admissions
515 Loudon Road
Loudonville, New York 12211-1462
(518) 783-2423; 888-AT-SIENA
Web Site: http://www.siena.edu

PURPOSE

This program offers an eight-year continuum of education that has a special emphasis on the humanities and on community service while providing a sound understanding of both the natural and social sciences.

REQUIREMENTS FOR ENTRANCE

Students are selected for this program during the senior year of high school. Both residents and nonresidents of New York are eligible to apply. Candidates for admission to the Siena/AMC program must have completed at least four years of high school math and science. Typically, successful candidates will have enrolled in, or completed, advanced-level courses by the end of their senior year in high school. A well-rounded background and demonstrated leadership experience are also important. Of equal significance is the student's proven concern for others and for their community. Applicants must take either the SAT I or ACT Assessment. Tests must be completed by the November testing date prior to the proposed September matriculation.

SELECTION FACTORS

Academic factors considered in offering admission to an applicant include the following: required and elective courses taken, grades earned, class standing, SAT I or ACT scores, honors received, letters of recommendation, and unique academic experiences. Of great importance to the admission committee are such factors as extracurricular activities, evidence of intellectual curiosity, and interest in the humanities and in the sciences. Students generally rank among the top 10 percent of their high school class. The 1999–200 entering class had an average score of 680 on the SAT Verbal and 710 on the SAT Math. An interview is required.

CURRICULUM

This program offers a coordinated eight-year curriculum of premedical and medical education. The undergraduate phase offers an equal distribution of science and nonscience courses. Students graduate in four years with a bachelor of arts degree in biology with a minor in the humanities. The undergraduate phase of the program also includes a required summer of human service in a health-related agency, usually in an urban ghetto or developing nation. Passage from the undergraduate college to the medical school requires achievement of a 3.40 GPA and a continued interest in the human service dimension of the program. The medical college has replaced the traditional two years of basic science and two years of clinical science with an integrated four-year curriculum. Emphasis is placed on the pivotal role of primary care. The summer between the sophomore and junior years is dedicated to medically related volunteer service, usually in a rural or inner city clinic.

Students are not required to take the MCAT for admission to Albany Medical College. Students are expected to take Step 1 and Step 2 of the USMLE.

EXPENSES

The tuition for 1999–2000 was $13,600 at Siena College, and $30,797 at Albany Medical College.

FINANCIAL AID

Applicants can receive more information by contacting Siena College, Financial Aid Office at (518) 783-2427; or Albany Medical College, Financial Aid Office at (518) 262-5435.

APPLICATION AND ACCEPTANCE POLICIES

Filing of application:
  Earliest date: Sept. 1
  Latest date: Dec. 15
Application fee: $40 (Siena);
  $75 (Albany Medical College)
Acceptance notice:
  Earliest date: March 15
  Latest date: until classes are filled
Applicant's response to acceptance offer:
  Maximum time: May 1
Deposit to hold place in class: $200; nonrefundable
Starting date: September

INFORMATION ON 1999–2000 ENTERING CLASS

Number of	*In-State*	*Out-of-State*	*Total*
Applicants	160	151	311
Applicants Interviewed	21	18	39
New Entrants	3	8	11

SUNY Stony Brook and SUNY Stony Brook School of Medicine

Stony Brook, New York

ADDRESS INQUIRIES TO:

The Honors College
Scholars for Medicine Program
SUNY at Stony Brook
3071 N. Melville Library
Stony Brook, New York 11794-3359

PURPOSE

The Scholars for Medicine Program offers conditional acceptance to the Stony Brook School of Medicine to a select number of outstanding and highly motivated students. In addition to acquiring a solid background in the sciences, accepted students have access to a wide array of liberal arts courses offered through the University and its Honors College. Students also have access to medical school programs in research and a series of health related seminars.

REQUIREMENTS FOR ENTRANCE

Students are selected for this program only during the senior year of high school. There are no state residency requirements. No specific courses are required. Applicants must take the ACT or SAT.

SELECTION FACTORS

To be considered for this program, applicants must have a minimum SAT score of 1350 and unweighted high school GPA of 93. The applicant's high school academic record, standardized test reports, history of interests and activities and required interview with the School of Medicine are factors taken into account in offering admission to an applicant.

CURRICULUM

This eight-year program leads to the baccalaureate and M.D. degrees granted by the State University of New York at Stony Brook. Students are expected to complete the requirements for any of the baccalaureate degrees awarded by the University. Undergraduate work taken must include courses required by the School of Medicine: one year each of biology, physics, inorganic chemistry, organic chemistry (all with lab), and one year of English. No specific major is required for the premedical undergraduate phase.

Admission to the School of Medicine is contingent upon maintaining a minimum GPA of 3.4. The MCAT is required and the student should attain cumulative scores comparable to the national average of medical school matriculants. The USMLE Steps 1 and 2 are required for promotion and graduation, respectively, from the School of Medicine.

EXPENSES

In 1999–2000, the undergraduate tuition for New York State residents was $1,700 and for non-residents, $4,150. Student fees were $370. Medical school tuition for New York State residents was 10,840 and 21,940 for non-residents. Required medical student fees were $250.

FINANCIAL AID

Applicants can receive more information by contacting The Office of Financial Aid and Student Employment at SUNY Stony Brook at (631) 632-6840 or visit the Web site at http://naples.cc.sunysb.edu/Prov/financial.nsf.

APPLICATION AND ACCEPTANCE POLICIES

Filing of application:
  Earliest date: October 1
  Latest date: January 15
Application fee: None
Acceptance notice:
  Earliest date: March 15
  Latest date: April 10
Applicant's response to acceptance offer:
  Maximum time: May 1
Deposit to hold place in class: $100; refundable
Starting date: September

INFORMATION ON 1999–2000 ENTERING CLASS

Number of	*In-State*	*Out-of-State*	*Total*
Applicants	188	222	410
Applicants Interviewed	18	1	19
New Entrants	5	1	6

CHAPTER 10

Sophie Davis School of Biomedical Education/ City University of New York

This entry was not updated this year and is reprinted from the 1999–2000 edition of this publication.

New York, New York

ADDRESS INQUIRIES TO:

Sophie Davis School of Biomedical Education
City University of New York
Office of Admissions
Y Building, Room 205N
138th Street and Convent Avenue
New York, New York 10031
(212) 650-7708

PURPOSE

The purposes of this combined-degree program are to train primary care physicians who will work in medically underserved urban areas and to increase the number of minority physicians.

REQUIREMENTS FOR ENTRANCE

Students are selected for this program in the senior year of high school. Only residents of New York are eligible to apply. Applicants are expected to have completed the following courses by the time they graduate from high school: two semesters each of chemistry and biology and six to eight semesters of mathematics. They must take the ACT Assessment and a local mathematics placement test.

SELECTION FACTORS

Academic factors taken into account in offering admission to an applicant are: the high school GPA, scores on the ACT Assessment, and scores on the New York State Regents Examinations. In the 1997–98 entering class, the high school grades averaged 91.9, and the subscore on the Mathematics ACT Assessment averaged 29. The SAT Mathematics average was 630 and the SAT Verbal average was 610. Personal qualities sought in applicants include interest in people, concern for others, initiative, and leadership. An interview is required.

CURRICULUM

This seven-year program leads to a baccalaureate degree granted by the City College of New York and to the M.D. degree awarded by one of seven New York medical schools (Albany Medical College, Mount Sinai School, New York Medical College, New York University, SUNY Downstate, SUNY Stonybrook, or SUNY Syracuse/Binghamton).

During the first five years of the program, students fulfill all requirements for the B.S. degree and study the preclinical portion of the medical school curriculum. After successfully completing the five-year sequence and passing Step 1 of the USMLE examinations, students transfer to one of the participating medical schools in New York for their final two years of clinical training. Students are expected to pass Steps 1 and 2 of the USMLE examinations to graduate.

There is a strong emphasis on humanities and social sciences courses. The introduction of community medicine courses with field work and medical biochemistry and anatomy during the undergraduate phase is an innovative feature of this program. Students also benefit from counseling and academic support services.

EXPENSES

In 1997–98, resident undergraduate tuition per year was $3,400. Student fees were $95. Tuition for the final two years of the program varies according to the medical school attended.

FINANCIAL AID

Pell Grants, New York State tuition assistance, and the City College of New York biomedical stipend are sources of financial aid. More information about aid is available from the City College Financial Aid Office.

APPLICATION AND ACCEPTANCE POLICIES

Filing of application:
  Earliest date: Fall
  Latest date: Jan. 15
Application fee: None
Acceptance notice: April 1
Applicant's response to acceptance offer:
  Maximum time: May 1
Deposit to hold place in class: None
Starting date: September

INFORMATION ON 1997–98 ENTERING CLASS

Number of	*Total*
Applicants	491
Applicants Interviewed	156
New Entrants	62

Union College and Albany Medical College

Schenectady, New York

ADDRESS INQUIRIES TO:

Associate Dean of Admissions
Union College
Schenectady, New York 12308
(518) 388-6112; 888-843-6688
E-mail: admissions@union.edu
Web Site: http://www.union.edu/

PURPOSE

The Leadership in Medicine/Health Systems Program is specifically designed for students who want to prepare for the challenge of medical leadership by taking advantage of additional educational opportunities as part of their undergraduate education. In addition to offering the standard course work required for attaining the degrees of B.S., M.S., and M.D., the integrated program will focus on three areas essential for future leaders in medicine: health policy and health management, the ethical challenge, and the leadership challenge.

REQUIREMENTS FOR ENTRANCE

Students are selected for this program during the senior year of high school. Residents of New York as well as nonresidents of the state are eligible to apply. Applicants are expected to have completed a challenging curriculum in high school, which must include biology, chemistry and physics. They must take either the ACT Assessment or the SAT I and three SAT IIs (writing, a math, and a science). Tests must be completed by the November testing date prior to the proposed September matriculation.

SELECTION FACTORS

Academic factors considered in offering admission to an applicant include the quality and nature of course work in high school, performance in those courses, rank in high school class, and standardized test scores. In the 1999–2000 entering class, the average score was 700 for SAT Verbal and 700 for SAT Mathematics. Personal qualities sought in applicants include motivation, maturity, and personal development. Interviews by Union College and Albany Medical College are required.

CURRICULUM

This program leads to B.S. and M.S. degrees awarded by Union College and an M.D. degree granted by Albany Medical College.

At Union College, students take 30 courses—15 science, 15 nonscience, and complete an interdepartmental major in the humanities or social sciences. A special bioethics program supplemented by a health services practicum, a term abroad, and a program in health care management at the Union College Graduate Management Institute are also an integral part of the educational experience.

The curriculum for the B.S., M.S., and M.D. degrees requires eight years to complete. Students take a course in health and human values during the summer before matriculation in the medical school. The medical college has replaced the traditional two years of basic science and two years of clinical science with an integrated four-year curriculum.

Students admitted to the program are not required to take the MCAT for admission to Albany Medical College. Students are expected to take Steps 1 and 2 of the USMLE while at Albany Medical College.

EXPENSES

The 1999–2000 tuition was $23,892 for study at Union College and $30,797 at Albany Medical College.

FINANCIAL AID

Sources of financial aid include various programs based on need, student loans through federal and state assistance, work-study, and merit scholarships. For more information contact the Financial Aid Office of Union College at (518) 388-6123 or Albany Medical College at (518) 262-5435.

APPLICATION AND ACCEPTANCE POLICIES

Filing of application:
 Earliest date: Sept. 1
 Latest date: Dec. 15
Application fee: $50 (Union College);
 $75 (Albany Medical College)
Acceptance notice:
 Earliest date: March
 Latest date: until class is filled
Applicant's response to acceptance offer:
 Maximum time: May 1
Deposit to hold place in class: $400; nonrefundable
Starting date: September

INFORMATION ON 1999–2000 ENTERING CLASS

Number of	*In-State*	*Out-of-State*	*Total*
Applicants	86	272	358
Applicants Interviewed	43	64	107
New Entrants	11	8	19

University of Rochester School of Medicine and Dentistry

Rochester, New York

ADDRESS INQUIRIES TO:

Rochester Early Medical Scholars Coordinator
University of Rochester
Undergraduate Admissions—Box 270251
Rochester, New York 14627–0251
(716) 275-3221 or (888) 822–2256; (716) 461–4595 (FAX)
Web Site: http://www.rochester.edu

PURPOSE

The Rochester Early Medical Scholars Program (REMS) provides conditional acceptance to the University of Rochester School of Medicine and Dentistry to a group of exceptionally talented and motivated students. REMS allows undergraduates the utmost flexibility in degree programs, mentoring relationships with medical school staff, and early exposure to medical school curriculum through a series of lectures and seminars.

REQUIREMENTS FOR ENTRANCE

Students are selected for this program during their senior year of high school from a national pool. A recommended high school curriculum includes two years of foreign language and four years each of English, social studies, mathematics, and science. A transcript that includes Honors or AP courses is preferable. Applicants are expected to take the SAT or ACT Assessment.

SELECTION FACTORS

Outstanding achievement in a challenging high school curriculum, character, interests, maturity, and motivation necessary for a career in medicine are required for consideration for entry into the REMS program. Interviews are required. In the 1999–2000 entering class, REMS students had an average SAT verbal score of 698 and a math score of 736. In order to take their place in the first-year medical school class, REMS students must carry at least a 3.3 overall GPA and a 3.3 premedical course GPA by the end of the sophomore year, and a 3.5 overall GPA by the time of undergraduate graduation.

CURRICULUM

The eight-year program leads to a baccalaureate degree and the M.D. degree, both granted by the University of Rochester. Students must complete the baccalaureate degree. The most popular major is biology, followed by Health and Society, and biomedical engineering. Undergraduates are encouraged to pursue a variety of academic disciplines in addition to completing their premedical course requirements. Completion of a major is required.

The University of Rochester Medical School features an exciting newly revised curriculum that emphasizes problem-based learning and early patient contact. See <http://www.rochester.edu/SMDBulletin/UME/index.html> for details.

The University of Rochester Medical School has pioneered the "biopsychosocial model" of medicine, which stresses approaching the patient as a complete person. The revised curriculum allows early and increased access to patients and closer relationships with medical school faculty.

EXPENSES

Undergraduate tuition in 1999–2000 was $22,300 per year and annual fees total $9,868. Medical school tuition was $26,900 with annual fees of $1,568.

FINANCIAL AID

University of Rochester scholarships and loans plus governmental loans are available. For more information, write the Office of Financial Aid, University of Rochester, Box 270261, Rochester, New York 14627–0261; or phone (716) 275-3226 or (800) 881-8234.

APPLICATION AND ACCEPTANCE POLICIES

Filing of application:
- Earliest date: Sept. 1
- Latest date: Jan. 6

Application fee: $50

Acceptance notice:
- Earliest date: March 22
- Latest date: May 1

Deposit to hold place in class: $400; nonrefundable

Starting date: September

INFORMATION ON 1999–2000 ENTERING CLASS

Number of	*In-State*	*Out-of-State*	*Total*
Applicants	178	422	600
Applicants Interviewed	13	26	39
New Entrants	2	11	13

Case Western Reserve University

Cleveland, Ohio

ADDRESS INQUIRIES TO:

Douglas Brown, *Associate Director of Undergraduate Admissions*
Case Western Reserve University
10900 Euclid Avenue
Cleveland, Ohio 44106-7055
(216) 368-4450; 386-5111 (FAX)
Web Site: http://www.cwru.edu/

PURPOSE

This program is intended to provide college students with a greater sense of freedom and choice in the pursuit of a premedical baccalaureate degree.

REQUIREMENTS FOR ENTRANCE

Students are selected for this program during the senior year of high school. Both residents and nonresidents of Ohio are considered for admission. Applicants are expected to have completed the following courses by the time they graduate from high school: one year each of biology, chemistry, and physics and four years of mathematics. They must take either the ACT Assessment or the SAT I and SAT II.

SELECTION FACTORS

The applicant's high school academic record, standardized test reports, history of interests and activities, and a required interview are factors taken into account in offering admission to an applicant. Evidence of strong interpersonal and leadership skills is also sought. In the 1999–2000 entering class, the average combined SAT scores ranged from 1440 to 1520. The average combined ACT score ranged from 30 to 34, and the average high school GPA was 4.31.

CURRICULUM

This eight-year program leads to the baccalaureate and M.D. degrees granted by Case Western Reserve University. Students are expected to complete the requirements for any of the baccalaureate degrees awarded by the colleges of the university. They are expected to satisfy all requirements of and earn a baccalaureate prior to matriculating in the School of Medicine. The work taken for the baccalaureate must include the studies specifically required of applicants by the School of Medicine: one year of biology, two years of chemistry including organic chemistry, one year of physics, and freshman expository writing. No specific major concentration is required for the premedical undergraduate phase. To date, the majors most commonly taken have been biology and biochemistry. Anthropology is the next most popular major.

The first four years of the program are devoted to study for the baccalaureate and the last four years to the curriculum for medicine. Students in the medical phase are required to pass Step 1 of the USMLE for promotion within the program and are required to pass Step 2 of the USMLE in order to graduate.

EXPENSES

In 1999–2000 the tuition for the undergraduate phase of the program was $19,200 per year, plus annual fees. Medical school tuition was $30,600, plus annual fees.

FINANCIAL AID

Sources of aid for the undergraduate phase include merit and need-based aid, college work-study, and university grants and scholarships. Merit-based scholarships for undergraduates begin at 1300 SAT/31 ACT and the top 15 percent in class rank. For information about aid contact the Office of University Financial Aid at (216) 368-4530.

APPLICATION AND ACCEPTANCE POLICIES

Filing of application:
Latest date: Dec. 15
Application fee: None
Acceptance notice:
Latest date: April 15
Applicant's response to acceptance offer:
Maximum time: May 1
Deposit to hold place in class: $200; nonrefundable
Starting date: Last week in August

INFORMATION ON 1999–2000 ENTERING CLASS

Number of	*In-State*	*Out-of-State*	*Total*
Applicants	294	307	601
Applicants Interviewed	26	35	61
New Entrants	11	6	17

Northeastern Ohio Universities College of Medicine (NEOUCOM)

Rootstown, Ohio

ADDRESS INQUIRIES TO:

R. Stephen Manuel, *Director of Admissions*
Northeastern Ohio Universities
College of Medicine
4209 State Route 44, P.O. Box 95
Rootstown, Ohio 44272-0095
(330) 325-6270; 325-8372 (FAX)
Web Site: http://www.neoucom.edu

PURPOSE

The mission of the Northeastern Ohio Universities College of Medicine (NEOUCOM) is to graduate qualified physicians oriented to the practice of medicine at the community level, with an emphasis on primary care: family medicine, internal medicine, pediatrics, and obstetrics-gynecology.

REQUIREMENTS FOR ENTRANCE

Students are selected for this program during the senior year of high school. Both residents and nonresidents of Ohio are eligible to apply; however, strong preference is given to in-state applicants. Applicants are expected to have pursued a solid college preparatory curriculum, including four years of mathematics and four years of science. They must take either the ACT or the SAT.

SELECTION FACTORS

The academic factors that are taken into account in offering admission to applicants include standardized test scores, high school GPA and science GPA, extracurricular involvement, medical exposure, course work, state of legal residence, and interview outcome. In 1999–2000, the mean high school GPA of matriculants was 3.88. The average test score for the ACT was 30, and SAT scores averaged 1330. Career maturity and emotional maturity are among the personal qualities weighed by the admissions committee. An interview is required by invitation only.

CURRICULUM

Students in this combined-degree program study for a baccalaureate degree granted by Youngstown State University, Kent State University, or the University of Akron and for the M.D. degree granted by NEOUCOM.

Students must complete requirements for a bachelor's degree with a major in integrated life sciences. The curriculum takes six or seven years to complete. Some of the educational innovations offered include an introduction to clinical medicine course taught at area family practice centers in the freshman and sophomore medical school years and a one-month primary care preceptorship course in the senior medical school year. Further, most of the basic science courses are taught in just one year (M 1) in contrast to the more traditional two-year sequence.

Students are expected to pass both Step 1 and Step 2 of the USMLE for graduation from Northeastern Ohio Universities College of Medicine.

EXPENSES

Tuition and fees for years 1 and 2 for 1999–2000 were determined by each undergraduate university.

FINANCIAL AID

Sources of aid are scholarships, grants, loans, and work. For more information on financial aid, contact Northeastern Ohio Universities College of Medicine, Financial Aid Office at (330) 325-2511; University of Akron, Financial Aid Office, (330) 972-7032; Kent State University, Financial Aid Office, (330) 672-2972; or Youngstown State University, Financial Aid Office, (330) 742-3505.

APPLICATION AND ACCEPTANCE POLICIES

Filing of application:
  Earliest date: Sept. 1
  Latest date: Dec. 15
Application fee: $25 or $30; varies with each undergraduate institution
Acceptance notice:
  Earliest date: April 1
  Latest date: June 20
Applicant's response to acceptance offer:
  Maximum time: 1 to 2 weeks
Deposit to hold place in class: None
Starting date: June or July

INFORMATION ON 1999–2000 ENTERING CLASS

Number of	*In-State*	*Out-of-State*	*Total*
Applicants	409	266	675
Applicants Offered Interviews	217	35	252
New Entrants	93	10	103

University of Cincinnati College of Medicine

Cincinnati, Ohio

ADDRESS INQUIRIES TO:

University of Cincinnati
College of Medicine
231 Bethesda Avenue, Room E-251
Cincinnati, Ohio 45267-0555
(513) 558-7314; 558-1165 (FAX)
Web Site: www.med.uc.edu

PURPOSE

The University of Cincinnati College of Medicine has a unique Dual Admissions Program, which accepts high school seniors into one of five undergraduate Ohio colleges and into the College of Medicine. The College of Medicine has established a partnership with the following Ohio universities: University of Dayton, John Carroll University, Miami University, Xavier University, University of Cincinnati College of Engineering, and the University of Cincinnati undergraduate campus. Each program will invite selected students already accepted into their university to apply for this program. Once accepted, students will receive an outstanding education while preparing for medical school and building the qualities and characteristics to become an excellent physician.

REQUIREMENTS FOR ENTRANCE

Both residents and nonresidents of Ohio are eligible to apply. Priority will be given to Ohio residents. Each university determines the academic requirements, but the ACT and/or SAT are required.

SELECTION FACTORS

Each university determines the academic requirements. The applicant's GPA is also taken into consideration when admission is offered. An interview is required for admission.

To apply or obtain additional information about each university please contact:

University of Dayton: JAMS Program: Dr. Larry Fox, (937) 229-4369.

John Carroll University: Dr. John Klein, (216) 397-4736.

Miami University: (513) 529-2531.

Xavier University: Dr. Carolyn Chambers or Suzette Combs, (513) 745-3691.

University of Cincinnati, College of Engineering—CONNECTIONS E, or Undergraduate Program—CONNECTIONS: Jennifer Rosichan, (513) 556-2166.

General information may also be obtained through the University of Cincinnati College of Medicine, Web Site: www.med.uc.edu/admissions/pathway.htm.

CURRICULUM

The course of study consists of four years at the undergraduate school, followed by four years in the College of Medicine. The University of Cincinnati College of Engineering is a nine-year program. Students are strongly urged to complete a baccalaureate degree. For most universities, there is no required major.

Students must take the MCAT in their junior year. The student must obtain a minimum score of at least 27, with a score of 9 or above on the Biological Sciences section, and not less than an 8 on one of the remaining subtests.

The student must pass Steps 1 and 2 of the USMLE in order to graduate. The USMLE Step 1 is administered at the completion of Year 2.

EXPENSES

The undergraduate portion of the tuition and fees varies with each undergraduate institution. In 1999–2000, medical school tuition for residents was $12,612, and nonresidents, $22,545, plus $561 for student fees.

FINANCIAL AID

For more information about financial aid, contact the Financial Aid Office of the specific undergraduate university listed above.

APPLICATION AND ACCEPTANCE POLICIES

Filing of application:
  Varies with undergraduate university
Application fee: None
Acceptance notice:
  Earliest date: April 15
Applicant's response to acceptance offer:
  Maximum time: May 1
Deposit to hold place in class: None
Starting date:
  Varies with undergraduate university

INFORMATION ON 1999–2000 ENTERING CLASS

Information varies at each undergraduate institution.

Lehigh University and MCP Hahnemann University School of Medicine

Bethlehem, Pennsylvania

ADDRESS INQUIRIES TO:

Office of Admissions
27 Memorial Drive West
Lehigh University
Bethlehem, Pennsylvania 18105
(610) 758-3100; 758-4361 (FAX)
Web Site: http://www.lehigh.edu

PURPOSE

This program gives gifted high school students who are certain that they want to become physicians the opportunity to obtain a liberal arts education and reduce their total educational cost.

REQUIREMENTS FOR ENTRANCE

Students are selected for this program during the senior year of high school. Residents and nonresidents of Pennsylvania are considered for this program. Applicants are expected to have completed the following courses by the time they finish high school: four years each of English and mathematics and two years each of history, science, and a foreign language. Applicants are expected to take the SAT. SAT II tests are not required but are highly recommended (i.e., math, English composition, and chemistry).

SELECTION FACTORS

Generally, a combined SAT score of 1360 (recentered), rank in the top 10 percent of the high school class, and a strong motivation for science are necessary for entrance in this program. In 1999–2000, matriculants had a high school GPA of 3.9, an SAT Verbal score of 722, and an SAT Math score of 726. Maturity, stability, scholarship, flexibility, independence, and service to others are personal characteristics sought among applicants. An interview is required. Once admitted to the program, students are expected to maintain an overall grade-point average of 3.45 or better with no grade less than a C in any course. Candidates are required to take the MCAT. It is required that the three numbered scores equal or exceed 9 on the same test.

CURRICULUM

This program, six or seven years in duration, allows students to obtain a bachelor's degree from Lehigh University and an M.D. degree from the MCP Hahnemann University School of Medicine. Students do have the flexibility of remaining three years rather than two at Lehigh, however, to pursue additional course work or study abroad.

Students are not required to complete work for a bachelor's degree; however, specific course requirements for the degree include two semesters of English, three semesters of math, eight semesters of natural and physical sciences, three semesters each of humanities and social sciences, a freshman seminar, a writing intensive, and four semesters of electives.

All students must pass USMLE Step 1 and Step 2 in order to graduate from medical school.

EXPENSES

In 1999–2000 tuition at Lehigh University was $23,150 per year.

FINANCIAL AID

Institutional scholarships and loans are available, as well as federal loan programs and armed services scholarships. More financial aid information can be obtained from the Financial Aid Office, Lehigh University, 218 W. Packer Avenue, Bethlehem, Pennsylvania 18015.

APPLICATION AND ACCEPTANCE POLICIES

Filing of application:
  Earliest date: Sept. 1
  Latest date: Dec. 1
Application fee: $50
Acceptance notice:
  Earliest date: April 1
  Latest date: April 15
Applicant's response to acceptance offer:
  Maximum time: May 1
Deposit to hold place in class: $500; nonrefundable
Starting date: August

INFORMATION ON 1999–2000 ENTERING CLASS

Number of	*Total*
Applicants	272
Applicants Interviewed	70
New Entrants	8

Pennsylvania State University and Jefferson Medical College of Thomas Jefferson University

University Park, Pennsylvania

ADDRESS INQUIRIES TO:

Undergraduate Admissions Office
201 Shields Building
Box 3000
Pennsylvania State University
University Park, Pennsylvania 16804-3000
(814) 865-5471

PURPOSE

This program, which began in 1963, is a cooperative effort between Pennsylvania State University and Jefferson Medical College of Thomas Jefferson University in Philadelphia. Students can earn both the B.S. and M.D. degrees in six calendar years after graduation from high school.

REQUIREMENTS FOR ENTRANCE

Students are selected for this program only during the senior year of high school. Both residents and nonresidents of Pennsylvania are considered for admission, but preference is given to qualified applicants from Pennsylvania. Applicants are expected to have completed the following courses by the time they graduate from high school: four units of English, one and one-half units of algebra, one unit of plane geometry, one-half unit of trigonometry, three units of science, and five units from social studies, humanities, and/or arts.

SELECTION FACTORS

To be considered for this program, applicants must be in the top 10 percent of their high school class and offer a combined SAT score of 1450 (recentered). In the 1999–2000 entering class, the average combined score on the SAT was 1510. Motivation, compassion, integrity, dedication, and performance in nonacademic areas are among the personal characteristics sought in applicants. An interview is required.

Special attention is given to the student's progress during each semester while at Pennsylvania State University. Students must take a full course load and maintain a minimum GPA of 3.5 in both science and nonscience courses. For subsequent admission to Jefferson Medical College, students in this combined-degree program must take the MCAT prior to matriculation into medical school.

CURRICULUM

This six-year program leads to a baccalaureate degree granted by Pennsylvania State University and to the M.D. degree awarded by Jefferson Medical College.

Students begin this program in June immediately after high school graduation. They spend two full years on the Pennsylvania State, University Park campus and then proceed to Jefferson Medical College for their regular four-year curriculum. The B.S. degree from Pennsylvania State University is awarded after successful completion of the sophomore year at Jefferson Medical College, and the M.D. degree is awarded after successful completion of the senior year at Jefferson. While at Jefferson students must take and pass Steps 1 and 2 of the USMLE .

EXPENSES

Annual undergraduate tuition at Pennsylvania State in 1999–2000 for residents of Pennsylvania was $3,081 and for nonresidents $6,639. Tuition for 1999–2000 at Jefferson Medical College was $28,376 for residents and nonresidents.

FINANCIAL AID

Scholarships, loans, and grants are the sources of financial assistance available. For more information write the Office of Student Financial Aid, Pennsylvania State University, University Park, Pennsylvania 16804-3000.

APPLICATION AND ACCEPTANCE POLICIES

Filing of application:
  Earliest date: July 1
  Latest date: Nov. 30
Application fee: $50
Acceptance notice:
  Earliest date: March 15
Applicant's response to acceptance offer:
  Maximum time: May 1
Deposit to hold place in class: $300;
  all but $100 refundable
Starting date: June

INFORMATION ON 1999–2000 ENTERING CLASS

Number of	*Total*
Applicants	420
Applicants Interviewed	84
New Entrants	22

Brown University

Providence, Rhode Island

ADDRESS INQUIRIES TO:

College Admission Office
Brown University
Box 1876
Providence, Rhode Island 02912
(401) 863-2378
College Web Site: http://www.brown.edu/
PLME Web Site: http://biomed.brown.edu/Medicine_Programs/PLME.html

PURPOSE

The Program in Liberal Medical Education (PLME) offers a unique experience in medical education. We seek to graduate physicians who are broadly and liberally educated, and who will view medicine as a socially responsible human service profession. Designed as an eight-year continuum, the PLME combines liberal arts and professional education. Great flexibility is built into the program. Each student develops an individualized educational plan in close collaboration with PLME faculty advisors. The PLME is the primary route of admission to the Brown University School of Medicine.

REQUIREMENTS FOR ENTRANCE

Students are selected for the PLME in the senior year of high school. The Brown Admission Office recommends that applicants should have pursued the following: four years of English, with significant emphasis on writing; three years of college preparatory mathematics; three years of a foreign language; two years of laboratory science above the freshman level; two years of history, including American history; at least one year of course work in the arts; and at least one year of elective academic subjects. Prospective science or engineering majors should have taken physics, chemistry, and advanced mathematics. Familiarity with computers is recommended for all applicants. Applicants must take the SAT I and three SAT IIs, or the ACT. (PLME applicants are encouraged to include a science SAT II test.)

SELECTION FACTORS

Students are selected on the basis of scholastic accomplishment and promise, intellectual curiosity, emotional maturity, character, motivation, sensitivity, caring, and particularly the degree to which they seem adapted to the special features of the program. In the 1999–2000 entering class, students on average were in the top two percent of their high school class and had achieved on the average a score of 710 Verbal and 720 Mathematics on the SAT I. An interview is not required.

CURRICULUM

The PLME leads to a baccalaureate degree and to the M.D. degree granted by Brown University School of Medicine. Students must complete a baccalaureate degree in the field of their choice. Each student's educational plan is highly individualized. The PLME has introduced several innovations in medical education, including a competency-based curriculum that defines nine abilities and a core knowledge base expected of all graduates in the M.D. class of 2000 and beyond.

EXPENSES

In 1999–2000 the undergraduate tuition at Brown University was $24,624 per year and the medical school tuition was $27,704.

FINANCIAL AID

For undergraduates in the first four years of the PLME, financial aid is awarded by the Financial Aid Office at Brown University as a package. Students are awarded monies via scholarships, work-study, and loans. During the last four years of the PLME, financial aid is administered by the Office of Admissions and Financial Aid of the school of medicine. Both loans and scholarships are available, although loans are the most common form of assistance.

APPLICATION AND ACCEPTANCE POLICIES

Filing of application:
  Earliest date: Nov. 1
  Latest date: Jan. 1
Application fee: $55
Acceptance notice:
  Earliest date: Dec. 15
  Latest date: April 3
Applicant's response to acceptance offer:
  Maximum time: May 1
Deposit to hold place in class: None
Starting date: Early September

INFORMATION ON 1999–2000 ENTERING CLASS

Number of	*In-State*	*Out-of-State*	*Total*
Applicants	40	1,555	1,595
New Entrants	3	53	56

East Tennessee State University

Johnson City, Tennessee

ADDRESS INQUIRIES TO:

Dr. Lattie F. Collins
Director, Premedical-Medical Program
Office of Medical Professions Advisement
East Tennessee State University
P.O. Box 70,592
Johnson City, Tennessee 37614-0592
(423) 439-5602; 439-6905 (FAX)

PURPOSE

The Premedical-Medical Program (PMMD Program) at East Tennessee State University is an eight-year coordinated curriculum (four years of undergraduate preparation followed by four years of medical education) leading to the award of both the B.A./B.S. and M.D. degrees. The PMMD Program is designed to (1) identify and accept promising students into medical education early in their college careers; (2) provide a strong liberal arts foundation emphasizing the humanities; (3) eliminate the redundancy of course work often present in the usual four-year premedical program, followed by four years of medical school; and (4) allow students the opportunity for personal growth and maximum benefit from their undergraduate experience by reducing the stress and anxiety associated with the standard medical school application process.

*The PMMD Program is **not** an accelerated program; eight full years are required from college entry until completion of the M.D. degree. The PMMD Program is **not** a transfer program; prospective applicants are expected to enter East Tennessee State University as beginning freshmen.*

REQUIREMENTS FOR ENTRANCE

Students are selected for the PMMD Program at the end of their freshman year on the East Tennessee State University (ETSU) campus, during which they enroll in an approved set of courses. This is not a transfer program; students who have earned more than 14 semester hours of college credit before entering ETSU are not eligible for selection. There are no state residency requirements, but residents of Tennessee will be given preference in the selection process. There are no specific high school course requirements. Applicants must have taken the ACT and/or SAT assessments.

SELECTION FACTORS

Applicants are expected to have graduated in the top 20 percent of their high school classes, and must have scored at or above the 85th percentile for college-bound high school seniors on the ACT and/or SAT. Students must maintain a GPA of 3.3/4.0 or better during their freshman year in order to be considered for admission. The average high school GPA for students admitted to the PMMD Program in summer 1999 was 3.8/4.0, and the average GPA for their freshman year was 3.7/4.0. Their average composite ACT assessment was 27.

Two or more interviews are required. Students are not required to take the MCAT for selection, but are required to take the MCAT and to perform at a satisfactory level prior to beginning the medical school component of the program.

CURRICULUM

The Premedical-Medical Program leads to a baccalaureate degree in the College of Arts and Sciences and the M.D. degree awarded by the James H. Quillen College of Medicine. All students in this program must complete an undergraduate major or minor in an approved humanities discipline and must participate in a special noncredit seminar on topics of current interest in medicine.

Students are required to pass Step 1 of the USMLE before entering the final year of clerkship studies. Students must pass Step 2 of the USMLE in order to graduate.

EXPENSES

In 1999–2000, the undergraduate tuition rate was $2,532 per year and the medical school tuition rate was $11,124 per year for Tennessee residents. The corresponding out-of-state tuition rates were $7,648 and $21,862.

FINANCIAL AID

For more information, contact the Office of Financial Aid, East Tennessee State University, P.O. Box 70,772, Johnson City, Tennessee 37614.

APPLICATION AND ACCEPTANCE POLICIES

Filing of application (end freshman year):
  Earliest date (typical): March 15
  Latest date (typical): April 1
Application fee: None
Acceptance notice:
  Earliest date: July 1
  Latest date: Aug. 1
Applicant's response to acceptance offer:
  Maximum time: 2 weeks
Deposit to hold place in class: None
Starting date: Aug. 15

INFORMATION ON 1999–2000 ENTERING CLASS

Number of	*In-State*	*Out-of-State*	*Total*
Applicants	19	0	19
Applicants Interviewed	19	0	19
New Entrants	14	0	14

CHAPTER 10

Fisk University
Meharry Medical College

Nashville, Tennessee

ADDRESS INQUIRIES TO:

Anthony E. Johnson, *Director*
Fisk University
Office of Admissions
1000 17th Avenue North
Nashville, Tennessee 37208
(800) 443-3475; (615) 329-8774 (FAX)
Web Site: www.fisk.edu

PURPOSE

The Joint Program in Biomedical Sciences is designed to address America's need to train bright young minorities who are dedicated to finding solutions to biomedical problems through research, and who will be future health care providers.

REQUIREMENTS FOR ENTRANCE

Students are selected at the end of their first semester of undergraduate course work on the Fisk University campus. There are no specific high school course requirements. Applicants must have taken the ACT and/or SAT assessments.

SELECTION FACTORS

The courses taken and grades earned at Fisk University, plus ACT and/or SAT scores are considerations for eligibility for this program. Applicants must rank in the top 20 percent of their high school class. Students must take the MCAT prior to admission into the clinical phase of the program, and a satisfactory score is required for medical school admission.

CURRICULUM

The Joint Program in Biomedical Sciences, seven years in duration, allows students to obtain a baccalaureate degree from Fisk University and an M.D. degree from Meharry Medical College.

Course requirements for the baccalaureate degree include 8 semesters of natural and physical sciences and 12 semesters each in the humanities and social sciences. Students are required to spend two summers in structured academic enrichment.

Students must take Steps 1 and 2 of the USMLE during the medical school portion of the program. Passing these examinations is a factor in promotion and graduation from medical school.

The most frequent major chosen by students is biology, followed by chemistry.

EXPENSES

The undergraduate tuition for 1999–2000 was $8,740 for residents and nonresidents, plus $300 in annual fees. Tuition for medical school was $21,824, plus $3,998 in annual fees.

FINANCIAL AID

Applicants and students can apply for institutional scholarships and grants, U.S. Department of Education Title IV Federal Student Aid (work study and loans, U.S. Department of Health and Human Services Student Aid Programs (loans and scholarships), Southern Regional Education Board Grants, and Tennessee Black Conditional Grants.

Meharry's Office of Student Financial Aid makes available most federal, regional and state financial aid applications and brochures on numerous funding opportunities. See Meharry's Web site, www.mmc.edu (index to financial assistance), for sources of financial aid. The Meharry Medical College Library, as well as local public libraries, has publications on most sources of student financial aid. Applicants can receive more information from the Office of Student Financial Aid, Meharry Medical College, 1005 D.B. Todd Boulevard, Nashville, Tennessee 37208.

APPLICATION AND ACCEPTANCE POLICIES

Filing of application:
  Earliest date: Feb. 1
  Latest date: Dec. 15
Application fee: None
Acceptance notice:
  Earliest date: Feb. 21
  Latest date: March 1
Applicant's response to acceptance offer:
  Maximum time: 1 week
Deposit to hold place in class: None
Starting date: Retroactive second semester, undergraduate year 1

INFORMATION ON 1999–2000 ENTERING CLASS

Number of	*Total*
Applicants	11
Applicants Interviewed	10
New Entrants	4

Rice University and Baylor College of Medicine

Houston, Texas

ADDRESS INQUIRIES TO:

Rice University
Office of Admissions—MS-17
6100 Main Street
Houston, Texas 77005
(713) 527-4036

PURPOSE

To promote the education of future physicians who are scientifically competent, compassionate, and socially conscious in order to apply insight from extensive study of liberal arts and other disciplines to the study of modern medical science.

REQUIREMENTS FOR ENTRANCE

Students are selected for this program during their senior year of high school. Both residents and nonresidents of Texas are considered for admission. Applicants are expected to have had a varied and rigorous high school program with high academic achievement. They must take the SAT I or ACT plus three SAT II subject tests.

SELECTION FACTORS

The high school academic record, standardized test scores, course selection, extracurricular activities, and letters of recommendation are some of the factors taken into account in offering admission to an applicant. In the 1999–2000 entering class, students averaged above the top five percent.

CURRICULUM

This is not an accelerated program; all students must complete four years of undergraduate education and four years of medical school.

Students earn a baccalaureate degree from Rice University, and are awarded an M.D. degree from Baylor College of Medicine. Minimum course requirements for this program include at least two semesters each in the humanities and social sciences, and eight semesters in the natural and physical sciences.

The medicine portion of the curriculum devotes roughly 1½ years to the basic sciences with clinical experience, and 2½ years to clinical science with some basic sciences.

The MCAT is not required for promotion or admission to the medical school. Students are required to take Step 1 of the USMLE in their sophomore or junior years. They are also required to take Step 2 of the USMLE, but passing these examinations is not a graduation requirement.

EXPENSES

In 1999–2000 the undergraduate tuition for all students was $15,350 per year plus $450 in student fees. The medical school tuition for residents was $6,550; for nonresidents it was $19,650 annually plus $1,792 in student fees.

FINANCIAL AID

Sources of aid include academic and athletic scholarships, and need-based loans. Applicants can receive more information from the Rice Admission Office, M.S. 17, 6100 Main Street, Houston, Texas 77035.

APPLICATION AND ACCEPTANCE POLICIES

Filing of application:
  Earliest decision plan deadline date: Nov. 1
  Latest date: Dec. 1
Application fee: $35
Acceptance notice:
  Latest date: Mid-April
Applicant's response to acceptance offer:
  Maximum time: May 1
Deposit to hold place in class: $100; nonrefundable
Starting date: Aug. 28

INFORMATION ON 1999–2000 ENTERING CLASS

Total number of applicants: 222

Number of	*In-State*	*Out-of-State*	*Total*
Applicants Interviewed	12	25	37
New Entrants	6	9	15

Texas A&M University System Health Science Center College of Medicine

College Station, Texas

ADDRESS INQUIRIES TO:

Texas A&M University
Office of Honors Programs and Academic Scholarships
College Station, Texas 77843-4233
(409) 845-1957; 845-0300 (FAX)
Web Site: http://hsc.tamu.edu/Admis/MSS.html

PURPOSE

The Medical Science Scholars/Baccalaureate-M.D. Degree Program offers highly qualified high school students multiple opportunities to broaden their educational and life experiences, and explore interdisciplinary programs and projects that take full advantage of our location on the campus of one of the nation's leading universities. Students who are selected and successfully complete an accelerated curriculum will earn both their baccalaureate and M.D. degrees in as few as six years.

REQUIREMENTS FOR ENTRANCE

To be considered for entrance, an applicant must be a National Merit, National Achievement, or National Hispanic Scholar. Admission is restricted to residents of Texas. All applicants must be recipients of one of the following four-year competitive academic scholarships from Texas A&M University: the President's Endowed, the Lechner, the McFadden, or the President's Achievement Award Scholarships, all administered through the Office of Honors Programs and Academic Scholarships.

SELECTION FACTORS

The College of Medicine will consider other factors, such as SAT I or ACT scores, high school class rank, leadership activities, health-related or research experiences, community involvement, two letters of recommendation, and personal interviews.

CURRICULUM

A student who is admitted to the Medical Science Scholars Program will need to meet certain requirements to progress to College of Medicine enrollment. These requirements include a minimum of 60 resident hours including the following prerequisite courses: General Biology, Advanced Biology, General Chemistry, Organic Chemistry, Physics, Calculus, and English totaling 44 credit hours.

The MCAT *is not required* of students in the program to enroll in the College of Medicine. Enrollment requires a minimum grade point average of 3.40 overall, and 3.40 in the chosen major, and no grade below a "C" in any of the medical prerequisite courses. In addition, the College of Medicine evaluates letters of recommendation from undergraduate faculty and physician mentors, participation in extracurricular activities, demonstrated leadership, community service, a realistic assessment of medicine as a career, and independent study or research.

EXPENSES

Undergraduate educational expenses for nine months at Texas A&M will vary according to personal needs and course of study. The undergraduate tuition and fees, books, supplies, transportation, room and board, incidental and living expenses total approximately $10,219. Residents pay $36 per semester credit hour with a minimum of $120 per semester or $60 per summer term.

The medical school tuition cost for Texas residents is $6,550 per year. Estimated annual costs, which include fees, room and board, books and supplies, transportation, and other personal expenses, for state residents in years 1 to 4 amount to approximately $24,000.

FINANCIAL AID

The financial aid program at Texas A&M is designed for all students who have demonstrated financial need for assistance to meet college expenses and who are making satisfactory academic progress, as defined by the Department of Student Financial Aid.

To apply for financial aid, students must submit the FAFSA. Financial aid applications are available from high school counselors, most college or university student financial aid offices, or directly from: Director of Financial Aid, Texas A&M University, College Station, Texas 77843-1252; (409) 845-3236 or 845-3987.

Sources of aid include grants, student part-time employment, the college work-study program, and loan programs.

APPLICATION AND ACCEPTANCE POLICIES

Filing of application:
  Earliest date: Sept. 1
  Latest date: Beginning of the second week of January
Application fee: $50
Acceptance notice:
  Earliest date: May 1
Applicant's response to acceptance offer:
  Maximum time: Two weeks
Deposit to hold place in class: None
Starting date: August

INFORMATION ON 1999–2000 ENTERING CLASS

Number of	*Total*
Applicants	44
Applicants Interviewed	35
New Entrants	22

Eastern Virginia Medical School

Norfolk, Virginia

ADDRESS INQUIRIES TO:

Office of Admissions
Eastern Virginia Medical School
721 Fairfax Avenue
Norfolk, Virginia 23507-2000
(757) 446-5812; 446-5896 (FAX)
Web Site: www.evms.edu

PURPOSE

We currently have combined programs with five universities—the College of William and Mary, Old Dominion University, Hampton University, Norfolk State University, and Hampden-Sydney College. The purpose of these programs is to enlist outstanding high school and undergraduate students into a track that provides great freedom and choice in the pursuit of a baccalaureate degree.

REQUIREMENTS FOR ENTRANCE

Depending on the undergraduate institution, students are selected during their senior year of high school or after their freshman year of college. Both residents and nonresidents of Virginia are eligible to apply. There are no specific high school course requirements, but students must take the SAT.

SELECTION FACTORS

Although the criteria for consideration into the program differs at each of the undergraduate institutions, all applicants are screened on the basis of their academic qualifications. Selected applicants are invited for an interview.

CURRICULUM

The eight-year curriculum leads to a baccalaureate degree awarded by the College of William and Mary, Old Dominion University, Hampton University, Norfolk State University, or Hampden-Sydney College. The M.D. degree is granted by Eastern Virginia Medical School. The course requirements for the baccalaureate degree vary at each undergraduate institution, but the most frequent major is biology. This early assurance program does, however, permit the student the opportunity for academic diversity. Students selected who have SAT scores greater than 1200 will not be required to take the MCAT. Step 1 of the USMLE must be taken at the completion of the second year of medical school. Students must pass Steps 1 and 2 of the USMLE to complete the program and receive the M.D. degree.

EXPENSES

In 1999–2000 the annual tuition for medical school for residents was $15,000 and for nonresidents it was $27,500. The student fees were $1,491 per year.

FINANCIAL AID

For information about financial aid during the undergraduate phase, contact the Office of Financial Aid at the undergraduate institutions outlined. Five programs are available: the College of William and Mary, Randolph A. Coleman, Ph.D., (757) 221-2476; Old Dominion University, Mark S. Elliott, Ph.D., (757) 683-4078; Hampton University, Harold Marioneaux, D.D.S., (757) 728-6897; Norfolk State University, Hollis Baker, Ph.D., (757) 823-2511; and Hampden-Sydney College, Anne Lund, Ph.D., (804) 224-6175. For information about financial aid during the medical school phase, contact the Office of Financial Aid at (757) 446-5813.

APPLICATION AND ACCEPTANCE POLICIES

Information varies at each undergraduate institution.
Application fee: $25

INFORMATION ON 1999–2000 ENTERING CLASS

Total number of applicants: 132

Number of	*Total*
Applicants Interviewed	39
New Entrants	8

CHAPTER 10

Virginia Commonwealth University

Richmond, Virginia

ADDRESS INQUIRIES TO:

Dr. Anne L. Chandler
Associate Director, University Honors Program
Virginia Commonwealth University
P.O. Box 843010
Richmond, Virginia 23284-3010
(804) 828-1803; 828-1355 (FAX)
E-mail: alchandl@vcu.edu
Web Site: www.vcu.edu/honors

PURPOSE

The Guaranteed Admission Program offers academically capable, highly focused students an opportunity to pursue diverse, intellectually challenging programs of study without the pressure of competing further for medical school admission. Close contact with the School of Medicine throughout the undergraduate program aids students in testing their career choice and in preparing for a lifelong commitment to learning in the profession.

REQUIREMENTS FOR ENTRANCE

Students are selected during their senior year of high school, and there are no residency restrictions. All candidates are considered. The specific high school course requirements are as follows: eight semesters of English; six semesters each of social sciences, mathematics, and sciences; a foreign language, or four semesters each of two languages. We also require standardized admissions tests such as the ACT≥29; or the combined SAT of 1270 in a single sitting with neither score below 530, and an unweighted GPA of 3.0 (4.0 scale).

SELECTION FACTORS

The academic factors considered in offering admission to an applicant are: GPA, letters of reference, test scores, well-rounded, rigorous academic preparation, health care-related experience, and written and oral communication skills. The GPA for the 1999–2000 entering class was 3.8 (unweighted scale of 4.0), and the average SAT was 1420. Selected applicants are invited for a required interview.

CURRICULUM

Students are required to complete a baccalaureate degree. The most frequent major is biology; the next most frequent is chemistry. Both are awarded by Virginia Commonwealth University. Specific course requirements vary depending upon the major. During medical school, there is, however, a longitudinal clinical experience (Foundation of Clinical Medicine) in a community, primary care practice that meets weekly for both of the first two years. Students are required to take Step 1 of the USMLE at the end of their second year. They must also take Step 2, but passing these examinations is not a graduation requirement. The Doctor of Medicine is also awarded at Virginia Commonwealth University. It takes eight years to fulfill the requirements for both degrees.

EXPENSES

Tuition for undergraduates in the 1999–2000 academic year was $2,492 for residents and $11,946 for nonresidents. The medical school tuition in 1999–2000 was $10,428 for residents and $26,734 for nonresidents. Student fees averaged $1,095 for undergraduates and $1,133 for medical students per year.

FINANCIAL AID

There are several sources of financial aid available to students—scholarships, loans, grants, and work-study. For more information contact the Virginia Commonwealth University, P.O. Box 842506, Richmond, Virginia 23284-2506; (804) VCU-MONY.

APPLICATION AND ACCEPTANCE POLICIES

Filing of application:
  Earliest date: Sept. 1
  Latest date: Dec. 15
Application fee: $25
Acceptance notice:
  Earliest date: April 1
Applicant's response to acceptance offer:
  Maximum time: May 1 (4 weeks)
Deposit to hold place in class: $100; nonrefundable
Starting date: Fall 2000

INFORMATION ON 1999–2000 ENTERING CLASS

Number of	*Total*
Applicants	135
Applicants Interviewed	43
New Entrants	17

University of Wisconsin Medical School

Madison, Wisconsin

ADDRESS INQUIRIES TO:

Medical Scholars Program
University of Wisconsin Medical School
1300 University Avenue, Room 1140 A
Madison, Wisconsin 53706
(608) 263-7561; 262-2327 (FAX)
Web Site: http://www.medsch.wisc.edu/education/msp/msp.html

PURPOSE

The Medical Scholars Program provides conditional admission to the University of Wisconsin Medical School for approximately 50 highly qualified Wisconsin high school seniors. Medical scholars are a part of the medical school community and may participate in specially designed basic science and clinical experiences.

REQUIREMENTS FOR ENTRANCE

Students are selected for this program during the senior year of high school. Only residents of Wisconsin are eligible to apply. Applicants are expected to have completed the following courses by the time they graduate from high school: eight semesters of mathematics, eight semesters of English, six semesters of science (at least one semester each of biology, chemistry, and physics), six semesters of social studies, and four semesters of a foreign language. They must take either the SAT or the ACT Assessment.

SELECTION FACTORS

To be eligible for application, students must have attained a minimum academic GPA of 3.8 (includes English, mathematics, science, social studies, and foreign language in grades 9 through 11), be ranked in the top five percent of their high school class or have a minimum combined SAT score of 1300 or a minimum composite score of 30 on the ACT Assessment. In the 1999–2000 entering class, the average GPA was 3.98, the average SAT Verbal score was 718, and the average composite score on the ACT Assessment was 32. An interview is not required.

CURRICULUM

This program, normally seven to nine years in duration, allows students to obtain a bachelor's degree from the University of Wisconsin—Madison and an M.D. degree from the University of Wisconsin Medical School.

Students are expected to complete work for the bachelor's degree. Requirements for that degree vary according to the major chosen, but all include course work in the humanities, social sciences, and natural and physical sciences. The most frequent major chosen by students in this program is molecular biology, followed by zoology.

Educational innovations offered include the following: (a) a wide range of experiences in medical science research and exposure to clinical medicine allowing students to integrate undergraduate and medical education; (b) the opportunity to major in any subject; (c) completion of the undergraduate program in three to five years; and (d) a semester or year studying in a foreign country.

Students are expected to take Step 1 of the USMLE at the end of the second year of medical school, with a passing score required in order to begin clinical work. Passing both Steps 1 and 2 is a graduation requirement.

EXPENSES

In 1999–2000, residents of Wisconsin paid $3,737.70 per year to attend the University of Wisconsin—Madison and $17,005.70 per year at the University of Wisconsin Medical School.

FINANCIAL AID

Scholarships and loans are available to students according to their need. More information can be obtained from the University of Wisconsin—Madison Financial Aid Office, 432 North Murray Street, Madison, Wisconsin 53706.

APPLICATION AND ACCEPTANCE POLICIES

Filing of application:
- Earliest date: Sept. 30
- Latest date: Jan. 15

Application fee: None

Acceptance notice:
- Earliest date: April 1
- Latest date: April 1

Applicant's response to acceptance offer:
- Maximum time: May 1

Deposit to hold place in class: None

INFORMATION ON 1999–2000 ENTERING CLASS

Number of	*Total*
Applicants	250
New Entrants	48

ASSOCIATION OF AMERICAN MEDICAL COLLEGES

United States Medical Schools

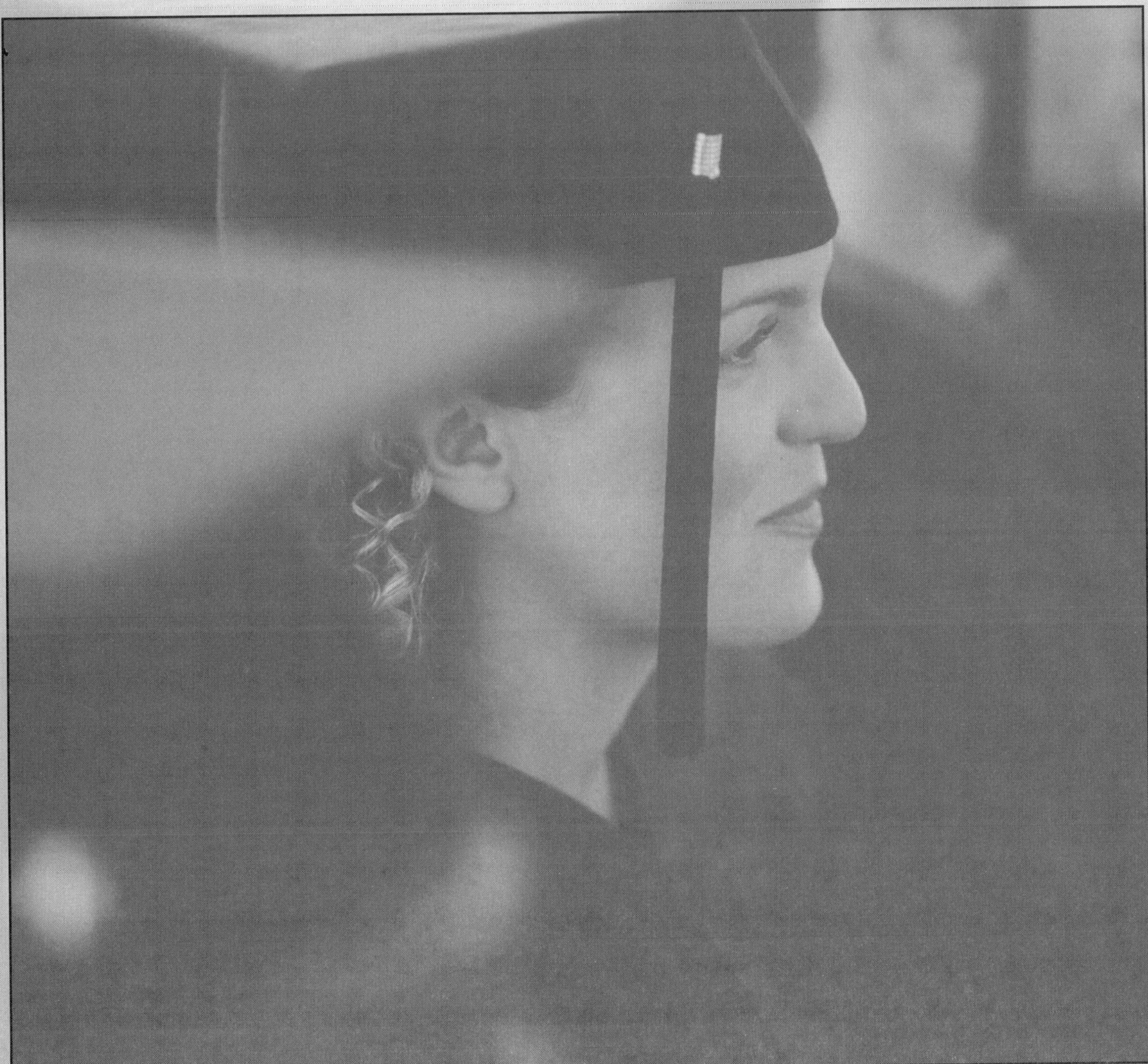

www.tomorrowsdoctors.org

MSAR

MEDICAL SCHOOL ADMISSION REQUIREMENTS

Information About U.S. Medical Schools

Accredited by the LCME

11

Information about individual medical schools is given in the following two-page entries for 122 schools in the United States and 3 schools in Puerto Rico that will be considering applications for fall 2000 entering classes. The schools presented here are fully accredited as of fall 1995 by the Liaison Committee on Medical Education (LCME), which is sponsored by the Association of American Medical Colleges (AAMC) and the American Medical Association (AMA).

The University of Minnesota—Duluth School of Medicine has a two-year basic medical science program; students transfer to the University of Minnesota Medical School—Minneapolis to complete their training. Individual school entries provide the tuition and student fees for a 1998–99 first-year student.

Each school entry provides statistics on the number of applicants, interviewed applicants, and new entrants (students entering medical school for the first time, excluding repeaters and reentrants) to the 1998–99 first-year class. These statistics are presented by residence status—in-state and out-of-state. Foreign nationals who do not have permanent resident status in the United States are included in the out-of-state figures.

ABBREVIATIONS

Listed below are the abbreviations used in the school entries in this chapter.

AMCAS—American Medical College Application Service

CLEP—College Level Examination Program

FAF—Financial Aid Form

FAFSA—Free Application for Federal Student Aid

GAPSFAS—Graduate and Professional School Financial Aid Service

GPA—Grade-point average

MCAT—Medical College Admission Test

VR—Verbal Reasoning

PS—Physical Sciences

WS—Writing Sample

BS—Biological Sciences

USMLE—United States Medical Licensing Examination

WICHE—Western Interstate Commission for Higher Education

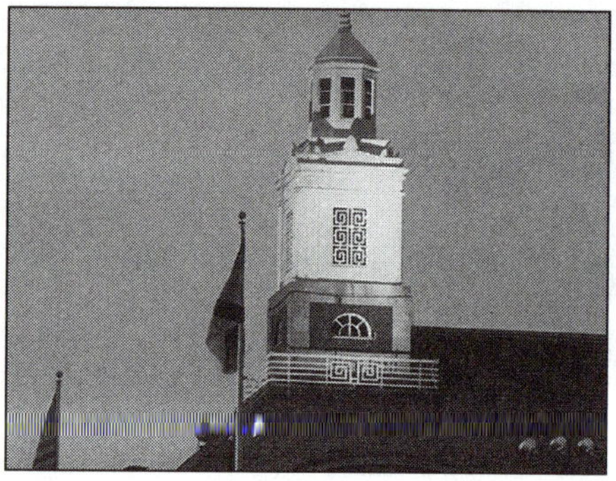

University of Alabama School of Medicine

Birmingham, Alabama

Dr. William B. Deal, *Dean*
Dr. George S. Hand, Jr., *Assistant Dean for Admissions*
Mark H. Martin, *Associate Director of Medical Student Services for Financial Aid*

ADDRESS INQUIRIES TO:

Office of Medical Student Services/Admissions
University of Alabama
School of Medicine
P-100 Volker Hall
1670 University Boulevard
Birmingham, Alabama 35294-0019
(205) 934-2330; 934-8724 (FAX)
E-mail: admissions@uasom.meis.uab.edu
Web Site: http://www.uab.edu/uasom/

MISSION STATEMENT

The School of Medicine is dedicated to the education of physicians and scientists in all of the disciplines of medicine and biomedical investigation for careers in practice, teaching, and research. Necessary to this educational mission are the provision of outstanding medical care and services and the enhancement of new knowledge through clinical and basic biomedical research.

GENERAL INFORMATION

The School of Medicine was founded in Mobile in 1859, shifted to the main campus of the University of Alabama in Tuscaloosa in 1920, and relocated to Birmingham in 1945. The University of Alabama School of Medicine, composed of the medical branches in Tuscaloosa, Birmingham, and Huntsville, was created in 1969. Birmingham is the main campus, and the Huntsville Program and the College of Community Health Sciences in Tuscaloosa are branch campuses.

CURRICULUM

The academic program consists of a four-year sequence that provides training in basic science and clinical areas. It emphasizes the fundamentals that underlie all medical practice. Consideration is given also to the emotional, cultural, and social characteristics of patients and to the need for adapting medical care to meet their needs. Initially, basic human biology, including anatomy, physiology, biochemistry, nutrition, behavioral sciences, and neurosciences, is emphasized. Second-year courses include microbiology, pharmacology, and pathology. The basic science years are completed by an integrative study of organ-system disorders and disease processes. All students are required to pass Step 1 of the USMLE at the end of the second year.

The third year and a part of the fourth year consist of required rotations through the clinical science disciplines (medicine, surgery, pediatrics, obstetrics-gynecology, family medicine/rural medicine, and psychiatry/neurology). This involves participation, under faculty supervision, in the care of patients both in the hospital and in ambulatory settings. The remainder of the fourth year is an elective or individualized experience program. All students are required to pass Step 2 of the USMLE prior to graduation.

Students complete two years of basic science course work in Birmingham; then, the clinical clerkships may be taken among the three clinical campuses during the third and fourth years. Students may choose to be assigned permanently to either Huntsville or Tuscaloosa for completion of the third and fourth years, but electives may be taken in a variety of locations.

The faculty and administration are strongly interested in attracting individuals who will train to be generalist physicians and give strong evidence of a willingness to practice in underserved areas.

An Early Medical School Acceptance Program (EMSAP) is available for outstanding Alabama high school seniors who have earned a 3.5 GPA or higher and have an ACT score of 30 or higher, and/or an SAT score of 1320 or higher. This is not an accelerated program nor is it a six-year program. EMSAP students will enter the University of Alabama at Birmingham for their undergraduate study and earn a baccalaureate degree before entering medical school.

REQUIREMENTS FOR ENTRANCE

At least 90 semester hours from an accredited institution and the MCAT are required. The MCAT should be taken during the spring before making application in early summer. A program leading to the bachelor's degree is highly recommended. Suitable major areas include the social sciences, humanities, and biological and physical sciences. It is strongly recommended that applicants also have some course work in the behavioral sciences. College work must include:

	Sem. hrs.
General biology or zoology	8
Inorganic chemistry (with lab)	8
Organic chemistry (with lab)	8
General physics (with lab)	8
College mathematics	6
English (composition and literature)	6

SELECTION FACTORS

Required interviews are arranged at the discretion of the Admission Committee. Alabama residents are given preference in the selection process, but nonresidents with superior academic credentials (GPA and BCPM of 3.5 or higher and MCAT scores of 10 or higher on each subtest along with superior essay scores) and demonstrated evidence of nonacademic success and commitment are encouraged to apply. Nonresident students with weaker credentials should not apply. Foreign applicants must have a permanent resident visa. Alabama residents from rural areas and from minority groups are especially encouraged to apply. Race, religion, national origin, age, handicap, and sex are not factors in consideration for admission.

Secondary applications are forwarded to all Alabama residents. Only selected nonresidents are forwarded secondary applications depending on the quality of their overall application. To receive a secondary application, nonresidents must meet the overall GPA and MCAT standards stated above, but not all qualified with these criteria are considered competitive. Final determination on nonresidents who receive a secondary application is made on the basis of MCAT scores, GPA, medical-related experiences, quality of curriculum, breadth of extracurricular activities, leadership ability, community service, and potential for success as a physician.

Acceptances were issued to 226 applicants to obtain a class of 160 entering students (including 8 M.D.-Ph.D. students). Class characteristics include: *mean GPA 3.62; mean MCAT: VR-9.7, PS-9.8, BS-10.1; 63 females; 11 African Americans; and 24 ethnic students. Undergraduate major*, 36 percent biology, 9 percent chemistry, 6 percent engineering, 9 percent biomedical sciences; 17 percent from other sciences and math with the remainder from a variety of fields including English, history, business, economics, and music. Students came from 55 colleges and universities.

Students in good academic standing may be transferred from other U.S. allopathic medical schools for compelling reasons. Available positions are limited to attrition. Applications are not accepted from individuals attending foreign medical schools or osteopathic medical schools.

FINANCIAL AID

About 78 percent of our students receive financial aid. Available loan funds are disbursed primarily on the basis of demonstrated financial need. State scholarships/loans are available in limited numbers to Alabama residents who can demonstrate economic need. Other scholarships are awarded on a merit basis. Students are advised not to seek outside employment. Summer research opportunities, supported by stipends and fellowships, are available.

INFORMATION FOR MINORITY STUDENTS

Through the Office of Minority Enhancement, the Admission Committee attempts to identify and provide academic counseling and information to minority students early in their college careers to facilitate application processes. The School of Medicine will consider the waiver of application fees for disadvantaged students, and some interviewing costs may be defrayed.

Public Institution

APPLICATION AND ACCEPTANCE POLICIES FOR 2001–2002 FIRST-YEAR CLASS

School participates in AMCAS. *See Chapter 6.*

Filing of AMCAS application
- Earliest date: June 1, 2000
- Latest date: Nov. 1, 2000

School application fee after screening: $65
Oldest MCAT scores considered: 1998
Does have Early Decision Program (EDP)
- For Alabama residents only
- EDP application period: June 1–Aug. 1, 2000
- EDP applicants notified by: Oct. 1, 2000

Acceptance notice to regular applicants
- Earliest date: Oct. 15, 2000
- Latest date: Until class is filled

Applicant's response to acceptance offer
- Maximum time: 15 days

Requests for deferred entrance considered: Yes
Deposit to hold place in class (applied to tuition): $50, due with response to acceptance offer (Residents only)
Deposit refundable prior to: May 15, 2001
Estimated number of new entrants: 160 (14 EDP)
Starting date: July 2001

TUITION AND STUDENT FEES PER YEAR FOR 1999–2000 FIRST-YEAR CLASS

Tuition
- Resident: $7,069
- Nonresident: $21,207

Student fees: $2,856

INFORMATION ON 1999–2000 FIRST-YEAR CLASS

Number of	*In-State*	*Out-of-State*	*Total*
Applicants	461	1,060	1,521
Applicants Interviewed	344	177	521
New Entrants*	141	19	160

*95% took the MCAT; 99% had baccalaureate degrees.

CHAPTER 11

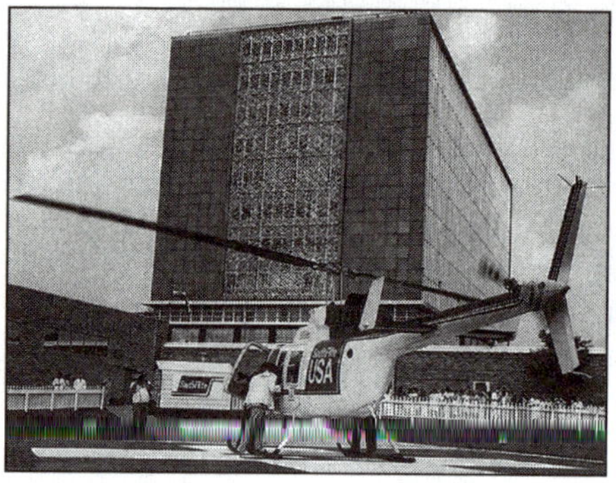

University of South Alabama College of Medicine

Mobile, Alabama

Dr. Robert A. Kreisberg, *Interim Dean*
Dr. Betsy Bennett, *Vice Dean, Student Affairs and Medical Education*
Mark Scott, *Director for Admissions*

ADDRESS INQUIRIES TO:

Office of Admissions, 2015 MSB
University of South Alabama
College of Medicine
Mobile, Alabama 36688-0002
(334) 460-7176; 460-6278 (FAX)

GENERAL INFORMATION

The College of Medicine of the University of South Alabama was approved by the Board of Trustees of the university in 1967; the legislature of the state of Alabama passed a resolution authorizing the college on August 19, 1967. The college admitted a charter class of 25 students in January 1973 and a full class of 64 students in September 1973. No increase or decrease in the number of entering students is planned. The basic medical sciences are housed on the university campus in a building that was completed in March 1974. The largest site for the clinical education program is the University of South Alabama Medical Center. Operating continuously since 1831, this hospital has provided medical education for more than a century. It functions as the major physician-staffed emergency facility in South Alabama and has been named a Level I trauma center by the Alabama Committee on Trauma. Other clinical training facilities include the U.S.A. Springhill Campus, U.S.A. Cancer Center and Clinical Building, U.S.A. Health Services Building, and Searcy Hospital. U.S.A. Knollwood and U.S.A. Children's and Women's Hospitals, our most recent additions, provide our students with state of the art clinical training facilities.

CURRICULUM

The first year is devoted to the basic sciences of anatomy, physiology, biochemistry, neuroanatomy, and embryology. However, opportunity for early introduction to clinical problems is afforded by courses such as Correlation Conferences and Medical Practice and Society. The second year includes pathology, physical diagnosis, microbiology-immunology, pharmacology, and behavioral science. Public health/epidemiology and medical genetics round out the second-year curriculum. All students are required to take and pass Step 1 of the USMLE at the end of the second year. The third year is composed of clinical clerkships in medicine, surgery, pediatrics, psychiatry, obstetrics-gynecology, and family practice. The fourth year is composed of 9 rotations of four weeks each. The student is required to select one rotation each in clinical neuroscience, surgical subspecialties, ambulatory care, primary care subspecialty in medicine, pediatrics, or obstetrics-gynecology, acting internship, and an in-house elective. Three of the rotations may be used for approved extramural experiences. Students are required to take and pass Step 2 of the USMLE in September of the fourth year. An A–F (A, B, C, D, F) grading system is used with the exception of the fourth year, during which an honors/pass/fail system is used.

The philosophy of the institution is to utilize all of the existing resources that provide opportunities for almost all of the experiences in clinical medicine. After acquiring a sound basis in scientific medicine, students then have the opportunity to select multiple tracks of study.

A combined M.D.-Ph.D. program in basic medical sciences is also offered.

REQUIREMENTS FOR ENTRANCE

The MCAT and three years of college are required; the baccalaureate degree is highly desirable. Each applicant must have at least 90 semester hours of acceptable credit from an accredited undergraduate institution. Required courses are:

	Sem. hrs.
General biology (with lab)	8
General chemistry (with lab)	8
Organic chemistry (with lab)	8
General physics (with lab)	8
Humanities	6
English composition and/or literature	6
College mathematics	8

Calculus is highly recommended.

The University of South Alabama College of Medicine does not accept pass/fail grades for required science courses, except in the rare instance in which an applicant's college assigns only pass/fail grades.

Applicants are strongly urged to take the MCAT in the spring of the year of application and to have their basic science requirements completed at the time of application. Required course work in process or fall MCAT scores delay the processing of an application.

SELECTION FACTORS

The Committee on Admissions will consider seriously all candidates whose undergraduate academic work and scores on the MCAT indicate that they will be able to handle the rigorous curriculum of the College of Medicine. However, consideration will be given to more than scholastic achievement alone. Applicants will be considered from the standpoint of their potential to become conscientious and capable physicians. The University of South Alabama provides equal educational opportunities and is open to all qualified students without regard to race, creed, national origin, sex, or handicap with respect to all of its programs and activities. Because the college is state-supported, preference is shown to Alabama residents; however, residents of the Mississippi Gulf Coast and Florida Panhandle qualify for in-state tuition.

Disadvantaged, rural, and minority residents of Alabama are strongly encouraged to apply. The application process consists of two stages: the preliminary AMCAS application and the final application sent when requested by the Committee on Admissions. This latter application requires recommendations, a photograph, and a $50 fee. After review of the final application, the committee will select those applicants to be invited to the campus for interviews. Fee waivers, based solely on economic need, are granted when documented.

The 65 members of the 1998 entering class came from 31 different undergraduate schools. The *average undergraduate GPA* was 3.70; *average MCAT scores,* VR-9.5, PS-10.0, BS-10.0; 90 percent *residents* of Alabama.

FINANCIAL AID

The Office of Financial Aid coordinates the programs of assistance available to medical students demonstrating financial need. Scholarships are also available for entering freshmen and medical students who have demonstrated academic excellence and/or financial need.

A limited number of state scholarships/loans are available to Alabama residents who can demonstrate economic need. After graduation, repayment may be made by cash or by the practice of medicine in certain areas of the state for the number of years stipulated by law.

The Medical Student Summer Research Program is available to entering first-year students and rising second-year students. The participants are paid a stipend and no previous research experience is necessary. Part-time employment is available; however, students are discouraged from accepting employment during academic periods.

INFORMATION FOR MINORITY STUDENTS

The school is committed to the enrollment and education of individuals from all disadvantaged groups. For information, write Dr. Hattie M. Myles, assistant dean of special programs and student affairs.

Public Institution

APPLICATION AND ACCEPTANCE POLICIES FOR 2001–2002 FIRST-YEAR CLASS

School participates in AMCAS. See Chapter 6.

Filing of AMCAS application
  Earliest date: June 1, 2000
  Latest date: Nov. 15, 2000
School application fee to all applicants: $50
Oldest MCAT scores considered: 1997
Does have Early Decision Program (EDP)
  For Alabama residents only
  EDP application period: June 1–Aug. 1, 2000
  EDP application notified by: Oct. 1, 2000
Acceptance notice to regular applicants
  Earliest date: Nov. 1, 2000
  Latest date: Until class is filled
Applicant's response to acceptance offer
  Maximum time: 2 weeks
Requests for deferred entrance considered: Yes
Deposit to hold place in class (applied to tuition):
  $50, due with response to acceptance offer
Deposit refundable prior to: May 15, 2001, if requested in writing
Estimated number of new entrants: 64 (10 EDP)
Starting date: Aug. 2001

TUITION AND STUDENT FEES PER YEAR FOR 1999–2000 FIRST-YEAR CLASS

Tuition
  Resident: $7,000
  Nonresident: $14,000

Student fees: $2,315

INFORMATION ON 1999–2000 FIRST-YEAR CLASS

Number of	*In-State*	*Out-of-State*	*Total*
Applicants	426	570	996
Applicants Interviewed	200	19	219
New Entrants*	59	5	64

*All took the MCAT and had baccalaureate degrees.

CHAPTER 11

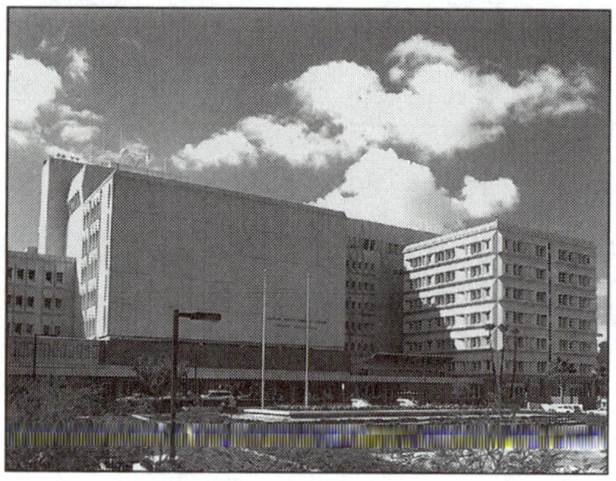

University of Arizona College of Medicine

Tucson, Arizona

Dr. James E. Dalen, *Vice President for Health Sciences and Dean, College of Medicine*
Dr. Shirley Nickols Fahey, *Associate Dean*
Maggie Gumble, *Program Coordinator Senior, Financial Aid*

ADDRESS INQUIRIES TO:

Admissions Office, Room 2209
University of Arizona
College of Medicine
P.O. Box 245075
Tucson, Arizona 85724-5075
(520) 626-6214; 626-4884 (FAX)
Web Site: http://www.medicine.arizona.edu

MISSION STATEMENT

The mission of the College of Medicine, as it pertains to medical students, is to provide medical students with the knowledge and skill basic to the practice of medicine, and inculcate them with the fundamental attitudes of compassionate patient care and a spirit and desire for lifelong independent learning and scholarship.

GENERAL INFORMATION

The College of Medicine enrolled its first class of students in 1967. As a professional and graduate college of the University of Arizona located adjacent to the main campus, its programs provide education and training for both the M.D. and Ph.D. degrees.

The University of Arizona Health Sciences Center complex consists of several interconnected buildings and adjoining structures on a 30-acre site north of the main campus (Arthritis Center, Basic Sciences Building, Clinical Sciences Building, Life Sciences Building, Outpatient Clinic, Arizona Health Sciences Library, University Medical Center, Children's Research Center, and Arizona Cancer Center). Under construction is a heart center. The colleges of nursing and pharmacy are located south of the Basic Sciences Building. A student wing of the Basic Sciences Building houses the multidisciplinary laboratories, anatomy laboratories, the learning resource center, lecture rooms, conference rooms, student lounge, and support facilities.

CURRICULUM

The overall purpose of the educational program is to give students the desire for lifelong learning in medicine by creating study habits that call for the continuous pursuit of knowledge and the capacity to modify previously acquired information. The program also aims to give students the skills to conduct patient care activities as well as the professional attitudes consonant with the charge to provide patients with preventive and curative advice and treatment.

Biologic, cultural, psychosocial, economic, and sociologic concepts and data are provided in the core curriculum. Increasing emphasis is placed on problem-solving ability, beginning with initial instruction and carried through to graduation. Excellence in performance is encouraged and facilitated. Awareness of the milieu in which medicine is practiced is also encouraged. The core curriculum comprises three years of required studies and one year of elective rotations. The learning environment encompasses lectures, small-group discussion and problem-solving sessions, independent study, clinical clerkships, practice in physical diagnosis, computer-based instruction, and a variety of other modes for the learner. Students learn in the classroom, conference room, laboratory, clinic and physician's office, bed units of hospitals, special sites for diagnostic and therapeutic maneuvers, University Medical Center, and a variety of inpatient and outpatient settings in Tucson, Phoenix, and throughout Arizona. All medical students will participate in an educational experience with an underserved population sometime during medical school. Upon graduation the physician is equipped to continue postgraduate education in general or specialty practice, teaching, or research. Combined M.D.-Ph.D. and M.D.-M.P.H. programs of study are also offered.

REQUIREMENTS FOR ENTRANCE

All applicants must be residents of Arizona or WICHE certified and funded residents of Alaska, Montana, or Wyoming. The MCAT and a minimum of three years of college are required. Each applicant must successfully complete at least 90 semester hours (135 quarter hours) at an accredited college or university, including 30 semester hours of upper division courses. A baccalaureate degree is preferred. Applicants educated outside the United States or Canada must have completed the same required courses as students in the U.S. or Canada, including 30 hours of upper division courses, prior to submitting an application. Postbaccalaureate students should have recent courses in the required science areas. The following specific courses are required:

	Sem./Qtr.
General biology or zoology	2/3
General chemistry	2/3

Organic chemistry	2/3
Physics	2/3
English (comp. and lit.)	2/3

CLEP or AP credits are not acceptable for the required courses. Applicants are strongly urged to take the MCAT in the spring of the year of application and to have their basic requirements completed at the time of application. All required courses must be completed by the spring semester prior to matriculation. Applicants are encouraged to take the required science courses that include laboratory experiences. No preference is given to any particular kind of undergraduate academic major, although applicants are encouraged to have a broad social science and/or humanities background.

Many Arizona residents and patients who receive care at the Arizona Health Sciences Center and its affiliated clinics and hospitals speak Spanish as their primary language, and it would be useful for our medical students to be conversant in Spanish.

SELECTION FACTORS

Applications are only considered from Arizona residents; highly qualified applicants who are WICHE certified and funded residents of Alaska, Montana, and Wyoming; and Native Americans who reside on reservations contiguous with the state of Arizona. Applicants from states other than these will not be considered. Applicants are chosen on the basis of their ability, motivation, integrity, emotional maturity, interpersonal skills, patient-related activity, and other personal characteristics, which the Admissions Committee regards as important for prospective medical students and the successful practice of medicine. In evaluating candidates, attention is given to the entire academic record, MCAT scores, college preprofessional committee evaluations, the AMCAS Personal Comments, other letters of recommendation, and personal interviews. Also considered is breadth of the undergraduate education, whether in the humanities, social sciences, or natural sciences. Applicants who meet the above qualifications will be interviewed at the College of Medicine. Acceptance is dependent on far more than academic achievement and is considered from the standpoint of the applicant's potential as a physician.

Accepted students for the 1999 entering class had the following characteristics: *mean GPA,* 3.55; *sex,* 45 percent women; *residence,* 100 percent from Arizona; *overall acceptance rate,* 23.7 percent of those seriously considered received acceptances; and 117 acceptances were offered out of 494 applicants considered. Disadvantaged, rural, and minority residents of Arizona are strongly encouraged to apply. The College of Medicine does not discriminate on the basis of sex, age, race, creed, national origin, or handicap in its admission policies.

FINANCIAL AID

Federal and local scholarships and loans are available to students with financial need. Eighty-seven percent of the students are receiving financial assistance. All determinations of need are made after an applicant is accepted for enrollment.

INFORMATION FOR MINORITY AND NONTRADITIONAL STUDENTS

The College of Medicine and the Office of Minority Affairs have an active program dedicated to the recruitment, admission, education, and graduation of an increased number of individuals from minority groups. The program offers the Minority Medical Education Program for premed students and a summer Preprofessional Program for entering medical students. Learning specialists work closely with students during all phases of their medical education. The Commitment to Underserved People (CUP) project provides numerous opportunities to participate in neighborhood clinic settings. Tutoring, counseling, and a variety of student support services are also available. Faculty members participate in all aspects of the program.

Public Institution

APPLICATION AND ACCEPTANCE POLICIES FOR 2001–2002 FIRST-YEAR CLASS

School participates in AMCAS. See Chapter 6.

Filing of AMCAS application
Earliest date: June 1, 2000
Latest date: Nov. 1, 2000
School application fee: None
Oldest MCAT scores considered: 1998
Does not have Early Decision Program
Acceptance notice to regular applicants
Earliest date: Jan. 26, 2001
Latest date: Until class is filled
Applicant's response to acceptance offer
Maximum time: 2 weeks
Requests for deferred entrance considered: Yes
Deposit to hold place in class: None
Estimated number of new entrants: 100
Starting date: July 2001

TUITION AND STUDENT FEES PER YEAR FOR 1999–2000 FIRST-YEAR CLASS

Tuition
Resident: $8,760
Nonresident: Not applicable

Student fees: $88

INFORMATION ON 1999–2000 FIRST-YEAR CLASS

Number of	*In-State*	*Out-of-State*	*Total*
Applicants	537	65	602
Applicants Interviewed	494	3*	497
New Entrants†	100	0*	100

*Certified WICHE applicants from Alaska, Montana, and Wyoming.
†All took the MCAT and had baccalaureate degrees.

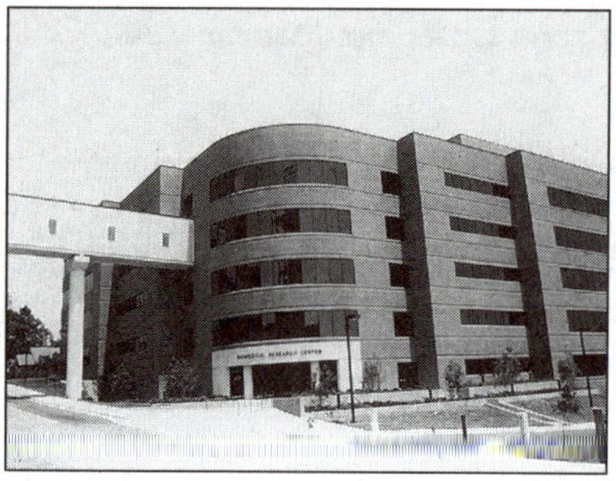

University of Arkansas College of Medicine

Little Rock, Arkansas

Dr. I. Dodd Wilson, *Dean*
Tom G. South, *Director, Admissions and Financial Aid*
Dr. Richard Wheeler, *Associate Dean, Student and Academic Affairs*

ADDRESS INQUIRIES TO:

Tom G. South
Student and Academic Affairs
University of Arkansas College of Medicine
4301 West Markham Street, Slot 551
Little Rock, Arkansas 72205-7199
(501) 686-5354; 686-5873 (FAX)
E-mail: SouthTomG@exchange.uams.edu
Web Site: http://www.uams.edu

MISSION STATEMENT

The mission of the University of Arkansas for Medical Sciences is to provide excellent educational opportunities for students of the health care professions in a stimulating environment of basic and clinical research, integrated with the delivery of superb comprehensive health care services.

In fulfilling its educational mission, the five academic units of the UAMS—the College of Medicine, Nursing, Pharmacy, Health Related Professions, and the Graduate School—as well as the University Hospital, the Area Health Education Center, the Arkansas Cancer Research Center, the Harvey and Bernice Jones Eye Institute, and the Donald W. Reynolds Center on Aging provide the environment and opportunities for students and practitioners alike to learn and maintain the knowledge and skills they need. These programs integrate the liberal arts with the biological, physical, and behavioral sciences, and emphasize lifelong learning for practitioners in the health professions.

UAMS is the principal biomedical research center for the state of Arkansas. In its programs of research, UAMS seeks to stimulate and support scholarly inquiry for both faculty and students aimed at maintaining and preserving knowledge, and making discoveries that address the health needs of the state, the nation, and the world.

The service mission is fulfilled by providing comprehensive health care services to meet both the educational needs of our students and the special health care needs of the state. As the only academic medical center in Arkansas, the unique role of UAMS is to provide services requiring highly specialized personnel and technology. These services are delivered in an interdisciplinary environment to all Arkansans, regardless of their ability to pay.

In addition, comprehensive services in health, wellness, and rehabilitation are offered in a statewide context. Our service mission is enhanced by affiliation with the Arkansas Children's Hospital, the John L. McClellan Memorial Veterans Administration Medical Center, the Arkansas Rehabilitation Institute, the Central Arkansas Radiation Therapy Institute, and the Arkansas State Hospital. Additional cooperative programs are offered with other hospitals and practitioners affiliated with the AHEC Programs.

The UAMS mission encompasses a responsibility to its alumni and other health care practitioners of Arkansas to help them continue to improve their professional knowledge and skills. All schools and departments offer lifelong learning opportunities as appropriate to their mission.

CURRICULUM

Along with the standard courses in anatomy, biochemistry, and physiology, the first year includes a program to introduce the student to clinical contacts and concepts. This is accomplished with formal lectures in medico-socioeconomic topics, small-group discussions, and faculty-supervised interviews with patients, and the extensive use of standardized patients.

The duration of the second-year program is nine months; the study consists of a standard but shortened curriculum.

The third year is a full 48 weeks with rotation through the major clinical services. This expanded clinical year provides substantial preparation for the predominantly elective fourth year, which consists of a minimum of 36 weeks to a maximum of 48 weeks of courses selected with the assistance of a faculty advisor. On- and off-campus electives are available to round out preparation for each student's career goals. The traditional grading system (A, B, C, D, F) is used throughout the first three years. Elective courses and a few selected ones in the first three years are graded as pass/fail. Opportunities are provided for students to engage in research activities and to pursue graduate courses leading to the M.S. and Ph.D. degrees.

REQUIREMENTS FOR ENTRANCE

The MCAT and at least 90 semester hours of college work are required; a baccalaureate degree is strongly recommended. The following courses must be completed prior to matriculation:

	*Semesters**
Biology	2
General chemistry	2
Organic chemistry	2
Physics	2

Mathematics 2
English 3
*Or equivalent.

No particular undergraduate field is given preference in the selection process; students from a variety of backgrounds are actively sought. While applicants are encouraged to follow their own interests in selecting college majors, courses such as embryology, genetics, quantitative analysis, psychology, history, and logic are also recommended.

Applicants must have taken the MCAT no earlier than April 1997 and prior to the November 1 application deadline. Students enrolled in graduate/professional programs must have an advisor submit a letter assuring graduation prior to medical college entry in August.

SELECTION FACTORS

Selection is based on scholastic attainment, performance on the MCAT, personal interviews with members of the faculty, and recommendations, particularly evaluations by college preprofessional advisory committees. Applicants should also demonstrate time and effort devoted to volunteerism and community service. Selection is made without regard to race, sex, creed, national origin, age, or handicap. Unsuccessful applicants may reapply without prejudice.

Matriculants for the 1999 entering class had the following profile: *mean GPA,* 3.57 (97 percent above 3.0); *sex,* 33 percent women; *undergraduate major,* 79 percent in science disciplines, *average MCAT score,* 9.0.

Although applications are accepted from students who are not residents of the state of Arkansas, preference must be given to qualified resident applicants. Nonresidents who do not have a GPA of at least 3.5 (based on a 4.0 scale) and above average scores on each section of the MCAT should not apply.

Qualified nonresidents will be considered if they can demonstrate strong ties to Arkansas. Students demonstrating strong ties to Arkansas will receive a supplemental application and information.

FINANCIAL AID

Approximately 85 percent of our medical students received financial aid. The average educational indebtedness for graduates in 1999 was $62,800. The financial status of applicants is not a factor in selection for admission.

The Community Match Program allows students who commit to practice primary care medicine in rural communities in Arkansas to receive up to $66,000 ($16,500 per academic year). The rural community provides one-half of the funds, and the remaining half is provided by the College of Medicine's Community Match Program. The student is obligated to return to the rural community following residency training and practice full time for the same number of years the student was assisted during medical school. For each year of service, one year of loans is forgiven until the debt is retired. A unique feature of the program allows alternates, who sign rural practice contracts, the opportunity to advance to the top of the alternate list. For additional details, contact the Financial Aid Office.

INFORMATION FOR MINORITY STUDENTS

Minority students are encouraged to apply for admission. The Office of Minority Student Affairs has developed an active recruitment and retention program. The Summer Science Program for Minority Students is available for five weeks during the summer and offers an introduction to the medical school curriculum, along with reading and study skill enrichment sessions designed to strengthen students in these areas. A prematriculation program is available, and has as its primary focus students who may have some problems mastering the medical college curriculum. Every effort is made by the faculty to assist students academically as these needs are identified.

Public Institution

APPLICATION AND ACCEPTANCE POLICIES FOR 2001–2002 FIRST-YEAR CLASS

School participates in AMCAS. See Chapter 6.

Filing of AMCAS application
Earliest date: June 1, 2000
Latest date: Nov. 1, 2000
School application fee to all applicants: $50
Oldest MCAT scores considered: 1997
Does not have Early Decision Program
Acceptance notice to regular applicants
Earliest date: Dec. 15, 2000
Latest date: Until class is filled
Applicant's response to acceptance offer
Maximum time: 2 weeks
Requests for deferred entrance considered: Yes
Deposit to hold place in class: None
Estimated number of new entrants: 150
Starting date: Aug. 2001

TUITION AND STUDENT FEES PER YEAR FOR 1999–2000 FIRST-YEAR CLASS

Tuition
Resident: $8,928
Nonresident: $17,856

Student fees: $175

INFORMATION ON 1999–2000 FIRST-YEAR CLASS

Number of	*In-State*	*Out-of-State*	*Total*
Applicants	294	353	647
Applicants Interviewed	290	25	315
New Entrants*	140	4	144

*All took the MCAT; 99% had baccalaureate degrees.

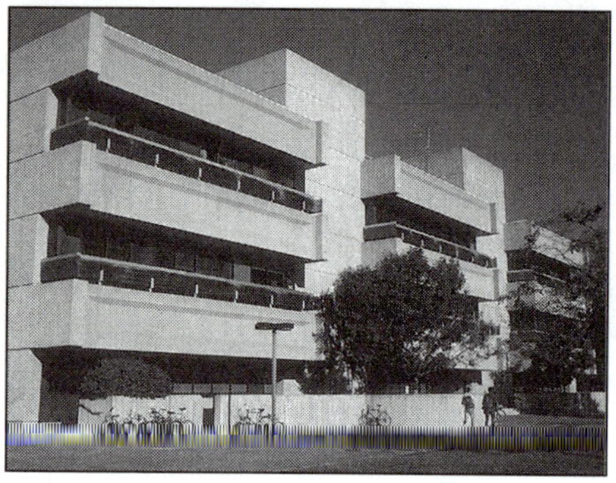

University of California, Davis School of Medicine

Davis, California

Dr. Joseph Silva, Jr., *Dean*
Ernest L. Lewis, *Associate Dean*
Edward D. Dagang, *Director of Admissions*

ADDRESS INQUIRIES TO:

Office of Admissions
School of Medicine
University of California
One Shields Avenue
Davis, California 95616-8661
(530) 752-2717
Web Site: http://www-med.ucdavis.edu/
E-mail: medadmisinfo@ucdavis.edu

MISSION STATEMENT

The mission of the School of Medicine at the University of California, Davis, involves four closely interwoven components: education, research, patient care, and public service. The school is firmly committed to excellence in all four components.

GENERAL INFORMATION

The School of Medicine, University of California, Davis, admitted its first class in 1968. The school provides its students with a foundation of medical knowledge upon which they may proceed to careers in primary care, specialty practice, research, public health, or administration.

CURRICULUM

The curriculum provides a balanced blend of basic and clinical sciences. Basic science courses are emphasized during the first year and continue into the second year with the integration of core clinical courses. Early clinical exposure is provided during the first year through a continuing course entitled Introduction to Patient Evaluation and continues into the second year in the Physical Diagnosis course. A strong emphasis is placed within the curriculum on problem solving and knowledge of essential concepts. The third and fourth years provide the predominant component of clinical training with required clerkships in the third year and expanding opportunity for flexibility in the fourth year. Most courses are departmental with overall governance by the Committee on Educational Policy of the Academic Senate. The curriculum undergoes constant reexamination for excellence and topicality. From the onset of the curriculum, students have the opportunity to take a broad range of elective courses, many with a heavy clinical emphasis.

The Davis campus affords opportunities for interaction with other schools, colleges, departments, and laboratories of the university. Research, teaching, and service are interrelated, and the biological and allied sciences are emphasized. Close relationships are enjoyed with the School of Veterinary Medicine, the California Primate Research Center, the Laboratory for Energy Related Health Research, and the Food Protection and Toxicology Center.

First- and second-year students attend preclinical science classes in the Tupper Hall complex in Davis. Very early in the student's training, use is made of the clinical facilities of the University of California, Davis, Medical Center, with a 453-bed main hospital, the Shriners Hospital for Children, and the extensive ambulatory clinic facilities of the Ellison Ambulatory Care Center. The Health System offers a full range of inpatient services, diagnostic services, an ambulatory care program with over 150 specialty clinics, and 24-hour major emergency medical service.

In addition to the doctor of medicine degree, UC Davis offers a variety of dual-degree programs through coordination with other graduate school divisions. These advanced degrees can couple the M.D. degree to the Ph.D., M.S., and M.A. degrees through the division of graduate studies of UC Davis. The M.D. degree can also be combined with an M.B.A. through the Graduate School of Management of UC Davis, with an M.P.H. degree through the School of Public Health, University of California, Berkeley.

REQUIREMENTS FOR ENTRANCE

The MCAT and three years (90 semester hours or 135 quarter hours) in an accredited college or university in the United States or Canada are required. Applicants are urged to take the MCAT in the spring but no later than the summer in which the application is made. A course of study leading to a bachelor's degree is recommended.

The school believes a medical student should have a sound background in the humanities and behavioral and social sciences as well as in the physical and biological sciences. Premedical requirements must be completed by June of the year of desired entry. The following college-level courses are required:

	Years
English	1
Biological sciences (with lab)	1
General chemistry (with lab)	1
Organic chemistry	1

If two or more undergraduate courses are offered, the more rigorous option is recommended.

Physics 1
Mathematics
Course work sufficient to satisfy prerequisites for integral calculus is required (1 semester or 2 quarters of college level calculus).

CLEP credit is not acceptable for prerequisite courses.

SELECTION FACTORS

The School of Medicine selects students for admission with a view to meeting the needs of society, of the medical profession, and of the school. Because the educational experience is enhanced by the interaction of students from various backgrounds, the school desires diversity in its student body. This is reflected in the school's commitment to expand opportunities in medical education for individuals from groups underrepresented in medicine as the result of social discrimination and to increase the number of physicians practicing in underserved areas. Therefore, the Admissions Committee, which is composed of individuals from a variety of cultural backgrounds representative of a broad spectrum of medical sciences, evaluates applicants in terms of all relevant factors. These include academic credentials, with due regard to how they may have been affected by disadvantage experienced by the applicant; such personal traits as character and motivation; experience in the health sciences and/or the community; career objectives; and the ability of the individual to make a positive contribution to society, the profession, and the school.

Factors considered are the applicant's scholastic record, MCAT performance, and reports of teachers and advisors regarding intellectual capacity, motivation, and emotional stability. Characteristics that may make such applicants particularly attractive to the Admissions Committee are outstanding nonacademic achievements, capability for independent study, maturity, and other factors that suggest good academic potential.

A personal interview will normally be required of each applicant who is accepted. Regional interviews are not normally available. Primary consideration for admission will be given to students who are legal residents of California. UCDavis School of Medicine participates in the WICHE Professional Student Exchange Program for applicants from certain western states that do not have medical schools.

FINANCIAL AID

A complete range of financial aid is available to medical students at the University of California, Davis: scholarships, fellowships, grants, and a variety of loans. The majority of financial aid is awarded based on demonstrated financial need. However, all accepted students are considered for university-awarded, merit- and need-based scholarships.

Historically, students at the School of Medicine have been able to receive full financial aid funding of their calculated financial need. Financial aid applications are available in December or early January. Students granted an interview can request an application by mail or pick up an application when they come to UC Davis for their interview. Early application for aid is strongly recommended. Questions should be directed to the Financial Aid Office at (530) 752-6618, or by e-mail at medfinancialaid@ucdavis.edu.

INFORMATION FOR DISADVANTAGED APPLICANTS

The Office of the Dean of Education offers a variety of supplemental assistance programs and services for medical students, premed undergraduates, and high school students. The mission is to ensure diversity amongst students and faculty through outreach, development, and support activities for individuals from educationally and socioeconomically disadvantaged backgrounds, as well as to ensure that all medical students are prepared to give the best care to the wide variety of people in California and beyond.

Public Institution

APPLICATION AND ACCEPTANCE POLICIES FOR 2001–2002 FIRST-YEAR CLASS

School participates in AMCAS. See Chapter 6.

Filing of AMCAS application
Earliest date: June 1, 2000
Latest date: Nov. 1, 2000
School application fee after screening: $40
Oldest MCAT scores considered: August 1997
Does not have Early Decision Program
Acceptance notice to regular applicants
Earliest date: Oct. 15, 2000
Latest date: Until class is filled
Applicant's response to acceptance offer
Maximum time: 2 weeks
Requests for deferred entrance considered: Yes
Deposit to hold place in class: None
Estimated number of new entrants: 93
Starting date: Sept. 2001

TUITION AND STUDENT FEES PER YEAR FOR 1999–2000 FIRST-YEAR CLASS

Tuition
Resident: None
Nonresident: $9,804

Student fees: $9,921

INFORMATION ON 1999–2000 FIRST-YEAR CLASS

Number of	*In-State*	*Out-of-State*	*Total*
Applicants	3,173	1,058	4,231
Applicants Interviewed	*	*	442
New Entrants†	93	0	93

*Data not available.
†All took the MCAT and had baccalaureate degrees.

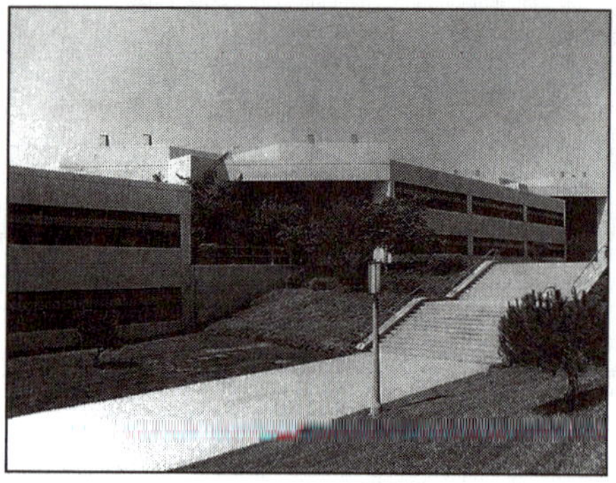

University of California, Irvine College of Medicine

Irvine, California

Dr. Thomas C. Cesario, *Dean*
Dr. Alberto Manetta, *Senior Associate Dean, Educational Affairs*
Dr. Ralph E. Purdy, *Associate Dean, Admissions and Outreach*

ADDRESS INQUIRIES TO:

Office of Admissions and Outreach
UCI-College of Medicine
802, Room 100—Medical Education Bldg.
Irvine, California 92697-4089
(949) 824-5388; (800) 824-5388;
(949) 824-2485 (FAX)
Web Site: http://www.com.uci.edu

GENERAL INFORMATION

The predecessor of the University of California, Irvine (UCI) College of Medicine began as a private institution in 1896. It became part of the University of California in 1965 and was relocated to a 122-acre site on the Irvine campus in 1968, admitting the first group of medical students the same year.

Since its establishment at UCI, the college has grown extensively, attaining national recognition. Approximately 380 medical students are enrolled at the college, and over 100 students are pursuing graduate degrees in the biomedical sciences. The faculty includes more than 450 full-time and 1,700 voluntary members in 20 academic departments. The faculty have expertise in a wide range of biomedical subjects. Research emphasized at the college includes the following multispecialty areas: the neurosciences, oncology, cardiovascular and pulmonary diseases, medical imaging, geriatric medicine, immunology, molecular biology and human genetics, and neonatology.

The UCI Clinical Services System consists of the UCI Medical Center, off-site outpatient facilities, and numerous affiliated hospitals and clinics that participate in the educational and research programs of the college.

CURRICULUM

The college offers a well-balanced curriculum in the clinical and basic sciences through educational and research programs in 20 academic departments. The curriculum consists of 16 instructional periods spread over four years, including a 10-week vacation period between the first and second years, and up to 12 weeks of vacation in the senior year. The core curriculum provides a body of knowledge and skills considered requisite for all those receiving the M.D. degree, regardless of their specific specialty choices.

The first two years of the curriculum are scheduled on a modified quarter system and concentrate on the sciences basic to clinical medicine and preclinical courses. The third and fourth years of the core curriculum consist of clinical clerkships and are scheduled according to 10-week quintiles. Students are also provided ample opportunity to participate in clinical and research elective courses of their choosing.

The focus of this curriculum is on active medical student participation toward the achievement of educational objectives. Demonstrations, small-group discussions, seminars, laboratory work by students, student projects oriented to problem solving, and exposure to clinical situations are integral parts of this focus. An honors/pass/fail grading system is used.

An ongoing Academic Monitoring Program beginning with enrollment is coordinated by the Office of Student and Resident Affairs to identify students in academic difficulty early in their course work and to ensure the availability of all resources before serious academic difficulties are encountered. Faculty advisors are assigned to all students to provide academic advice through their medical school years. A Peer Tutoring Program is available to all medical students to provide tutorial assistance in the basic and clinical sciences. Study skills training and USMLE review courses are also provided.

A combined M.D.-Ph.D. degree is available through the Medical Scientist Program for highly qualified students who have the required academic background, research experience, and strong commitment to a career in biomedical research. Applicants to the Medical Scientist Program must notify the College of Medicine and complete a supplemental application form. In applying for the program, students must meet the admission requirements of both the College of Medicine and the Office of Research and Graduate Studies, as well as the specific admission requirements of the individual graduate program they select.

In addition, students who meet the requirements also have the opportunity to complete the M.B.A. degree offered by UCI's Graduate School of Management.

REQUIREMENTS FOR ENTRANCE

The MCAT and a minimum of three full years of undergraduate college course work are required; however, almost all students accepted in recent years have obtained their bachelor's degrees. The latest MCAT that can be accepted is that given in August of the year before anticipated admission.

Minimum requirements include the successful completion of the following courses with a grade of C or better:

	Sem. hrs.
Biology and/or zoology	12
Must include one year of lower division biology and/or zoology plus one-half year of upper division courses, excluding botany.	
General chemistry	8
Organic chemistry	8
Physics	8
Calculus	(1 qtr.)
Biochemistry	3

Applicants who do not meet these requirements or who do not indicate that these subjects will be completed by the date of entrance will not be considered for admission.

The Admissions Committee desires to admit students with diverse backgrounds, and no specific undergraduate major is required; however, demonstrated ability in the sciences is of great importance.

SELECTION FACTORS

The UCI College of Medicine seeks to admit students who are highly qualified to receive training in the practice of medicine, and whose backgrounds, talents, and experiences contribute to the college's goal of achieving a broad spectrum of diversity in the student body. The Admissions Committee carefully reviews all applicants whose undergraduate record and scores on the MCAT indicate that they will be able to handle the rigorous curriculum of medical school. Careful consideration is given to applicants from disadvantaged backgrounds (that is, disadvantaged through social, cultural, and/or economic conditions). In addition to scholastic achievement, attributes deemed desirable in prospective students include indications of leadership ability and participation in extracurricular activities, such as research and medically related experience, as well as community service. Preference is given to California residents and consideration is given only to those applicants who are either U.S. citizens or permanent residents.

The AMCAS application is used for preliminary screening. Upon decisions of the Admissions Committee, applicants may be asked to submit additional information. Invitations for personal interviews are extended. The UCI College of Medicine does not provide funds for interview trips; however, interview reports from other medical schools may be submitted in place of on-campus interviews.

The Admissions Committee reviews the academic records, letters of recommendation, and the results of personal interviews before making its final selections.

The 1999 entering class had the following statistics: *mean science GPA*, 3.65; *mean GPA*, 3.67, *mean MCAT*, 10.59.

FINANCIAL AID

The Office of Medical Student Financial Aid offers a variety of aid programs (scholarships, grants, and loans) to assist medical students. To qualify for assistance from most of these programs, an applicant must demonstrate financial need. Currently, 87 percent of the entering students receive aid of some type. For further information, call (949) 824-6476.

INFORMATION FOR DISADVANTAGED APPLICANTS

Qualified applicants from disadvantaged backgrounds are encouraged to apply. The application fee may be waived to individuals granted a fee waiver by AMCAS. Programs for the recruitment and retention of disadvantaged students have been developed through the Office of Admissions and Outreach. For further information, call (949) 824-8930.

Public Institution

APPLICATION AND ACCEPTANCE POLICIES FOR 2001–2002 FIRST-YEAR CLASS

School participates in AMCAS. See Chapter 6.

Filing of AMCAS application
  Earliest date: June 1, 2000
  Latest date: Nov. 1, 2000
School application fee after screening: $40
  Oldest MCAT scores considered: 1998
Does not have Early Decision Program
Acceptance notice to regular applicants
  Earliest date: Nov. 15, 2000
  Latest date: Until class is filled
Applicant's response to acceptance offer
  Maximum time: 2 weeks
Requests for deferred entrance considered: Yes
Deposit to hold place in class: None
Estimated number of new entrants: 92
Starting date: Sept. 2001

TUITION AND STUDENT FEES PER YEAR FOR 1999–2000 FIRST-YEAR CLASS

Tuition
  Resident: None
  Nonresident: $9,804

Academic fees: $10,805

INFORMATION ON 1999–2000 FIRST-YEAR CLASS

Number of	*In-State*	*Out-of-State*	*Total*
Applicants	3,393	390	3,783
Applicants Interviewed	421	8	429
New Entrants*	92	0	92

*All took the MCAT and had baccalaureate degrees.

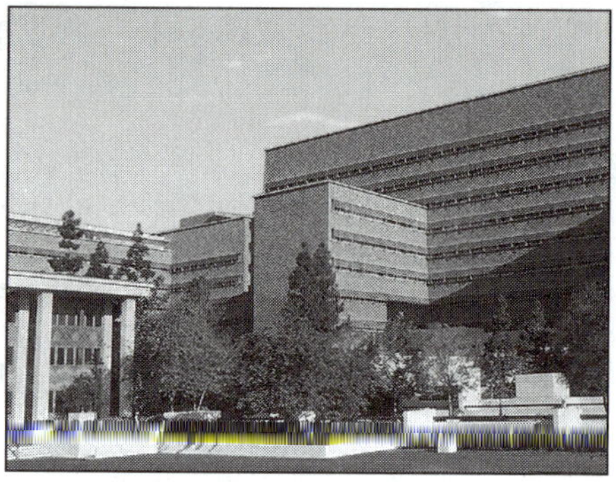

University of California, Los Angeles UCLA School of Medicine

Los Angeles, California

Dr. Gerald Levey, *Dean*
Dr. Neil Parker, *Dean for Admissions and Students*
Lili Fobert, *Director of Admissions*

ADDRESS INQUIRIES TO:

UCLA School of Medicine
Office of Admissions, Box 957035
Los Angeles, California 90095-7035
(310) 825-6081
Web Site: http://www.medstudent.ucla.edu/admissions

GENERAL INFORMATION

The UCLA School of Medicine graduated its first class in 1955. The medical school is situated on the UCLA campus. The University Medical Center, UCLA Ambulatory Medical Plaza, UCLA Childrens Hospital, and Stein Eye Institute are adjacent to the school. These institutions, together with the Santa Monica Hospital and the School of Dentistry, Nursing, and Public Health, are integral parts of the School of Medicine and the Center for the Health Sciences. Close affiliation exists between the UCLA School of Medicine and the Los Angeles County Harbor/UCLA Medical Center, the Veterans Administration Medical Centers at West Los Angeles and Sepulveda, Cedars-Sinai Medical Center, and Olive View Medical Center.

CURRICULUM

The first two years of a four-year curriculum present a thorough knowledge of the sciences basic to medicine. An integrated approach to basic and clinical sciences is enhanced through problem-based learning in small-discussion groups in most courses of the first- and second-year curricula. Students are introduced to a holistic approach to patient care from the beginning of medical school and throughout the curriculum, through the innovative and nationally recognized doctoring courses. The second year centers on the processes of disease, with emphasis on organ-system oriented instruction. The third year has a core curriculum of clinical clerkships encompassing the areas of internal medicine, surgery, obstetrics and gynecology, pediatrics, psychiatry, family practice, radiology, neurology, head and neck, orthopedics, urology, and ophthalmology. The school is moving to a special focus in the fourth year to provide a meaningful clinical and educational experience. Electives in the clinical continuum are designed to give students a foundation on which to develop and fulfill their personal interests, broaden their clinical knowledge, and give them an educational advantage in securing the clinical training calculated to best prepare them for postgraduate medical training. In 1993, UCLA initiated a pass-fail grading system with letters of distinction possible for outstanding performance.

Students are encouraged to participate in school and student organized activities. During the school year, students run clinics at the Salvation Army Homeless Center, Health Fairs, and DOC/STATS, which teach high school students about preventive health. Summers are filled with research projects, clinic and community work, as well as educational endeavors and opportunities such as international electives.

A Medical Scientist Training Program, leading to both M.D. and Ph.D. degrees, is available for a limited number of students who desire careers in medical research. This program requires six to seven years to complete and provides rigorous research training in addition to the medical curriculum. Stipends are available for some of the students in this program.

New programs leading to the M.D.-M.B.A. and M.D.-M.P.H. over a five-year period are available.

DREW/UCLA MEDICAL PROGRAM

Approximately 24 of the 145 students admitted each year have been admitted to the Drew/UCLA Medical Program. This program is designed to attract students who have an interest in addressing the concerns of underserved populations. Students will spend their first two years at the UCLA campus and their second two years at the Drew campus. Interested applicants should contact: Charles R. Drew University of Medicine and Science, 1621 East 120th Street, Los Angeles, California 90059; or call (323) 563-4960.

UCR/UCLA BIOMEDICAL SCIENCES PROGRAM

An additional 24 students are admitted to the UCLA School of Medicine through participation in the UCR/UCLA Biomedical Sciences Program, a cooperative venture with the University of California, Riverside (UCR). Students follow an integrated course of study through five years on the UCR campus and the final two years of clinical studies at the UCLA School of Medicine. Interested high school students should write to: Division of Biomedical Sciences; University of California, Riverside; Riverside, California 92521-0121.

REQUIREMENTS FOR ENTRANCE

The MCAT and three years of college are required. Ordinarily a baccalaureate degree is required, but in exceptional instances those who have completed three full academic years at an approved college or university will be considered. The required courses are:

	Years
English and composition	1
College physics (with lab)	1
Chemistry (with lab)	2
(Must include study of inorganic chemistry and organic chemistry)	
Biology	1
(One year of general biology with lab)	
College mathematics	1

Study of introductory calculus and statistics is required.

Spanish, computer skills, and humanities are recommended.

Candidates are urged to take the MCAT in the spring rather than in the summer of the year of application.

SELECTION FACTORS

The Admissions Committee gives preference to those applicants who present evidence of broad training and high achievement in their college education and possess, in the greatest degree, those traits of personality and character essential to success in medicine. Applicants whose records are judged by the Admissions Committee to qualify them for further consideration will receive a supplemental application. The completed applications are reviewed on the basis of letters of recommendation, supplemental applications, personal comments, GPA, and MCAT scores. Qualified applicants will receive an interview with members of the Admissions Committee.

In the 1999 entering class, accepted students had the following profile: *mean science GPA,* 3.64; *mean nonscience GPA,* 3.73. Applicants to the 1999 class had the following profile: *mean overall science GPA,* 3.31; *mean nonscience GPA,* 3.47.

Selections are made on the basis of individual qualifications and not on the basis of race, sex, creed, age, sexual orientation, national origin, or handicap. A third application is discouraged.

FINANCIAL AID

Scholarships and loan funds from private, state, and federal sources are available to all U.S. citizens and are awarded on the basis of need and/or scholarship. The school makes every effort to provide as much aid as possible. Outside employment is not prohibited but is discouraged.

DISADVANTAGED APPLICANTS

The UCLA School of Medicine Admissions Committee is composed of subcommittees, one of which is devoted exclusively to the consideration of applicants who have had a disadvantaged educational or financial background. This admissions subcommittee, which is composed of faculty and medical students, makes recommendations for action to be taken on disadvantaged applicants, although final decisions are made by the full Admissions Committee.

ADDITIONAL INFORMATION

The decision of which medical school to attend is extremely important. In addition to the school of medicine brochure, which is located on our Web site, we hope to provide the applicant with critical information through our School of Medicine and Student Affairs Web sites. Additionally, students may check their application status on the Admission Web page. Students invited for interviews will have the opportunity to have student-led tours and meet with faculty, staff, and members of the Admissions Committee.

Public Institution

APPLICATION AND ACCEPTANCE POLICIES FOR 2001–2002 FIRST-YEAR CLASS

School participates in AMCAS. See Chapter 6.

Filing of AMCAS application
  Earliest date: June 1, 2000
  Latest date: Nov. 1, 2000
School application fee after screening: $40
Oldest MCAT scores considered: 1998
Does not have Early Decision Program
Acceptance notice to regular applicants
  Earliest date: Jan. 15, 2001
  Latest date: Aug. 1, 2001
Applicant's response to acceptance offer
  Maximum time: 2 weeks
Requests for deferred entrance considered: Yes
Deposit to hold place in class: None
Estimated number of new entrants: 145 (121 UCLA, 24 Drew/UCLA, 24 UCR/UCLA)
Starting date: Aug. 2001

TUITION AND STUDENT FEES PER YEAR FOR 1999–2000 FIRST-YEAR CLASS

Tuition
  Resident: None
  Nonresident: $9,804

Academic fees: $9,993

INFORMATION ON 1999–2000 FIRST-YEAR CLASS

Number of	*In-State*	*Out-of-State*	*Total*
Applicants	3,434	2,083	5,517
Applicants Interviewed	483	152	635
New Entrants*	96	25	121

*All took the MCAT and had baccalaureate degrees.

CHAPTER 11

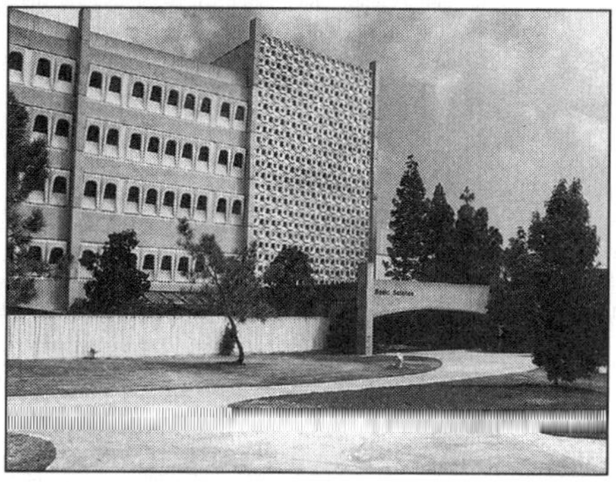

University of California, San Diego School of Medicine

La Jolla, California

Dr. David N. Bailey, *Dean*
Dr. Robert Resnik, *Associate Dean for Admissions*
Linda Whitson, *Director of Admissions*

ADDRESS INQUIRIES TO:

Office of Admissions, 0621
Medical Teaching Facility
University of California, San Diego
School of Medicine
9500 Gilman Drive
La Jolla, California 92093-0621
(858) 534-3880; 534-5282 (FAX)
Web Site: http://www.medicine.ucsd.edu

GENERAL INFORMATION

The simultaneous development of the School of Medicine and the general campus at the University of California, San Diego (UCSD), has fostered implementation of innovative programs enabling the medical students to benefit from the diversity of university faculty, from a wide variety of laboratory teaching facilities, and from a broad spectrum of clinical opportunities. Located on the main campus of the university at La Jolla, the School of Medicine is surrounded by learning resources and research institutions representing all disciplines. Unusual opportunities exist for integrating instruction in medical and related sciences with the natural sciences and disciplines centering on man in his social milieu. Clinical instruction is carried on at University of California Medical Center, Veterans Administration Hospital, Naval Regional Medical Center, and eight other affiliated hospitals and clinics.

CURRICULUM

The goal of the medical curriculum and faculty-student interactions is to develop critical, objective, conscientious physicians prepared for changing conditions of medical practice and continuing self-education.

The curriculum is divided into two major components: the core curriculum and the elective programs. These are pursued concurrently, with the core curriculum predominating in the early years. The core curriculum includes those aspects of medical education deemed essential for every medical student regardless of background or ultimate career direction. The integrated core curriculum of the first two years is designed to provide each entering student with an essential understanding of the fundamental disciplines underlying modern medicine. The core curriculum of the last two years is composed of the major clinical specialties taught in hospital settings, outpatient situations, and relevant extended-care facilities.

Each student is required to plan and complete an Independent Study Project in consultation with a member of the faculty. A written document is required in all projects. Other components are devised by the student and faculty member.

A Medical Scientist Training Program has been designed to provide the opportunity to earn both the M.D. and Ph.D. degrees over a six- to seven-year period of study for a limited number of students.

A Medical Scholars Program (B.S.-M.D.) is available for outstanding California high school seniors planning careers in medicine. A maximum of twelve students accepted to UCSD undergraduate school will also be provisionally accepted into the School of Medicine to begin their medical studies following receipt of their undergraduate degree. This is not an accelerated program.

REQUIREMENTS FOR ENTRANCE

The MCAT is required. A minimum of three years of college is required, including one full-time year at an accredited U.S. four-year university; the baccalaureate degree is preferred. It is recommended that students take their course of study in the most demanding curricular environment possible. Minimal requirements are successful completion of the following courses with a grade of C or better:

Biology: One year of college-level biology (excluding botany and biochemistry (8 sem. hrs.).
Chemistry: Two years of college-level chemistry; must include one year of organic chemistry (16 sem. hrs.).
Physics: One year of college-level general physics (8 sem. hrs.).
Mathematics: One year of course work; only calculus, statistics, or computer science will be considered (8 sem. hrs.).
English: Competence in speaking and writing English is required.

A broad base of knowledge is advantageous in preparing for the many roles of a physician and may include courses in: behavioral sciences, the biology of cells and development, genetics, biochemistry, English, or social sciences. Proficiency in a foreign language, such as Spanish, is considered highly desirable.

The Admissions Committee will only consider applicants who have taken the MCAT and completed the academic prerequisites.

SELECTION FACTORS

The Admissions Committee selects applicants who have demonstrated intelligence, maturity, integrity, and dedication to the ideal of service to society and who are best suited for an educational curriculum designed to prepare students for care of the total patient either in preparation for primary care specialization or as a groundwork for other fields of medicine. The school is seeking a student body with a broad diversity of backgrounds and interests reflecting our diverse population. The Admissions Committee has no preference as to undergraduate major but does prefer students with evidence of broad training and in-depth achievement in a particular area of knowledge, whether in the humanities, social sciences, or natural sciences.

Preference is necessarily afforded to California residents, and consideration is given only to applicants who are either U.S. citizens or permanent residents. Candidates are evaluated on the nature and depth of scholarly and extracurricular activities undertaken, their academic record, performance on the MCAT, letters of recommendation, and personal interviews. The Admissions Committee interview evaluates the applicant's abilities and skills necessary to satisfy the nonacademic or technical standards established by the faculty and the personal and emotional characteristics that are necessary to become an effective physician. The UCSD School of Medicine participates in the WICHE Professional Student Exchange Program for applicants from certain western states without medical schools. The School of Medicine does not accept transfer students.

Accepted students for the 1999 entering class had the following credentials: *mean GPA,* 3.65; *sex,* 39 percent women; *residence,* 98 percent from California; *undergraduate major,* 50 percent in biology or chemistry, with the remainder in the physical sciences, humanities, and social sciences; overall formal application and acceptance rates, 55 percent of those students interviewed received acceptances, and 287 acceptances were offered to obtain a class of 122 students.

FINANCIAL AID

Financial aid in the form of scholarships, grants, loans, and work opportunities is offered to help students in need of financial assistance. Approximately 90 percent of the students receive financial assistance during their four years of study. Medical Scientist Training Program participants may receive full tuition and a stipend for up to six years. An application form for financial aid is sent to every accepted student upon request.

DISADVANTAGED APPLICANTS

The UCSD School of Medicine is committed to expanding the educational opportunities for applicants coming from disadvantaged educational or economic backgrounds. This institutional commitment is expressed through a prematriculation summer program, tutorial support programs, and financial aid assistance.

Since the inception of the School of Medicine, it has been a national leader in maintaining a diverse student body and providing outreach programs for socioeconomically disadvantaged students at grade school through high school levels. The School of Medicine recognizes that disadvantaged students are under represented in the medical profession and regards a diverse student body among its highest priorities.

Public Institution

APPLICATION AND ACCEPTANCE POLICIES FOR 2001–2002 FIRST-YEAR CLASS

School participates in AMCAS. See Chapter 6.

Filing of AMCAS application
- Earliest date: June 1, 2000
- Latest date: Nov. 1, 2000

School application fee after screening: $40
Oldest MCAT scores considered: 1998
Does not have Early Decision Program
Acceptance notice to regular applicants
- Earliest date: Oct. 15, 2000
- Latest date: Until class is filled

Applicant's response to acceptance offer
- Maximum time: 2 weeks

Requests for deferred entrance considered: Yes
- Deposit to hold place in class: None

Estimated number of new entrants: 122
Starting date: Aug. 2001

TUITION AND STUDENT FEES PER YEAR FOR 1999–2000 FIRST-YEAR CLASS

Tuition
- Resident: None
- Nonresident: $9,804

Academic fees: $10,324

INFORMATION ON 1999–2000 FIRST-YEAR CLASS

Number of	*In-State*	*Out-of-State*	*Total*
Applicants	3,278	1,309	4,587
Applicants Interviewed	470	48	518
New Entrants*	119	3	122

*All took the MCAT; 99% had baccalaureate degrees.

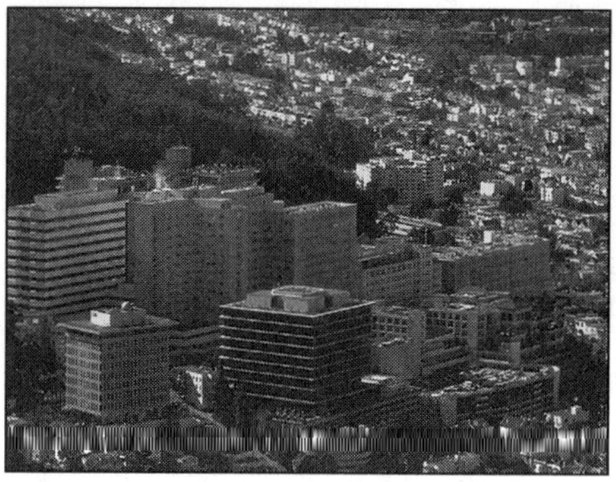

University of California, San Francisco School of Medicine

San Francisco, California

Dr. Haile T. Debas, *Dean*
Dr. Michael V. Drake, *Associate Dean for Admissions*
Kathleen Ryan, *Admissions Officer*

ADDRESS INQUIRIES TO:

School of Medicine, Admissions
C-200, Box 0408
University of California, San Francisco
San Francisco, California 94143
(415) 476-4044
Web Site: http://www.som.ucsf.edu

MISSION STATEMENT

The educational mission of the University of California, San Francisco (UCSF) School of Medicine is to provide a supportive and challenging educational environment in which students of diverse backgrounds prepare themselves for careers characterized by commitment to excellence, lifelong learning, and service to others through patient care, research, and teaching.

CURRICULUM

During the first two years, the primary focus is integrated core instruction in the basic, behavioral, social, and clinical sciences, and clinical experiences is introduced within the first weeks of classes. Emphasis is placed on small-group teaching. Students begin longitudinal patient experiences during the foundations of patient care course. In the last two years the various clinical departments provide 44 weeks of core clerkships, which teach students the basic skills of clinical medicine.The third-year core includes additional weeks of advanced integration of basic and behavioral science experiences, including clinical intersessions. An additional 42 weeks of clinical and basic science courses must be elected from a wide range of offerings at UCSF medical center and other hospitals.

The grading system is pass/not pass. Honors recognition is assigned on an individual basis in third- and fourth-year courses of three units or more.

There are numerous opportunities for students to engage in research. They include the joint-degree programs, Student Research Fellowship Program, research electives, and various opportunities offered at UCSF and other institutions. Students who wish to do research should consult with the director of student research.

Special programs are available for students who wish to earn the M.D. degree jointly with the M.S., M.P.H., or Ph.D. degree. In addition, through the Medical Scientist Training Program, approximately six to eight students in each class may obtain the M.D. and Ph.D. degrees in six or more years of study.

The Joint Medical Program, sponsored by the University of California at Berkeley and San Francisco, is a five-year graduate and professional program leading to M.S. and M.D. degrees. The goal of the graduate segment (three years at Berkeley) is to develop students' abilities to approach problems of health and disease that require in-depth training in a variety of disciplines. Basic science and introductory clinical courses are enriched by individually structured master's degree programs in selected areas of the medical sciences or in the social sciences pertinent to health care. Upon the student's completion of the Berkeley phase of the program, including a master's thesis, an M.S. degree in health and medical sciences is awarded. Students then transfer to UCSF for the remainder of their training for the M.D. degree. The size of each class is limited to 12 students. Details are available from: Graduate Office, Health and Medical Sciences Program, 570 University Hall, #1190 University of California, Berkeley, California 94720; telephone (510) 642-5671.

REQUIREMENTS FOR ENTRANCE

The MCAT and a minimum of three years of college are required. A baccalaureate degree is strongly recommended but not required. The MCAT must be taken within three years of application but no later than August of the year prior to matriculation. However, applicants are strongly urged to take the test the preceding spring rather than the summer.

Applicants must complete 135 quarter units (90 semester units) of acceptable transfer college credit by June of the year of desired entry. These courses must be completed at an accredited institution; moreover, only 105 acceptable quarter units may be transferred from a junior college. Courses must include:

	Qtr. hrs.
Biology or zoology (with lab)	12
Must include vertebrate zoology.	
General chemistry (with lab)	12
Organic chemistry	8
Physics (with lab)	12

Survey courses in the sciences are not acceptable as fulfilling the requirements in science.

It is to the applicant's advantage to complete the above prerequisites before taking the MCAT and filing an application.

SECONDARY APPLICATION INFORMATION

Upon receipt of the AMCAS application, applicants are sent a preliminary acknowledgment card. All files are reviewed on a rolling basis, therefore supporting documents should not be sent unless specifically requested to do so. Any letters of recommendation received prior to UCSF requesting them will be destroyed.

Applicant files pass through two screening processes within 8 to 12 weeks, and applicants are notified by the receipt of a secondary application or a letter of denial. Applicants sent a secondary application are asked to submit a minimum of three letters of recommendation, including two letters from the applicant's instructors. A maximum of five letters is preferred. If the applicant's undergraduate school has a premedical committee or its equivalent (an office that gathers all letters), letters must be sent from that committee or office.

Applications to the Medical Scientist Training Program and the UC Berkeley/UC San Francisco Joint Medical Program are included in the secondary application materials. Applicants may apply to the regular medical program and one or both of these programs at that time.

MEDICAL SCHOOL ADMISSIONS INFORMATION

Selection is based on an appraisal of both intellectual and personal characteristics, which the Admissions Committee regards as desirable for prospective medical students and physicians. Based on these considerations, a limited number of applicants (500) are selected for interview. Personal interviews are required of applicants who pass the second screening. Regional interviews are not available.

Successful applicants tend to have strong academic records; firm and clear motivation for medicine, which is manifested in their work experience, activities, or interests; and outstanding personal qualities. Academic performance is evaluated in relation to background, with the aim of determining the influence of external factors on this parameter. Since preference is given to California residents, only nonresidents with superior qualifications are encouraged to apply. Foreigners who are not permanent residents of the United States should not apply unless they have superior qualifications and adequate funding for their medical education and living expenses. The School of Medicine does not accept transfer students at any level, except for those students in the D.D.S.-M.D. program.

The School of Medicine has a long-standing commitment to increasing the number of physicians who are members of minority groups. As a result, over the last 30 years UCSF has had one of the highest minority enrollment and graduation rates of continental U.S. medical schools. In addition, the medical school welcomes applications from socioeconomically disadvantaged persons.

The UCSF School of Medicine does not discriminate on the basis of race, color, national origin, disability, religion, sex, sexual orientation, or age in any of its policies, procedures, or practices.

Some statistics of the 1999 entering class were: *mean cumulative GPA,* 3.75; *mean science GPA,* 3.77; *mean MCAT scores, VR*-11, *PS*-12, *BS*-12; 56 percent women; *nonwhite ethnic groups,* 54 percent; *underrepresented minority groups,* 17 percent.

FINANCIAL AID

A limited number of scholarships are awarded to entering students on the basis of scholarship and/or need. General financial support is awarded through the Student Financial Services Office. Aid packages consist of a combination of loans, grants-in-aid, and scholarships. Financial aid is only available to U.S. citizens or permanent residents of the United States.

Public Institution

APPLICATION AND ACCEPTANCE POLICIES FOR 2001–2002 FIRST-YEAR CLASS

School participates in AMCAS. See Chapter 6.

Filing of AMCAS application
  Earliest date: June 1, 2000
  Latest date: Nov. 1, 2000
School application fee after screening: $40
Oldest MCAT scores considered: 1998
Does not have Early Decision Program
Acceptance notice to regular applicants
  Earliest date: Dec. 15, 2000
  Latest date: Until class is filled
Applicant's response to acceptance offer
  Maximum time: 2 weeks
Requests for deferred entrance considered: Yes
Deposit to hold place in class: None
Estimated number of new entrants: 141
Starting date: Sept. 2001 (June 2001 for UCB-UCSF Joint Medical Program)

TUITION AND STUDENT FEES PER YEAR FOR 1999–2000 FIRST-YEAR CLASS

Tuition
  Resident: None
  Nonresident: $9,804

Academic Fees: $10,188

INFORMATION ON 1999–2000 FIRST-YEAR CLASS

Number of	*In-State*	*Out-of-State*	*Total*
Applicants	2,630	2,473	5,103
Applicants Interviewed	*	*	500
New Entrants†	105	36	141

*Data not available.
†All took the MCAT and had baccalaureate degrees.

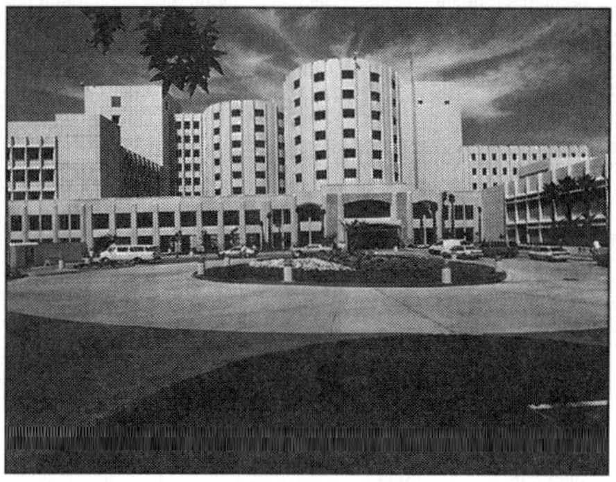

Loma Linda University School of Medicine

Loma Linda, California

Dr. Brian S. Bull, *Dean*
Dr. John Thorn, *Associate Dean for Admissions*
Verdell Schaefer, *Financial Aid Officer*

ADDRESS INQUIRIES TO:

Associate Dean for Admissions
Loma Linda University
School of Medicine
Loma Linda, California 92350
(909) 558-4467; 558-0359 (FAX)
Web Site: http://www.llu.edu
E-mail: ledwards@som.llu.edu

MISSION STATEMENT

Our overriding purpose is the formation of Christian physicians, educated to serve as generalists or specialists providing whole-person care to individuals, families, and communities.

GENERAL INFORMATION

The School of Medicine was organized in 1909 at Loma Linda. The campus is composed of basic science facilities and Loma Linda University Medical Center, which includes the Children's Hospital and the Loma Linda University Community Medical Center. Also used for clinical instruction are Loma Linda Behavioral Medicine Center, Jerry L. Pettis Memorial Veterans Hospital, Riverside County Regional Medical Center, and the White Memorial Medical Center in Los Angeles. San Bernardino County General Hospital, Kaiser Foundation Hospital, and Glendale Adventist Medical Center are also affiliated with the School of Medicine and are utilized for undergraduate and postgraduate clinical training.

Objectives of the School of Medicine include providing the student with a solid foundation of medical knowledge, assisting the student in the attainment of professional skills, and motivating investigative curiosity and a desire to participate in the advancement of knowledge. The school endeavors to reinforce interest in the practical application of Christian principles through service to humanity.

CURRICULUM

The major objective of the School of Medicine is to prepare students who will be well grounded in the science and art of medicine and who also will be prepared after further training for the practice of general medicine or any specialty.

The first two years are primarily devoted to the study of the basic medical sciences, including the relationship to pathology and clinical application, and the introduction to physical diagnosis and human behavior. The last two years provide clinical rotations in the major areas of medical practice: surgery, internal medicine, pediatrics, obstetrics-gynecology, family medicine, emergency medicine, ambulatory care, and psychiatry, as well as didactic and practical experience in preventive medicine. Elective time is available for various types of additional educational experience in the clinical or research areas to prepare students in their selection of postgraduate medical education.

Qualified students interested in a career in academic medicine may earn an M.S. or Ph.D. degree along with the M.D. degree. Six to seven years are required to complete this program.

Performance of students is evaluated by means of standard or scaled scores. The grading system is on a pass/fail basis.

REQUIREMENTS FOR ENTRANCE

The MCAT and a minimum of three years (90 semester hours or 135 quarter hours) of collegiate preparation in an accredited college or university in the United States or Canada are required. Preference is given to applicants who will have completed the baccalaureate degree prior to matriculation. No major is preferred, but a broad educational background is encouraged; however, demonstrated ability in the sciences is important. Rejected applicants may reapply and usually will receive the same consideration as first-time applicants.

Required courses are:

	Sem./Qtr. hrs.
General biology or zoology (with lab)	8/12
General or inorganic chemistry (with lab)	8/12
Organic chemistry (with lab)	8/12
Physics (with lab)	8/12
English	

Equivalent to satisfy baccalaureate degree requirement.

Biochemistry is strongly recommended.

Additionally, keyboard and computer skills are considered essential; further, an introductory course in basic statistics is recommended.

CLEP and pass/fail performances are not acceptable for the required courses.

Applicants are urged to take the MCAT in the spring of the year of application and to have the basic requirements completed at the time of application.

SELECTION FACTORS

The Admissions Committee seeks candidates who have demonstrated the greatest potential for becoming capable physicians. A strong academic background is needed in preparation for medical studies. While special attention is given to the performance in science courses, candidates should also have a solid foundation in the humanities, social sciences, and human behavior.

The Admissions Committee looks for applicants who demonstrate problem-solving skills, critical judgment, and the ability to pursue independent study and thinking. In evaluating academic achievements, the Admissions Committee considers such factors as the difficulty of the program, the need to work, social and cultural hardship, and participation in meaningful extracurricular activities. For nonacademic qualifications, the committee looks for a commitment to medicine, judgment, a positive attitude, ability to make decisions, emotional stability, and integrity.

The School of Medicine is owned and operated by the Seventh-day Adventist church; therefore, preference for admission is given to members of this church. However, it is a firm policy of the Admissions Committee to admit each year a number of nonchurch-related applicants who have demonstrated a strong commitment to Christian principles. No candidate is accepted on the basis of religious affiliation alone. The school does not discriminate on the basis of race, sex, age, or handicap.

After receipt of the AMCAS application, each applicant is requested to submit the supplementary form and supply preprofessional faculty evaluations and/or personal letters of recommendation. Invitations for an interview are extended to selected applicants on the medical school campus and on a regional basis at selected locations throughout the country.

Applicants with an outstanding academic record and with a particular interest in Loma Linda University School of Medicine are encouraged to apply through the Early Decision Program (EDP). Contact the associate dean for admissions prior to submitting AMCAS application.

Final selection is made by the Admissions Committee on the basis of overall scholastic record, personal character qualifications, and promise of success as a physician. Matriculated students for the class of 1999 had a *mean overall GPA* of 3.66.

FINANCIAL AID

The School of Medicine has limited loan funds available through the Student Finance Office. All aid is awarded on the basis of a uniform needs analysis. Financial aid information is provided to all accepted students. In view of the costs of a medical education, students are urged to plan their financial program carefully.

Private Institution

APPLICATION AND ACCEPTANCE POLICIES FOR 2001–2002 FIRST-YEAR CLASS

School participates in AMCAS. See Chapter 6.

Filing of AMCAS application
  Earliest date: June 1, 2000
  Latest date: Nov. 1, 2000
School application fee to all applicants: $75
Oldest MCAT scores considered: 1998
Does have Early Decision Program (EDP)
  EDP application period: June 1–Aug. 1, 2000
  EDP applicants notified by: Oct. 1, 2000
Acceptance notice to regular applicants
  Earliest date: Dec. 15, 2000
  Latest date: Until class is filled
Applicant's response to acceptance offer
  Maximum time: 30 days
Requests for deferred entrance considered: Yes
Deposit to hold place in class (applied to tuition):
  $100, due with response to acceptance offer
Deposit refundable prior to: May 15, 2001
Estimated number of new entrants: 159 (9 EDP)
Starting date: Aug. 2001

TUITION AND STUDENT FEES PER YEAR FOR 1999–2000 FIRST-YEAR CLASS

Tuition: $25,959 Student fees: $1,145

INFORMATION ON 1999–2000 FIRST-YEAR CLASS

Number of	*In-State*	*Out-of-State*	*Total*
Applicants	1,777	1,974	3,751
Applicants Interviewed	202	174	376
New Entrants*	82	78	160

*All took the MCAT; 97.5% had baccalaureate degrees.

CHAPTER 11

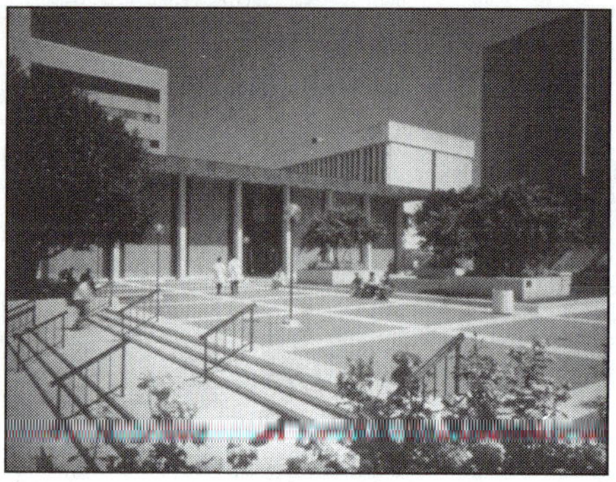

Keck School of Medicine of the University of Southern California

Los Angeles, California

Dr. Stephen J. Ryan, *Dean*
Dr. Erin A. Quinn, *Associate Dean for Admissions*
Robert J. Winikowski, *Director of Admissions*

ADDRESS INQUIRIES TO:

Office of Admissions
Keck School of Medicine of the
University of Southern California
1975 Zonal Avenue (KAM 100-C)
Los Angeles, California 90033
(323) 442-2552; 442-2433 (FAX)
E-mail: medadmit@hsc.usc.edu
Web Site: http://www.usc.edu/schools/medicine

MISSION STATEMENT

It is the mission of the Keck School of Medicine of the University of Southern California (USC) to improve society through the cultivation and enrichment of the human mind and spirit; to prevent and cure diseases and advance the science that makes this possible; and to lead in medical education, biomedical research, and health care delivery. Its highest priorities are to educate the next generation of physicians and biomedical scientists utilizing principles of research-based health care delivered with compassion, and according to the highest ethical and moral standards, to train students to be leaders in clinical medicine and basic science, and to instill in students the desire to pursue excellence throughout their lives.

GENERAL INFORMATION

USC, a privately supported, nondenominational, coeducational university, established its School of Medicine in 1885. The 31-acre campus is located directly across the street from its chief teaching hospital, the Los Angeles County+USC Medical Center. In addition to the Medical Center, which is one of the largest teaching centers in the United States, patient-care facilities include the 284-bed USC University Hospital, USC/Norris Cancer Center and Hospital, Doheny Eye Institute, Childrens Hospital Los Angeles, Rancho Los Amigos Medical Center, Hospital of the Good Samaritan, Barlow Respiratory Hospital, California Medical Center, Huntington Memorial Hospital, Presbyterian Intercommunity Hospital, House Ear Institute, Veterans Administration Outpatient Clinic, and White Memorial Medical Center.

CURRICULUM

Students are progressively involved in patient care beginning with patient contact during the first semester of the first year. An important feature is Introduction to Clinical Medicine, a course that begins in the freshman year and runs through the sophomore year. Doctor-patient relationships and interviewing are presented during the first year and physical diagnosis and history-taking are taught in the second. Groups of approximately six to seven students are led by a faculty member who serves as clinical tutor to these students for their first two years.

Basic sciences are taught largely in an organ system approach with increasing emphasis on case-based and computerized education. Appropriate material in the basic sciences is presented during the study of these systems; patients are observed and examined for clinical illustration of the subject under discussion. In this way, the student is better able to understand and retain the basic scientific principles of medicine.

In the second year the student studies the pathologic aspects of medicine, also predominantly in an organ system approach. In addition, a student may begin an investigative project sponsored by a department. The final two years are designed as a continuum of two academic calendar years. Each student's program is individually designed to include 52 weeks of required clerkships (i.e., medicine, general surgery, obstetrics-gynecology, pediatrics, psychiatry, neurology, family medicine, and surgical specialties), 12 weeks of selective clerkships at USC, 16 weeks of free electives, and a one-week clinical orientation program. In addition, 4 weeks are set aside for a required Physician in Society course.

Grading is on an honors, satisfactory, and unsatisfactory basis. Required clerkships include a near honors grading category.

SPECIAL PROGRAMS

Students have an opportunity to engage in clinical or basic research through voluntary participation in a summer fellowship program between the freshman and sophomore years.

The school sponsors an M.D.-Ph.D. program for those interested in obtaining these degrees jointly. A special fifth-year option is available for students who wish to pursue a research project and may be considering a career in academic medicine. A baccalaureate-M.D. program is offered and described in Chapter 10.

REQUIREMENTS FOR ENTRANCE

The MCAT and a minimum of four full years or 120 semester hours of academic work at an accredited college or university at the time of matriculation. Course work must include the following subjects:

	Sem./Qtr.
General Biology (with lab)	2/3
Organic chemistry (with lab)	1/2
General physics (with lab)	2/3
Biochemistry	1/1

Additionally, a course in basic molecular biology and 30 semester hours (or quarter equivalent) of course work in the social sciences, humanities, and English composition are required. Facility in the principles of college mathematics or calculus and in the use of computers as a tool for independent learning is recommended.

Applicants are strongly urged to take the MCAT in the spring of the year of application and to have their basic science requirements completed at the time of application.

Foreign students must have completed at least one year of study in an accredited university or college in the United States prior to application.

Individuals who have discontinued studies in medical school for academic reasons are not eligible to apply.

Applications for admission with advanced standing into the third year are accepted only from full-time medical students currently enrolled, or on approved leave-of-absence, and in good standing at an LCME-accredited medical school.

SELECTION FACTORS

The Admissions Committee seriously considers candidates whose academic achievement and MCAT performance indicate their ability to satisfactorily complete the rigorous curriculum of the medical school. Favorable consideration also reflects additional factors including motivation and evidence of qualities deemed desirable for the study and practice of medicine, significant achievements in nonacademic pursuits, and demonstrated commitment to service and community. The School of Medicine does not discriminate on the basis of race, creed, gender, nationality, residency, age, or handicap.

Receipt of the application from AMCAS is acknowledged. All candidates are requested to complete the supplemental application and arrange for submission of letters of recommendation. Interview selection is based upon careful evaluation of the application and all supporting documentation. Interviews are required of all applicants under serious consideration and are granted only by invitation of the Admissions Committee.

The 1999 entering class had a *mean GPA* of 3.50 and *mean MCAT* scores of 9.7 in Verbal Reasoning, 10.8 in Physical Sciences, and 10.9 in Biological Sciences. Women comprised 41 percent of the class, which came from 53 colleges and universities and 17 states. The mean age was 24 (range 20-34 years).

FINANCIAL AID

A variety of university scholarships and loans are available to supplement federal and state programs. Awards are based on need as demonstrated through a financial statement. Approximately 75 percent of students receive some type of financial assistance. Student employment during the academic year is discouraged. For additional information, contact Linda Lewis, director of financial aid, (323) 442-1016.

INFORMATION FOR MINORITY STUDENTS

The Office of Diversity provides supportive services to minority medical students, including organized tutorial assistance and group and individual counseling. Volunteer positions in various community clinics may be coordinated through the Office of Diversity. It also serves to create a warm environment where all students feel a sense of belonging. For more information, call (323) 442-1050.

Private Institution

APPLICATION AND ACCEPTANCE POLICIES FOR 2001–2002 FIRST-YEAR CLASS

School participates in AMCAS. See Chapter 6.

Filing of AMCAS application
  Earliest date: June 1, 2000
  Latest date: Nov. 1, 2000
School application fee to all applicants: $70
Oldest MCAT scores considered: 1998
Does have Early Decision Program (EDP)
  EDP application period: June 1–Aug. 1, 2000
  EDP applicants notified by: Oct. 1, 2000
Acceptance notice to regular applicants
  Earliest date: Jan. 1, 2001
  Latest date: Until class is filled
Applicant's response to acceptance offer
  Maximum time: 10 days
Requests for deferred entrance considered: Yes
Deposit to hold place in class (applied to tuition):
  $100, due with response to acceptance offer
Deposit refundable prior to: May 15, 2001
Estimated number of new entrants: 150
Starting date: Aug. 2001

TUITION AND STUDENT FEES PER YEAR FOR 1999–2000 FIRST-YEAR CLASS

Tuition: $32,266 Student fees: $1,108

INFORMATION ON 1999–2000 FIRST-YEAR CLASS

Number of	*In-State*	*Out-of-State*	*Total*
Applicants	*	*	5,466
Applicants Interviewed	*	*	500
New Entrants†	*	*	150

*Data not available.
†All took the MCAT and had baccalaureate degrees.

Stanford University School of Medicine

Stanford, California

Dr. Eugene A. Bauer, *Dean*
Dr. Gabriel Garcia, *Associate Dean of Admissions*
Charlene Hamada, *Director of Admissions*

ADDRESS INQUIRIES TO:

Office of Admissions
Stanford University School of Medicine
251 Campus Drive, Suite 309
Stanford, California 94305-5404
(650) 723-6861; 725-4599 (FAX)
Web Site: http://www.stanford.edu/

GENERAL INFORMATION

The school is part of the Stanford University Medical Center and consists of 26 departments. The major clinical teaching facilities are: Stanford University Hospital (663 beds), Lucile Packard Children's Hospital (152 beds), Santa Clara County Valley Medical Center (791 beds), and the Palo Alto Veterans Administration Hospital (1,000 beds). This association of hospitals provides facilities for comprehensive clinical training, and the school offers opportunities in many areas of fundamental and clinical research. Lane Medical Library has one of the largest collections of medical books in the West. SUMMIT (Stanford University Medical Media and Information Technologies) produces faculty- and student-authored programs.

CURRICULUM

The goals of the curriculum are to develop outstanding clinical skills in all students as well as the capacity for leadership in the practice of scientific medicine, and to prepare as many students as possible for careers in research and teaching. Stanford's flexible curriculum is its major innovative approach to medical education. This curriculum was designed to create an environment that encourages intellectual diversity and to provide opportunities for students to develop as individuals. While traditional courses and clerkships are required for graduation, the duration of study leading to the M.D. degree may vary from four to six years. Students have flexibility in sequencing courses and clerkships, and they may be exempt from basic science courses by demonstrating competency through examination. This curriculum stimulates self-directed learning, and it provides students time to pursue an investigative project, obtain teaching experience, perform community service, explore special interests, or obtain advanced degrees.

The required curriculum includes work in the basic medical sciences and clinical experiences in medicine, surgery, pediatrics, gynecology-obstetrics, and psychiatry. All M.D. candidates must satisfactorily complete at least 13 quarters of academic work. Fees for additional quarters are nominal. Students are encouraged to plan for a five-year course of study in order to include research activities, teaching assistantships, and a variety of elective courses both in the medical school and in other schools of the university in their educational enrichment plans. Thus, the time spent in medical school may vary with the individual student's background and study plans. Courses are graded pass/fail.

Stanford offers many opportunities for study in depth in the preclinical and clinical disciplines. Students with strong interests in careers in medical research should inquire from the Office of Admissions about the Medical Scientist Training Program (MSTP) or the training programs in cancer biology, immunology, medical information sciences, neurosciences, or pharmacology. These federally funded programs enable selected students to pursue research and course work leading to both the M.D. and Ph.D. degrees. Students request MSTP application forms on the supplementary application to the School of Medicine. Applications for other programs are also supplied on request to the specific department.

The medical school offers a summer matriculation program for new matriculants from disadvantaged backgrounds.

REQUIREMENTS FOR ENTRANCE

The MCAT is required, preferably taken in the spring but no later than late summer of the year of application. A baccalaureate degree is preferred but not required. Applicants seeking admission under unusual circumstances should contact the Office of Admissions. The minimal entry requirements are:

	Years
Biological science (with lab)	1
Chemistry, including organic chemistry (with labs)	2
Physics (with lab)	1

Courses in calculus, physical chemistry, behavioral sciences, and particularly in biochemistry are strongly recommended.

An undergraduate major in any field is acceptable, provided the candidate presents a record of outstanding achievement. Breadth of education and/or experience in the humanities and social sciences and knowledge of a foreign language are desirable.

SELECTION FACTORS

Stanford's educational milieu fosters rigorous scholarship and encourages students to develop investigative and innovative approaches to problems in medicine. The school seeks applicants who have a strong humanitarian commitment and whose originality, creativity, and independent critical thinking best equip them for this environment.

Stanford does not discriminate against applicants on the basis of race, religion, national origin, sex, marital status, age, or disability. The applicant's state of residence is irrelevant in the selection process. No preference is given to California residents. Foreign applicants must have completed a minimum of one year of study in a U.S., Canadian, or United Kingdom accredited college or university.

Acceptances are based upon standards of merit, and no quotas of any kind play a role in the evaluation or selection process.

In recent years, applicants granted admission have had a *mean GPA* of about 3.7 and *mean MCAT* scores as follows: *VR*-10, *PS*-11, *BS*-11. Applicants whose MCAT scores are below the national mean are highly unlikely to be admitted to the medical school.

The application fee applies to students who return the supplemental application and will be waived for applicants who have obtained a fee waiver from AMCAS. Otherwise, fee waiver requests must be accompanied by a supporting statement from the dean or financial aid officer.

Application during the summer or very early fall is strongly encouraged.

Transfer Students: For information on the transfer policy, you may contact the Office of Admissions at (650) 723-6861.

FINANCIAL AID

Acceptance is independent of the applicant's financial status, and Stanford makes every effort to ensure that students are not excluded from admission to the school for financial reasons. Approximately 70 percent of students receive some form of financial assistance. Available loan and grant funds are awarded to students on the basis of demonstrated need, as determined by a needs analysis. For federal aid, students are considered independent. For university-based aid, students are considered dependent, and the school will consider the student's parents' ability to contribute to the cost of financing the student's education in determining eligibility for university loans and grants. This applies regardless of your age, marital status, other graduate degrees, or the fact that you have been self-supporting for a number of years. Eligibility for aid is assessed according to the cost of attendance, and the student budget is standardized. Other approved expenses (outside the standard budget) will be met with a loan.

Foreign students who are not U.S. citizens or permanent residents are not eligible for federal or university-based aid. Foreign students must complete a certification of finances reflecting an escrow account of funds to cover their cost of education for the M.D. degree.

Teaching and research assistantships, for which students receive salary and tuition credit, can be used to offset loans, and may reduce the indebtedness of students on financial aid. However, these positions are not guaranteed, and should not be viewed as a way to meet expenses.

Applicants should complete the FAFSA at www.fafsa.ed.gov and the needs analysis at www.accessgrp.org as soon as possible after February 1 so that, if requested, a preliminary estimate of the financial aid award can be provided by the Office of Student Financial Services. The Supplemental Financial Aid application forms will be made available to all applicants who reach the interview stage. For additional information about financial aid, contact the Office of Student Financial Services at (650) 724-3181.

INFORMATION FOR MINORITY STUDENTS

Stanford has a student body that is highly qualified and diverse, which is essential to the education of physicians. With its strong belief in diversity, Stanford especially encourages applications from minorities, as well as from others whose background and experience provide additional dimensions to enhance the school's program. An early matric program, which includes preclinical course work and research opportunities, exists for students from disadvantaged backgrounds.

Private Institution

APPLICATION AND ACCEPTANCE POLICIES FOR 2001–2002 FIRST-YEAR CLASS

School participates in AMCAS. See Chapter 6.

Filing of AMCAS application
Earliest date: June 1, 2000
Latest date: Nov. 1, 2000
School application fee after screening: $55
Oldest MCAT scores considered: 1998
Deadline for complete application: Dec. 15, 2000
Does have Early Decision Program (EDP)
EDP application period: June 1–Aug. 1, 2000
EDP applicants notified by: Oct. 1, 2000
Acceptance notice to regular applicants
Earliest date: Oct. 15, 2000
Latest date: Until class is filled
Applicant's response to acceptance offer
Maximum time: 2 weeks
Requests for deferred entrance considered: Yes
Deposit to hold place in class: None
Estimated number of new entrants: 86 (2 EDP)
Starting date: Sept. 2001

TUITION AND STUDENT FEES PER YEAR FOR 1999–2000 FIRST-YEAR CLASS

Tuition: $28,548 Student fees: $694

INFORMATION ON 1999–2000 FIRST-YEAR CLASS

Number of	*In-State*	*Out-of-State*	*Total*
Applicants	2,328	4,102	6,430
Applicants Interviewed	303	316	619
New Entrants*	41	45	86

*All took the MCAT and had baccalaureate degrees.

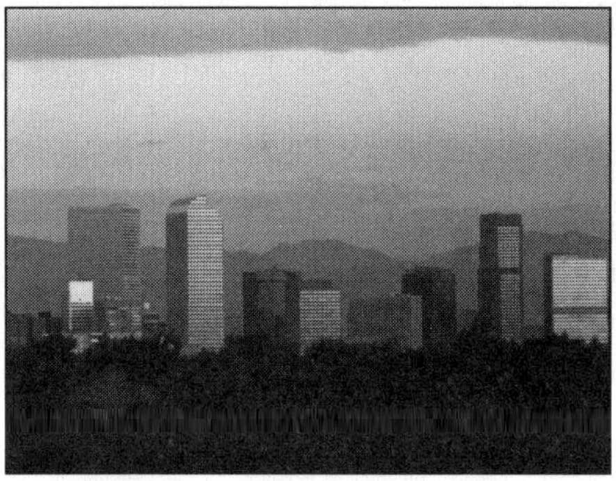

University of Colorado School of Medicine

Denver, Colorado

Dr. Richard D. Krugman, *Dean*
Dr. Maureen L. Garrity, *Associate Dean for Admissions*
Jane Nakata, *Director of Financial Aid*

ADDRESS INQUIRIES TO:

Medical School Admissions
University of Colorado
School of Medicine
4200 East 9th Avenue, C-297
Denver, Colorado 80262
(303) 315-7361; 315-8494 (FAX)
E-mail: somadmin@uchsc.edu
Web Site: http://www.uchsc.edu

MISSION STATEMENT

The mission of the University of Colorado School of Medicine is to provide Colorado, the nation, and the world with programs of excellence in:

- Education—through the provision of educational programs to medical students, allied health students, graduate students and housestaff, practicing health professionals, and the public at large;
- Research—through the development of new knowledge in the basic and clinical sciences, as well as in health policy and health care education;
- Clinical Care—through state-of-the-art clinical programs, which reflect the unique educational environment of the university, as well as the needs of the patients it serves; and,
- Community Service—through sharing the school's expertise and knowledge to enhance the broader community, including our affiliated institutions, other health care professionals, alumni and other colleagues, and citizens of the state.

GENERAL INFORMATION

The University of Colorado School of Medicine admitted its first students in 1883. The School of Medicine is a part of the University of Colorado Health Sciences Center, located in Denver. The Health Sciences Center also includes the schools of dentistry, nursing, pharmacy, and the graduate school. Basic science and clinical opportunities for the medical students are located throughout the Denver area in a number of hospitals and clinics, and rural health experiences are found throughout the state of Colorado. Although no official student housing is provided, the school is located in a neighborhood with a wide range of housing choices.

The medical school is home for approximately 1,200 full-time and 2,000 volunteer faculty members. In addition to educating students and participating in research, the faculty assumes considerable responsibility for patient care. Opportunities for student research and a variety of extracurricular activities are available.

CURRICULUM

The curriculum is designed to provide the scientific and clinical background to prepare graduates for the practice of medicine. Most of the basic science courses are taught during the first two years. Primary Care I, II, and III are longitudinal courses, taught over the first three years, and are designed to introduce students to clinical problems early in their medical education. Students spend two to three days each month with a physician/preceptor who is practicing in one of the primary care areas. The third and fourth years consist of clinical clerkships with required clerkships primarily in the third year and electives primarily in the fourth year.

REQUIREMENTS FOR ENTRANCE

The MCAT and a baccalaureate degree or at least 120 semester hours of college credit with a major leading to a degree are required. The MCAT must be taken before the November 1 application deadline. The following courses are required:

	Sem. hrs.
General biology or zoology (with lab)	8
General chemistry (with lab)	8
Organic chemistry (with lab)	8
General physics (with lab)	8
College mathematics Should include at least college-level algebra and trigonometry or the equivalent by means of advanced placement.	6
English literature, composition, or equivalent	9

In addition to these required courses, the following information may be helpful as applicants plan their pre-medical coursework. In choosing from among the available courses, our experience indicates that a good basis in molecular biology and genetics will be helpful. Although biochemistry is not a specific requirement, many of our students have reported that this course was useful as a preparation.

Although a strong background in science is important, a broad-based education and experiences in other areas such as humanities and social sciences are also important assets for the future physician.

In order to receive credit for any advanced placement, the subject matter credited must be listed on the official college transcript.

Starting with the class entering in the fall of 2001, each student will be required to have a personal computer. Specifics related to this requirement will be provided to all students when they are offered a place in the class.

SELECTION FACTORS

Places are offered to the applicants who appear to the Committee on Admissions to be the most highly qualified in terms of intelligence, achievement, character, motivation, maturity, and emotional stability. For this assessment, college grades, MCAT scores, recommendations, and personal interviews are used. Interviews are offered to selected applicants, and no applicant will be accepted without a personal interview.

Of the approximately 130 places in each class, more than 85 percent will be awarded to Colorado residents. Colorado residents from rural areas and from minority groups are especially encouraged to apply. Thereafter, preference will be given to applicants from certain western states participating in the WICHE program and to applicants from other states who have high GPAs and MCAT scores.

A wide variety of undergraduate majors are considered acceptable in the selection of applicants, and no special preferences are given to science majors over nonscience majors. However, demonstration of good performance in the required science courses is essential. Accepted students for the 1999 entering class had the following statistics: *mean GPA,* 3.6; *mean MCAT,* 10.1; *mean age,* 26 years; 53 percent women; 8 percent minorities.

The medical school has an active M.D.-Ph.D. combined-degree program for qualified applicants who combine medical school with intensive scientific training. Information about this program may be obtained by calling (303) 315-8986. Graduate study and research for the doctoral degree are pursued after the student has completed the basic science curriculum in the first two years. Medical students not in the combined-degree program may also be provided with research opportunities in the basic science or clinical departments.

Colorado residents and nonresidents from U.S. medical schools are considered for transfer into the sophomore or junior year if they are in good standing at their current school and if the curriculum is similar to the University of Colorado School of Medicine curriculum. Applicants from osteopathic or foreign medical schools are considered only if they are Colorado residents. These applicants are considered for transfer into the sophomore class after successful completion of two years in their school and receipt of a passing score on the USMLE Part I. Applications are available after March 1 for entrance that fall.

The University of Colorado School of Medicine does not discriminate on the basis of race, sex, creed, national origin, age, or disability. Financial status is not a factor in the selection of applicants.

FINANCIAL AID

The medical school participates in the federal aid programs and has a number of other scholarship and loan funds that are distributed on the basis of financial need. Colorado student grant funds are available for Colorado residents. Financial aid questions should be directed to (303) 315-8364.

INFORMATION FOR MINORITY STUDENTS

The University of Colorado encourages applications from qualified minority group students. Acceptance is determined by the Committee on Admissions based on the same criteria applied to nonminority applicants. Some disadvantaged students may have interview costs defrayed. Detailed information may be obtained from the Campus Office of Diversity at (303) 315-8558.

Public Institution

APPLICATION AND ACCEPTANCE POLICIES FOR 2001–2002 FIRST-YEAR CLASS

School participates in AMCAS. See Chapter 6.

Filing of AMCAS application
- Earliest date: June 1, 2000
- Latest date: Nov. 1, 2000

School application fee to all applicants: $70
Oldest MCAT scores considered: 1997
Does not have Early Decision Program
Acceptance notice to regular applicants
- Earliest date: Oct. 15, 2000
- Latest date: Varies

Applicant's response to acceptance offer
- Maximum time: 2 weeks

Requests for deferred entrance considered: Yes
Deposit to hold place in class (applied to tuition, fees, or other student obligations during last term): $200, due with response to acceptance offer
Deposit refundable prior to: July 1, 2001
Estimated number of new entrants: 125
Starting date: Aug. 2001

TUITION AND STUDENT FEES PER YEAR FOR 1999–2000 FIRST-YEAR CLASS

Tuition
- Resident: $11,182
- Nonresident: $54,576

Student fees: $2,174

INFORMATION ON 1999–2000 FIRST-YEAR CLASS

Number of	*In-State*	*Out-of-State*	*Total*
Applicants	651	1,683	2,334
Applicants Interviewed	397	204	601
New Entrants*	122	17	139

*All took the MCAT; 99% had baccalaureate degrees.

CHAPTER 11

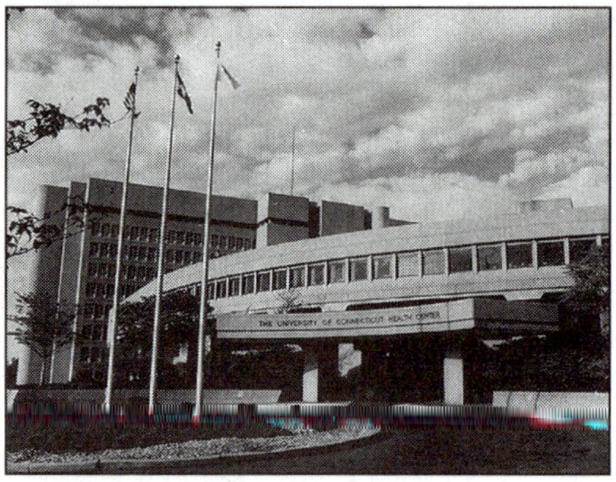

University of Connecticut School of Medicine

Farmington, Connecticut

Dr. Peter J. Deckers, *Dean*
Keat Sanford, *Assistant Dean for Admissions and Director of Student Services Center*
Patricia Lawson, *Director of Financial Assistance*

ADDRESS INQUIRIES TO:

Admissions Center
University of Connecticut
School of Medicine
263 Farmington Avenue, Rm. AG-062
Farmington, Connecticut 06030-1905
(860) 679-4713; 679-1282 (FAX)
E-mail: sanford@nso1.uchc.edu
Web Site: http://www.uchc.edu

GENERAL INFORMATION

Established in 1968 as a unit of the University of Connecticut, the School of Medicine occupies the University of Connecticut Health Center complex in Farmington. The Health Center includes under one roof the School of Medicine and School of Dental Medicine, the 204-bed University Hospital and Ambulatory Unit, and the 160,000-volume Stowe Library. Clinical training programs exist in eight affiliated hospitals in the greater Hartford area and 11 allied community hospitals.

CURRICULUM

The curriculum plan for medical students is based on a multidepartmental approach. Basic medical sciences are taught from an organ-system approach. Normal structure/function is presented first, followed by pathophysiology and therapeutic approaches. Patient contact begins in Year 1 as part of the clinical medicine course. Students learn medical history taking, physical diagnosis, and various other aspects of the physician-patient relationship. In addition, students participate in a longitudinal ambulatory clinical experience throughout all four years. In the third year, the students rotate through ambulatory and in-patient activities in each of the major clinical disciplines. In the fourth year, students complete clinical rotations in emergent and urgent care and have five months of electives. To aid individual development, students are assigned significant amounts of free time during the first two years and a wide choice of elective subjects in the clinical years. The NBME examinations are required of all students. The grading system is strictly pass/fail; there are no class rank scales or class standing. The third-year grading system is honors and pass/fail.

REQUIREMENTS FOR ENTRANCE

The MCAT and three years of college are required; four years of college and the baccalaureate degree are recommended. Prerequisite courses are:

	Sem. hrs.
General biology or zoology (with lab)	8
General chemistry (with lab)	8
Organic chemistry (with lab)	8
General physics (with lab)	8

The level of these required courses should be equal to courses for those majoring in these respective fields.

The School of Medicine supports the view that a broad liberal arts education provides the best background for those entering the medical profession. It will be difficult for students to master the programs in medicine unless they are adept in the use of the English language and in the handling of quantitative concepts. It is strongly recommended, therefore, that students include courses in their undergraduate curriculum that will provide them with a broad liberal arts background and aid them in the future development of their communicative and quantitative skills.

SELECTION FACTORS

The aim of the University of Connecticut School of Medicine is to accept qualified Connecticut residents, with special effort to include those at a disadvantage by reason of economic background or race. This assumes that places will be offered only to those whose achievements and/or capabilities are consistent with the rigor and high standards of the school's educational programs. A few exceptionally qualified out-of-state residents will be considered. An Early Assurance Program is available. Occasionally, a couple of transfer positions are available in the third year.

The factors considered by the Admissions Committee are the applicant's career and clinical specialty interests, achievements, ability, motivation, and character. The applicant's GPA and MCAT scores are considered along with difficulty of the academic program, evidence of academic achievement beyond the regular course work, and evidence of intellectual growth and development. Additional consideration is given for nonacademic activities and involvements and for letters of recommendation.

Requests to consider MCAT scores older than three years are handled individually. Personal interviews are arranged only at the request of the Admissions Committee. The 1999 entering class had a *mean GPA* of 3.62 and a *mean MCAT* of 30.6.

The University of Connecticut policy prohibits discrimination in education, in employment, and in the provision of services on account of race, religion, sex, age, marital status, national origin, ancestry, sexual orientation, disabled veteran status, physical or mental disability, mental retardation, other specifically covered mental disabilities, and criminal records that are not job related, in accordance with provisions of the Civil Rights Act of 1964, Title IX Education Amendments of 1972, the Rehabilitation Act of 1973, the Americans with Disabilities Act, and other existing federal and state laws and executive orders pertaining to equal rights.

FINANCIAL AID

Financial aid is available in three forms: scholarships; long-term, low-interest loans; and short-term, no-interest emergency loans. Eligibility for all programs is primarily based on demonstrated need. Approximately 80 percent of the students receive financial aid during the four-year educational period. Financial need is not considered relevant to the admissions process. A student's financial need is assessed after admission, and every effort is made to meet the student's minimum financial requirements. Further information is available from Patricia Lawson, director of financial aid.

MINORITY AFFAIRS

The School of Medicine recruits minority groups and disadvantaged applicants nationally through the Department of Health Careers Opportunity Programs (HCOP). Minority applications are reviewed by the same general procedure for all applications and by the full Admissions Committee. Candidates for admission receive a full and sensitive review and are selected on a competitive basis. Minority candidates invited for an interview meet with the staff of the HCOP Department who answer questions in an informal setting. The School of Medicine has developed summer enrichment programs for high school and college students from groups traditionally underrepresented in American medicine in order to expand the pool of minority applicants to medical school. Information about enrichment programs may be obtained by writing to the HCOP Department or by calling at (860) 679-3483.

Tutorial and counseling assistance is available to all students. The financial aid package is constructed on the basis of individual need, and every effort is made to meet this need. Application fees may be waived for disadvantaged students.

Public Institution

APPLICATION AND ACCEPTANCE POLICIES FOR 2001–2002 FIRST-YEAR CLASS

School participates in AMCAS. See Chapter 6.

Filing of AMCAS application
Earliest date: June 1, 2000
Latest date: Dec. 15, 2000
School application fee to all applicants: $60
Oldest MCAT scores considered: 1997
Does have Early Decision Program (EDP)
EDP application period: June 1–Aug. 1, 2000
EDP applicants notified by: Oct. 1, 2000
Acceptance notice to regular applicants
Earliest date: Oct. 15, 2000
Latest date: Until class is filled
Applicant's response to acceptance offer
Maximum time: 3 weeks
Requests for deferred entrance considered: Yes
Deposit to hold place in class (applied to tuition): $100, due with response to acceptance offer
Deposit refundable prior to: May 15, 2001
Estimated number of new entrants: 80 (8 EDP)
Starting date: Aug. 2001

TUITION AND STUDENT FEES PER YEAR FOR 1999–2000 FIRST-YEAR CLASS

Tuition
Resident: $9,375
Nonresident: $21,320
New England Regional: $14,060

Student fees: $3,835

INFORMATION ON 1999–2000 FIRST-YEAR CLASS

Number of	*In-State*	*Out-of-State*	*Total*
Applicants	336	1,824	2,160
Applicants Interviewed	225	175	400
New Entrants*	60	17	77

*All took the MCAT and had baccalaureate degrees.

CHAPTER 11

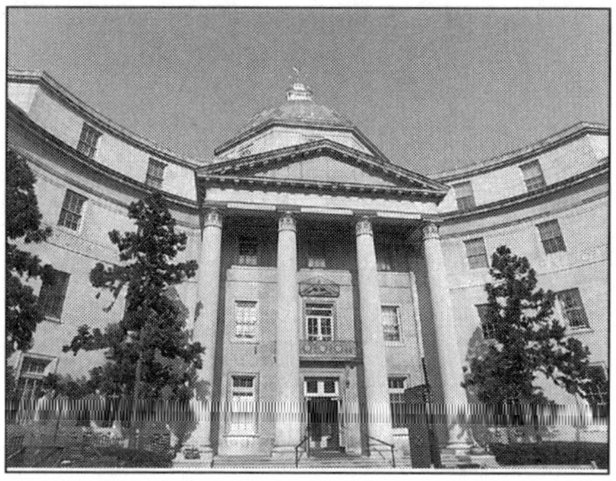

Yale University School of Medicine

New Haven, Connecticut

Dr. David A. Kessler, *Dean*
Dr. Thomas L. Lentz, *Assistant Dean for Admissions*
Pamela J. Nyiri, *Director of Financial Aid*

ADDRESS INQUIRIES TO:

Office of Admissions
Yale University
School of Medicine
367 Cedar Street
New Haven, Connecticut 06510
(203) 785-2643; 785-3234 (FAX)
E-mail: medical.admissions@yale.edu
Web Site: http://info.med.yale.edu/medadmit

MISSION STATEMENT

The aim of the Yale University School of Medicine is to produce physicians who will be among the leaders in their chosen field, whether it be in the basic medical sciences, academic clinical medicine, or medical practice in the community. Belief in the maturity and responsibility of the students is emphasized by creating a flexible educational program, through anonymous examinations, eliminating grades, and by encouraging independent study and research. The ideal Yale physician is a highly competent and compassionate practitioner of the medical arts, schooled in the current state of knowledge of both medical biology and patient care.

GENERAL INFORMATION

The Yale University School of Medicine was established by passage of a bill in the Connecticut General Assembly in 1810 granting a charter for the Medical Institution of Yale College. The Yale-New Haven Medical Center is composed of the School of Medicine, the School of Nursing, and the Yale-New Haven Hospital. The West Haven Veterans Hospital, Connecticut Mental Health Center, Yale Psychiatric Institute, Hospital of St. Raphael, and Waterbury Hospital are also used for instruction. The Yale Medical Library has an extensive collection of current and historical medical literature.

CURRICULUM

The educational objective of the School of Medicine is to develop physicians who are highly competent and compassionate practitioners of the medical arts, schooled in the current state of knowledge of both medical biology and patient care. It is hoped that Yale-trained physicians will establish a lifelong process of learning the medical, behavioral, and social sciences by independent study. The aim is to produce physicians who will be among the leaders in their chosen field, whether it be in the basic medical sciences, academic clinical medicine, or medical practice in the community. The program allows considerable freedom for planning according to the ability and interests of the student.

The first two years of the Yale School of Medicine are spent building a foundation in the basic sciences. The first year emphasizes normal biological form and function. The second-year curriculum emphasizes the study of disease. Throughout both years, a patient-doctor course meets weekly to teach physical diagnosis and the art of talking with patients. The third year is almost entirely devoted to clinical clerkships with 45 weeks of study in clerkships required for graduation. The fourth year is devoted to electives, a required primary care clerkship, and completion of the thesis work.

The thesis, a requirement since 1839, is an essential part of the curriculum and is designed to develop critical judgment, habits of self-education, and application of the scientific method to medicine. The thesis, based on original research in an area of the student's choosing, gives students the opportunity to work closely with faculty who are distinguished scientists, clinicians, and scholars.

A combined M.D.-Ph.D. Program is available for qualified applicants with a strong motivation toward a career in academic medicine and the biomedical sciences. Support is made available through the Medical Scientist Training Program. The M.D.-Ph.D. Program is flexible and normally takes seven to eight years to complete. Joint M.D.-J.D., M.D.-M.P.H., and M.D.-M.BA. programs are also available.

REQUIREMENTS FOR ENTRANCE

It is recommended that students enter medical school after four years of study in a college of arts and sciences or institute of technology. Students holding advanced degrees in science or other fields are also considered. Foreign students must complete one year of study and the pre-medical requirements in an American college or university prior to application. Students who have been refused admission on three prior occasions are ineligible to apply for admission to the first-year class. The MCAT and satisfactory completion of the following courses are required.

	Sem. hrs.
General biology or zoology (with lab)	6–8
General or inorganic chemistry (with lab)	6–8
Organic chemistry (with lab)	6–8
General physics (with lab)	6–8

Acceptable courses in these subjects usually extend over one year and are given credit for six to eight semester hours. The medical faculty has no preference as to a major field for undergraduate study but recommends that students advance beyond the elementary level in their field of study. Students entering college with a strong background in the sciences, as demonstrated by advanced placement, are encouraged to substitute advanced science courses for the traditional requirements listed above.

The secondary application for Yale may be completed in hard copy or at the listed Web address and forwarded to the Office of Admissions electronically.

SELECTION FACTORS

The Committee on Admissions in general seeks to admit students who best suit the philosophies and goals of the school, which include providing an education in the scholarly and humane aspects of medicine and fostering the development of leaders who will advance medical practice and knowledge. It also seeks to ensure an adequate representation of women and minority groups and a diversity of interests and backgrounds. The class entering in 1999 has 45 percent women, 22 percent underrepresented minority, and 21 percent Asian American and other minority students. Yale University School of Medicine does not discriminate on the basis of race, sex, religion, national origin, age, handicap, or sexual orientation.

All secondary applications are read and screened by members of the Admissions Committee. In considering applicants, the committee views the individual as a whole, taking into consideration each student's academic record, MCAT scores, pre-medical committee evaluations, letters of recommendation, outside accomplishments, personal qualities, and suitability for Yale.

Interviews are arranged only by invitation of the admissions committee. A large number of applicants have attained a high level of academic achievement as indicated by grades and test scores. Activities and accomplishments are of considerable importance in distinguishing candidates as individuals and demonstrating the ability to make significant independent contributions. The admissions committee also considers personal attributes thought to be important in a physician and suitability for the Yale program of medical education.

FINANCIAL AID

The school discourages excessive outside work and provides scholarship awards and loans for those who have serious financial needs. Financial aid applications will be mailed on or around January 1. All applicants for financial aid will be required to participate in FAFSA. A supplemental needs analysis will be required for students applying for institutional funds. This application will require student, spouse, and family financial statements.

INFORMATION FOR MINORITY STUDENTS

Yale University School of Medicine seeks to obtain an adequate representation of all minority groups and encourages qualified minority students to apply. Applicants invited for interviews will have the opportunity to meet with minority students and faculty to learn about the school. The Committee on Admissions includes minority members.

Further information may be obtained from Dr. Forrester Lee, assistant dean for multicultural affairs.

Private Institution

APPLICATION AND ACCEPTANCE POLICIES FOR 2001–2002 FIRST-YEAR CLASS

School participates in AMCAS. See Chapter 6.

Filing of AMCAS application
  Earliest date: June 1, 2000
  Latest date: Oct. 15, 2000
School application fee to all applicants: $65
Oldest MCAT scores considered: 1997
Does have Early Decision Program (EDP)
  EDP application period: June 1–Aug. 1, 2000
  EDP applicants notified by: Oct. 1, 2000
Acceptance notice to regular applicants
  Earliest date: March 15, 2001
  Latest date: Until class is filled
Applicant's response to acceptance offer
  Maximum time: 3 weeks
Requests for deferred entrance considered: Yes
Deposit to hold place in class (applied to tuition):
  $100, due with response to acceptance offer
Deposit refundable prior to: May 15, 2001
Estimated number of new entrants: 104 (1–3 EDP)
Starting date: Aug. 2001

TUITION AND STUDENT FEES PER YEAR FOR 1999–2000 FIRST-YEAR CLASS

Tuition: $29,200   Student fees: $200

INFORMATION ON 1999–2000 FIRST-YEAR CLASS

Number of	*In-State*	*Out-of-State*	*Total*
Applicants	150	2,319	2,469
Applicants Interviewed	41	709	750
New Entrants*	8	97	105

*All took the MCAT and had baccalaureate degrees.

CHAPTER 11

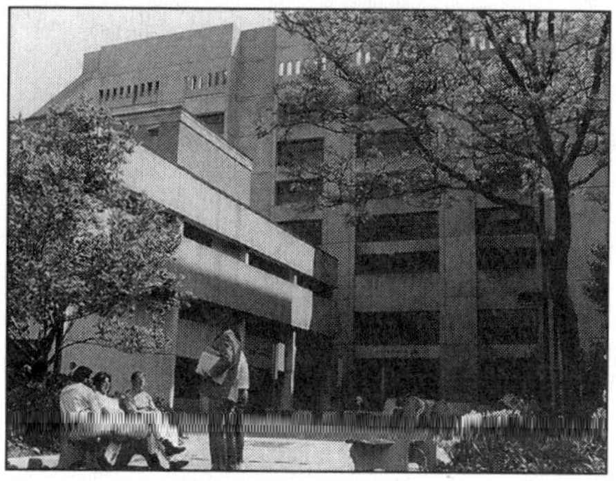

George Washington University School of Medicine and Health Sciences

Washington, D.C.

Dr. John F. Williams, *Vice President for Health Affairs and Dean, School of Medicine and Health Sciences*
Dr. Brian L. McGrath, *Assistant Dean for Admissions*
Diane P. McQuail, *Director of Admissions*

ADDRESS INQUIRIES TO:

Office of Admissions
George Washington University
School of Medicine and Health Sciences
2300 Eye Street, N.W., Room 716
Washington, D.C. 20037
(202) 994-3506
E-mail: medadmit@gwu.edu
Web Site: http://www.gwumc.edu/edu/admis/

MISSION STATEMENT

With a vision to be the preeminent health institution in the Washington Metropolitan area, George Washington University School of Medicine is dedicated to improving the health and well-being of our local community and beyond. We are committed to the highest quality of care and health services to the public, excellence and innovation in education, and research that expands the frontiers of science and knowledge. As a leader in health services, education, and research we strive to set standards of excellence by providing exemplary and innovative teaching programs that produce health professionals trained and prepared for the future; by generating and expanding health knowledge through superior programs in basic science, health policy, and applied research; by delivering compassionate, high quality, and patient-focused clinical care and health plan services; and by improving the health and well-being of our local, regional, national, and international community. To achieve our mission we are committed to the principles of altruism, collaboration, communication, compassion, innovation, integrity, respect, and service excellence.

GENERAL INFORMATION

Classes were first held in the School of Medicine of the George Washington University (GWU) in 1825. By 1973, modern facilities, including Ross Hall (a research and basic sciences center) and a medical library, were in operation near the University Hospital and clinics. The University Hospital provides clinical teaching and research opportunities; the clinics provide ambulatory experience in the medical and surgical specialties. The teaching services of the Children's Hospital National Medical Center, Fairfax Hospital, Holy Cross Hospital, National Naval Medical Center, St. Elizabeths Hospital, Veterans Administration Hospital, and Washington Hospital Center are available to students, under the direction of the faculty.

CURRICULUM

The curriculum is designed to provide students a medical education comprehensive enough to prepare them for generalist careers and offer them the exposure on which to base career selection. The faculty's objectives include imparting to students a substantial body of information, while stressing the attitude of compassion, the skill of problem solving, the habit of self-education, and a high regard for the acquisition of new knowledge, both basic and applied. Emphasis is placed on education through cooperative effort, not through competition.

Introduced in the fall of 1993, Practice of Medicine (POM) integrates the building blocks of a traditional medical education—a strong foundation of basic and clinical sciences—by interweaving them throughout the four-year curriculum. The first phase of this course places every student with a practicing clinician every other week throughout Years I and II. On alternate weeks, clinical assessment skills (including learning to take a history and do the core physical examination) will be taught and evaluated.

Clinical clerkships begin in the third year. Choice of courses is largely elective during the fourth year. The honors/pass/conditional/fail system is used for grading.

A joint program offered through GW's Columbian College and Graduate School of Arts and Sciences and the School of Medicine and Health Sciences is the Seven-Year Integrated B.A.-M.D. program. This program is designed for high school honor students of high ability and maturity who have already decided to become physicians and want to accomplish that goal in a shorter time and at a lower overall cost without seriously sacrificing the breadth of knowledge gained from a liberal arts education. Another joint program—an eight-year integrated engineering M.D. program—is available through the School of Engineering and the School of Medicine and Health Sciences. An early selection program is available to George Washington sophomores in their second semester.

Both M.D.-M.P.H. and M.D.-Ph.D. programs are available to medical students. Course work for the M.P.H. can begin the summer preceding medical school matriculation.

Transfer applications for the second- and third-year classes are accepted beginning in January.

REQUIREMENTS FOR ENTRANCE

The MCAT and 90 semester hours of credit applicable toward a B.A. or B.S. from an accredited U.S. or Canadian college is the minimal requirement. (Most students have completed four years of college.)

Required courses must be completed by July 2001:

	Sem. hrs.
Biology and/or zoology (with lab)	8
Inorganic chemistry (with lab)	8
Organic chemistry (with lab)	8
Physics (with lab)	8
English composition and literature	6

With the exception of these specific requirements, applicants are urged to follow their personal interests in developing a premedical course of study. Applicants with an undergraduate emphasis in the arts, humanities, and social sciences are welcomed.

SELECTION FACTORS

The first step in the selection procedure is an overall evaluation based on data contained in the AMCAS and supplemental applications. This evaluation screens applicants on the basis of grades (taking into account the college of origin as well as improvement in performance in later years); MCAT scores; extracurricular, health related, and/or research experiences; work experiences; and evidence of non-scholastic accomplishments. Evidence of good performance in recent, relevant course work is to an applicant's advantage. Some additional consideration is given to applicants from the District of Columbia and its metropolitan area as well as to applicants from the university's undergraduate school. The next phase of the selection procedure depends on careful examination of personal comments and letters of recommendation. The most promising applicants are then invited for a personal interview either at the school or with a regional interviewer. The last phase includes the review by the Committee on Admissions of the entire dossier. This phase is designed to select students with motivational and personal characteristics that the committee considers important in future physicians and who are academically well prepared. Many qualified reapplicants are accepted each year. There is no discrimination in the selection process because of race, gender, religion, age, marital status, sexual orientation, disability, or national or regional origin.

The 151 members of the 1999 entering class came from 68 different undergraduate schools. The *mean undergraduate GPA* was 3.57, although there was great variability about the average. Some other characteristics of the 1999 entering class were: *undergraduate major,* 34 percent in nonscience fields; *graduate degrees,* 35 students; *gender,* 71 women; *geographic,* generally proportional to applications from across the country.

FINANCIAL AID

Information regarding financial aid is available at the time of interview. Although responsibility for arranging the financing of a medical education must rest with the student, the financial aid officer will provide information and assistance to try to help students meet their needs. Merit-based admissions scholarships are available.

Because of the restrictions placed on funds, financial aid can rarely be obtained by non-U.S. citizens. This fact will have to play a role in the Committee on Admissions' deliberations on such candidates. Ability to pay expenses is not a consideration for U.S. citizens and permanent residents.

INFORMATION FOR MINORITY STUDENTS

Qualified minority applicants are invited and encouraged to apply.

Private Institution

APPLICATION AND ACCEPTANCE POLICIES FOR 2001–2002 FIRST-YEAR CLASS

School participates in AMCAS. See Chapter 6.

Filing of AMCAS application
  Earliest date: June 1, 2000
  Latest date: Dec. 1, 2000
School application fee to all applicants: $80
Oldest MCAT scores considered: 1998
Does have Early Decision Program (EDP)
  EDP application period: June 1–Aug. 1, 2000 (AMCAS applications are due in the Admissions Office by August 1, 2000.)
  EDP applicants notified by: Oct. 1, 2000
Acceptance notice to regular applicants
  Earliest date: Oct. 15, 2000
  Latest date: Until class is filled
Applicant's response to acceptance offer
  Maximum time: 2 weeks
Requests for deferred entrance considered: Yes
Deposit to hold place in class: $100, deposit is due between May 1–May 15, 2001; a tuition prepayment of $3,000 is required by July 1, 2001
Deposit is refundable prior to: May 15, 2001
Estimated number of new entrants: 150 (2 EDP)
Starting date: Aug. 2001

TUITION AND STUDENT FEES PER YEAR FOR 1999–2000 FIRST-YEAR CLASS

Tuition: $32,800   Student fees: $1,035

INFORMATION ON 1999–2000 FIRST-YEAR CLASS

Number of	*D.C.*	*Out-of-State*	*Total*
Applicants	46	9,626	9,672
Applicants Interviewed	11	1,053	1,064
New Entrants*	3	148	151

*All had baccalaureate degrees and took the MCAT.

CHAPTER 11

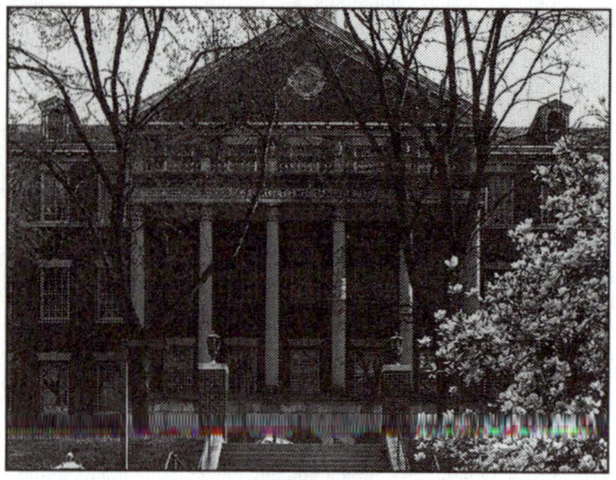

Georgetown University School of Medicine

Washington, D.C.

Dr. Carolyn B. Robinowitz, *Academic Dean*
Dr. Russell T. Wall III, *Associate Dean for Admissions and Student Services*
Eugene T. Ford, *Director of Admissions*

ADDRESS INQUIRIES TO:

Georgetown University
School of Medicine
3900 Reservoir Road, N.W.
Washington, D.C. 20007
(202) 687-1154
Web Site: http://www.dml.georgetown.edu/schmed

MISSION STATEMENT

The Georgetown School of Medicine was established in 1851 and is a part of the oldest Catholic and Jesuit-sponsored university in the United States. Georgetown seeks to educate and produce future physicians who possess a strong general foundation of basic and clinical science knowledge; well-developed clinical skills; the ability to make decisions based on scientific evidence; address care for the community, as well as individuals; and engage in continuous self-directed learning. The School of Medicine encourages attitudes and values that reflect the importance of ethical, spiritual, psychological, social, and cultural aspects of compassionate care and healing of the whole patient—a foundation that will equip Georgetown medical graduates for the pursuit of any one of the many possible avenues for medical practice in the twenty-first century, including specialization and subspecialization.

Our educational approach involves excellent basic science and clinical faculty who are committed to providing first-rate scientific information in an environment conducive to learning and application. All of our students participate in experimental small group and independent learning, including PBL and other forms of clinical decision-making/problem-solving, and utilize computer-based educational program supplements. Students also contribute heavily to our educational planning and evaluation activities and are valued members of all medical education committees.

GENERAL INFORMATION

The School of Medicine works in association with the 389-bed Georgetown University Hospital and 9 affiliated federal and community hospitals in the Washington metropolitan area. The medical center includes a Concentrated Care Center and Outpatient Surgical Center with state-of-the-art emergency, x-ray, and transplant facilities. The campus also contains a modern health science library and classroom and laboratory facilities dedicated to basic and preclinical science and research. Adjacent to the hospital is the Vincent T. Lombardi Cancer Research Center providing both research and clinical care. The school is near the National Institutes of Health and other internationally prominent health care and research facilities.

Georgetown also offers opportunities for the overall development of its student body. The Reverend Gerard F. Yates, S.J., Memorial Field House offers swimming facilities, jogging tracks, many athletic programs, and the availability of multi- and single-purpose courts. In the nearby Thomas and Dorothy Leavey Center a variety of dining establishments and guest quarters complement space for conferences and the performing arts.

CURRICULUM

Georgetown's curriculum combines diverse teaching modalities. Courses in the first two years focus on the development of fundamental knowledge concerning the body's normal and altered structure and functions. Small-group teaching and exposure to patient assessment and care begin early. In the third year, clinical clerkships in hospitals and ambulatory care settings stress the skills required to acquire and interpret patient-based data, while the fourth year further develops skills in patient management. Twenty-four weeks of electives are available during this final year, four of which may be used for vacation.

At Georgetown, the grading system consists of honors, high pass, pass, and fail.

A research track for medical students and a combined M.D.-Ph.D. program are also available; the Ph.D. may be taken in a basic medical science department or in philosophy-bioethics. Students may also apply for a five-year combined M.D.-M.B.A. program.

REQUIREMENTS FOR ENTRANCE

In general, Georgetown requires the MCAT and a minimum of three years of college (90 semester hours) for consideration of admission to the School of Medicine. The baccalaureate degree is highly desirable. The minimum specific course requirements are:

	Sem./Qtr.
Biology (with lab)	2/3
Inorganic chemistry (with lab)	2/3
Organic chemistry (with lab)	2/3
General physics (with lab)	2/3
English	2/3
Mathematics/statistics	(3 credits)

While a solid preparation in the basic sciences is essential, a broad background in the humanities and computer science is also important. Biochemistry is strongly recommended and can be substituted for second-semester organic chemistry.

Applicants should take the MCAT in the spring of the year they intend to apply and make sure that required courses will be completed. Georgetown allows six to eight hours of prerequisites to be taken during the application year. Applicants are cautioned that files are not reviewed until MCAT scores are received; a delay in the receipt of such credentials may delay consideration of an application.

SELECTION FACTORS

The Committee on Admissions selects students on the basis of academic achievements, character, maturity, and motivation. There are no geographical quotas. In rendering its decisions, the Committee on Admissions evaluates the applicant's entire academic record, performance on the MCAT, college premedical advisory committee evaluations, letters of recommendation, and personal interviews.

For the 1999 entering class, 8,323 candidates applied from over 719 undergraduate colleges. The applicants who enrolled had the following characteristics: *mean science GPA,* 3.60; *undergraduate major,* 66 percent in the biological sciences, 6 percent in the physical sciences, 14 percent in social sciences, 14 percent in various humanities and other majors; 46.2 percent *women.*

Georgetown requires personal interviews. These interviews are conducted on the medical center campus, and applicants are not invited to interview until all their credentials have been received and reviewed by the Committee on Admissions. A secondary application and essay are required for all applicants. Applicants are urged to submit their applications and supporting credentials as early as possible. The School of Medicine does not discriminate on the basis of race, sex, creed, age, handicap, or national or ethnic origin.

The School of Medicine has an Early Assurance Program with its undergraduate institution. Generally, applicants for transfer are considered only from LCME-accredited medical schools.

FINANCIAL AID

Georgetown's medical school participates in federal financial aid programs and awards school-administered grants, scholarships, and low-interest loans to students on the basis of financial need. Parents' financial information is required for students seeking school-administered aid.

Medical students at Georgetown are expected to take responsibility for their financial affairs in meeting deadlines for both tuition payment as well as in applying for financial aid. Loan indebtedness counseling is an important function of the Office of Student Financial Planning as a majority of students at the School of Medicine incur substantial educational debt. Candidates for admission are strongly encouraged to contact that office with questions about financial aid.

INFORMATION FOR MINORITY STUDENTS

In 1999 the School of Medicine had a minority enrollment, (including African American, Mexican American, mainland Puerto Rican, and native American students) totaling 8 percent of the entering class. Questions about programs and opportunities for qualified minority applicants should be addressed to the director, Office of Programs for Minority Student Development. The Georgetown Experimental Medical Studies (GEMS) Program is a one-year postbaccalaureate program for qualified minority and disadvantaged students. Priority consideration is given to residents of the District of Columbia. For more information, write or telephone the GEMS program coordinator, at (202) 687-1406.

Private Institution

APPLICATION AND ACCEPTANCE POLICIES FOR 2001–2002 FIRST-YEAR CLASS

School participates in AMCAS. See Chapter 6.

Filing of AMCAS application
  Earliest date: June 1, 2000
  Latest date: Nov. 1, 2000
School application fee to all applicants: $95
Oldest MCAT scores considered: 1997
Does not have Early Decision Program
Acceptance notice to regular applicants
  Earliest date: Oct. 15, 2000
  Latest date: Until class is filled
Applicant's response to acceptance offer
  Maximum time: 3 weeks
Requests for deferred entrance considered: Yes
Deposit to hold place in class (applied to tuition):
  $100, due March 15, 2001 or within 3 weeks of acceptance
Deposit refundable prior to: May 1, 2001
Partial tuition prepayment due: June 1, 2001
Estimated number of new entrants: 165
Starting date: Aug. 2001

TUITION AND STUDENT FEES PER YEAR FOR 1999–2000 FIRST-YEAR CLASS

Tuition: $29,940 Student Fees: $43

INFORMATION ON 1999–2000 FIRST-YEAR CLASS

Number of	*D.C.*	*Out-of-State*	*Total*
Applicants	41	8,282	8,323
Applicants Interviewed	16	965	981
New Entrants*	9	162	171

*All had baccalaureate degrees; 94% took the MCAT.

CHAPTER 11

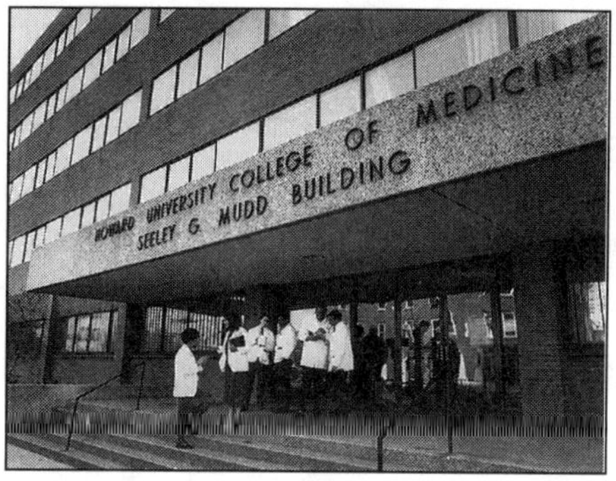

Howard University College of Medicine

Washington, D.C.

Dr. Floyd J. Malveaux, *Dean*
Dr. Dawn L. Cannon, *Assistant Dean for Student Affairs and Admissions*
Ann Finney, *Admissions Officer*

ADDRESS INQUIRIES TO:

Office of Admissions, Office of the Dean
Howard University
College of Medicine
520 W Street, N.W.
Washington, D.C. 20059
(202) 806-6270; 806-7934 (FAX)
Web Site: http://www.med.howard.edu/

GENERAL INFORMATION

The Howard University College of Medicine is the oldest and largest historically black medical school in the United States and the 36th oldest of all 125 medical schools in this country. Initially established as a medical department, the college opened in 1868 with eight students and seven faculty members. The medical department's primary goal then remains the college's today: to train students to become competent, compassionate physicians who will provide care in medically underserved communities.

In 1871, Howard University graduated its first medical class, consisting of two black men and three white men. One woman was graduated the following year. Subsequent classes throughout the College of Medicine's history have been similarly cosmopolitan in accordance with the spirit and intention of Howard University's founders. The college proudly cites its long history of training men and women of all races and ethnic origins, religions, creeds, nationalities, and economic backgrounds.

The college has more than 4,000 living alumni, including approximately 25 percent of all black practicing physicians in this country. During the first half of this century, the college contributed nearly half of the black physicians in the United States.

The 321-bed Howard University Hospital was completed in 1975. It is the college's primary teaching hospital for medical students and is used for postgraduate training in the various specialties of medicine. Medical students also serve clerkships at the District of Columbia General Hospital, St. Elizabeths Hospital, Walter Reed Army Medical Center, U.S. Naval Medical Center, the Washington Veterans Administration Medical Center, Providence Hospital, the National Rehabilitation Hospital, the Washington Hospital Center, and Prince George's Hospital Center.

CURRICULUM

The curriculum is designed to provide a firm basis for the science and art of medicine and to provide effective integration of basic science concepts, clinical application, and research. Students are presented the essential knowledge and skills necessary for the practice of medicine in courses that are required of all medical students. In addition, time is provided in the schedule for students to pursue areas of their interest through elective courses.

The required disciplines of the first and second years include gross and developmental anatomy, histology, biochemistry, physiology, pathology, pharmacology, medical genetics, psychiatry and biometrics, and epidemiology. In addition to these, several interdisciplinary courses are offered in the first two years: basic neuroscience, introduction to patient care I, immunology/medical microbiology/infectious diseases, pathophysiology of organ systems, and the principles of physical diagnosis in introduction to patient care III.

The third and fourth years consist of blocks of instruction in a continuum of clerkships and examinations in various clinical subjects. During the fourth year, opportunity is available for additional clinical or research experience through 20 or 24 weeks of required electives.

A five-year curriculum is offered to students who demonstrate during their first semester of enrollment or by the end of the January neuroscience course that they are having difficulty meeting the demands of the four-year curriculum and need additional time to meet the requirements for satisfactory performance. This curriculum, which does not require additional courses, includes changes in the scheduling of courses in the four-year curriculum to accommodate the one-year extension.

Satisfactory performance is required in all courses for promotion and graduation. Students are required to pass Step 1 of the USMLE for promotion to the third year. Passing Step 2 of the USMLE is required for graduation. Grades in the College of Medicine are reported as H (honors), S (satisfactory), or U (unsatisfactory).

A combined B.S.-M.D. program was initiated in 1974 for students enrolling in the Howard University College of Arts and Sciences from high school. Both degrees may be obtained in a six-year period.

An M.D.-Ph.D. degree program is available in anatomy, human genetics, microbiology, biochemistry, pharmacology, physiology, biology, and chemistry.

REQUIREMENTS FOR ENTRANCE

The MCAT is required. It is recommended that all applicants take the MCAT in the spring rather than in the fall of the year in which they apply. A minimum of 62 semester hours at an accredited U.S. or Canadian university or college is required. Course work should include:

	Sem. hrs.
Biology or zoology	8
General chemistry	8
Organic chemistry	8
General physics	8
College mathematics	6
English	6

SELECTION FACTORS

There are four major criteria used in the selection of applicants for admission to the College of Medicine: (1) character and discernible motivation for a career in medicine, (2) scholastic record, (3) results of the MCAT, and (4) letters of recommendation from preprofessional advisors and faculty. Candidates for admission and alternates are selected from those applicants who satisfy the criteria and who are most likely to serve in communities needing physician services. MCAT scores and GPAs are used for initial screening.

An invitation for an interview may be extended to an applicant after the Committee on Admissions has made a preliminary examination of the applicant's credentials and has decided that an interview is desirable. Although the total student is evaluated, the Committee on Admissions gives strongest consideration to those who have GPAs of 3.0 and above.

There are no residence restrictions. All applicants will be evaluated regardless of their sex, race, religion, national or ethnic origin, age, marital status, or handicap.

A nonrefundable $150 enrollment fee (due with response to acceptance) is required of accepted students who have never previously enrolled at Howard University. This is in addition to the $100 refundable good faith deposit.

FINANCIAL AID

Approximately 85 percent of the students enrolled in the College of Medicine receive some sort of financial assistance. Financial aid applicants must submit the FAFSA. Students with demonstrated need may receive school-based scholarships and loans, and those who qualify are recommended for federally guaranteed and private educational loans. Some merit awards are offered to outstanding entering freshmen and for exceptional academic performance in the medical curriculum. Some students receive scholarships and loans funded by the U.S. Public Health Service or by the military.

Private Institution

APPLICATION AND ACCEPTANCE POLICIES FOR 2001–2002 FIRST-YEAR CLASS

School participates in AMCAS. See Chapter 6.

Filing of AMCAS application
  Earliest date: June 1, 2000
  Latest date: Dec. 15, 2000
School application fee to all applicants: $45
Oldest MCAT scores considered: 1997
Does not have Early Decision Program
Acceptance notice to regular applicants
  Earliest date: Oct. 15, 2000
  Latest date: Until class is filled
Applicant's response to acceptance offer
  Maximum time: 30 days (5–7 days after June 1)
Requests for deferred entrance considered: Yes
Deposit to hold place in class (applied to tuition):
  $100, due with response to acceptance offer
Deposit refundable prior to: May 15, 2000
Estimated number of new entrants: 110
Starting date: Aug. 2000

TUITION AND STUDENT FEES PER YEAR FOR 1999–2000 FIRST-YEAR CLASS

Tuition: $16,950 Student fees: $948

INFORMATION ON 1999–2000 FIRST-YEAR CLASS

Number of	*D.C.*	*Out-of-State*	*Total*
Applicants	35	5,278	5,313
Applicants Interviewed	14	535	549
New Entrants*	3	110	113

*All took the MCAT; 97.3% had baccalaureate degrees.

CHAPTER 11

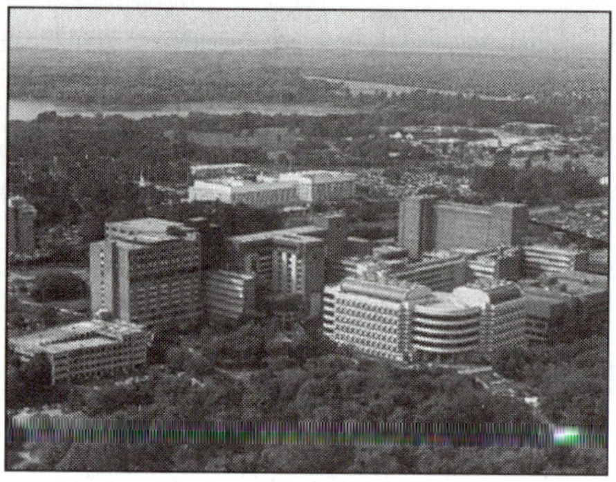

University of Florida College of Medicine

Gainesville, Florida

Dr. Kenneth I. Berns, *Dean*
Dr. Josepha A. Cheong, *Chair, Medical Selection Committee*
Eileen M. Parris, *Coordinator of Financial Aid*

ADDRESS INQUIRIES TO:

Chair, Medical Selection Committee
Box 100216
UF Health Sciences Center
University of Florida
College of Medicine
Gainesville, Florida 32610–0216
(352) 392-4569; 846-0622 (FAX)
Web Site: http://www.med.ufl.edu/

GENERAL INFORMATION

The College of Medicine, a component college of the University of Florida Health Science Center, admitted the first class in September 1956. Situated at the southeast corner of the 2,000-acre campus of the University of Florida, the College of Medicine enjoys the benefit of strong ties with other programs within the university as well as a close relationship to the other Health Science Center colleges (dentistry, health professions, nursing, pharmacy, and veterinary medicine). The University of Florida Health Science Center complex also includes the Chandler A. Stetson Medical Science Building, the Communicore Building (library, teaching laboratories, and classrooms), the Academic Research Building, the Cancer Research Building, Shands Hospital, the Brain Institute, and the Veterans Administration Medical Center, located across the street from the Health Science Center. The University of Florida Health Science Center—Jacksonville is our urban campus. Formal educational affiliations have also been established in Ft. Lauderdale, Miami, Orlando, and Pensacola.

CURRICULUM

The curriculum is divided into three blocks of time—preclinical basic sciences (first two years), clinical clerkships (third year), and postclerkship electives and required courses (fourth year). The required clinical clerkship rotations provide the students with experiences in eight general areas of medicine—anesthesiology, family medicine, medicine, neurology, psychiatry, obstetrics and gynecology, surgery, and pediatrics. The rotations include a 12-week interdisciplinary clerkship, which includes ambulatory clinical experience in family medicine, medicine, and pediatrics. Another 12-week clerkship includes medicine, anesthesiology, geriatrics, neurology, and advanced cardiac life support. The fourth year includes four weeks of required medicine, pediatrics, or family medicine, four weeks of required advanced pharmacology, and four weeks of required surgery. The remainder of the senior year is devoted to elective course work. Students' performance in academic course work will be evaluated by letter grades. However, some courses use a pass-fail system.

During the first summer and the elective period, students may choose involvement in biomedical or clinical research. Students may also delay a clerkship rotation to the fourth year.

Students may elect the option of taking preclinical basic science courses over a three-year period. This option might provide an opportunity for research or be advantageous to students from nonscience or disadvantaged backgrounds and who would benefit from a more moderately paced schedule.

MEDICAL SCIENTIST TRAINING PROGRAM (M.D.-PH.D.)

This program offers an opportunity for students who are motivated toward an academic career in the medical sciences. The M.D.-Ph.D. program is designed to be intensive, yet flexible, and to provide a smooth interface between clinical and research training. Candidates for this program must satisfy admission requirements for the college of medicine and the graduate school and have significant research experience.

JUNIOR HONORS MEDICAL PROGRAM

Students accepted into the Junior Honors Medical Program at the end of their second year of college enroll in basic medical science seminars and undergraduate courses during their third year. They become full-time medical students during their fourth year and receive a B.S. degree at the end of their fourth year from the College of Liberal Arts and Sciences. Although primarily intended for students in their second year at the University of Florida, applications from students enrolled at other colleges and universities will be considered. Further information may be obtained by writing to the admissions office.

REQUIREMENTS FOR ENTRANCE

Only U.S. citizens and permanent resident aliens will be considered. The MCAT is required and must be taken within three years before matriculation (1998, 1999, 2000), and before the December 1 application deadline. The student should complete the requirements for a bachelor's degree at an accredited American college or university prior to matriculation. In exceptional instances students upon whom the degree has not been conferred may be admitted. College work must include:

	Sem. hrs.
Biochemistry (with lab)	4
Biology (with lab)	8
Inorganic chemistry (with lab)	8
Organic chemistry (with lab)	4
General physics (with lab)	8

SELECTION FACTORS

Applicants will be appraised on the basis of personal attributes, academic record, evaluation of past activities, the MCAT, and letters of recommendation. A personal interview is required to complete the application process and is granted at the discretion of the Medical Selection Committee. The school does not discriminate on the basis of race, sex, age, disability, creed, or national origin. Although Florida residents are given preference in admission, a limited number of nonresidents are considered each year. Nonresident applicants must demonstrate superior qualifications. The College of Medicine welcomes applications from minorities and from persons who demonstrate a clear, long-standing commitment to underserved populations.

Students matriculating into the 1999 entering class had the following characteristics: *mean GPA,* 3.72; *MCAT,* 29.5; *female,* 45 percent; 6 percent *minorities.*

FINANCIAL AID

Financial assistance is available to all enrolled students who show need. The College has scholarships and low interest loans available. Applications are mailed to all accepted applicants. Summer and school-year research fellowships are also available.

FLORIDA STATE UNIVERSITY PROGRAM IN MEDICAL SCIENCES (PIMS)

The Program in Medical Sciences is an inter-university program between Florida State University and the University of Florida College of Medicine. Thirty first-year medical students are selected by the Program Selection Committee to complete the first year of basic medical sciences curriculum at Florida State University. The program is open to all residents of Florida who complete a baccalaureate degree and fulfill the usual prerequisite course requirements, which include two semesters of biochemistry and two semesters of organic chemistry. Application is through AMCAS. Early selection is open to outstanding applicants from Florida State University, University of West Florida, and Florida Agricultural and Mechanical University. The program is especially interested in selecting students who have a likelihood of practicing medicine in primary care medical specialties. Students from rural areas, minorities, and applicants who demonstrate a dedication to service to others are encouraged to apply. During this first-year experience, students gain clinical skills by serving in local health clinics, working with primary care physicians who serve as their preceptors, and completing a semester-long preceptorship at the Family Practice Residency Program at Tallahassee Memorial Regional Medical Center. Students complete the remaining three years of medical education at the University of Florida College of Medicine upon successful completion of the first-year curriculum. For further information write: Program in Medical Sciences, Florida State University, Tallahassee, Florida 32306-4051; or phone: (850) 644-1855.

Public Institution

APPLICATION AND ACCEPTANCE POLICIES FOR 2001–2002 FIRST-YEAR CLASS

School participates in AMCAS. See Chapter 6.

Filing of AMCAS application
  Earliest date: June 1, 2000
  Latest date: Dec. 1, 2000
School application fee: None
Oldest MCAT scores considered: 1998
Does not have Early Decision Program
Acceptance notice to regular applicants
  Earliest date: Oct. 15, 2001
  Latest date: Until class is filled
Applicant's response to acceptance offer
  Maximum time: 2 weeks
Requests for deferred entrance considered: Yes
Deposit to hold place in class: None
Estimated number of new entrants: 73
Starting date: Aug. 2001

TUITION AND STUDENT FEES PER YEAR FOR 1999–2000 FIRST-YEAR CLASS

Tuition	Student fees
Resident: $9,684	Resident: $1,268
Nonresident: $27,335	Nonresident: $2,150

INFORMATION ON 1999–2000 FIRST-YEAR CLASS

Number of	*In-State*	*Out-of-State*	*Total*
Applicants	1,045	952	1,997
Applicants Interviewed	292	22	314
New Entrants*	73	0	73

*All took the MCAT and had baccalaureate degrees.

CHAPTER 11

University of Miami School of Medicine

Miami, Florida

Dr. John G. Clarkson, *Senior Vice President for Medical Affairs and Dean, School of Medicine*
Dr. R.E. Hinkley, *Associate Dean for Admissions and Enrollment Management*
Laura L. Horsley, *Assistant Dean for Student Financial Assistance*

ADDRESS INQUIRIES TO:

Office of Admissions
University of Miami
School of Medicine
P.O. Box 016159
Miami, Florida 33101
(305) 243-6791; 243-6548 (FAX)
E-mail: med.admissions@miami.edu
Web Site: http://www.miami.edu/medical-admissions

MISSION STATEMENT

The University of Miami has four interrelated missions: patient care, teaching, research, and community service.

GENERAL INFORMATION

The University of Miami School of Medicine is the largest and oldest medical school in the state of Florida. Since its founding in 1952, the School of Medicine has experienced a remarkable growth rate and has been the catalyst in the development of one of the largest and most comprehensive health care centers in the nation. In 1999 the school had a full-time faculty of 960, an annual budget of $460 million, research expenditures of $159 million, and a total of more than 5,200 graduates.

The School of Medicine is located on the medical campus next to Jackson Memorial Hospital in the Civic Center area of Miami. Classrooms used by students during the first two years, as well as administrative offices and research laboratories, are located in the Rosenstiel Medical Sciences Building and the Glaser Medical Research Building. Jackson Memorial Hospital and the Veterans Affairs Medical Center provide the primary settings in which third- and fourth-year students acquire and hone their clinical skills. Six hospitals are located on the medical campus and provide a complete spectrum of clinical experiences.

Also located on the medical campus and affiliated with the University of Miami School of Medicine are the Mailman Center for Child Development, the Bascom Palmer Eye Institute and Anne Bates Leach Eye Hospital, the Applebaum Magnetic Resonance Imaging Center, the Ambulatory Care Center, the UM Hospitals and Clinics, the Diabetes Research Institute, and the Ryder Trauma Center. The Sylvester Comprehensive Cancer Center is the only facility in the state of Florida to be designated as a comprehensive center by the National Cancer Institute. The Lois Pope LIFE Center and Batchelor Pediatric Institute are scheduled to open in 2000 and will add 270,000 square feet of research and clinic space to the medical campus.

CURRICULUM

The curriculum is a well-balanced educational program, and its goal is to educate students to be knowledgeable and compassionate physicians. The first two years are devoted primarily to the basic sciences and are taught in a "block" format. The Community Clinical Experience is a course that provides students with extensive direct patient contact and hospital experience throughout the first two years of the curriculum.

Clinical teaching in the third and fourth years is primarily at the bedside and is supported by small-group conferences. Required clerkships include medicine, generalist primary care, obstetrics, pediatrics, psychiatry, surgery, neurology, family medicine, anesthesia, and geriatrics. Much of the fourth year is spent in selective and elective clerkships.

The School of Medicine has two B.S.-M.D. programs for residents of Florida only. Information about these special programs may be obtained from the Office of Undergraduate Admissions at (305) 284-4323. The school sponsors an M.D.-Ph.D. program, which is not limited to residents of Florida.

REQUIREMENTS FOR ENTRANCE

The School of Medicine only accepts U.S. citizens and permanent residents of the United States who have completed a minimum of 90 semester hours of college work. Credits earned at foreign institutions are not accepted. Courses specifically required are:

	Sem. hrs.
English	6
Chemistry (with lab)	8
Organic chemistry (with lab)	8
Physics (with lab)	8
General biology or zoology	6
Other science courses*	6

*These may be distributed in the biological sciences, chemistry, physics, or mathematics. A course in biochemistry is strongly recommended and can be substituted for one semester of organic chemistry.

AP credit may be used as part of the 90-semester-hour total, but the credits listed above should be graded credits. CLEP credits are not accepted.

All applicants must take the MCAT exam no later than the fall preceding the year in which they hope to enroll in the School of Medicine.

SELECTION FACTORS

Florida residents are given preference in all admissions decisions. Residents of other states are encouraged to apply only if they have a truly superior academic record and MCAT scores or have other unique qualifications that the Committee on Admissions would find desirable. Foreign students are not accepted. Applications of Florida residents who have at least a 3.0 GPA (on a 4.0 scale), or a post-bac or graduate GPA of at least 3.4 (minimum of 13 credits) are reviewed. Secondary applications are sent to those who appear to be most competitive. Applications from non-Florida residents are reviewed only if they have a science GPA and cumulative GPA of at least 3.4. The Committee gives careful consideration to many factors when evaluating candidates for admission. Some of these factors are preparedness to study medicine, MCAT scores, and personal factors such as maturity, dedication, motivation, interpersonal skills, and leadership ability. The 1999 entering class (143 new entrants) had the following profile: *mean GPA*, 3.65 (3.4-3.9); *mean MCAT scores*: VR-9.6 (7-13), PS-9.6 (7-13), BS-10.2 (6-14); 56 percent *women*, 10 percent minorities; 70 percent *biology or chemistry* majors; *undergraduate colleges*, 38 represented. Applicants' files are reviewed without regard to race, creed, sex, national origin, age, or handicap. A personal interview is required to complete the application process. Interviews are arranged only at the initiative of the Admissions Office and are held on the medical campus. Applicants should reapply only if they have significantly improved their overall credentials.

Applications for transfer are accepted **only** from Florida residents who did their undergraduate work in the United States and who are currently enrolled and in good academic standing at a medical school accredited by the World Health Organization. Further information about transfer applications may be obtained by calling or E-mailing the Office of Admissions.

FINANCIAL AID

Eighty percent of all medical students receive some kind of financial aid. In 1999–2000 the amount awarded totaled about $18 million. The school participates in all major federal and state programs. Several scholarships are awarded each year for academic promise and for proven financial need. Information concerning financial assistance and student budgets may be obtained by calling the Office of Student Financial Assistance at (305) 243-6211.

INFORMATION FOR MINORITY STUDENTS

The Minority Students Health Careers Motivation Program is a special seven-week summer program that provides premedical undergraduates with the opportunity to gain first-hand knowledge of the requirements of a medical education. The program gives participants a "mini" medical school experience and consists of courses in human anatomy, biochemistry, and microbiology, along with a specialized course in reading and study skills, and an MCAT prep course. Books, supplies, meals, and housing are provided by the program and all accepted students receive a stipend. Applications and information may be obtained by calling (305) 243-5998.

Private Institution

APPLICATION AND ACCEPTANCE POLICIES FOR 2001–2002 FIRST-YEAR CLASS

School participates in AMCAS. See Chapter 6.

Filing of AMCAS application
  Earliest date: June 1, 2000
  Latest date: Dec. 15, 2000
School application fee after screening: $55
Oldest MCAT scores considered: 1997
Does not have Early Decision Program (EDP)
Acceptance notice to regular applicants
  Earliest date: Oct. 15, 2000
  Latest date: Until class is filled
Applicant's response to acceptance offer
  Maximum time: 2 weeks
Requests for deferred entrance considered: Yes
Deposit to hold place in class (applied to tuition): $100
Deposit refundable prior to: May 15, 2001
Estimated number of new entrants: 140
Starting date: Aug. 2001

TUITION AND STUDENT FEES PER YEAR FOR 1999–2000 FIRST-YEAR CLASS

Tuition
  Resident: $25,670
  Nonresident: $35,670

Student fees: $120

INFORMATION ON 1999–2000 FIRST-YEAR CLASS

Number of	*In-State*	*Out-of-State*	*Total*
Applicants	1,209	937	2,146
Applicants Interviewed	283	5	288
New Entrants*	142	1	143

*All took the MCAT; 84% had baccalaureate degrees.

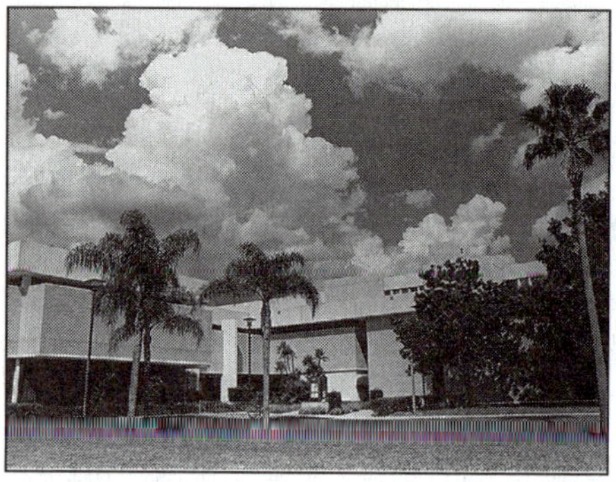

University of South Florida College of Medicine

Tampa, Florida

Dr. Randolph Manning, *Associate Dean, Student Affairs*
Jay S. Layman, *Director of Admissions*
Carolyn Nicolosi, *Director of Student Affairs*

ADDRESS INQUIRIES TO:

Office of Admissions
Box 3
University of South Florida
College of Medicine
12901 Bruce B. Downs Boulevard
Tampa, Florida 33612-4799
(813) 974-2229; 974-4990 (FAX)
Web Site: http://www.med.usf.edu

GENERAL INFORMATION

The College of Medicine, one of the three Colleges of the University of South Florida (USF) Health Sciences Center, admitted the first class of medical students in 1971. At present, the freshman class consists of 96 new students each year. In addition to the three colleges, the Health Sciences Center includes a medical science area, auditorium, cafeteria, medical library, and medical clinics. Clinical instruction for College of Medicine students is in large part based in Tampa at the USF Medical Clinics, Tampa General Hospital, James A. Haley Veterans Hospital, Tampa Unit Shriners Hospital for Crippled Children, H. Lee Moffitt Cancer Center and Research Institute, University Psychiatry Center, University Diagnostic Institute, Genesis Clinic, USF Eye Institute, USF Dialysis Center, and the 17 Davis Pediatric Ambulatory Care Centers. Clinical instruction is also provided at All Children's Hospital, Bayfront Medical Center, Bay Pines Veterans Hospital in St. Petersburg, and the Orlando Regional Medical Center.

CURRICULUM

The four-year curriculum is designed to permit the student to learn the fundamental principles of medicine, to acquire skills of critical judgment based on evidence and experience, and to develop an ability to use principles and skills wisely in solving problems of health and disease. It includes the sciences basic to medicine, the major clinical disciplines, and other significant elements such as behavioral science, medical ethics, and human values.

The intent is to foster in students the ability to learn through self-directed, independent study throughout their professional lives. Using both ambulatory and hospital settings, students are given increasing responsibility for patient care in preparation to enter graduate medical education residencies.

Some students begin medical school with future plans such as primary care practice, clinical research, or preventive medicine and public health. For these students, special opportunities are available in medical school. For students seriously considering primary care, there are special opportunities to test and to reinforce this interest through a variety of existing and newly developed programs. Special programs are available for a select few students interested in an intense research career or to acquire both the M.D. and Ph.D. degrees in less time than would ordinarily be required for each separately. Likewise, it is possible for a student interested in public health, preventive medicine, epidemiology, health care systems, and related areas to achieve both an M.D. and master's in public health (M.P.H.) degree with minimal additional time. The M.P.H. degree is awarded through the College of Public Health. A new program in the dual M.D.-M.B.A. gives medical students the opportunity to earn a master's degree in business administration while training to be physicians.

PREMEDICAL HONORS PROGRAM

This is an integrated program in which the College of Medicine will reserve certain places in the first-year medical class for superior students who satisfy the requirements for both university honors and admission to the study of medicine. All questions concerning the premedical options in university honors should be addressed to: Director of Honors; CPR 107; University of South Florida; Tampa, Florida 33620; the telephone number is (813) 974-3087.

REQUIREMENTS FOR ENTRANCE

The MCAT is required. Students applying should plan to complete the requirements for a bachelor's degree at an accredited university or college by the time of matriculation. Required courses are as follows:

	Semesters
General biology (with lab)	2
General chemistry (with lab)	2
Organic chemistry (with lab)	2
General physics (with lab)	2
Mathematics	2
English	2

Applicants are strongly urged to take the MCAT in the spring of the year of application and to have their basic science requirements completed at the time of application. No applicant will be considered for admission until the application materials are complete and received in the Admissions Office. Applications from individuals who wait to take the MCAT in the spring of the year in which they anticipate matriculating will not be considered.

SELECTION FACTORS

The selection of students of medicine is based on character, integrity, motivation, academic achievement, emotional maturity, stability, and the applicant interview. In addition, course load and types of courses taken will be evaluated and will constitute a factor in the overall evaluation.

Although the selection process is essentially competitive, with evaluation of students by their college faculty being a significant factor, there are some general guidelines on suitability of an applicant to the college. Because the University of South Florida is a state institution, preference is given to Florida residents. In those instances where residency is in question, for tuition purposes, an applicant is requested to submit a Declaration of Domicile. *Nonresidents are discouraged from applying.*

Applicants requesting an application should clearly indicate whether or not they are Florida residents.

To be considered, Florida residents should have an OGPA and SGPA of 3.0 or better on a 4.0 scale and an overall MCAT average of 8 or better with not more than one score of 7 in any area.

The 1999 entering class profile was: *mean SGPA,* 3.8; *mean MCAT scores, OGPA*-3.8; *VR*-9.7, *PS*-10.1, *BS*-10.2; *minorities,* 8.3 percent; *sex,* 46.9 percent female.

The Admissions Office may at its discretion invite the applicant to come for a personal interview. An invitation for an interview means only that the initial evaluation is sufficiently high to warrant further consideration by the Medical Student Selection Committee. Eligibility for admission will be determined without regard to race, creed, sex, age, religion, national origin, or handicap.

FINANCIAL AID

The financial status of applicants does not affect their acceptance. Limited funds are available for loans and scholarships.

First-year students are not permitted to engage in outside employment. There are employment opportunities in Tampa and the surrounding area for spouses.

Questions may be addressed to Michele Williamson, director of financial aid, by telephoning (813) 974-2068.

INFORMATION FOR MINORITY STUDENTS

Events, activities, programs, and facilities of the University of South Florida are available to all without regard to race, sex, religion, national origin, Vietnam or disabled veteran status, handicap, or age, as provided by law and in accordance with its respect for personal dignity. Qualified minority applicants who are Florida residents are strongly encouraged to apply; the telephone number is (813) 974-3609.

Public Institution

APPLICATION AND ACCEPTANCE POLICIES FOR 2001–2002 FIRST-YEAR CLASS

School participates in AMCAS. See Chapter 6.

Filing of AMCAS application
 Earliest date: June 1, 2000
 Latest date: Dec. 1, 2000
School application fee to all applicants: $20
Oldest MCAT scores considered: 1997
Does have Early Decision Program (EDP)
 For Florida residents only
 EDP application period: June 1–Aug. 1, 2000
 EDP applicants notified by: Oct. 1, 2000
Acceptance notice to regular applicants
 Earliest date: Oct. 15, 2000
 Latest date: Until class is filled
Applicant's response to acceptance offer
 Maximum time: 2 weeks
Requests for deferred entrance considered: Yes
Deposit to hold place in class: None
Estimated number of new entrants: 96 (29 EDP)
Starting date: Aug. 2001

TUITION AND STUDENT FEES PER YEAR FOR 1999–2000 FIRST-YEAR CLASS

Tuition	Student fees
Resident: $9,684	Resident: $1,257
Nonresident: $27,335	Nonresident: $2,140

INFORMATION ON 1999–2000 FIRST-YEAR CLASS

Number of	*In-State*	*Out-of-State*	*Total*
Applicants	1,227	384	1,611
Applicants Interviewed	296	0	296
New Entrants*	96	0	96

*All took the MCAT and had baccalaureate degrees.

CHAPTER 11

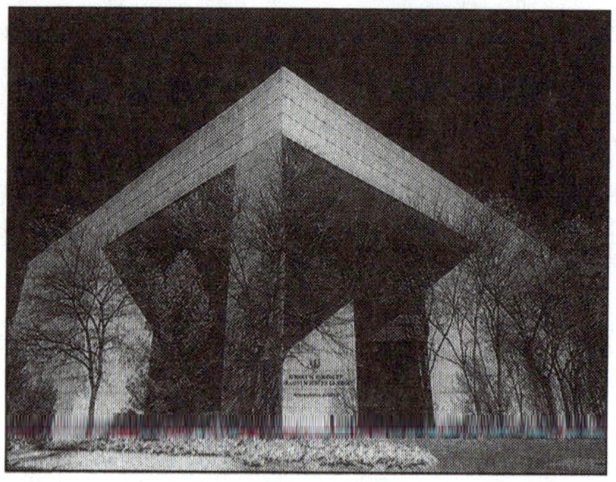

Emory University School of Medicine

Atlanta, Georgia

Dr. Thomas J. Lawley, *Dean*
Dr. J. William Eley, *Assistant Dean and Director of Admissions*
Dr. Jonas A. Shulman, *Executive Associate Dean for Medical Education/Student Affairs*

ADDRESS INQUIRIES TO:

Medical School Admissions, Room 115
Woodruff Health Sciences Center
Administration Building
Emory University
School of Medicine
Atlanta, Georgia 30322-4510
(404) 727-5660; 727-5456 (FAX)
E-mail: medschadmiss@medadm.emory.edu
Web Site: http://www.emory.edu/WHSC/

MISSION STATEMENT

Emory University School of Medicine is committed to providing leaderhsip in medicine and science through the development of recognized programs of excellence and innovation in medical education, biomedical research, and patient care.

GENERAL INFORMATION

The Emory University School of Medicine, a private school, was founded in 1915, resulting from several reorganizations dating from 1854 when the Atlanta Medical College was founded. Students spend the first two years primarily on the university campus. The last two years are spent in the school's teaching hospitals, in which there are more than 3,000 beds and large outpatient clinics.

Emory University is accredited by the Commission on Colleges of the Southern Association of Colleges and Schools.

CURRICULUM

The curriculum is intended to lay a comprehensive foundation for a career in practice, teaching, research, or other medical areas. The first two years consist primarily of basic health sciences and incorporate multimedia teaching aids. Recent curricular changes include a reduction in lecture hours, a parallel increase in small-group/problem-based learning, and introduction to patients in the first year of medical school. Courses are often interdisciplinary, for example, neurobiology, molecular and human genetics, medical problem solving, patient-doctor, and human values in medicine. In the second year, students complete their basic science background and spend a major portion of their time in integrated courses in pathology, pathophysiology, and clinical methods, which extend broadly into the various clinical fields. The third and fourth years are devoted exclusively to instruction in all major clinical subjects, including primary care. The 19-month period of actual coursework includes time for elective clerkships that encompass a large variety of studies at both local and distant sites.

A combined M.D.-Ph.D. degree program is available for highly qualified students interested in careers in academic medicine. This six- to eight-year program provides the in-depth clinical experience and biomedical research training necessary for future medical scientists. A five-year dual-degree M.D.-M.P.H. program is also available to prepare medical students for leadership roles in public health.

REQUIREMENTS FOR ENTRANCE

The MCAT and a minimum of three years of college are required. Ninety semester or 135 quarter hours in arts and sciences at an institution accredited by its regional association must be completed to be eligible for enrollment.

The premedical program should be aimed toward a balanced liberal education and should ensure thorough grounding in the stated requirements. Majors in the sciences or non-sciences are equally acceptable. The latter must show competence in the natural sciences and mathematics. Majors in the natural sciences or mathematics should always include subjects of broad educational value in their premedical curricula.

Specific minimum requirements are:

	Sem. hrs
Biology (with lab)	8
Inorganic chemistry (with lab)	8
Organic chemistry (with lab)	8
Physics (with lab)	8
English	6
Humanities, social and/or behavioral sciences	18

Biochemistry is highly recommended.

Undergraduate degree credit that has been granted to the student on the basis of CLEP will be accepted provided (1) the credit appears on the official transcript and (2) CLEP credits are not the sole fulfillment of any specific course requirement listed above. CLEP credit in excess of 25 percent of a student's total undergraduate credit will not be accepted.

SELECTION FACTORS

Students are selected on the basis of scholastic achievement, fitness and aptitude for the study of medicine, and personal qualifications, without regard to race, sex, sexual orientation, age, disability, creed, veteran status, or national origin. About half of these students are residents of Georgia. All applicants must (a) present a level of scholarship above average (GPA of 3.6 or above is recommended for non-Georgians); (b) take the MCAT preferably in the spring, but no later than the fall of the year of application; (c) apply through AMCAS and submit the required Emory supplemental application form and fee (this form is sent immediately upon receipt of the AMCAS application); (d) have the required evaluation(s) submitted; and (e) appear for a personal interview before the Admission Committee if invited. Applications are screened for possible interview only after all required items have been received. Interview is by invitation and is conducted only at Emory University. Students from foreign schools must have completed at least one year of academic work in an accredited U.S. or Canadian institution. It is anticipated anyone enrolled in a graduate-degree program will have completed all required work for the degree by the date of matriculation. Only students enrolled in U.S. LCME-accredited medical schools are eligible to apply for transfer to Emory's third-year class. Advanced standing is not given for work completed in other professional or graduate schools.

The 1999 class had the following credentials at the time of application: *mean GPA,* 3.75; *mean MCAT scores, VR*-10.1, *PS*-10.8, *WS*-P, *BS*-10.8; *undergraduate major,* 42 percent in biology, 16 percent in chemistry, 23 percent in humanities and social/behavioral sciences, 8 percent in a nonscience combined with biology/chemistry or physics, and 11 percent in other disciplines. Other characteristics of the entering class of 111 students were: *sex,* 47 percent women; *non-white ethnic groups,* 20 percent; *minority groups,* 8.1 percent.

FINANCIAL AID

A limited number of scholarships and loans are available through the Financial Aid Office of Emory University. Approximately 79 percent of all the enrolled medical students receive scholarships and loans through Emory University. Most scholarships and loans are awarded on the basis of documented financial need. Application information may be requested prior to acceptance from the university Financial Aid Office. Approximately two percent of the students receive U.S. Armed Forces scholarships. A limited number of highly qualified students in the first-year class are awarded merit scholarships. Foreign citizens who are not permanent residents of the United States must provide and document their own funding for tuition, fees, and living expenses. Although foreign citizens are not eligible for any federally based aid, they may be considered for merit scholarships and loans from sources outside of Emory. The university's Financial Aid Office may be reached at 1-800-727-6039.

Seven Robert Woodruff Fellowships, not based on need, are awarded yearly to entering students. Additional information on this competitive, merit-based program is available from the Medical School Admissions Office.

INFORMATION FOR MINORITY STUDENTS

Emory University School of Medicine is strongly committed to increasing opportunities for minority students. The Office of Minority Affairs works in conjunction with the Admission Committee and the Office of Student Affairs in the recruitment, selection, and retention of qualified minority students. Further inquiries may be addressed to Dr. Robert Lee, director of minority affairs.

Private Institution

APPLICATION AND ACCEPTANCE POLICIES FOR 2001–2002 FIRST-YEAR CLASS

School participates in AMCAS. See Chapter 6.

Filing of AMCAS application
  Earliest date: June 1, 2000
  Latest date: Oct. 15, 2000
School application fee to all applicants: $60
Oldest MCAT scores considered: 1991
Does not have Early Decision Program
Acceptance notice to regular applicants
  Earliest date: Oct. 15, 2000
  Latest date: Mid-March 2001
Applicant's response to acceptance offer
  Maximum time: 2 weeks
Requests for deferred entrance considered: Yes
Deposit to hold place in class: None
Estimated number of new entrants: 110
Starting date: Late July/Aug. 2001

TUITION AND STUDENT FEES PER YEAR FOR 1999–2000 FIRST-YEAR CLASS

Tuition: $27,059   Student fees: $400

INFORMATION ON 1999–2000 FIRST-YEAR CLASS

Number of	*In-State*	*Out-of-State*	*Total*
Applicants	563	6,270	6,833
Applicants Interviewed	137	625	762
New Entrants*	43	68	111

*All took the MCAT and had baccalaureate degrees.

CHAPTER 11

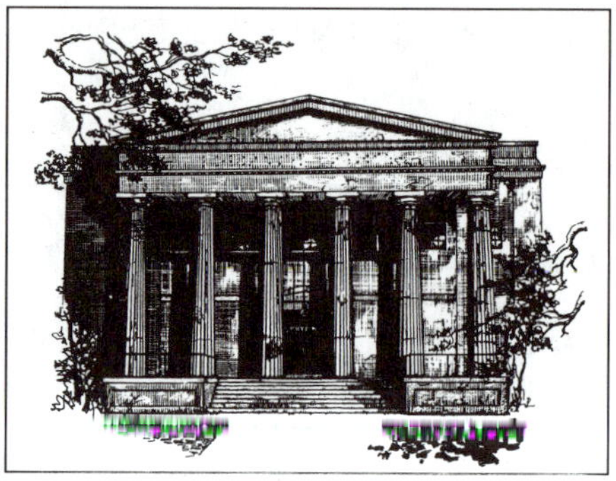

Medical College of Georgia School of Medicine

Augusta, Georgia

Dr. Darrell G. Kirch, *Dean*
Dr. Gary C. Bond, *Associate Dean for Admissions*
Sandra D. Fowler, *Director of Student Financial Aid*

ADDRESS INQUIRIES TO:

Dr. Gary C. Bond
Associate Dean for Admissions
School of Medicine
Medical College of Georgia
Augusta, Georgia 30912-4760
(706) 721-3186; 721-0959 (FAX)
E-mail: stdadmin@mail.mcg.edu
Web Site: http://www.mcg.edu

MISSION STATEMENT

As a unit of the University System of Georgia, the Medical College of Georgia is committed to cultural, ethnic, racial, and gender diversity in the faculty, staff, and student body, supported by practices and programs that embody the ideas of an open, democratic, and global society.

As an academic health center and research university, the Medical College of Georgia is committed to a shared responsibility for meeting the health care needs of a widely dispersed and highly diverse population.

GENERAL INFORMATION

The School of Medicine of the Medical College of Georgia was founded in 1828 and is the nation's 11th oldest medical school. The institution is a separate university under the Georgia Higher Education System and consists of five schools: medicine, allied health, dentistry, graduate studies, and nursing.

The Medical College of Georgia Hospital and Clinics is the primary clinical teaching facility. Other hospitals in Augusta and in cities throughout the state have affiliate agreements with the Medical College of Georgia to provide clinical teaching facilities.

CURRICULUM

During the first year (Phase I), students study the structure and functions of the human body through courses in anatomy, histology and development, biochemistry and genetics, neuroscience, physiology, psychiatry, ethics and health promotion. Courses in ethics, community medicine, behavioral science/psychiatry, and the patient-doctor clinical experience introduce students to ethical and interpersonal aspects of the practice of medicine. Contact with patients begins with physical diagnosis I and patient-doctor courses during the first year.

The second year (Phase II) emphasizes the pathophysiologic basis of clinical medicine with courses in pathology, pharmacology, clinical microbiology, reproductive endocrinology, introduction to clinical medicine, ethics, disease prevention, problem-based learning, and physical diagnosis II. A student-led, faculty-facilitated, problem-based learning course emphasizes skills of case-based and self-directed learning, development of information retrieval and analysis skills, group dynamics, and evaluation.

Interdepartmental cooperation and clinical relevance are stressed throughout the first two years. During part of the first year, two afternoons a week are available for electives.

During Phase III, students are required to take 18 months of academic work, which must include 12 months of basic clerkships in the departments of medicine, surgery, obstetrics and gynecology, family medicine, pediatrics, and neuroscience. The remaining 6 months consist of an acting internship, emergency medicine/surgical subspecialties, and electives. Students are required to pass Step 1 of the USMLE at the end of their second year and Step 2 of the USMLE prior to graduation.

REQUIREMENTS FOR ENTRANCE

The MCAT and three years of undergraduate college work leading to a baccalaureate degree in an institution accredited by its regional association are required. However, preference is given to students who will have completed the baccalaureate degree prior to enrollment at the School of Medicine.

College work must include:

	Years
Biology or zoology (with lab)	1
Inorganic chemistry (with lab)	1
Advanced chemistry (with lab)	1
Must include one semester or two quarters of organic chemistry.	
Physics (with lab)	1
English (sufficient to satisfy baccalaureate degree requirements.)	

Biochemistry is highly recommended.

These required courses must be taken on a letter or number grading system (not pass/fail) if at all possible.

SELECTION FACTORS

Applicants for admission to the School of Medicine are evaluated on a competitive basis. Information used for assessing an individual's academic accomplishments, personal attributes, and interests includes, but is not limited to, the applicant's responsibilities prior to application to medical school; involvement in extracurricular and community activities; ethnic, socioeconomic, and cultural background; region of residence with respect to its health professional needs; commitment to practice in an underserved area of Georgia; letters of recommendation by the premedical advisor and two personal references; motivation and potential for serving as a physician; personal interviews; performance on the Medical College Admission Test; and college grades including undergraduate, graduate, and postbaccalaureate. In addition, the medical school faculty has specified nonacademic (technical) standards, which all students must meet in order to participate effectively in the medical education program and in the practice of medicine.

Preference is given to residents of Georgia. A maximum of five percent of the entering class may be nonresidents of Georgia.

Application through the Early Decision Program is encouraged for Georgia residents interested in attending the Medical College of Georgia. Early Decision applicants must take the MCAT prior to making application. All other applicants must take the MCAT no later than the fall of the year application is made.

Interviews are by invitation and are with members of the Admissions Committee, faculty, students, and/or individuals from the community. About 500 applicants are interviewed each year. Regional interviews are not available.

Applicants must have received at least the last two years of their education at an accredited U.S. or Canadian college or university in order to be considered. Transfer admission with advanced standing is on a space-available basis, and only students who are currently in good academic standing in an LCME-accredited medical school may be considered for transfer admission. Anyone enrolled in a graduate-degree program is expected to complete all requirements for that degree prior to the date of matriculation.

The Medical College of Georgia does not discriminate on the basis of age, race, sex, creed, or national origin in its admissions process.

FINANCIAL AID

The Office of Financial Aid coordinates the programs of assistance that are available to medical students.

An applicant's financial status does not affect acceptance for admission. Information and applications may be obtained by writing the Office of Financial Aid.

INFORMATION FOR MINORITY STUDENTS

The School of Medicine at the Medical College of Georgia seeks to enroll qualified minority students. One of the primary recruiting mechanisms is a summer program designed for undergraduate college students who show academic promise and desire to study medicine. Students may apply for this program by writing to Dr. R. Allen-Noble, associate dean for special academic programs. For further information, please contact Special Academic Programs, School of Medicine (AA-153), Medical College of Georgia, Augusta, GA 30912-1900; (706) 721-2522.

GENERALIST PHYSICIAN INITIATIVE

The Generalist Physician Initiative at the Medical College of Georgia, funded in part by the Robert Wood Johnson Foundation, is an effort to graduate more physicians who choose to practice family medicine, general internal medicine, or general pediatrics. The initiative involves all aspects of medical education, from pre-entry through undergraduate and residency education, to practice entry and support of generalist physicians. It is anticipated that ultimately 50 percent of MCG graduates will select generalist residency and generalist practice.

Public Institution

APPLICATION AND ACCEPTANCE POLICIES FOR 2001–2002 FIRST-YEAR CLASS

School participates in AMCAS. See Chapter 6.

Filing of AMCAS application
  Earliest date: June 1, 2000
  Latest date: Nov. 1, 2000
School application fee: None
Oldest MCAT scores considered: 1998
Does have Early Decision Program (EDP)
  For Georgia residents only
  EDP application period: June 1–Aug. 1, 2000
  EDP applicants notified by: Oct. 1, 2000
Acceptance notice to regular applicants
  Earliest date: Oct. 15, 2000
  Latest date: Until class is filled
Applicant's response to acceptance offer
  Maximum time: 2 weeks
Requests for deferred entrance considered: Yes
Deposit to hold place in class (applied to tuition):
  $50, due with response to acceptance offer
Deposit refundable prior to: Aug. 2001 (Orientation)
Estimated number of new entrants: 180 (55 EDP)
Starting date: Aug. 2001

TUITION AND STUDENT FEES PER YEAR FOR 1999–2000 FIRST-YEAR CLASS

Tuition
  Resident: $5,542
  Nonresident: $22,168

Student fees: $483

INFORMATION ON 1999–2000 FIRST-YEAR CLASS

Number of	*In-State*	*Out-of-State*	*Total*
Applicants	793	702	1,495
Applicants Interviewed	438	10	448
New Entrants*	178	2	180

*All took the MCAT; 99% had baccalaureate degrees.

CHAPTER 11

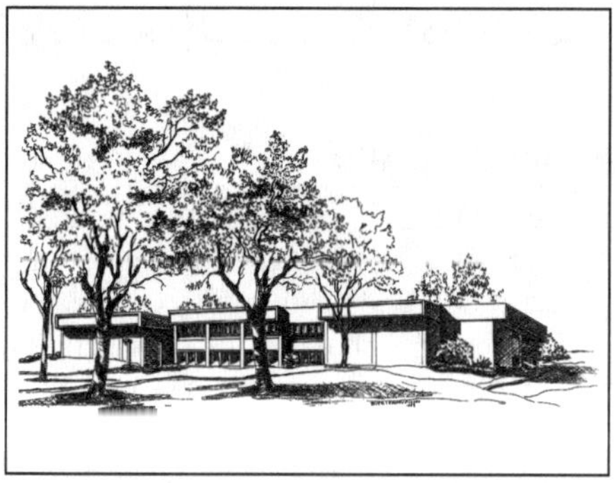

Mercer University School of Medicine

Macon, Georgia

Dr. W. Douglas Skelton, *Senior Vice President for University Research and Health Affairs, Dean School of Medicine*
Dr. Roger W. Comeau, *Associate Dean for Admissions and Student Affairs/Registrar*
Youvette D. Hudson, *Director for Financial Aid*

ADDRESS INQUIRIES TO:

Office of Admissions and
Student Affairs
Mercer University
School of Medicine
Macon, Georgia 31207
(912) 301-2524; 301-2547 (FAX)
E-mail: kothanek.j@gain.mercer.edu
Web Site: http://www.mercer.edu/

GENERAL INFORMATION

Mercer University School of Medicine (MUSM) admitted its charter class in August 1982. The school's mission is to educate physicians to meet the health care needs of rural and other underserved areas of Georgia. The program's educational format is that of problem-based, student-centered learning.

The medical education building located on the campus of Mercer University serves as the primary center for learning during the first two years. Mercer Health Systems, a 40-room ambulatory care facility, the Medical Center of Central Georgia, in Macon, and the Memorial Medical Center, in Savannah, serve as the primary affiliate clerkship sites. Clinical teaching is also provided at the Floyd Medical Center in Rome, Phoebe Putney Memorial Hospital in Albany, the Medical Center in Columbus, and several rural hospitals throughout Georgia.

CURRICULUM

While the major emphasis during the first two years is placed on the acquisition and practical application of basic science knowledge, there are also programs in bioethics and those that are designed to prepare the students for contact with patients in various inpatient, outpatient, community, and rural settings.

The Biomedical Problems Program is the educational vehicle for motivating students to obtain and apply the basic scientific knowledge germane to the practice of medicine. The onus of gathering this knowledge is on the individual student through a program of self-directed learning. The application occurs in small-group tutorials in which theme-based cases are discussed.

In the Clinical Skills Program students learn the basic skills necessary for interaction with patients. These skills include interview/medical history and physical examination techniques. Students interview and examine actual and "standardized" patients. The latter group is composed of persons who have been trained to portray specific medical problems and behavioral roles, and to give constructive feedback to students.

The Community Office Practice Program (COPP) provides students with the opportunity to learn and experience current administrative practices while observing and participating in the clinical aspects of a community-oriented, primary care medical practice. Students become familiar with the nature of a primary care practice in rural Georgia, while being educated on the health needs of individuals, families, and communities in the Community Science Program. It extends throughout the four years and culminates in a 4-week senior rural clerkship.

The third year consists of required clinical rotations in internal medicine, surgery, pediatrics, obstetrics-gynecology, ambulatory family medicine, and psychiatry. In addition, there are weekly programs in radiology. The fourth year is devoted to advanced clinical work, which includes 20 weeks of electives and required clerkships in acute or critical care, surgery subspecialties, rural and community medicine, and substance abuse.

REQUIREMENTS FOR ENTRANCE

The MCAT and the equivalent of three academic years or a minimum of 90 semester hours in an approved college or university are required for admission. Students are advised to balance their work in the biological sciences with courses in the social sciences and humanities. In addition, they are urged to follow their own inclinations in choosing a subject to pursue as a major. Required courses are:

	Years
General biology (with lab)	1
General or inorganic chemistry (with lab)	1
Organic chemistry or organic/biochemistry sequence (with lab)*	1
General physics (with lab)	1

**Must include one semester or two quarters of organic chemistry. Biochemistry is highly recommended.*

SELECTION FACTORS

The Admissions Committee has accepted only applicants who are legal residents of Georgia. Each applicant must also show promise of learning effectively in Mercer's curriculum and show strong potential of practicing a medical specialty commensurate with the health care needs of rural and other underserved areas of Georgia.

In addition to the AMCAS application, a supplementary application is required of applicants who meet preliminary selection criteria. This application has a $25 fee and requests the following: two letters of recommendation or one premedical committee evaluation, a personal history (a chronological list of residences and activities since the beginning of high school), certification of Georgia residency, and a list of the required premedical courses.

Interviews are by invitation only and are held at the medical school. In making the final decisions for acceptance or rejection, the Admissions Committee considers all criteria but emphasizes strongly an applicant's potential for complying with the mission of the institution. The committee does not discriminate on the basis of race, sex, creed, national origin, age, or handicap.

The 54 students that matriculated in 1999 consisted of 32 men and 22 women, 1 minority student, and the average age was 23.

FINANCIAL AID

Financial aid in the form of loans and scholarships is available. Awards are made on the basis of need and merit, with 88 pecent of the students receiving aid. Students can be approved for up to 15 hours of employment. Although acceptance to MUSM is not based on an applicant's ability to pay, the responsibility for adequate funding rests with the student. The financial aid officer conducts financial management conferences and assists students in obtaining needed support. An MUSM Faculty-Staff Emergency Loan Fund for students is also available.

INFORMATION FOR MINORITY STUDENTS

The school is committed to the recruitment of qualified individuals from minority groups and disadvantaged backgrounds.

Private Institution

APPLICATION AND ACCEPTANCE POLICIES FOR 2001–2002 FIRST-YEAR CLASS

School participates in AMCAS. See Chapter 6.

Filing of AMCAS application
  Earliest date: June 1, 2000
  Latest date: Nov. 1, 2000
School application fee after screening: $25
Oldest MCAT scores considered: 1998
Does have Early Decision Program (EDP)
  For Georgia residents only
  EDP application period: June 1–Aug. 1, 2000
  EDP applicants notified by: Oct. 1, 2000
Acceptance notice to regular applicants
  Earliest date: Oct. 15, 2001
  Latest date: Until class is filled
Applicant's response to acceptance offer
  Maximum time: 2 weeks
Requests for deferred entrance considered: Yes
Deposit to hold place in class (applied to tuition):
  $100, due with response to acceptance offer
Deposit refundable prior to: May 15, 2001
Estimated number of new entrants: 56 (12 EDP)
Starting date: Aug. 2001

TUITION AND STUDENT FEES PER YEAR FOR 1999–2000 FIRST-YEAR CLASS

Tuition and student fees: $21,778

INFORMATION ON 1999–2000 FIRST-YEAR CLASS

Number of	*In-State*	*Out-of-State*	*Total*
Applicants	546	468	1,014
Applicants Interviewed	182	0	182
New Entrants*	54	0	54

*All took the MCAT and had baccalaureate degrees.

CHAPTER 11

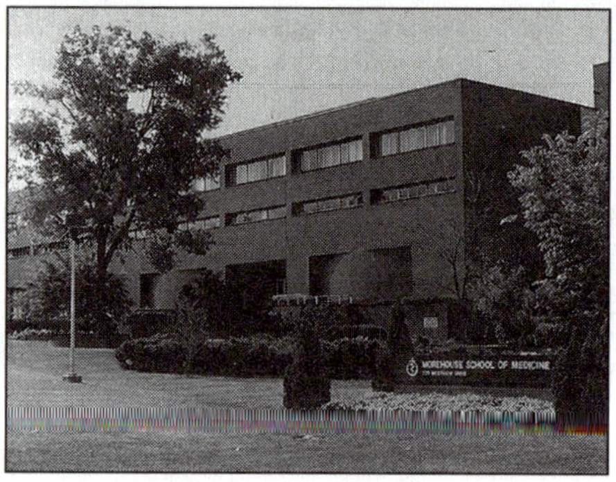

Morehouse School of Medicine

Atlanta, Georgia

Dr. Angela Walker Franklin, *Associate Dean for Student Affairs*
Karen A. Lewis, *Assistant Director of Admissions*
Cynthia Handy, *Director of Student Fiscal Affairs*

ADDRESS INQUIRIES TO:

Admissions and Student Affairs
Morehouse School of Medicine
720 Westview Drive, S.W.
Atlanta, Georgia 30310-1495
(404) 752-1650; 752-1512 (FAX)
Web Site: http://www.msm.edu

MISSION STATEMENT

Morehouse School of Medicine's main mission is to recruit and train minority and other students as physicians, biomedical scientists, and public health practitioners committed to meeting the primary health care needs of the underserved.

GENERAL INFORMATION

Morehouse School of Medicine is one of three medical schools in the nation founded by historically black institutions and is the first such medical school begun in this century. The School of Medicine admitted its first students to a two-year basic medical science curriculum in September 1978. The inaugural M.D. degree class graduated in May 1985.

Basic science teaching facilities are located in the lecture halls and multidisciplinary laboratories of the Basic Medical Sciences Building, which also houses research laboratories, preclinical departments, and administrative offices. The medical education building, dedicated in May 1987, houses clinical and preclinical departments, research laboratories, study areas, and the library. In May 1996, the new Multidisciplinary Research Center was dedicated.

Clinical instruction takes place in affiliated hospitals and clinics, including Grady Memorial Hospital and Southwest Community Hospital. The school also administers the Area Health Education Center Program.

CURRICULUM

An educational experience focusing both on scientific medicine and on meeting more effectively the primary health care needs of underserved inner-city and rural patients is offered. The concept of the patient as a whole person is fostered through a variety of teaching experiences that relate social, environmental, emotional, and cultural factors to medical disorders.

The first two years of the curriculum emphasize an understanding of the principles, concepts, and major factual background of the basic medical sciences. Exposure to clinical medicine begins in the first year through assignment to a preceptor and increases in the second year with introduction to clinical medicine. Clinical education is continued through core clerkships during the third and fourth years with 20 weeks of electives in the senior year. The major strengths of the curriculum include small class size, a highly diversified faculty, and courses that are taught by departmental and/or interdisciplinary faculty.

All students are required to pass Step 1 and Step 2 of the USMLE for promotion and graduation respectively. Student performance is evaluated primarily by letter grade. Promotion into the next year's class is recommended by the Student Academic Progress and Promotions Committee.

First-year classes begin in early July with a required summer program. Learning resources and other support services are available to all students throughout their four years. Morehouse School of Medicine also offers the Ph.D. in Biomedical Sciences and Master of Public Health degrees.

REQUIREMENTS FOR ENTRANCE

The MCAT and completion of a baccalaureate degree are required. It is highly recommended that the MCAT be taken in the spring of the year in which the application is made.

The faculty has no preference as to the major field of undergraduate study; students should determine their fields of major study according to their personal interest. Applicants are expected to present a sound, well-balanced academic background with evidence of competency in the stated requirements. Specific minimum requirements are:

	Year
Biology (with lab)	1
Inorganic or general chemistry (with lab)	1
Organic chemistry (with lab)	1
Physics (with lab)	1
College mathematics	1
English (including composition)	1

Course work in behavioral sciences is strongly recommended.

SELECTION FACTORS

Selection of students for admission is made by the Committee on Admissions after careful consideration of many factors. These include MCAT scores, the undergraduate academic record, the extent of academic improvement, balance and depth of academic program, difficulty of courses taken, and other indicators of maturation of learning ability. Additional factors considered by the committee include the nature of extracurricular activities, hobbies, the need to work, research projects and experiences, evidence of activities that indicate concurrence with the school's mission, and evidence of pursuing interests and talents in depth. Finally, the committee looks for evidence of those traits of personality and character essential to success in medicine: compassion, integrity, motivation, and perseverance.

All information available about each applicant is considered without assigning priority to any single factor. Students are admitted on the basis of individual qualifications regardless of sex, age, race, creed, national origin, or handicap. Preferential consideration is given to qualified applicants who are residents of the state of Georgia. However, all well-qualified applicants are encouraged to apply.

After receipt and preliminary screening of the AMCAS application, qualified applicants will be invited to submit a supplementary application and letters of evaluation. After review of all submitted materials, applicants who are competitive in this stage of the admissions process are invited to Atlanta for a personal interview. Interviews are arranged only by invitation of the Committee on Admissions.

Medical education requires that the accumulation of scientific knowledge be accompanied by the simultaneous acquisition of skills and professional attitudes and behavior. Technical standards have been established as a prerequisite for admission and graduation from the Morehouse School of Medicine. All courses in the curriculum are required in order to develop essential skills required to become a competent physician.

A candidate for the M.D. degree must have aptitude, abilities, and skills in five areas: observation, communication, motor, conceptual integrative and quantitative, and behavior and social.

Morehouse School of Medicine's Technical Standards for Medical School Admissions and Graduation are provided in the supplemental application packets.

Applicants are not considered for admission who have been dismissed from another medical school for academic or disciplinary reasons. Transfer applications are considered only from students in good standing at an LCME-accredited U.S. or Canadian medical school (foreign medical schools, osteopathic, veterinary, or dental schools are not acceptable). Transfers are allowed into the second year only on a space-available basis. Transfer application deadline is May 1.

FINANCIAL AID

A broad financial aid program is available. In addition to federally insured loan programs, a number of scholarships and loans are available. Scholarships and loans are awarded on the basis of documented financial need as determined by the College Scholarship Service needs analysis system (see Part 1). Applicants with an AMCAS fee waiver can waive the $45 school application fee. Accepted applicants are eligible to apply for financial aid to the Office of Student Fiscal Affairs. Approximately 94 percent of the students receive some form of financial aid during a part or all of their four years of study. Students are discouraged from accepting outside employment because of the lack of available time during a heavy academic schedule.

Private Institution

APPLICATION AND ACCEPTANCE POLICIES FOR 2001–2002 FIRST-YEAR CLASS

School participates in AMCAS. See Chapter 6.

Filing of AMCAS application
  Earliest date: June 1, 2000
  Latest date: Dec. 1, 2000
School application fee to all applicants: $45
Oldest MCAT scores considered: 1998
Does have Early Decision Program (EDP)
  For URM residents of Georgia only
  EDP application period: June 1–Aug. 1, 2000
  EDP applicants notified by: Oct. 1, 2000
Acceptance notice to regular applicants
  Earliest date: Dec. 20, 2000
  Latest date: Until class is filled
Applicant's response to acceptance offer
  Maximum time: 2 weeks
Requests for deferred entrance considered: Yes
Deposit to hold place in class (applied to tuition):
  $100, due with response to acceptance offer
Deposit refundable prior to: May 15, 2001
Estimated number of new entrants: 40 (1 EDP)
Starting date: July 2001

TUITION AND STUDENT FEES PER YEAR FOR 1999–2000 FIRST-YEAR CLASS

Tuition: $19,200 Student fees: $2,574

INFORMATION ON 1999–2000 FIRST-YEAR CLASS

Number of	*In-State*	*Out-of-State*	*Total*
Applicants	305	2,542	2,847
Applicants Interviewed	74	129	203
New Entrants*	26	14	40

*All took the MCAT and had baccalaureate degrees.

CHAPTER 11

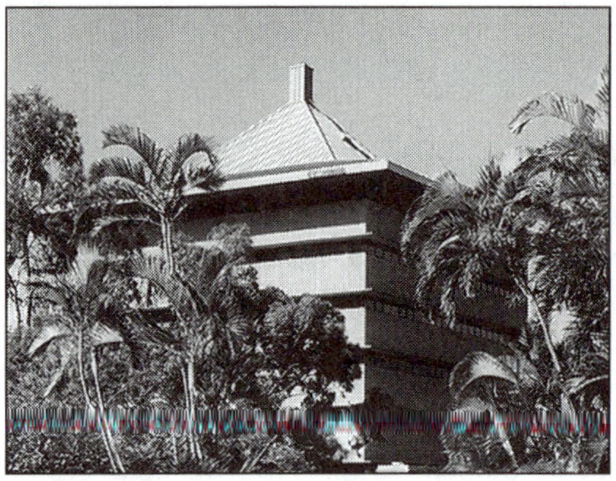

University of Hawai'i at Mānoa John A. Burns School of Medicine

Honolulu, Hawaii

Dr. Edwin C. Cadman, *Dean*
Dr. Satoru Izutsu, *Associate Dean/Chair, Admissions Committee*
Marilyn M. Nishiki, *Admissions Officer/Registrar*

ADDRESS INQUIRIES TO:

Office of Admissions
University of Hawai'i at Mānoa
John A. Burns School of Medicine
1960 East-West Road
Honolulu, Hawaii 96822
(808) 956-8300; 956-9547 (FAX)
E-mail: nishikim@jabsom.biomed.hawaii.edu
Web Site: http://medworld.biomed.hawaii.edu

MISSION STATEMENT

The school's basic mission is the teaching and training of high-quality physicians, biomedical scientists, and allied health workers for Hawaii and the Pacific.

GENERAL INFORMATION

The University of Hawai'i at Mānoa John A. Burns School of Medicine is in the College of Health Sciences and Social Welfare, which also includes schools of public health, nursing, and social work. The School of Medicine is located on the Mānoa campus of the university in Honolulu and has some elements at nearby Leahi Hospital. It also has teaching facilities in affiliated community hospitals and primary care clinics throughout the state.

CURRICULUM

The school employs a problem-based learning curriculum, in which basic sciences are learned in the context of understanding and managing clinical problems. There are no required discipline-specific courses in the first two years. Clinical work, including principles of history taking and physical diagnosis, behavioral science, and community medicine, begins in the first year.

Special features of the program include the following: an emphasis on primary care medicine and cross-cultural psychiatry; clinical training in community hospitals and primary care clinics (by medical school faculty); interdisciplinary training in community medicine together with students of public health, nursing, and social work; and opportunities for preceptorships in rural areas of the Hawaiian Islands and other areas of the Pacific Basin.

Beginning in September 1992, 15 students who entered the freshman class experienced about 30 percent of their academic and clinical training at community sites. This program, known as the Academic Community Partnership in Health Professions Education and previously funded by the Kellogg Foundation, is at the Waianae Coast Comprehensive Health Center, the Kalihi-Palama Clinic, and the Queen Emma Clinics at the Queen's Medical Center. It will eventually involve other health care facilities around the state of Hawaii.

An honors/credit/no credit grading system is used along with individual evaluations of student performance by faculty.

REQUIREMENTS FOR ENTRANCE

The MCAT (taken within three years of the expected date of matriculation and no later than August of the year of application) and at least 90 college credits are required. Course work must include:

	Sem. hrs.
Biology (with lab)	8
Chemistry (with lab)	4
Molecular and Cell Biology (with lab)	4
Biochemistry	3
Physics (with lab)	8

These courses should be rigorous and the type acceptable for students majoring in these areas and where indicated should include laboratory experience. Additional enrichment in the biological social sciences is encouraged (e.g., immunology, genetics, microbiology, human anatomy, physiology, embryology, psychology, and sociology). Applicants also must be fully competent in reading, speaking, and writing the English language.

SELECTION FACTORS

All applicants are considered without discrimination as to age, sex, race, creed, national origin, or handicap. The school admits 62 students to its regular freshman class. The University of Hawai'i at Mānoa John A. Burns School of Medicine's first priority is to admit applicants with strong ties to the state of Hawaii. Applications go through two screens. The first admissions screen determines an applicant's ties to the State of Hawaii. This screen reviews an applicant's state or country of a) legal residence, b) birthplace, c) high school graduated, d) college attended, and e) parents' legal residence. An applicant who meets three of the five categories demonstrates ties to the state of Hawaii. The second admissions screen is the academic screen in which a resident or nonresident candidate must pass in order to be invited for interviews. Selection depends upon the prospective medical student's character, scholarship, ideals, motivation, and aptitude. An evaluation of what the potential student might contribute to the health profession in the Pacific is an integral part of the selection process. For the limited number of applicants who reach a secondary screening level, interviews are conducted in Hawaii. All interviewed applicants are reviewed and rated by the Admissions Committee. Acceptance, alternate, and rejection letters are mailed by late April. Offers of acceptance are sent out to the top-ranked applicants to fill the entering first-year class. Nonresident candidates must be highly ranked, preferably with some ties to Hawaii, to be accepted. No additional supplemental materials are requested of applicants on the alternate list.

The 1999 regular entering class had the following profile: *mean cumulative GPA,* 3.57; *mean MCAT scores, VR*-9.38, *PS*-9.87, *BS*-10.26.

Some candidates for the M.D. degree may also work toward master's or Ph.D. degrees within the university. Such joint programs require the explicit permission of the associate dean for student affairs, the university's Graduate Division, and the appropriate graduate faculty. Separate applications must be made to the Graduate Division and to the medical school. Applicants are accepted independently by the respective degree programs.

FINANCIAL AID

Financial status is not a factor in considering applicants for acceptance. Although financial aid is limited, efforts are made to assist medical students in obtaining loans and scholarships wherever possible. Loan funds from federal sources are only available to U.S. citizens. In general, students are discouraged from seeking outside employment. Approximately 70 percent of the student body currently receive financial assistance.

INFORMATION FOR MINORITY STUDENTS

The student body and faculty are cosmopolitan and include African Americans, Caucasians, Chinese, Filipinos, Hawaiians, Japanese, Koreans, Micronesians, Samoans, and others.

The John A. Burns School of Medicine is actively involved in the recruitment, admission, and retention of students from disadvantaged backgrounds, who are interested in pursuing an M.D. degree. The school provides a range of student services and faculty development programs through its Native Hawaiian Center of Excellence. In addition the school offers the Imi Hó ola Postbaccalaureate Program for students whose medical school applications were rejected, but who are deemed capable of succeeding in medical school. The curriculum emphasizes the integration of concepts and principles in the sciences and humanities, and further develops communication and learning skills. Interested persons are encouraged to contact Dr. Nanette L.K. Judd, Project Director, Imi Hó ola Postbaccalaureate Program, 1960 East-West Road, Honolulu, Hawaii 96822; or call (808) 956-3466.

Public Institution

APPLICATION AND ACCEPTANCE POLICIES FOR 2001–2002 FIRST-YEAR CLASS

School participates in AMCAS. See Chapter 6.

Filing of AMCAS application
  Earliest date: June 1, 2000
  Latest date: Dec. 1, 2000
School application fee after screening: $50
Oldest MCAT scores considered: 1998
Does have Early Decision Program (EDP)
  For residents of Hawaii only
  EDP application period: June 1–Aug. 1, 2000
  EDP applicants notified by: Oct. 1, 2000
Acceptance notice to regular applicants
  Earliest date: Oct. 15, 2000
  Latest date: Until class is filled
Applicant's response to acceptance offer
  Maximum time: 2 weeks
Requests for deferred entrance considered: Yes
Deposit to hold place in class: None
Estimated number of new entrants: 62 (1 EDP)
Starting date: Aug. 2001

TUITION AND STUDENT FEES PER YEAR FOR 1999–2000 FIRST-YEAR CLASS

Tuition
  Resident: $12,840
  Nonresident: $25,776
Student fees: $107

INFORMATION ON 1999–2000 FIRST-YEAR CLASS

Number of	*In-State*	*Out-of-State*	*Total*
Applicants	198	898	1,096
Applicants Interviewed	155	51	206
New Entrants*	55	7	62

*All took the MCAT; 98% had baccalaureate degrees.

CHAPTER 11

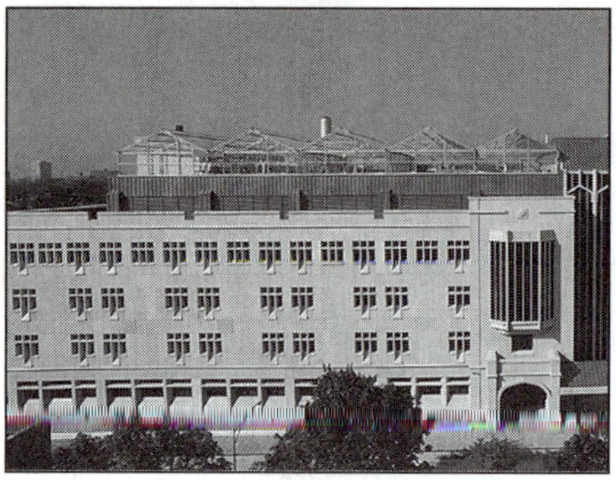

University of Chicago Pritzker School of Medicine

Chicago, Illinois

Dr. Glenn D. Steele, *Dean, Division of Biological Sciences and Pritzker School of Medicine*
Dr. Norma Wagoner, *Dean of Students*
Sylvia Robertson, *Director of Admissions*

ADDRESS INQUIRIES TO:

Office of the Dean of Students
Medical School Admissions
Pritzker School of Medicine
924 E. 57th Street, BLSC 104
Chicago, Illinois 60637-5416
(773) 702-1937; 702-2598 (FAX)
Web Site: http://pritzker.bsd.uchicago.edu

MISSION STATEMENT

The mission of the Division of the Biological Sciences of the University of Chicago is to discover and create new knowledge of living systems, to preserve and communicate knowledge through education, and to nurture and sustain a community of scholars. These scholars pursue this mission through research; through education of basic scientists, physicians, and others interested in living things; and through the enlightened and compassionate care of patients in a humane, academic environment. This faculty is oriented by values that include the responsibility to reduce human suffering, the desire to enhance human potential, and the obligation to be responsive to the rights and needs of both the individual and the community.

GENERAL INFORMATION

The University of Chicago is located on the south side of Chicago in the ethnically diverse community of Hyde Park, just 12 minutes from downtown Chicago. Organized into four major divisions—biological sciences, physical sciences, humanities, and social sciences—the university is made up predominantly of graduate and professional students. In addition to the four major divisions are six professional schools including the Pritzker School of Medicine, all on one campus. Nationally, Pritzker School of Medicine is unique in that it is a part of an academic Division of the Biological Sciences. As an integral part of a world-class university, it offers medical students diverse opportunities for interdisciplinary learning, clinical training, and research. In this environment, the school's mission is to train academic physicians. Over 90 percent of all students engage in some form of scholarly activity prior to completing the M.D. degree, and nearly 20 percent pursue combined M.D.-Ph.D. degrees. Of graduates from 1978–87, 19.1 percent became faculty members, a figure which is consistently among the highest.

CURRICULUM

The Pritzker School of Medicine is engaged in two major activities for education in the remainder of this century and the next. The first one was the completion of the Biological Sciences Learning Center and the Jules Knapp Institute for Molecular Medicine. This combined teaching and research facility serves as a visible sign of the linkages among science, teaching, and medicine in achieving the institution's mission. The Learning Center provides students and faculty a place to creatively use new methods and technologies. The Knapp Institute for Molecular Medicine houses research facilities for immunology, neurobiology, human genetics, molecular cardiology, and molecular oncology. The second one is curricular innovation. First-year students are taught clinical skills through an introduction to history taking and interviewing using standardized patients and small-group settings. In addition, students have the opportunity to explore the social, cultural, and ethical issues facing medicine with physicians from the McLean Center for Clinical Medical Ethics.

Basic science course work is horizontally integrated during the first two years, and the clinical skills course serves to bring about vertical integration with the patient as a focus. The third year is all clinical at three major sites: the University of Chicago Hospitals, Weiss Hospital, and MacNeal Hospital. Increased opportunities in primary care now include five months of outpatient and family practice medicine. The majority of the fourth year is elective. Pritzker is on a pass/fail grading system and does not require students to pass the USMLE for graduation.

A select number of students can pursue the M.D. and Ph.D. degrees in basic science areas with funding from the Medical Scientist Training Program or the NIH Pediatrics Growth and Development Training Grant. Other funding opportunities exist. The Ph.D. programs in Medicine, Arts, and Sciences (MAS) encourage students to pursue graduate studies in one of the arts and social sciences related to medicine. The M.B.A. or J.D. can be obtained if one is accepted to those schools.

REQUIREMENTS FOR ENTRANCE

The MCAT is required of all applicants. Applicants are required to have completed at least 90 credit hours of college-level work, although a four-year baccalaureate degree is preferable. Pritzker's academic program is rigorous, and applicants are encouraged to obtain a strong course foundation in general education (English composition, mathematics, social sciences, and humanities), as well as the required science courses. The specific course requirements for admission are:

	Years
Biology or zoology (with lab)	1
Inorganic chemistry (with lab)	1
Organic chemistry (with lab)	1
Physics (with lab)	1

Pritzker has a rigorous graduate-level curriculum in biochemistry, and applicants are encouraged to have a working knowledge of biochemical principles prior to matriculation. Biochemistry with lab may be substituted for one half of the organic chemistry requirement.

SELECTION FACTORS

Applicants are selected solely on the basis of their ability, achievement, motivation, and humanistic qualities. Pritzker does not discriminate on the basis of race, sex, creed, national origin, age, or handicap. The Committee on Admissions carefully selects between 500 and 600 applicants from among its large applicant pool for interviews on the Pritzker campus from mid-September through March. There are no residency restrictions, but about 35 percent of the entering class come from the state of Illinois. Students in the 1999 entering class had the following academic profile: average *GPA–science,* 3.60; *cumulative,* 3.61; *average MCAT*, 10.1; 10.8; 10.7.

During most application cycles the University of Chicago has a very small number (1-3) of positions available for transfer into the second- and third-year classes. Students who are successful in achieving transfer have compelling personal reasons to be in the Chicago area and academic and extracurricular credentials, which match those of the class they seek to enter. Transfer applications are available after February 1, 2001, for entry in 2001.

A University of Chicago supplementary application is mailed to every applicant who submits an application through AMCAS. The deadline for submission of the completed supplementary application, for entry in 2001, is January 5, 2001. Letters of recommendation are required as part of the application. Once the application materials are complete, the Admissions Committee reviews the candidate's total file. The decision is then made of whether or not to extend an interview invitation. Personal characteristics and learning skills are as important as demonstrated excellence in academic performance. There must be evidence of commitment, not only to acquire an excellent knowledge base but also to develop learning and problem-solving skills, which will sustain the individual for lifelong learning.

FINANCIAL AID

The Pritzker School of Medicine believes no student should be denied admission or be unable to attend for financial reasons. Scholarships and low-interest loans are made available to all students who have demonstrated need. There are both federally subsidized loans and low or no interest loans from the university. Approximately 82 percent of students receive some form of financial assistance. Current levels of indebtedness for Pritzker students are below the national mean for private institutions. Financial aid packets are mailed to all accepted applicants after January 1. Financial aid resources for international applicants are extremely limited.

INFORMATION FOR MINORITY STUDENTS

Pritzker is particularly interested in seeking diversity among its students and is sensitive to society's needs for increasing the representation of minority men and women among physicians. Minority medical students who have attended Pritzker often assume strong leadership roles, both within their class and at the national level.

Private Institution

APPLICATION AND ACCEPTANCE POLICIES FOR 2001–2002 FIRST-YEAR CLASS

School participates in AMCAS. See Chapter 6.

Filing of AMCAS application
  Earliest date: June 1, 2000
  Latest date: Nov. 15, 2000
School application fee after screening: $60
Oldest MCAT scores considered: 1998
  Does have Early Decision Program (EDP)
  EDP application period: June 1–Aug. 1, 2000
  EDP applicants notified by: Oct. 1, 2000
Acceptance notice to regular applicants
  Earliest date: Oct. 15, 2000
  Latest date: Until class is filled
Applicant's response to acceptance offer
  Maximum time: 30 days
Requests for deferred entrance considered: Yes
Deposit to hold place in class (applied to tuition):
  $100, due with response to acceptance offer
Deposit refundable prior to: July 1, 2001
Estimated number of new entrants: 104 (2 EDP)
Starting date: Sept. 2001

TUITION AND STUDENT FEES PER YEAR FOR 1999–2000 FIRST-YEAR CLASS

Tuition: $25,074   Student fees: $1,326

INFORMATION ON 1999–2000 FIRST-YEAR CLASS

Number of	*In-State*	*Out-of-State*	*Total*
Applicants	1,020	6,423	7,443
Applicants Interviewed	157	420	577
New Entrants*	40	64	104

*All took the MCAT and had baccalaureate degrees.

CHAPTER 11

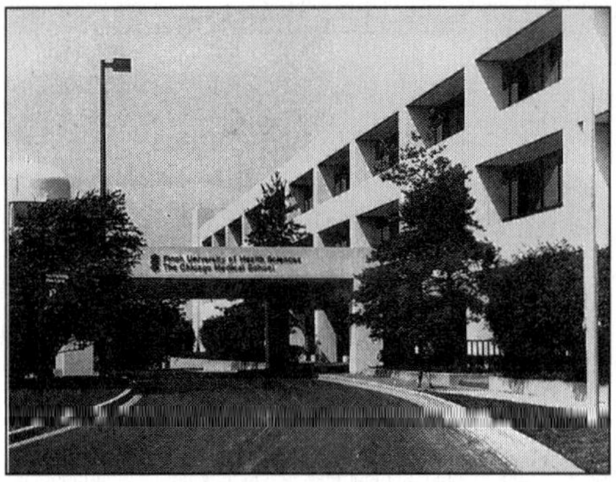

Finch University of Health Sciences/ Chicago Medical School

North Chicago, Illinois

Dr. Robert M. Suskind, *Dean, Chicago Medical School*
Kristine A. Jones, *Director of Admissions and Registrar*
Maryann DeCaire, *Director of Financial Aid*

ADDRESS INQUIRIES TO:

Office of Admissions
Chicago Medical School
3333 Green Bay Road
North Chicago, Illinois 60064
(847) 578-3206/3207
E-mail: jonesk@finchcms.edu
Web Site: http://www.finchcms.edu/

MISSION STATEMENT

The mission of Finch University of Health Sciences/ Chicago Medical School is to acquire, preserve, enhance, and communicate knowledge of the health sciences for the welfare of humanity and improvement of the environment. The school is dedicated to the education and training of professionals in the health sciences at all levels of training and experience. These goals are continually evaluated in terms of the school nurturing education, research, and health care delivery.

GENERAL INFORMATION

The Chicago Medical School, founded in 1912, is part of the Finch University of Health Sciences, which is located in North Chicago, Illinois. It is a private, nonsectarian, coeducational institution chartered by the state of Illinois and administered by a Board of Trustees. The Chicago Medical School is the core component of three allied units. One unit is the School of Graduate and Postdoctoral Studies, which grants degrees at the master and doctoral levels in the major basic science areas, as well as the doctorate in clinical psychology. The School of Related Health Sciences currently offers programs in physical therapy, medical technology, healthcare management, nutrition, and physician assistant practice, leading to DPT, baccalaureate, and master's degrees. In addition, the university has a B.S.–M.D. honors program in engineering/medicine, in conjunction with the Illinois Institute of Technology. Clinical training at various levels is provided at Cook County Hospital, Edward Hines Veterans Affairs Medical Center, Christ Hospital, Mt. Sinai Hospital, North Chicago Veterans Affairs Medical Center, Illinois Masonic Medical Center, Swedish Covenant Hospital, Norwalk (CT) Hospital, and Lutheran General Hospital.

CURRICULUM

To meet the changing needs of the future physician, the content of the curriculum is under continual evaluation and revision. The curriculum offers students a strong foundation in both the science and practice of medicine by providing an interface between basic science and clinical science.

Currently, the four-year curriculum consists of 13 terms. Of the 6 terms of basic science, the first 3 are devoted primarily to the study of the structure and function of the human body. Many courses, including medical ethics, genetics, and biostatistics, are offered in didactic and small-group sessions. The following 3 terms are devoted to the study of disease etiology, processes, therapy, and prevention. Concomitantly, there is extensive training in physical diagnosis, medical interviewing, and history-writing. Of the last 7 terms, 48 weeks are devoted to junior clinical rotations and 36 weeks are spent in senior clinical selectives, electives, and/or basic science courses. The required junior clinical clerkships include medicine, surgery, obstetrics-gynecology, psychiatry, family medicine, pediatrics, emergency medicine, and ambulatory care medicine. The senior requirements include a medical subinternship and a neurology clerkship, plus 28 weeks of approved electives (14 of which must be done on campus). The elective period gives students an opportunity, through both intramural and extramural experiences, to explore and strengthen their personal career interests.

Along with passing all courses and clerkships, students are required to pass Step 1 and Step 2 of the USMLE as a requisite for graduation.

All students are required to complete the first two years within three academic years; clinical clerkships and electives are to be completed within 2½ years. Thus, students must complete their education at the Chicago Medical School in no more than 5½ years, unless enrolled in a combined-degree program, or on an approved extended program, or on an approved leave of absence.

Combined M.D.-Ph.D. degree programs are available for students interested in biomedical or clinical research. These programs provide an opportunity for a limited number of students to pursue a program of individualized course work and research leading to the M.D. and Ph.D. degrees. Candidates who complete their Ph.D. degrees may receive full tuition scholarships for all four years of medical school and their graduate studies. Applications and additional information are available from the director, combined M.D.-Ph.D. degree program.

REQUIREMENTS FOR ENTRANCE

The MCAT and three years of college (minimum of 135 quarter hours) are required; the baccalaureate degree is preferred. The college work must include the following:

	Years
Biology or zoology (with lab)	1
Inorganic chemistry (with lab)	1
Organic chemistry (with lab)	1
General physics (with lab)	1

Science courses beyond those required will be helpful in preparing for study in medical school; however, the applicant is expected to have a broad foundation in general education, and any major field of interest is acceptable.

SELECTION FACTORS

Students are selected on the basis of various criteria, including scholarship, character, motivation, and educational background without regard to race, creed, religion, sex, sexual orientation, disability, age, or national origin. One's potential for the study and practice of medicine will be evaluated on the basis of academic achievement, MCAT results, personal appraisals by a preprofessional advisory committee or individual instructors, and a personal interview, if requested by the Student Admissions Committee.

Successful applicants for the 1999 entering class had the following credentials: *mean GPA,* 3.29; *residence,* 37 percent from Illinois, with the remainder from 18 other states; *undergraduate major,* 44 percent in biology or chemistry, with the remainder from a variety of fields. Approximately 31 percent of those seriously considered matriculated.

Applicants working on advanced degrees will be considered on the same basis as all other applicants. Applicants who have not been accepted previously and who make reapplication will be treated on the same basis as first-time applicants.

Finch University offers other programs that produce applicants who are considered for admission by the Chicago Medical School. Acceptance of graduates from the MS Applied Physiology program and others may effectively reduce the number of places available for general AMCAS applicants.

FINANCIAL AID

Limited university-administered financial aid is available to students who are unable to meet school costs through family resources and major financial aid programs. Awards are made to eligible students based on the availability of funds and demonstrated financial need (expenses minus resources). The university utilizes FAFSA to uniformly measure student resources. Approximately 75 percent of the medical students receive financial assistance. An average award through university-administered funds is $2,500 for full-need medical students.

INFORMATION FOR MINORITY STUDENTS

The school maintains an extensive recruitment and retention program for minority students. Application fees may be waived for financially disadvantaged students. Deceleration of basic science curriculum is an option available to all students with demonstrated need.

Private Institution

APPLICATION AND ACCEPTANCE POLICIES FOR 2001–2002 FIRST-YEAR CLASS

School participates in AMCAS. See Chapter 6.

Filing of AMCAS application
  Earliest date: June 1, 2000
  Latest date: Nov. 15, 2000
School application fee to all applicants: $85
Oldest MCAT scores considered: 1998
Does have Early Decision Program (EDP)
  EDP application period: June 1–Aug. 1, 2000
  EDP applicants notified by: Oct. 1, 2000
Acceptance notice to regular applicants
  Earliest date: Oct. 15, 2000
  Latest date: Until class is filled
Applicant's response to acceptance offer
  Maximum time: 2 weeks
Requests for deferred entrance considered: Yes
Deposit to hold place in class (applied to tuition):
  $100, due with response to acceptance offer
Deposit refundable prior to: May 15, 2001
  Estimated number of new entrants: 165 (3 EDP)
Starting date: July 2001

TUITION AND STUDENT FEES PER YEAR FOR 1999–2000 FIRST-YEAR CLASS

Tuition: $33,527 Student fees: $100

INFORMATION ON 1999–2000 FIRST-YEAR CLASS

Number of	*In-State*	*Out-of-State*	*Total*
Applicants	1,150	7,912	9,062
Applicants Interviewed	146	384	530
New Entrants*	61	105	166

*All took the MCAT and had baccalaureate degrees.

UIC The University of Illinois at Chicago

Chicago-Peoria-Rockford
Urbana/Champaign

University of Illinois at Chicago College of Medicine

Chicago, Illinois

Dr. Gerald S. Moss, *Dean*
Dr. Jorge A. Girotti, *Associate Dean and Director, College of Medicine Admissions*
James Mendez, *Associate Director of Financial Aid*

ADDRESS INQUIRIES TO:

Medical College Admissions
Room 165 CME M/C 783
University of Illinois
College of Medicine
808 South Wood Street
Chicago, Illinois 60612-7302
(312) 996-5635; 996-6693 (FAX)
Web Site: http://www.uic.edu/depts/mcam

GENERAL INFORMATION

Founded in 1881 as the College of Physicians and Surgeons of Chicago, the name was changed to the University of Illinois College of Medicine in 1900. Following a reorganization of college structure approved by the Board of Trustees in 1982, the College of Medicine programs are now conducted on two educational tracks at four geographic sites. The College of Medicine at Chicago is located at the Health Sciences Center of the university. The College of Medicine at Urbana-Champaign offers a four-year medical curriculum integrated with the programs of a comprehensive campus. The College of Medicine at Peoria includes facilities in each of the hospitals in that community and a modern downtown campus. The College of Medicine at Rockford has a centrally located campus and conducts programs in each of the Rockford hospitals and in several nearby smaller communities.

CURRICULUM

There are two separate curricular tracks within the College of Medicine. Students assigned to the Chicago campus will pursue their full four-year program of undergraduate medical education under the supervision of the faculty at that site. Students assigned for their first year of instruction to the Urbana-Champaign campus either will remain assigned to that site for the last three years or will transfer to Peoria or Rockford for the three remaining years of the program. Once students begin in either Chicago or Urbana-Champaign, transfers between curricular tracks will be limited.

Each clinical curriculum presents techniques and information necessary for examination and care for the patient, and each provides supervised experiences in a wide variety of clinical settings under direction of the faculty. Through college-level faculty committees consisting of representation from all sites, the standards of quality are regularly evaluated for admissions, instruction student appraisal, and student promotion.

The college also offers a number of special programs. The Medical Scholars Program on the Urbana-Champaign campus links the medical school with over 40 other academic units, including the natural and biological sciences, social sciences, humanities, business administration, and law, so that students can earn a combined graduate and medical degree. A combined-degree program on the Chicago campus enables medical students to carry out graduate work in the basic medical sciences and public health. The Chicago, Rockford, and Peoria campuses offer independent study programs through which medical students can design their own curricula and carry out in-depth studies of health care topics in which they have a special interest.

REQUIREMENTS FOR ENTRANCE

All candidates must take the MCAT no later than the fall test period of the academic year in which application is made. The Committee on Admissions uses in its evaluation the highest MCAT scores reported of three previous years.

Applicants must be citizens of the United States or permanent legal residents in order to apply.

Applicants must receive the baccalaureate degree prior to matriculation in the College of Medicine. Students may elect any major field of interest. Biology, chemistry (through organic), physics or biophysics, and behavioral science will be particularly helpful in preparing for study in the college. However, the undergraduate major may be chosen from the humanities, fine arts or behavioral, biological, or physical sciences. Mathematics through calculus is useful for those anticipating advanced work in basic or clinical research.

The following courses are required:

	Semesters
Biology or equivalent (with lab)	2
Inorganic chemistry or equivalent (with lab)	2
Organic chemistry (with lab)	2
(Note: introductory biochemistry may substitute for a semester of organic chemistry)	
General physics or equivalent	2
Social science with an emphasis in the behavioral sciences	3

A minimum of two semesters must be taken in a sequence within the same department and an additional semester within the social sciences. Letters of recommendation are required of all applicants.

SELECTION FACTORS

All candidates apply to the Committee on Admissions, and admitted applicants are given their choices of study sites insofar as places permit. Prospective and admitted students are provided with detailed information to help in their selection of sites.

The College of Medicine endeavors to select applicants who in the judgment of the Committee on Admissions demonstrate best the academic achievement, emotional stability, maturity, integrity, and motivation adjudged necessary for successful study and practice of medicine. The committee is interested in evidence of the applicant's capacity for mature and independent scholarship, while discouraging rigid patterns of course work. The committee will consider the quality of work of each applicant in all subject areas, the breadth of education, achievement in advanced projects, and work and extracurricular experiences that demonstrate the applicant's imagination, initiative, and creativity. The College of Medicine does not discriminate against applicants on the basis of race, creed, sex, religion, national origin, age, disability, or status as a disabled veteran or veteran of the Vietnam era.

Selection of students is based on a critical evaluation of all available data on each applicant and on the changing needs of society. The Committee on Admissions gives strong preference to candidates who are Illinois residents and who also: (1) possess a GPA of B or better, (2) have attained an MCAT score above the national mean, and (3) meet the safety and technical standards set by the college. Candidates whose formal education has been interrupted are reviewed with respect to their potential contribution to the practice of medicine and to their competitive status with other applicants. An interview of selected candidates will be required.

FINANCIAL AID

Entering students are encouraged to provide timely application through the College of Medicine's Office of Student Financial Aid for loan funds and grant-in-aid scholarship assistance based on need. Grants and scholarships to meet proven financial need are awarded each year to students from all classes. Financial aid consultation and information can be obtained by calling (312) 413-0127.

INFORMATION FOR MINORITY AND RURAL CANDIDATES

The College of Medicine has developed programs to encourage applications from qualified individuals from medically underserved areas of Illinois. The college maintains a professional staff to provide guidance and counseling to motivated students from minority ethnic groups (African American, Hispanic, American Indian) and resident candidates whose backgrounds indicate potential for rural Illinois practice. The Committee on Admissions reviews all applications, and students are accepted on the basis of their potential for successfully meeting all college standards leading to the M.D. degree.

Public Institution

APPLICATION AND ACCEPTANCE POLICIES FOR 2001–2002 FIRST-YEAR CLASS

School participates in AMCAS. See Chapter 6.

Filing of AMCAS application
- Earliest date: June 1, 2000
- Latest date: Dec. 31, 2000

School application fee after screening: $40
Oldest MCAT scores considered: 1998
Does have Early Decision Program (EDP)
- For Illinois residents only
- EDP application period: June 1–Aug. 1, 2000
- EDP applicants notified by: Oct. 1, 2000

Acceptance notice to regular applicants
- Earliest date: Oct. 15, 2000
- Latest date: Until class is filled

Applicant's response to acceptance offer
- Maximum time: 2 weeks

Requests for deferred entrance considered: Yes
Deposit to hold place in class: None
Estimated number of new entrants: 300 (10 EDP)
Starting date: Aug. 2001

TUITION AND STUDENT FEES PER YEAR FOR 1999–2000 FIRST-YEAR CLASS

Tuition
- Resident: $16,294
- Nonresident: $39,826

Student fees: $1,560

INFORMATION ON 1999–2000 FIRST-YEAR CLASS

Number of	*In-State*	*Out-of-State*	*Total*
Applicants	1,677	2,483	4,160
Applicants Interviewed	638	91	729
New Entrants*	275	25	300

*All took the MCAT and had baccalaureate degrees.

CHAPTER 11

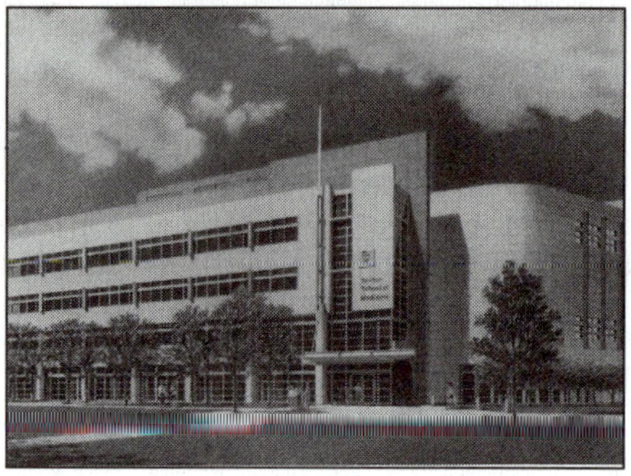

Loyola University Chicago Stritch School of Medicine

Maywood, Illinois

Dr. Stephen Slogoff, *Acting Dean*
LaDonna E. Norstrom, *Assistant Dean, Admissions*
Donna J. Sobie, Director, *Financial Aid*

ADDRESS INQUIRIES TO:

Loyola University Chicago
Stritch School of Medicine
Office of Admissions
2160 South First Avenue
Maywood, Illinois 60153
(708) 216-3229

GENERAL INFORMATION

Loyola University Chicago is a private university founded in 1870 by the Jesuits. It is one of the largest Catholic universities in the United States. By 1920 the university had organized several small medical colleges into a new medical school. In 1948 the school was named in honor of Samuel Cardinal Stritch, Archbishop of Chicago. In 1969 the university opened the Loyola University Medical Center, built on land given by the Veterans Administration, in Maywood, a suburban community located 12 miles west of the Chicago Loop. The medical center houses both the Stritch School of Medicine and the Foster G. McGaw Hospital. Students receive their clinical training at the 541-bed McGaw Hospital, at the 639-bed Hines Veterans Administration Hospital, and at a number of affiliated hospitals in the Chicago area.

CURRICULUM

The primary purpose of the Stritch School of Medicine is to train physicians who will care for their patients with skill, respect, and compassion. The personal and intellectual development of each student is promoted through close contact with members of the faculty and administration. Students are exposed to the operation of a large medical center, as well as to VA and community offices and hospitals, where they learn in an atmosphere of cooperation and mutual assistance. The first year of the curriculum concentrates on the basic principles and processes related to the normal structure, function, and regulation of the human body. In addition, the first year includes instruction in health promotion/disease prevention, health care finance and access, medical ethics, medical/legal issues, and the doctor/patient relationship. Students also have the opportunity to visit ambulatory care sites to experience the delivery of medical care in the ambulatory setting. The second year of the curriculum focuses on basic science principles related to the mechanisms of human disease, neuroscience, and the therapeutic approach to disease. Additionally, students have the opportunity to continue to develop their knowledge about human behavioral science, physical examination skills, basic clinical skills, evidence-based clinical decision making, and medical ethics and humanities. The third and fourth years are organized into clinical clerkships. The core curriculum includes medicine (12 weeks), critical-care experiences (4 weeks), sub-internship (4 weeks), surgery (12 weeks), pediatrics (6 weeks), psychiatry (6 weeks), family medicine (6 weeks), neurology (4 weeks), and obstetrics and gynecology (6 weeks). Students also take between 26 and 34 weeks of electives during the fourth year. Through these electives, they anticipate their residency training and prepare for careers in medicine suited to their particular interests and talents.

Special features of the curriculum include the Medical Humanities Program, which extends from the basic science semesters through clinical training, a Mentor Program, and the Dual Degree Program, whereby medical students can earn M.D. and Ph.D. degrees in order to prepare for careers as medical scientists and teachers.

REQUIREMENTS FOR ENTRANCE

A bachelor's degree and the MCAT, preferably taken by the spring but no later than the fall of the year of application, are required. The following courses are required:

	Years
Biology or zoology (with lab)	1
Inorganic chemistry (with lab)	1
Organic chemistry (with lab)	1
Physics (with lab)	1

A semester or quarter of biochemistry can be substituted for part of the organic chemistry requirement.

Any undergraduate major is acceptable. Applicants are expected to take challenging course work in the humanities and social sciences, and they should be able to speak and write the English language correctly.

Applicants must be U.S. citizens or hold a permanent resident visa. As a rule, applicants are limited to applying no more than twice. Applicants enrolled in advanced-degree programs must expect to complete their degrees prior to matriculation.

SELECTION FACTORS

The academic record will be evaluated for both depth and breadth of study. Circumstances, such as need to work, which affect a student's academic performance will be taken into account when the record is evaluated. The 1999 entering class had a mean GPA of 3.60. Applicants who present academic credentials that indicate they are capable of succeeding in the rigors of a medical education will be evaluated for evidence of the personal qualifications they can bring to the medical profession. Essential characteristics include an interest in learning, integrity, compassion, and the ability to assume responsibility. Of particular concern will be an applicant's exploration of the field of medicine and the nature of the motivation to enter this career. Each year approximately 600 applicants are invited to interviews with members of the Committee on Admissions. These interviews are conducted only at the medical center campus.

At least 50 percent of each entering class are residents of Illinois. Approximately 45 percent of each entering class are women, and the age range of accepted applicants is quite broad. Early submission of the AMCAS application and prompt return of all supporting material will enhance an applicant's chance of being offered a place in the class.

Loyola University does not discriminate on the basis of race, religion, national origin, sex, age, or handicap. The Committee on Admissions attempts to select students with diversified backgrounds for the contributions they can make to the educational process and the medical profession. Members of minority groups are encouraged to apply.

FINANCIAL AID

Over 90 percent of Stritch students receive some form of financial aid during the four years of medical school. Student aid is primarily in the form of loans, but limited scholarship and grant money is also available. Some students have found it possible to work during their first two years, often in jobs at the medical center. The school's financial aid office attempts to keep student debt at a manageable level through workshops on budgeting and financial planning. Applicants should receive a preliminary financial aid award approximately two months after submitting financial aid forms.

TRANSFER/ADVANCED STANDING

Medical students who wish to transfer to Stritch for their third year must be enrolled in an allopathic medical school located in the United States that is accredited by the Liaison Committee on Medical Education. Space for transfer students depends on attrition; consequently few, if any, spaces are available each year.

Students who wish to transfer to Stritch may contact our Admissions Office beginning March 1 to request a special application; submission deadline for all materials is May 1. Applicants must take Step 1 of the United States Medical Licensing Examination (USMLE) under the sponsorship of their present medical school.

INFORMATION FOR MINORITY STUDENTS

Minority Medical Education program (MMEP)

The Loyola University Chicago Stritch School of Medicine is a participant in the Minority Medical Education Program through the Chicago Summer Science Enrichment Program. The MMEP was developed by the Robert Wood Johnson Foundation and is supported by it in conjunction with the Association of American Medical Colleges. This six-week, intensive summer enrichment program provides highly motivated minority students with an integrated, science-oriented curriculum designed to strengthen their competitiveness for medical school admission. The Chicago Summer Science Enrichment Program uses the resources of Loyola and three other Chicago-area medical schools to provide educational experiences uniquely directed toward the needs and preparatory background of participants who are enrolled in all years of undergraduate college. Applications are available in the fall annually. Further information is available from MMEP@aamc.org or juana@prufrock.bsd.uchicago.edu.

Private Institution

APPLICATION AND ACCEPTANCE POLICIES FOR 2001–2002 FIRST-YEAR CLASS

School participates in AMCAS. See Chapter 6.

Filing of AMCAS application
  Earliest date: June 1, 2000
  Latest date: Nov. 15, 2000
School application fee after screening: $50
Oldest MCAT scores considered: 1997
Does not have Early Decision Program
Acceptance notice to regular applicants
  Earliest date: Oct. 15, 2000
  Latest date: Until class is filled
Applicant's response to acceptance offer
  Maximum time: 2 weeks
Requests for deferred entrance considered: Yes
Deposit to hold place in class: None
Estimated number of new entrants: 130
Starting date: July 2001

TUITION AND STUDENT FEES PER YEAR FOR 1999–2000 FIRST-YEAR CLASS

Tuition: $28,800   Student fees: $655

INFORMATION ON 1999–2000 FIRST-YEAR CLASS

Number of	*In-State*	*Out-of-State*	*Total*
Applicants	1,372	6,500	7,872
Applicants Interviewed	251	334	585
New Entrants*	65	65	130

*All took the MCAT and had baccalaureate degrees.

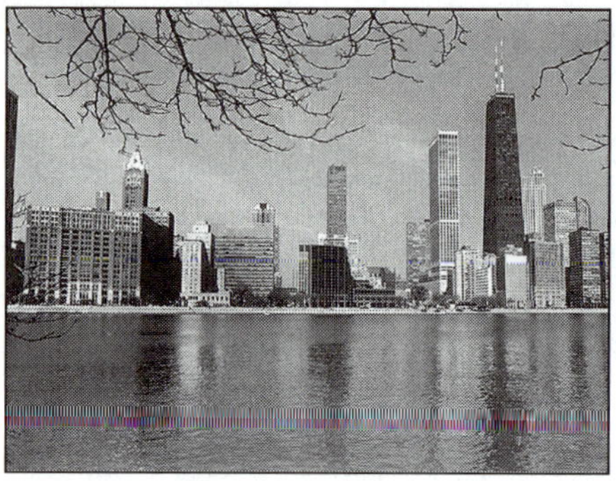

Northwestern University Medical School

Chicago, Illinois

Dr. Lewis Landsberg, *Interim Dean*
Dolores G. Brown, *Associate Dean for Admissions*
Effie N. Barnett, *Director of Financial Aid*

ADDRESS INQUIRIES TO:

Northwestern University Medical School
303 East Chicago Avenue
Chicago, Illinois 60611
(312) 503-8206
E-mail: med-admissions@nwu.edu
Web Site: http://www.nums.nwu.edu/viewbook/mdprog.htm

MISSION STATEMENT

Students graduated from Northwestern University Medical School are well grounded scientifically and clinically. Committed to the ethical and humane practice of medicine, they learn how to approach patients, perform physical examinations, and formulate a plan of investigation for optimal health management. Beyond diagnosis and treatment, they appreciate the importance of disease prevention, utilizing the skills of allied health professionals, and ascertaining the role of the patient's relationships with family, friends, and the community in producing and alleviating symptoms. Students become life-long learners, understanding that knowledge at any time is only a prologue to new facts and concepts. They are well prepared for their choice of careers in either the practice of medicine, or for a research-oriented career in academic medicine.

GENERAL INFORMATION

Founded in 1859, the Medical School is located on the university's lakefront Chicago campus. Medical students may live on campus at Abbott Hall or Lake Shore Center. More than 2,400 full-time, part-time, and contributed services faculty members offer instruction in the basic sciences and clinical medicine. The school also offers opportunities in basic science research and clinical research. The McGaw hospitals at which students gain clinical experience—a group of urban, suburban, specialized, and general hospitals—are Northwestern Memorial, Children's Memorial, Evanston, and Glenbrook hospitals; Rehabilitation Institute of Chicago; and VA Chicago Health Care System—Lakeside Division.

CURRICULUM

Northwestern medical students are trained through an integrated, organ system-based curriculum that contains the essential basic science and the biopsychosocial foundations of medicine. There are two hours of lecture and two hours of directed, independent, active learning (problem-based learning, laboratories, small-group discussions, student presentations, and group projects) each morning.

The first year integrates biochemistry, cell and molecular biology, genetics, cell physiology, gross and microscopic anatomy, physiology, and neuroscience, while the second year combines immunology, microbiology, infectious diseases, pharmacology, pathology, and pathophysiology. Three short blocks of time are devoted to Medical Decision Making, which develops a student's abilities in information analysis and management, dealing with uncertainty and clinical decision making, and refining learning skills.

In the first two years, students also take Patient, Physician, and Society (PPS), which meets two afternoons a week. Each student participates as a member of one of four colleges, led by a mentor faculty member. Designed to facilitate student collaboration, faculty-student interaction, and active patient contact, the course involves learning skills physicians should possess to practice medicine (e.g., interviewing and physical examination skills, communication skills, and an understanding of human behavior) and prepares the students to confront and learn to deal with attitudes and knowledge reflecting the interface of medicine with society. These include such topics as ethics and human values, epidemiology, preventive medicine, health care economics, and organized medicine.

In the third and fourth years, students learn from attending physicians and residents during clinical clerkships in medicine, surgery, neurology, psychiatry, pediatrics, obstetrics and gynecology, dermatology, orthopedic surgery, ophthalmology, otolaryngology, primary care, urology, and physical medicine and rehabilitation. A subinternship of the student's choice and electives round out the curriculum.

NUMS offers three combined-degree programs: M.D.-Ph.D., M.D.-M.M., and M.D.-M.P.H. The M.D.-Ph.D. (Medical Scientist Training Program), offered by the medical school in cooperation with the graduate school, prepares students for careers in academic medicine. Inquiries about the M.D.-Ph.D. program should be directed to the MSTP Program Office, Ward 6-204, 303 East Chicago Avenue, Chicago, IL 60611-3008.

The M.D.-M.M. program with the Kellogg Graduate School of Management enables students to obtain both medical and business degrees in five calendar years. Students apply to the M.D.-M.M. program after their first year of medical school. The M.D.-M.P.H. program provides students with a broader and deeper experience in public health and enables students to obtain both degrees in four years. Inquiries should be directed to the M.D.-M.P.H. Office at 680 North Lake Shore Drive, Suite 1102, Chicago, IL 60611-4402. Special research, clinical, and other programs have been arranged to meet individual student interests.

HONORS PROGRAM

One of the oldest combined baccalaureate-M.D. programs in the country, the Honors Program in Medical Education (HPME) each year selects approximately 40 highly motivated, talented high school graduates for a course of study leading to baccalaureate and M.D. degrees in seven years. Inquiries should be directed to the Office of Undergraduate Admission, P.O. Box 3060, Evanston, Illinois 60204-3060.

REQUIREMENTS FOR ENTRANCE

Northwestern requires the MCAT and 135 quarter hours (90 semester hours) of undergraduate course work from an accredited college or university in the United States or Canada. Applicants may have chosen any field of study for their major, however, year-long courses in biology, general and organic chemistry, and physics are recommended as preparation for the MCAT and for medical school. Significant clinical experience is considered to be an important asset.

Candidates are expected to take the Spring MCAT and to have completed at least their baccalaureate degree requirements prior to medical school matriculation.

SELECTION FACTORS

Reviewers look for evidence of emotional maturity, motivation, past achievement, and character as well as academic excellence. A premium is placed on breadth and depth of the academic program, life experiences of the individual, and clinical and research exposure. Applicants should be liberally educated men and women who have studied in some depth subjects beyond the conventional premedical sciences. Panel interviews are required of all students considered seriously for acceptance; interview invitations are issued solely upon the request of the Admissions Committee and are conducted at the medical school.

Some characteristics of the 1998 entering class were: *GPA,* 3.7; *MCAT scores* averaging about the 85th percentile nationally; *average age,* 23 (range 19-46); *sex,* 46 percent women.

The Medical School faculty has established technical performance standards. Candidates for admission should demonstrate the mental capability, moral integrity, and physical skills required to function effectively in a broad variety of laboratory and clinical situations. Northwestern University does not discriminate on the basis of race, religion, national origin, sex, age, or handicap in its educational programs or activities in accordance with civil rights legislation.

FINANCIAL AID

Financial considerations do not influence admissions decisions. More than 60 percent of the student body have received financial aid. Support is provided primarily through national and local loan programs. Northwestern University offers a loan program to international students who have a co-signer on the loan.

Accepted applicants wishing to receive further information may write to the assistant director for financial aid, 850 N. Lake Shore Drive, Room 209, Chicago, Illinois 60611.

INFORMATION FOR MINORITY STUDENTS

The Medical School is committed to diversity in the student body, and makes a concerted effort to recruit, admit, and graduate students from minority groups. Minority groups are also represented in the admissions committee, interview committee, and faculty.

Private Institution

APPLICATION AND ACCEPTANCE POLICIES FOR 2001–2002 FIRST-YEAR CLASS

School participates in AMCAS. See Chapter 6.

Filing of AMCAS application
  Earliest date: June 1, 2000
  Latest date: Oct. 15, 2000
School application fee after screening: $60
Oldest MCAT scores considered: 1997
Does not have Early Decision Program
Acceptance notice to regular applicants
  Earliest date: Dec. 15, 2000
  Latest date: Varies
Applicant's response to acceptance offer
  Maximum time: 2 weeks
Requests for deferred entrance considered: Yes
Deposit to hold place in class: None
Estimated number of new entrants: 162
Starting date: Sept. 2001

TUITION AND STUDENT FEES PER YEAR FOR 1999–2000 FIRST-YEAR CLASS

Tuition: $30,417 Student fees: $1,000

INFORMATION ON 1999–2000 FIRST-YEAR CLASS

Number of	*In-State*	*Out-of-State*	*Total*
Applicants	1,092	7,549	8,641
Applicants Interviewed	85	527	612
New Entrants*	42	128	170

*All took the MCAT and had baccalaureate degrees (excluding the HPME entrants).

CHAPTER 11

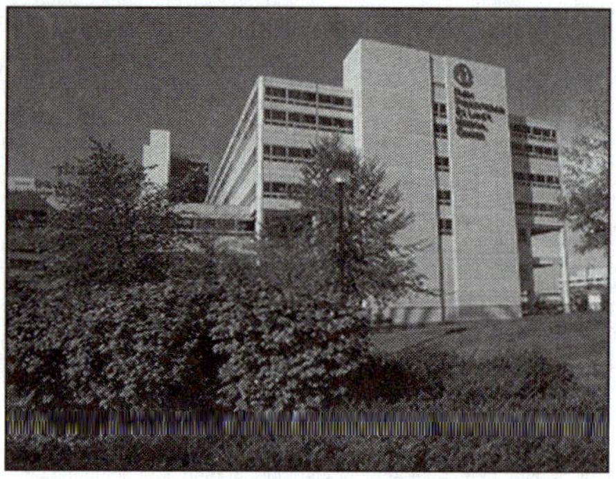

Rush Medical College of Rush University

Chicago, Illinois

Dr. Erich E. Brueshke, *Dean*
Jan L. Schmidt, *Director of Admissions*
Robert Dame, *Director of Student Financial Aid*

ADDRESS INQUIRIES TO:

Office of Admissions
524 Armour Academic Center
Rush Medical College of Rush University
600 South Paulina Street
Chicago, Illinois 60612
(312) 942-6913; 942-2333 (FAX)
Web Site: http://www.rush.edu
E-mail: medcol@rush.edu

MISSION STATEMENT

The purpose of Rush University is to educate students as practitioners, scientists, and teachers who will become leaders in advancing health care and to further the advancement of knowledge through research. As a major component of Rush-Presbyterian-St. Luke's Medical Center, the university integrates patient care, education, and research through the practitioner-teacher model. Rush University encourages the growth of its students by committing itself to the pursuit of excellence, to the advancement of knowledge, to free inquiry, and to the highest intellectual and ethical standards.

GENERAL INFORMATION

Rush Medical College, founded in 1837, is the oldest component of Rush University. The original medical college graduated over 10,000 physicians before closing in 1942. Rush Medical College, a private school, reopened in 1971 and is part of Rush University.

Through the academic and health care network of more than a dozen affiliated hospitals and a neighborhood health center, Rush-Presbyterian-St. Luke's Medical Center serves 1.5 to 2 million people. Thus, the students of Rush University train in urban, suburban, and rural areas in a variety of socioeconomic and ethnic settings.

CURRICULUM

Rush Medical College provides a firm background in the science of medicine and a balanced introduction to the practice of clinical medicine in a four-year curriculum designed to provide educational flexibility. A major goal of the college and its faculty is to create an environment that fosters commitments to competent and compassionate patient care and to attitudes of inquiry and lifelong learning.

Beginning in 2001, Rush Medical College will introduce a single, unified curriculum for all 120 students. The basic science curriculum will place an increased emphasis on small-group and self-directed learning. The Curriculum Renewal Committee is working with the Curriculum Committee to develop the framework for this new curriculum, which will emphasize the knowledge, skills, attitudes, and behaviors that are expected in future practitioners of medicine. The Generalist Curriculum, which was implemented in 1996, will serve as the core around which the basic sciences are taught. The three Generalist Curriculum courses are Physical Diagnosis, Interviewing and Communication, and Primary Care Preceptorship. These courses are taught throughout the preclinical years. The Primary Care Preceptorship is a longitudinal experience designed to provide students with an opportunity to observe and interact with physicians and their patients in an outpatient, primary care setting.

The third and fourth years consist of required core clerkships in internal medicine, surgery, obstetrics and gynecology, pediatrics, psychiatry, family practice, and neurology; a required subinternship in internal medicine, pediatrics, or family practice; and a minimum of 18 weeks of elective clerkships. Many students spend some of their elective clerkship experience in foreign countries.

Rush University offers qualified students who aspire to careers in academic medicine and research the opportunity to enroll in a combined M.D.-Ph.D. program. Ph.D. programs are offered in the Graduate College in the following areas: anatomical sciences, biochemistry, immunology, microbiology, medical physics, neurosciences, pharmacology, and physiology. Students in concurrent programs must meet the full conditions and requirements of the Graduate College, Graduate Division, and the Medical College.

Upon entering Rush Medical College, each student is assigned an academic advisor to help define goals, aid in the selection of courses of study, provide other counseling, and serve as role model and friend. This advisor will continue with the student as the student progresses through school.

REQUIREMENTS FOR ENTRANCE

The MCAT and 90 semester hours of undergraduate work in an accredited college are required. College work must include the following science areas:

	Sem. hrs.
Biology or zoology	8
Inorganic chemistry	8

Organic chemistry 8
General physics 8

Four semester hours of biochemistry may be substituted for the second semester of organic chemistry.

Sound preparation in the basic sciences is essential, but a broad background in the humanities and wide exposure to people and their problems are equally necessary.

Applicants are strongly urged to take the MCAT in the spring of the year of application; however, those who take it in the fall will also be considered.

SELECTION FACTORS

Students who enter the Rush Medical College program are carefully selected for their intellectual and social maturity and represent a wide variety of educational and social backgrounds. Problem-solving skills, critical judgment, and the capability to pursue independent study are considered important. Majors in science and majors in other areas with demonstrated excellence in the required science courses are considered equally appropriate to a medical education at Rush Medical College. All applicants to Rush are invited to complete the supplemental application and submit letters of recommendation. The Committee on Admissions looks for objective evidence that the applicant will be able to handle the academic demands of the medical curriculum. In evaluating academic achievement, the committee does consider factors such as the degree of difficulty of the program, the need to work, social and cultural backgrounds, and other factors that may affect the record. In the nonacademic realm, maturity, a balanced education, personal integrity, and motivational factors are considered essential determinants.

Undergraduate academic achievement, recommendations of premedical committees and/or undergraduate faculty, performance on the MCAT, and personal interviews (which are requested of those applicants who are considered competitive candidates by the Committee on Admissions) are considered in the evaluation of applicants. Interviews are held only on the Rush campus and strong preference is given to residents of Illinois. Only applications from U.S. citizens or permanent residents are considered. The average GPA and MCAT scores approximate those of nationally accepted applicants. All applicants are considered without regard to sex, religion, race, age, handicap, or national origin. Applicants from minority groups are encouraged to apply. Rush will waive its application fee for applicants who receive an AMCAS fee waiver.

FINANCIAL AID

Determination of a financial aid award is made after acceptance into medical school. The financial aid package will consist primarily of loans. Due to limited institutional scholarship assistance, scholarship eligibility is based on parents' resources regardless of the student's age or status. Students are awarded financial aid packages to meet 100 percent of the demonstrated financial need during each year of their medical education. Approximately 80 percent of the medical students receive financial assistance from state, federal, institutional, or other sources outside the family.

TRANSFER

Only those students who are currently enrolled and in good academic standing at LCME-accredited medical schools are considered eligible to apply for transfer. Students must also pass USMLE Step 1 at the conclusion of their second year of medical studies. The number of positions available for transfer is strictly limited by attrition.

Private Institution

APPLICATION AND ACCEPTANCE POLICIES FOR 2001–2002 FIRST-YEAR CLASS

School participates in AMCAS. See Chapter 6.

Filing of AMCAS application
  Earliest date: June 1, 2000
  Latest date: Nov. 15, 2000
School application fee to all applicants: $55
Oldest MCAT scores considered: 1997
Does have Early Decision Program (EDP)
  EDP application period: June 1–Aug. 1, 2000
  EDP applicants notified by: Oct. 1, 2000
Acceptance notice to regular applicants
  Earliest date: Oct. 15, 2000
  Latest date: Until class is filled
Applicant's response to acceptance offer
  Maximum time: 2 weeks
Requests for deferred entrance considered: Yes
Deposit to hold place in class (applied to tuition):
  $100, due with response to acceptance offer
Deposit refundable prior to: May 15, 2000
Estimated number of new entrants: 120 (10 EDP)
Starting date: Sept. 2000

TUITION AND STUDENT FEES PER YEAR FOR 1999–2000 FIRST-YEAR CLASS

Tuition: $27,120 Student fees: $1,104

INFORMATION ON 1999–2000 FIRST-YEAR CLASS

Number of	*In-State*	*Out-of-State*	*Total*
Applicants	1,433	3,109	4,542
Applicants Interviewed	322	155	477
New Entrants*	95	24	119

*All took the MCAT and had baccalaureate degrees.

CHAPTER 11

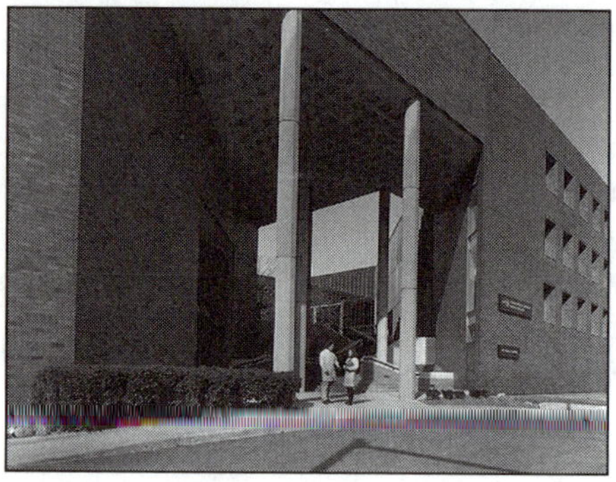

Southern Illinois University School of Medicine

Springfield, Illinois

Dr. Carl J. Getto, *Dean and Provost*
Erin L. Graham, *Director of Admissions*
Nancy Calvert, *Director of Financial Aid*

ADDRESS INQUIRIES TO:

Office of Admissions
Southern Illinois University
School of Medicine
P.O. Box 19624
Springfield, Illinois 62794-9624
(217) 524-6013; 785-5538 (FAX)
E-mail: egraham@siumed.edu
Web Site: www.siumed.edu

GENERAL INFORMATION

Southern Illinois University School of Medicine was established in 1969 and graduated its first class in 1975. Students spend the first 12 months of the program at the medical education facilities on the Carbondale campus and the remaining three years at the Medical Center in Springfield.

CURRICULUM

SIU School of Medicine conducts its four-year program on two campuses. The first year occurs on SIU's Carbondale campus and takes advantage of the basic science faculty and facilities located there. The remaining three years are spent at the Medical Center in Springfield. In the summer of 2000, Southern Illinois University School of Medicine will implement a major curriculum revision. The overall focus of the new curriculum will be on student-directed learning in a small group setting, with close integration of basic science and clinical information throughout the four-year course of study. Continuity clinic assignments will allow students to follow a patient group over time beginning in the first year.

Another major change in Curriculum 2000 is the addition of a Mentored Professional Enrichment Project, which will be an optional experience between the first and second years that allows students to work with a mentor over the course of 12 weeks to complete a project that allows them to increase their knowledge in a wide variety of areas ranging from rural practice to population and/or community health to academic medicine to bench research.

The first two years of the curriculum will engage students in case-based learning, with much student time spent in small group learning activities. Basic sciences will be emphasized, and clinical activities will center on building basic clinical skills and enhancing the learning of basic science concepts in a clinical context. Thirty to fifty percent of students' scheduled time will be spent in clinical activities during these first two years. An increased emphasis on issues such as community health care and the psychosocial issues of medicine will continue SIU School of Medicine's emphasis on caring while curing—treating patients as people, rather than medical conditions.

The third year will consist of a series of multidisciplinary clinical rotations, with emphasis on both hospital-based and ambulatory practice. These activities will take place at various locations throughout the state. Basic sciences will be re-emphasized throughout the third year as students work with patients.

The fourth year will comprise a series of "pathways" designed to help students with final preparations for residency. Pathways currently under consideration are primary care, rural care, surgical specialties, emergency medicine, and research. Basic sciences will again be re-emphasized as a part of patient care.

Curriculum 2000 is designed to prepare students for careers as professionals in the rapidly changing field of health care while providing a means for developing the knowledge and skills necessary for licensure, residency, and future accreditation examinations. Its development offers students and faculty an opportunity to enter the new millennium as participants in an innovative medical school known for a medical education program that trains the best possible physicians and scientists.

The grading system is honors/pass/fail.

The school also offers a six-year M.D.-J.D. program.

REQUIREMENTS FOR ENTRANCE

Applications for the M.D. program are accepted from Illinois residents who are U.S. citizens and those foreign citizens possessing a permanent resident visa. A minimum of 90 semester hours of undergraduate work in an accredited degree-granting college or university are required. Foreign students are advised to have completed at least 60 semester hours of course work in the United States. The M.D.-J.D. program is open to out-of-state applicants. Applicants are expected to have a good foundation in the natural sciences, social sciences, and humanities and to demonstrate facility in writing and speaking the English language.

To perform well on the MCAT, it is advisable to have had a minimum of two years of college chemistry (including organic), one year of physics, one year of biological or life sciences, mathematics (including statistics), and one year of English composition.

SELECTION FACTORS

Preference is given to those with sufficient recent academic activity to demonstrate the potential for successful completion of the rigorous educational program and to those who demonstrate the necessary noncognitive characteristics of a successful medical student and physician. Although the Admissions Committee establishes no quotas, an effort is made to recruit qualified applicants from groups that have been underrepresented in the medical profession. Applicants are selected for interview according to their strengths in academics, extracurricular activities, employment, and volunteer experiences, in addition to area of residence with preference given to central and southern Illinois residents. Selected applicants are interviewed in either Springfield or Carbondale; an interview is a prerequisite to acceptance.

The School of Medicine does not discriminate on the basis of race, religion, age, sex, handicap, or national or ethnic origin in administration of its education policies, admissions policies, scholarship and loan programs, and other school-administered programs.

FINANCIAL AID

Southern Illinois University School of Medicine participates in all major Federal Student Aid programs. Students receive financial aid on the basis of their need as calculated on the FAFSA. Scholarship and grant aid is generally limited to students who demonstrate exceptional need.

The financial aid office provides short-term emergency loans as well as loan indebtedness counseling and assistance with securing outside loans and scholarships. Accepted applicants may contact the Office of Student Affairs—Financial Aid at (217) 785-2224 for additional information.

INFORMATION FOR DISADVANTAGED STUDENTS

The School of Medicine sponsors the Medical/Dental Education Preparatory Program (MEDPREP) for disadvantaged undergraduate or postbaccalaureate students, as well as underrepresented, rural, or low-income students. MEDPREP is a non-degree-granting program located on the Carbondale campus. Students who are admitted to the program must begin their matriculation during the fall. The MEDPREP curriculum is designed to meet students' individual preparatory needs. It consists of developmental and enrichment tutorials in small class format, preparation for the MCAT, and medical school application assistance. Additionally, students enroll in preprofessional courses offered by other departments on the campus. Personal, academic, and career counseling is also provided. MEDPREP does not offer a guarantee of eventual acceptance to the School of Medicine or to any other medical school, but MEDPREP students who meet the criteria established for the MEDPREP Alliance are offered acceptance to the S.I.U. School of Medicine. Careful consideration will be given to MEDPREP participant applicants by the School of Medicine and those selected medical schools working cooperatively with MEDPREP. Inquiries should be addressed to: Director, MEDPREP, Southern Illinois University School of Medicine, Carbondale, Illinois 62901-4323.

Public Institution

APPLICATION AND ACCEPTANCE POLICIES FOR 2001–2002 FIRST-YEAR CLASS

School participates in AMCAS. See Chapter 6.

Filing of AMCAS application
  Earliest date: June 1, 2000
  Latest date: Nov. 15, 2000
School application fee after screening: $50
Oldest MCAT scores considered: 1998
Does not have Early Decision Program
Acceptance notice to regular applicants
  Earliest date: Nov. 2000
  Latest date: Until class is filled
Applicant's response to acceptance offer
  Maximum time: 2 weeks
Requests for deferred entrance considered: Yes
Deposit to hold place in class (applied to tuition):
  $100, due with response to acceptance offer
Deposit refundable prior to: May 15, 2000
Estimated number of new entrants: 72
Starting date: Aug. 2001

TUITION AND STUDENT FEES PER YEAR FOR 1999–2000 FIRST-YEAR CLASS

Tuition
  Resident: $10,028
  Nonresident: $30,084

Student fees: $1,064

INFORMATION ON 1999–2000 FIRST-YEAR CLASS

Number of	*In-State*	*Out-of-State*	*Total*
Applicants	1,039	430	1,469
Applicants Interviewed	285	3	288
New Entrants*	72	0	72

*All had baccalaureate degrees and took the MCAT.

CHAPTER 11

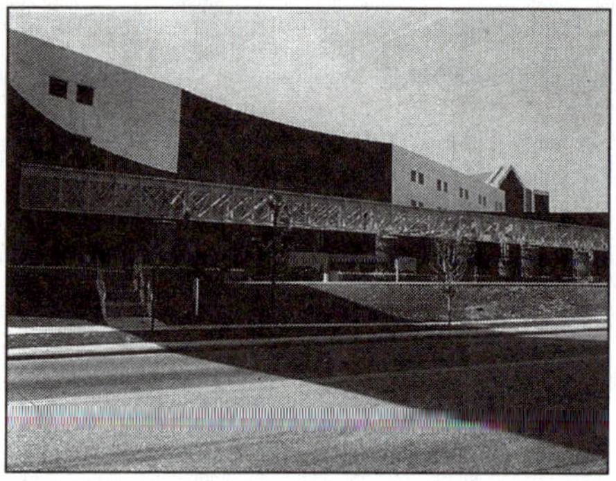

Indiana University School of Medicine

Indianapolis, Indiana

Dr. Robert W. Holden, *Dean*
Dr. George T. Lukemeyer, *Chair, Admissions Committee*
Robert M. Stump, Jr., *Director of Admissions*

ADDRESS INQUIRIES TO:

Medical School Admissions Office
Fesler Hall 213
Indiana University
School of Medicine
1120 South Drive
Indianapolis, Indiana 46202-5113
(317) 274-3772
Web Site: http://www.medicine.iu.edu/home.html

MISSION STATEMENT

The goal of the Indiana University School of Medicine is the education of physicians, scientists, and other health professionals in an intellectually rich environment with research as its scientific base. In education, we are committed to imparting a fundamental understanding of both clinical practice and the basic scientific knowledge upon which it rests, to provide a firm foundation for lifelong learning. In research, we are committed to the advancement of knowledge. In patient care, we are committed to the highest standards of medical practice in an atmosphere of respect and empathy for our patients. Education, research, and delivery of health care are inseparable components of our mission. Excellence can only be achieved when all components are of highest quality, well integrated, and mutually supportive.

GENERAL INFORMATION

Indiana University School of Medicine, founded in 1903, is the sole institution responsible for providing medical education in the state of Indiana and operates the Indiana Statewide Medical Education System. The school has centers for medical education at Bloomington, Evansville, Fort Wayne, Gary, Lafayette, Muncie, South Bend, and Terre Haute, where students may spend their first two years of medical school. The Medical Center in Indianapolis has students enrolled in all four years of the medical curriculum.

In addition to its role and responsibilities in teaching, patient care, and service, Indiana University School of Medicine is a major academic research center.

Indiana University School of Medicine utilizes a number of integrated teaching hospitals on or near the medical center campus, as well as other affiliated hospitals in Indianapolis and throughout the state.

CURRICULUM

The basic medical sciences are presented in the first two years. In addition, a multidisciplinary course, Introduction to Clinical Medicine, spans the first two years. Students' skills, knowledge, and attitudes about patient care begin to take shape in this course as they encounter patients for the first time.

The Northwest Center for Medical Education's Regional Center Alternative Pathway utilizes problem-based learning methods, including small-group, case-based tutorial sessions, laboratories, and a few optional lectures to fully prepare medical students for their clinical medical education.

A 12-month clinical clerkship program at the medical center in Indianapolis occupies the third year and includes units in family medicine, internal medicine, surgery, obstetrics and gynecology, pediatrics, and psychiatry. In the fourth year, students complete clerkships in neurosensory science, radiology, and surgical specialties, and select six one-month elective units from an approved list of hundreds of choices. With the permission of the faculty, students may arrange for elective experiences around the country and abroad.

Students interested in research or academic medicine may enroll in the combined-degree program and pursue a Ph.D. degree in addition to the M.D. degree.

In Indianapolis, the School of Medicine's basic science departments offer combined-degree programs in nine basic science disciplines. A special Indiana Medical Scientist Program offers financial support and research opportunities for outstanding students.

The Medical Sciences Program in Bloomington offers studies in anatomy, biochemistry, pathology, pharmacology, and physiology. Also available to combined-degree students in Bloomington are studies in the humanities, law, and social and behavioral sciences as well as in the biological and physical sciences.

In cooperation with Purdue University, combined-degree programs are offered in engineering, medicinal chemistry, molecular biology, and neuroscience at the Lafayette Center for Medical Education.

REQUIREMENTS FOR ENTRANCE

The School of Medicine recommends that students preparing for the study of medicine take a variety of courses commonly included in a traditional liberal arts and sciences curriculum.

The MCAT and a minimum of three college years (90 semester hours) are required. Physical education and ROTC courses will not be accepted as part of the 90 semester hours. The undergraduate course work must include:

	Years
Biology (with labs)	1
General chemistry (with labs)	1
Organic chemistry (with labs)	1
Physics (with labs)	1

Applicants should take the MCAT in the spring prior to making application.

The Admissions Committee shows preference to applicants who will have at least a baccalaureate degree prior to matriculation in medical school.

There is a graduate program in the medical sciences for disadvantaged and minority students whose applications show promise, but are not quite competitive for admission to medical school.

All applications are reviewed by the full Admissions Committee, which accepts students on an individual basis according to their potential and promise for medical school and for service as physicians. For additional information, please contact the Admissions Office.

SELECTION FACTORS

Students are offered places in the class on the basis of scholarship, character, personality, references, residence, interview, and performance on the MCAT. In addition, the medical school faculty has specified non-academic criteria (technical standards), which all applicants must meet in order to participate effectively in the medical education program and the practice of medicine.

Because the School of Medicine is state-supported, the Admissions Committee shows preference to Indiana residents in selecting the class. Nevertheless, a number of nonresidents are offered acceptances each year (59 for the 1999 entering class). The applications of nonresidents who have significant ties to the state of Indiana may be given greater consideration.

The average GPA of the 1999 entering class was 3.68/4.0. Average MCAT scores were: *VR*-9.5, *PS*-9.7, *WS*-0, *BS*-10.0.

The School of Medicine does not discriminate on the basis of race, sex, age, handicap, creed, or national origin.

FINANCIAL AID

Scholarships and long-term, low-interest loans are available to students with financial need. There are also scholarships for students who have demonstrated academic excellence.

There is a significant scholarship for Indiana residents who commit to practicing primary care medicine in a medically underserved location.

INFORMATION FOR MINORITY STUDENTS

Applications from disadvantaged individuals and members of minority groups are encouraged.

The school recruits capable minority college students and provides counseling for high school and college students interested in the health professions.

The School of Medicine has instituted a pre-matriculation program. Selected students are invited to participate in a two-week medical preparatory program prior to the medical school's orientation activities.

Public Institution

APPLICATION AND ACCEPTANCE POLICIES FOR 2001–2002 FIRST-YEAR CLASS

School participates in AMCAS. See Chapter 6.

Filing of AMCAS application
  Earliest date: June 1, 2000
  Latest date: Dec. 15, 2000
School application fee after screening: $35
Oldest MCAT considered: 1997
Does have Early Decision Program (EDP)
  EDP application period: June 1–Aug. 1, 2000
  EDP applicants notified by: Oct. 1, 2000
Acceptance notice to regular applicants
  Earliest date: Oct. 15, 2000
  Latest date: Varies
Applicant's response to acceptance offer
  Maximum time: 3 weeks
Requests for deferred entrance considered: Yes
Deposit to hold place in class: None
Estimated number of new entrants: 280 (25 EDP)
Starting date: Aug. 2001

TUITION AND STUDENT FEES PER YEAR FOR 1999–2000 FIRST-YEAR CLASS

Tuition
  Resident: $13,245
  Nonresident: $30,330

Student fees: $1,352

INFORMATION ON 1999–2000 FIRST-YEAR CLASS

Number of	*In-State*	*Out-of-State*	*Total*
Applicants	631	1,528	2,159
Applicants Interviewed	568	277	845
New Entrants*	265	15	280

*All took the MCAT and had baccalaureate degrees.

CHAPTER 11

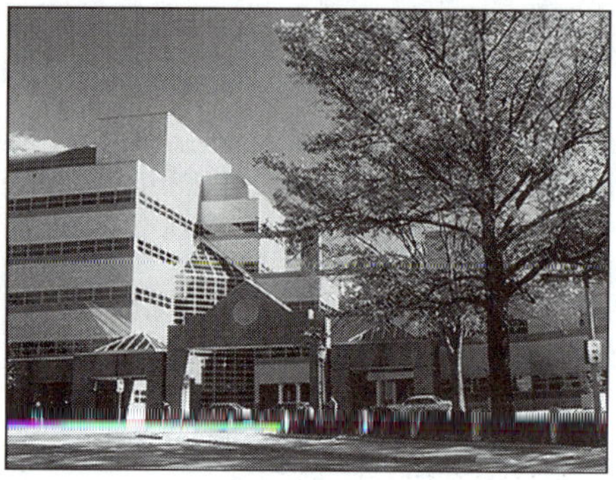

University of Iowa College of Medicine

Iowa City, Iowa

Dr. Robert P. Kelch, *Dean*
Catherine M. Solow, *Director of Admissions*
Linda G. Bissell, *Director of Financial Aid*

ADDRESS INQUIRIES TO:

Director of Admissions
University of Iowa
College of Medicine
100 Medicine Administration Building
Iowa City, Iowa 52242-1101
(319) 335-8052; 335-8049 (FAX)
E-mail: medical-admissions@uiowa.edu
Web Site: http://www.medicine.uiowa.edu

MISSION STATEMENT

The College of Medicine has three inextricably linked missions: education, research, and service. The college aspires to be responsive to the needs of society, and in particular the citizens of Iowa, through the excellence of its educational programs in the health professions and biomedical sciences, by the outstanding quality of its research, and through the provision of innovative and comprehensive health care and other services.

GENERAL INFORMATION

The College of Medicine originated in 1868 and has evolved into a major health center serving the entire state and region. The health sciences campus includes the University of Iowa Hospitals and Clinics; Veterans Administration Hospital; Hardin Health Sciences Library; and medical college, basic sciences, dental, nursing, and pharmacy buildings. A new Medical Education and Biomedical Research Facility is under construction on the Health Sciences campus. The new facility (approximately 203,000 square feet) will provide teaching, research, and student spaces. The medical school has a full-time teaching faculty.

CURRICULUM

The new curriculum, introduced with the 1995 entering class, is intended to more efficiently incorporate advances in medical knowledge, to better prepare students to address developing health care issues, to enable students to utilize current health care delivery patterns, and to allow students and faculty to take advantage of improved instructional approaches. Case-based and self-directed learning, clinical correlation, computer-based learning, small-group activities, and vertical integration of material are emphasized.

Year 1 is devoted to the investigation of the normal structure and function of the human body. Core material from the traditional basic science disciplines is presented in the first semester. The second semester is devoted to an integrated, interdisciplinary core of material arranged on an organ system basis. Year 2 is devoted to the investigation of abnormal structure and function. Discipline-specific courses are utilized to present core material in the first half of the year. Early patient contact, an introduction to medical history taking and physical diagnosis, and coverage of emerging topic areas such as continuity of care and behavioral medicine are presented in the Foundations of Clinical Practice, a course that runs concurrently throughout the first two years of the curriculum. In the fourth semester, introduction to the clinical disciplines provides students with a foundation in clinical medicine that will prepare them to perform effectively in the clinical arena.

The two clinical years of the curriculum afford a broad base of clinical experiences and training to provide the student with the essential skills and knowledge required to enter residency training. A generalist core, which includes community-based primary care experiences as well as exposure to the generalist specialties and required selective segments in a variety of other specialty areas, is a feature of the clinical years. Ample time for electives is provided.

In order to prepare academicians in medicine, a Medical Scientist Training Program is offered, which leads to both the M.D. and Ph.D. degrees over a six- to seven-year period.

REQUIREMENTS FOR ENTRANCE

The MCAT and a minimum of 94 semester hours, including the general graduation requirements, in an approved college are required. Completion of four years of college, including the requirements for the baccalaureate degree, is preferred. The college curriculum must include the following course work with appropriate laboratory experiences:

Biological sciences: A complete introductory course in the principles of animal biology or zoology and botany (but not botany alone) and one advanced course in biology.

Chemistry: A complete introductory course in organic chemistry, which would ordinarily follow a complete introductory course in modern general chemical principles.

Physics: A complete introductory course.

Mathematics: College algebra and trigonometry or advanced college mathematics when college algebra and trigonometry were completed in high school.

The remaining hours are chosen by the student. It is assumed that rhetoric, literature, social and behavioral science, and historical culture are generally among the courses taken as requirements for a baccalaureate degree. A natural science major is not required as the college recognizes the value of a broadly educated student body.

Applicants for admission to the College of Medicine must demonstrate the capability to complete the entire medical curriculum, which requires proficiency in a variety of cognitive, problem-solving, manipulative, communicative, and interpersonal skills.

SELECTION FACTORS

The Admissions Committee selects those applicants best qualified for the study and practice of medicine. To be eligible for admission, the applicant must have attained at least a 2.5 GPA (based on a 4.0 scale) for all college work undertaken. Fulfillment of the basic requirements does not guarantee admission. The major factors considered are:

1. Overall undergraduate academic record as reflected in the GPA: 3.6 class average.
2. Science GPA: 3.6 class average.
3. MCAT: 9–10 class average on each sub-test.
4. Residence: Preference is given to Iowa residents with high scholastic standing. Consideration is also given to outstanding nonresidents. Only citizens or permanent residents of the United States are eligible to apply.
5. Personal characteristics: Evaluated by means of specially designed evaluation forms completed by evaluators who are chosen by the applicant, and from information on the AMCAS application.
6. On-site personal interviews (by invitation).

Applications for transfer or admission with advanced standing are generally not considered.

FINANCIAL AID

Applicants are selected without consideration of their ability to meet the expenses of attending medical school. Students receive financial aid solely on the basis of need as calculated using the FAFSA. Limited scholarship assistance is also available.

While students are responsible for their own financial support, the college provides information and advice on locating sources of funds. Loan and grant funds from private, state, collegiate, and federal sources are available through the college.

INFORMATION FOR DISADVANTAGED APPLICANTS

The College of Medicine provides financial and academic assistance to educationally and economically disadvantaged students and those underrepresented in American medicine. Financial aid packages are designed individually on the basis of need. Grant assistance is available for financially disadvantaged students. A prefreshman summer program includes orientation, case-based learning experences, study skills, and introduction to first-year courses. Tutorial assistance and mentor programs exist to assist students in successfully completing the curriculum. The application fee and admission deposit may be defrayed for financially disadvantaged students.

Public Institution

APPLICATION AND ACCEPTANCE POLICIES FOR 2001–2002 FIRST-YEAR CLASS

School participates in AMCAS. See Chapter 6.

Filing of AMCAS application
  Earliest date: June 1, 2000
  Latest date: Nov. 1, 2000
School application fee after screening: $30
Oldest MCAT scores considered: 1991
Does have Early Decision Program (EDP)
  EDP application period: June 1–Aug. 1, 2000
  EDP applicants notified by: Oct. 1, 2000
Acceptance notice to regular applicants
  Earliest date: Oct. 15, 2000
  Latest date: Aug. 2001
Applicant's response to acceptance offer
  Maximum time: 2 weeks
Requests for deferred entrance considered: Yes
Deposit to hold place in class (applied to tuition):
  $50, due March 1, 2001, or within 2 weeks of acceptance offer if accepted after March 1, 2001
Deposit refundable prior to: June 15, 2001
Estimated number of new entrants: 157
Starting date: Aug. 2001

TUITION AND STUDENT FEES PER YEAR FOR 1999–2000 FIRST-YEAR CLASS

Tuition
  Resident: $9,840
  Nonresident: $26,356

Student fees: $869

INFORMATION ON 1999–2000 FIRST-YEAR CLASS

Number of	*In-State*	*Out-of-State*	*Total*
Applicants	339	2,148	2,487
Applicants Interviewed	235	275	510
New Entrants*	118	39	157

*All took the MCAT and had baccalaureate degrees.

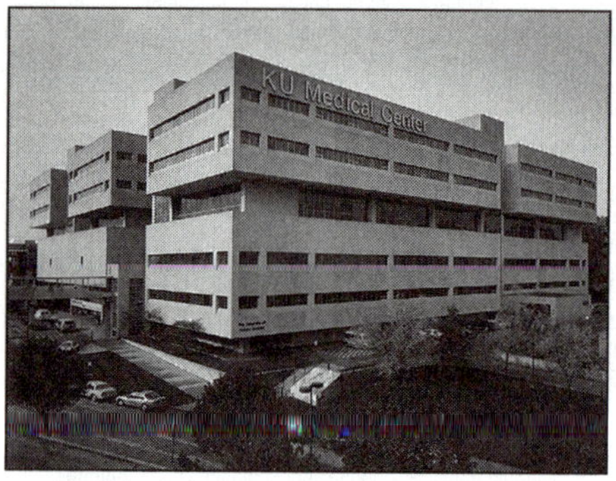

University of Kansas School of Medicine

Kansas City, Kansas

Dr. Deborah E. Powell, *Executive Dean*
Sandra J. McCurdy, *Assistant Dean for Admissions*
Sara Honeck, *Director of Student Financial Aid*

ADDRESS INQUIRIES TO:

Assistant Dean for Admissions
University of Kansas
School of Medicine
3901 Rainbow Boulevard
Kansas City, Kansas 66160-7301
(913) 588-5245; 588-5259 (FAX)
Web Site: http://www.kumc.edu/som/som.html

MISSION STATEMENT

The University of Kansas School of Medicine is dedicated to excellence in educating physicians and scientists to serve the health needs of Kansas; in providing high-quality care for patients throughout the state, region, and nation; and in discovering and applying new knowledge through basic and clinical research.

GENERAL INFORMATION

The University of Kansas School of Medicine was established in 1899 with a two-year program, which expanded to four years in 1906. It is located on the Medical Center campus in Kansas City, Kansas, which also houses the schools of nursing, allied health, and graduate studies. There are 1,500 faculty members in the School of Medicine, including 450 full-time faculty members in general and specialty medicine and the basic sciences. Full-time members actively participate in the teaching, service, and research mission of the school. Facilities at the Medical Center include the Archie R. Dykes Library of the Health Sciences; the Orr-Major basic sciences facility, containing classrooms, laboratories, an auditorium, and a learning resources center; the Ernst F. Lied Biomedical Research Building; and the University Hospital. This 485-bed hospital offers complete primary and tertiary care for patients of all ages and care for a wide range of problems from traumatic injuries to specialized care for those with chronic conditions.

The School of Medicine-Wichita campus was accredited in 1974, and a portion of every class completes clinical training at four Wichita hospitals.

CURRICULUM

The School of Medicine's curriculum ensures a sequential and interdisciplinary medical education with an emphasis on a generalist approach to the diagnosis, treatment, and management of patients' illnesses. This curriculum is designed to assist students in their acquisition of the knowledge, skills, and attitudes needed to become highly competent and caring physicians.

The first two years of the curriculum provide the basic biomedical and social sciences foundation essential to the practice of medicine. Didactic and self-directed learning are balanced between small-group activities and lectures of no more than 12 hours per week. In addition, first- and second-year medical students are paired with a mentoring physician in a longitudinal ambulatory clinical experience.

During years three and four, students participate in the delivery of health care in ambulatory and hospital settings, both in the community and at the KU Medical Center. The curriculum consists of required clerkships in the core clinical areas as well as a one-month preceptorship with a practicing Kansas physician. Students also choose from a large selection of basic science and clinical electives to complete a well-rounded educational program. Seminars facilitate continuing student discussion of issues raised during their first two years of study, and a comprehensive advising system assists medical students with academic, personal, and professional development.

A five-level grading system of superior, high satisfactory, satisfactory, low satisfactory, or unsatisfactory is utilized. Students must pass the USMLE Step 1 to continue their clinical training and Step 2 to graduate from the School of Medicine.

A combined M.D.-Ph.D. program in basic medical sciences is also offered. Further information and application forms may be obtained from the Office of Graduate Studies at (913) 588-5241.

REQUIREMENTS FOR ENTRANCE

The MCAT is required. Applicants must complete a course of study leading to a baccalaureate degree, which will be conferred prior to the planned date of enrollment in medical school. The degree requirement may be modified under exceptional circumstances. Specific minimum course work requirements are:

	Sem. hrs.
General biology (with lab)	8
Inorganic chemistry (with lab)	8
Organic chemistry or organic chemistry/ biochemistry sequence (with lab)	8
Physics (with lab)	8

Calculus, statistics, or computer science 3
English 3-6
(sufficient credit to meet the prerequisites for a liberal arts degree)

Undergraduate courses should be rigorous and, in general, equivalent to courses taken by students majoring in those subject areas. The Admissions Committee does not give preference to a major field of study, and students are strongly advised to balance their work in the natural sciences with courses in the social sciences and humanities. No other specific courses are required.

SELECTION FACTORS

Applicants are strongly encouraged to submit their AMCAS applications no later than September 1, 2000. Early application allows sufficient time for preliminary screening, for mailing of secondary applications, and for the subsequent screening for invitation to interview. Qualified residents of Kansas are given strong first preference for receipt of secondary applications, for interview, and for selection to the entering class. Successful nonresident applicants are those who have significant ties to Kansas or who will add breadth to the class.

The selection of students is made after careful consideration of the entire application, letters of evaluation, and a personal interview. Each applicant's scholarship is evaluated, but it is recognized that individual capabilities and professional promise cannot always be completely measured by traditional systems of grading. Trends in academic performance, the AMCAS personal statement, impressions gained from the interview, and the record of extracurricular activities and involvement in community affairs will be assessed in considering the applicant's candidacy. The University of Kansas does not discriminate on the basis of race, sex, religion, sexual orientation, national origin, age, or handicap.

The 1998 entering class was made up of 88 percent *Kansans*, 42 percent *women*, and 14 percent *minorities*, and 27 percent of the class were 25 years of age or older. The *mean GPA* was 3.6 with *MCAT scores* above the 60th percentile.

Applications for transfer are taken only upon the rare occasion of an available position in the third-year class. Kansas residents with a compelling need to transfer are given highest priority.

FINANCIAL AID

Numerous loans and scholarships are available for students attending the University of Kansas School of Medicine. The majority are based on financial need, determined by filing a Free Application for Federal Student Aid. Over 90 percent of students receive some type of financial assistance.

A major source of assistance is the Kansas Medical Student Loan Program, which provides payment of tuition and a stipend of up to $1,500 per month. Recipients may receive loan forgiveness by practicing primary care medicine in a small town or rural area in Kansas. Application forms and additional information can be obtained by contacting the Office of Student Financial Aid at (913) 588-5170.

INFORMATION FOR MINORITY STUDENTS

The School of Medicine has an active program dedicated to the recruitment, admission, retention, education, and graduation of increased numbers of individuals from minority groups. Several scholarships are available for qualified minority students. For additional information contact the associate dean for cultural enhancement and diversity at (913) 588-5292.

Public Institution

APPLICATION AND ACCEPTANCE POLICIES FOR 2001–2002 FIRST-YEAR CLASS

School participates in AMCAS. See Chapter 6.

Filing of AMCAS application
  Earliest date: June 1, 2000
  Latest date: Oct. 15, 2000
School application fee after screening: $40 for nonresidents who are invited to complete secondary application.
Oldest MCAT scores considered: 1998
Does have Early Decision Program (EDP)
  EDP application period: June 1–Aug. 1, 2000
  EDP applicants notified by: Oct. 1, 2000
Acceptance notice to regular applicants
  Earliest date: Dec. 1, 2000
  Latest date: Varies
Applicant's response to acceptance offer
  Maximum time: 2 weeks
Requests for deferred entrance considered: Yes
Deposit to hold place in class (applied to tuition): $50, due with response to acceptance offer
Deposit refundable prior to: May 15, 2001
Estimated number of new entrants: 175 (30 EDP)
Starting date: Aug. 2001

TUITION AND STUDENT FEES PER YEAR FOR 1999–2000 FIRST-YEAR CLASS

Tuition
  Resident: $9,664
  Nonresident: $23,334
Student fees: $310

INFORMATION ON 1999–2000 FIRST-YEAR CLASS

Number of	*In-State*	*Out-of-State*	*Total*
Applicants	415	977	1,392
Applicants Interviewed	305	71	376
New Entrants*	154	21	175

*All took the MCAT and had baccalaureate degrees.

CHAPTER 11

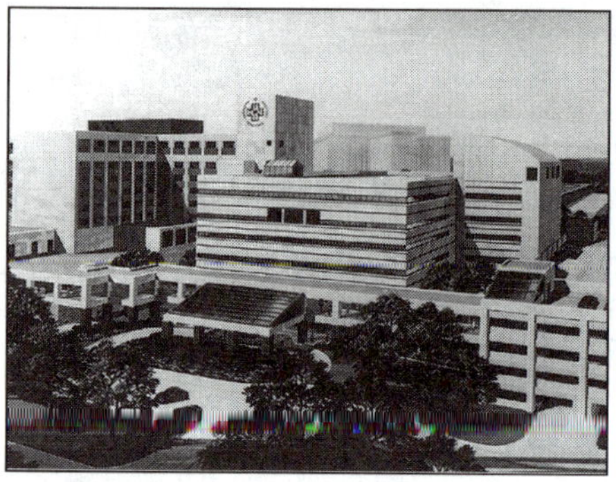

University of Kentucky College of Medicine

Lexington, Kentucky

Dr. Emery A. Wilson, *Dean*
Dr. Carol L. Elam, *Assistant Dean for Admissions*
Linda A. Gilbert, *Financial Aid Coordinator*

ADDRESS INQUIRIES TO:

Admissions, Room MN-102
Office of Academic Affairs
University of Kentucky College of Medicine
Chandler Medical Center
800 Rose Street
Lexington, Kentucky 40536-0298
(859) 323-6161; 323-2076 (FAX)
Web Site: http://www.comed.uky.edu/medicine

MISSION STATEMENT

The mission of the College of Medicine is to assume a leadership role in addressing the health care needs of the Commonwealth of Kentucky and to be preeminent among medical schools in selected areas of education, research, and service.

GENERAL INFORMATION

Established in 1956 by the Commonwealth of Kentucky and the University of Kentucky Board of Trustees, the University of Kentucky College of Medicine admitted its first class in 1960. The College of Medicine is part of the University of Kentucky Chandler Medical Center located on the university campus in Lexington.

The medical center comprises five colleges: medicine, nursing, pharmacy, dentistry, and allied health professions. The majority of on-site clinical teaching occurs at the 473-bed University of Kentucky Hospital, the 662-bed Veterans Affairs Medical Center, and the Kentucky Clinic. Hospitals throughout Lexington and across the Commonwealth hold affiliation agreements with the college for clinical teaching and patient service.

Basic science teaching areas for lecture, laboratory, and small-group instruction, as well as the Medical Center Library, are located in the Medical Sciences Building. Adjacent are the Health Science Learning Center, Critical Care Center, Sanders-Brown Center on Aging, Lucille Parker Markey Cancer Center, Mills-Davis Magnetic Resonance Imaging and Spectroscopy Center, and University of Kentucky Student Health Service.

CURRICULUM

In a new curriculum designed to integrate basic and clinical sciences, medical students are taught the fundamental problems of human biology, how to recognize the causes of these problems, and how to prevent disease and treat patients. Year 1 of the Kentucky medical curriculum focuses on normal function of the human body (human structure, cellular structure and function, neurosciences, and human function). First-year students receive early exposure and experience in patient care through the study of interviewing, history taking, physical examination skills, and clinical decision making. In the first two years, medical students also explore principles of prevention and assess the impact of social, ethical, legal, economic, and psychological factors using case studies and small-group discussions. Year 2 exposes students to abnormal functions of the human body as related to disease processes. Course work is designed to integrate studies of infectious disease, immunology, pathology, and pharmacology. Computer-based instruction reinforces basic science studies and provides linkages to clinical applications.

Clinical students work with patients in both inpatient hospital and outpatient clinic settings and are required to take medical histories, perform physical examinations on patients, and monitor laboratory tests. Year 3 of the Kentucky medical curriculum includes an integrated women's maternal and child health clerkship, along with clinical neurosciences, primary care, internal medicine, and surgery. Year 4 is highlighted by required rotations in emergency medicine, clinical pharmacology, rural medicine, two acting internships, and a three-month elective period.

Third-year medical students may apply for the accelerated residency programs in family medicine and general internal medicine. These programs combine the fourth year of medical school with the first year of residency.

Selected students may opt to pursue a combined M.D.-Ph.D. in anatomy and neurobiology, biochemistry, microbiology and immunology, pharmacology, or physiology and biophysics. Combined-degree programs are also available in preventive medicine, nutritional sciences, toxicology, and biomedical engineering.

REQUIREMENTS FOR ENTRANCE

Applicants are expected to have a broad foundation in the natural sciences, social sciences, and humanities and should demonstrate facility in writing and speaking the English language.

Applicants are strongly urged to complete their baccalaureate degrees. The MCAT is required for admission. Applicants are strongly encouraged to take the spring exam. Specific course requirements are:

	Semesters
Biology (with labs)	2
General chemistry (with labs)	2
Organic chemistry (with labs)	2
Physics (with labs)	2
English	2

Emphasis is placed on written and spoken communication.

SELECTION FACTORS

The University of Kentucky College of Medicine gives preference to qualified applicants who are residents of Kentucky. Determination of state residence is made by the registrar's office. Applicants' files are reviewed without regard to race, sex, creed, national origin, age, or handicap. Secondary applications are sent to all Kentucky residents and to those nonresidents with undergraduate GPA's of 3.75 or higher and MCAT scores of 10 or higher on each subscale. Selected candidates are invited for interviews conducted at the University of Kentucky College of Medicine.

Necessary personal attributes of applicants include time management abilities, interpersonal skills, leadership, and demonstrated service to others. Admission decisions are made based upon review of academic and nonacademic factors including scholastic excellence, MCAT performance, personal attributes, breadth of experience, exposure to the profession, premedical recommendations, and admission interviews.

The students enrolled in the 1998 entering class had the following profile: *mean GPA*, 3.54; *women*, 37 percent; residence, 93 percent; *undergraduate major*, 79 percent in the natural sciences with the remainder from the social and behavioral sciences, engineering, and liberal arts. Transfers from USMLE-accredited schools only are considered on a space-available basis. The University of Kentucky College of Medicine does not discriminate on the basis of race, sex, creed, national origin, age, or handicap.

FINANCIAL AID

A limited number of scholarship grants are awarded to selected students with exceptional achievement. Approximately 85 percent of the student body receives financial assistance through loans and scholarships. Institutional loan/scholarship assistance is available for eligible resident and nonresident students. Kentucky residents who plan to practice in rural Kentucky may receive aid from the Rural Kentucky Medical Scholarship Fund.

The Office of Academic Affairs provides financial aid counseling and assists students in applying for aid. Only in rare circumstances are students given permission to seek employment.

INFORMATION FOR MINORITY STUDENTS

The University of Kentucky College of Medicine is committed to the recruitment and retention of underrepresented and disadvantaged students. Interested applicants are encouraged to contact the admissions office.

Public Institution

APPLICATION AND ACCEPTANCE POLICIES FOR 2001–2002 FIRST-YEAR CLASS

School participates in AMCAS. See Chapter 6.

Filing of AMCAS application
  Earliest date: June 1, 2000
  Latest date: Nov. 1, 2000
School application fee after screening: $30
Oldest MCAT scores considered: Aug. 1998
Does have Early Decision Program (EDP)
  EDP application period: June 1–Aug. 1, 2000
  EDP applicants notified by: Oct. 1, 2000
Acceptance notice to regular applicants
  Earliest date: After interview
  Latest date: Until class is filled
Applicant's response to acceptance offer
  Maximum time: 2 weeks
Requests for deferred entrance considered: Yes
Deposit to hold place in class (applied to tuition):
  $100, due with response to acceptance offer
Deposit refundable prior to: March 1, 2001
Estimated number of new entrants: 95 (25 EDP)
Starting date: Aug. 2001

TUITION AND STUDENT FEES PER YEAR FOR 1999–2000 FIRST-YEAR CLASS

Tuition
  Resident: $9,890
  Nonresident: $25,280

Student fees: $494

INFORMATION ON 1999–2000 FIRST-YEAR CLASS

Number of	*In-State*	*Out-of-State*	*Total*
Applicants	460	903	1,363
Applicants Interviewed	260	41	301
New Entrants*	87	8	95

*All took the MCAT; 99% had baccalaureate degrees.

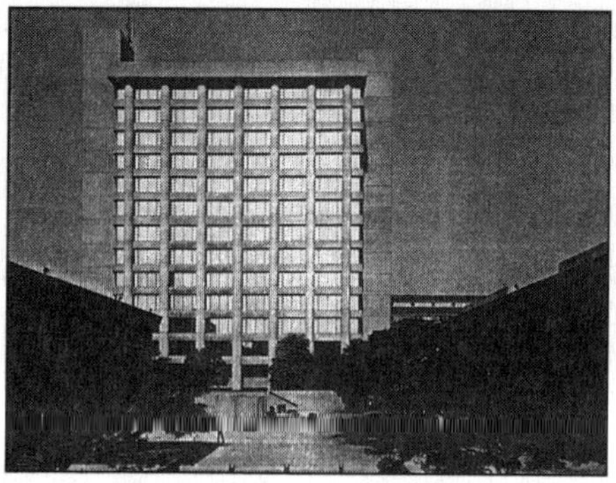

University of Louisville School of Medicine

Louisville, Kentucky

Dr. Joel Kaplan, *Vice President for Hospital Affairs and Dean*
Libby Sklare, *Director of Admissions*
Leslie Kaelin, *Director of Financial Aid*

ADDRESS INQUIRIES TO:

Office of Admissions
School of Medicine
Abell Administration Center
323 East Chestnut
University of Louisville
Louisville, Kentucky 40202-3866
(502) 852-5193
Web Site: http://www.louisville.edu

MISSION STATEMENT

The University of Louisville School of Medicine has a mandated statewide mission to meet the educational, research, and patient-care needs of the Commonwealth of Kentucky, within the resources available, and to cooperate with other health sciences center schools and colleges in educating health care teams. The educational program is designed to train physicians who are sensitive to medical ethics and who will meet the diverse health care needs of the Commonwealth of Kentucky.

GENERAL INFORMATION

The School of Medicine was established at the Louisville Medical Institute in 1833 and became affiliated with the University of Louisville in 1846. In 1970 the university became a member of the state system of higher education. The School of Medicine is part of the modern Health Sciences Center located near downtown Louisville that also includes the Schools of Dentistry, Nursing, and Allied Health Sciences. A new medical research building is currently under construction.

The major clinical teaching activities take place in the 404-bed acute and trauma care University Hospital. Within one or two blocks are four formally affiliated hospitals, which include the only full-service children's hospital in the state of Kentucky—Kosair-Children's Hospital, Jewish Hospital, Norton Hospital, and the Veterans Administration Medical Center. Other facilities include the world-renowned Kentucky Lions Eye Research Institute; James Brown Cancer Center; the Child Evaluation Center; Amelia Brown Fazier Rehabilitation Center; and the Trover Clinic, an off-campus teaching center located in Madisonville, Kentucky.

CURRICULUM

At the University of Louisville School of Medicine, an educational program has been developed that provides an efficiently organized, penetrating presentation of the general information considered essential for all physicians, yet has sufficient flexibility to allow effective development of a student's individual abilities and interests. The major components of this program are the Core Curriculum, the Preclinical Elective Program, the Clinical Elective Program, and combined study.

The purpose of the Core Curriculum, which extends over the four-year course of study, is to provide each student with the general education and training considered essential to all physicians. It stresses understanding of concepts and general principles instead of a superficial knowledge of details. It provides opportunity for correlation among the sciences so that information received in one subject can reinforce ideas and build upon concepts developed in another. The incorporation of clinical correlation into the first two years demonstrates how knowledge of the basic sciences applies directly to the solution of problems of human disease. The Core Curriculum, for the first two academic years, is divided into four quarters (one-half-semester intervals) of nine weeks each. Within these smaller subdivisions it is possible to vary the balance of departmental activities to accommodate a better integrated presentation of subject matter.

The Core Curriculum for the last two years follows a track system of clerkships and electives, which exposes students to all of the major clinical fields of medicine. The newly revised curriculum includes an emphasis on primary care and ambulatory health care delivery sites. Students are also required to complete rotations at rural or urban AHEC sites in the third and fourth years. The schedule provides considerable flexibility and opportunities for selecting elective courses.

The purpose of the Preclinical Elective Program is to allow each student to extend his/her education in certain areas of scientific knowledge. The electives make it possible to construct a program of medical education that best meets the needs, abilities, and goals of the individual student. Students also are permitted to take courses as electives in divisions of the University of Louisville other than the School of Medicine, class schedule permitting. In addition to the courses listed, students with a research interest are permitted to participate in an approved research activity for credit. Elective courses constitute an integral part of the student's total program in medical school. Second-year students take two credit hours of elective courses.

In the Clinical Elective Program, the student selects a faculty member who works in a preceptorial relationship in the area of the student's interest. Virtually every member of the full-time clinical faculty participates in the program, as do many members of the basic science faculty. Students may select intensive exposure to any of the clinical areas or research experience in any of the basic science or clinical areas. During this time, a student also may select courses from the second-year elective program.

Especially capable students enrolled in the School of Medicine may work toward an M.S. or Ph.D. degree while pursuing the M.D. degree. A certain number of core and elective courses may be used to fulfill requirements for these degrees. By enrolling in the Graduate School at or near the beginning of medical school and using elective time, it is possible for a student to receive an M.S. degree at the same time the M.D. degree is granted. A five-year M.D.-M.B.A. program is also available.

REQUIREMENTS FOR ENTRANCE

The MCAT is required. A bachelor's degree is recommended and most successful candidates have earned the bachelor's degree by the time they enroll in the medical school. Required courses are:

	Sem. hrs.
Biology (with lab)	8
General or inorganic chemistry (with labs)	8
Organic chemistry (with labs)	8
Physics (with labs)	8
College mathematics	8
Or one semester of calculus	
English	8

Proficiency in written and oral English is required.

SELECTION FACTORS

Because the University of Louisville is a state institution, the School of Medicine gives preference to qualified residents of Kentucky. Applicants are selected on the basis of their individual merits without bias concerning sex, race, creed, national origin, age, or handicap.

Applicants are chosen on the basis of intellect, integrity, maturity, and the ability to interact with sensitivity with others. In the selection of applicants, consideration is given to the past academic record, evaluations of college preprofessional committees or faculty letters of recommendations, extracurricular activities, and personal interviews. The interviews are given considerable weight and are held at the medical school.

Some characteristics of students in the 1998 entering class were: *mean MCAT* 9, *mean GPA,* 3.6; *sex,* 47 percent women; *minority,* 10 percent.

FINANCIAL AID

Financial needs of the applicant are not a consideration in the selection process. After acceptance, every effort is made to assist students in meeting their financial requirements. Approximately 85 percent of the student body receive some degree of financial aid during the academic year. Scholarships are available on a limited basis and are granted according to demonstrated financial need and scholastic and professional promise. Student Research Scholarships are available to qualified students during the summer months.

INFORMATION FOR MINORITY STUDENTS

Applications from disadvantaged individuals and members of minority groups are encouraged. The School of Medicine has a prematriculation program. Applicants are reviewed by the full Admissions Committee, which accepts students on an individual basis according to their potential and promise of medical school and service as physicians.

Public Institution

APPLICATION AND ACCEPTANCE POLICIES FOR 2001–2002 FIRST-YEAR CLASS

School participates in AMCAS. See Chapter 6.

Filing of AMCAS application
  Earliest date: June 1, 2000
  Latest date: Nov. 1, 2000
School application fee to all applicants: $25
Oldest MCAT scores considered: 1998
Does have Early Decision Program (EDP)
  EDP application period: June 1–Aug. 1, 2000
  EDP applicants notified by: Oct. 1, 2000
Acceptance notice to regular applicants
  Earliest date: Oct. 1, 2000
  Latest date: April 30, 2001
Applicant's response to acceptance offer
  Maximum time: 2 weeks
Requests for deferred entrance considered: Yes
Deposit to hold place in class (applied to tuition):
  $100, due with response to acceptance offer
Deposit refundable prior to: March 1, 2001
Estimated number of new entrants: 141 (20 EDP)
Starting date: Aug. 2001

TUITION AND STUDENT FEES PER YEAR FOR 1999–2000 FIRST-YEAR CLASS

Tuition
  Resident: $9,890
  Nonresident: $25,280

Student fees: $286

INFORMATION ON 1999–2000 FIRST-YEAR CLASS

Number of	*In-State*	*Out-of-State*	*Total*
Applicants	447	1,006	1,453
Applicants Interviewed	265	35	300
New Entrants*	124	17	141

*All took the MCAT and had baccalaureate degrees.

CHAPTER 11

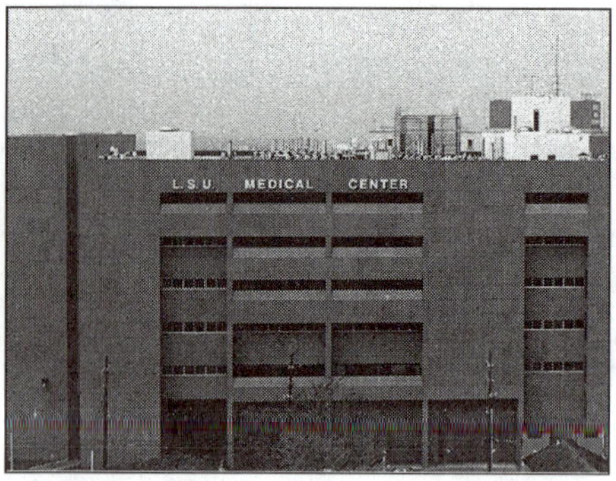

Louisiana State University School of Medicine in New Orleans

New Orleans, Louisiana

Dr. Robert L. Marier, *Dean*
Dr. Sam G. McClugage, *Assistant Dean for Admissions*
Patrick Gorman, *Director of Student Financial Aid*

ADDRESS INQUIRIES TO:

Admissions Office
Louisiana State University
School of Medicine in New Orleans
1901 Perdido Street, Box P3-4
New Orleans, Louisiana 70112-1393
(504) 568-6262; 568-7701 (FAX)
E-mail: ms-admissions@lsumc.edu
Web Site: http://www.medschool.lsuhsc.edu/admissions

MISSION STATEMENT

The Louisiana State University (LSU) School of Medicine in New Orleans is dedicated to providing the opportunity for an excellent medical education to all Louisiana applicants who are prepared to benefit from its curriculum and instruction. To this end, the Admissions Committee will strive to recruit and admit residents from Louisiana from every geographic, economic, social, and cultural dimension of the state of Louisiana.

GENERAL INFORMATION

The LSU School of Medicine in New Orleans was established in 1931 by authorization provided in the charter of Louisiana State University and Agricultural and Mechanical College adopted in 1877. The original building was constructed at 1542 Tulane Avenue, adjacent to the Medical Center of Louisiana at New Orleans (Charity Hospital). Over the years, additions were added to the original structure, and new buildings were erected as the school expanded, including a Residence Hall and Student Center at 1900 Perdido Street, a Medical Education Building at 1901 Perdido Street, and the Lions-LSU Clinics Building at 2020 Graver Street. A new Clinical Sciences Building is currently under construction. The School of Medicine is one component of the LSU Health Sciences Center in New Orleans, which includes Schools of Allied Health, Dentistry, Graduate Studies, and Nursing.

The major teaching hospitals are the Medical Center of Louisiana in New Orleans and University Hospital. Other hospitals in the city are also used for clinical instruction and residency training. Also, some residency programs and clerkships are available at the University Medical Center in Lafayette, and the Earl K. Long Hospital in Baton Rouge.

A student housing facility is available. Furnished and unfurnished apartments are available for married and single students, and regular dormitory-type space is also available.

CURRICULUM

The first two years of the medical school curriculum emphasize several basic sciences and their relevancy to clinical medicine. Clinical experiences begin in the first year in courses such as Introduction to Clinical Medicine. The second year of medical school utilizes an integrated approach to the teaching of basic science and preclinical courses within an environment that fosters an early exposure to patient care. Clerkships begin in the third year where students rotate through the various clinical disciplines. In the fourth year, students are given several months for electives in addition to required rotations in Ambulatory Medicine, Acting Internships, etc. Some of these rotations can be completed at the institutions associated with the LSU School of Medicine throughout the state or at other approved institutions outside the state or country.

Computer-assisted instruction is an important component of the curriculum. Each medical school class is provided access to state-of-the-art computer laboratories, which are located in buildings where the students are taking courses.

Although major emphasis is placed on training primary care physicians, there are many opportunities for research and the pursuit of more specialized training. There are several Centers of Excellence that provide opportunities for research and training in such areas as cancer, neuroscience, genetics, alcohol and drug abuse, and asthma.

The Honors Programs at LSUHSC supplements the regular curriculum and is designed to challenge the exceptional student while stimulating the interests of the individual. It entails an independent research program that encompasses basic and clinical sciences in the pursuit of a problem of scientific interest.

The M.D.-Ph.D. program is available for highly motivated students interested in academic medicine. Only applicants who are first accepted to medical school can be considered for this program. Information can be obtained by calling the School of Graduate Studies, (504) 568-2211.

Students are required to pass Step 1 of the USMLE before progressing to the third year. They must pass Step 2 prior to graduation.

The curriculum is under constant evaluation and review by both faculty and students.

REQUIREMENTS FOR ENTRANCE

The MCAT is required and must be taken at a time that enables scores to be received by the Admissions Office prior to the November application deadline to be considered for admission the following August. Applicants are strongly urged to complete the regular four-year undergraduate curriculum and take the appropriate recommended courses before entering the study of medicine. The school encourages a balance between the natural sciences, social sciences, and the humanities.

Specific course requirements are:

	Sem. hrs.
Biology or zoology (with lab)	8
General or inorganic chemistry (with lab)	8
Organic chemistry (with lab)	8
Physics (with lab)	8

Demonstrated proficiency in spoken and written English is required.

Current policy precludes acceptance of advanced placement courses for credit toward fulfilling specific requirements in the sciences (biology, chemistry, and physics). The School of Medicine does not accept pass/fail grades for required science courses.

SELECTION FACTORS

The Admissions Committee will evaluate all applicants who are residents of the state of Louisiana using any or all of several criteria. Some of these are: academic factors such as grades and test scores, strength of the letters of recommendation, strength of the interviews, employment history and whether or not the applicant had to work to go to college, demonstrated history of leadership, demonstrated history of community service, an assessment of all extracurricular activities in which the applicant participated, special honors that have been awarded to the applicant, hobbies and interests, socioeconomic background, where in the state the applicant was raised, and whether there were any factors in the applicant's background that may have hindered him/her from achieving a higher level of academic achievement. There is no discrimination because of race, religion, sex, age, handicap, national origin, or financial status. Transfer students from U.S. medical schools who are nonresidents may be considered for upper-level classes. Interviews are arranged by invitation and are conducted at the medical campus in New Orleans.

FINANCIAL AID

Financial assistance is available for students through several different methods. There are direct scholarship programs, scholarships for disadvantaged students, state and federal loan programs, work-study programs, and employment opportunities in the New Orleans area for students in their third and fourth years. Financial assistance information is available from the Student Financial Aid Office at (504) 568-4820.

INFORMATION FOR MINORITY STUDENTS

Members of minority groups are encouraged to apply. The School of Medicine's Office of Community and Minority Health Education actively recruits minority students and provides counseling for high school and college students.

Further information may be obtained by contacting Dr. Edward Helm, Associate Dean for Community and Minority Health Education, at (504) 568-8501 or at the address listed on the previous page.

Public Institution

APPLICATION AND ACCEPTANCE POLICIES FOR 2001–2002 FIRST-YEAR CLASS

School participates in AMCAS. See Chapter 6.

Filing of AMCAS application
  Earliest date: June 1, 2000
  Latest date: Nov. 15, 2000
School application fee after screening: $50
Oldest MCAT scores considered: Aug. 1997
Does have Early Decision Program (EDP)
  For Louisiana residents only
  EDP application period: June 1–Aug. 1, 2000
  EDP applicants notified by: Oct. 1, 2000
Acceptance notice to regular applicants
  Earliest date: Oct. 15, 2000
  Latest date: Varies
Applicant's response to acceptance offer
  Maximum time: 2 weeks
Requests for deferred entrance considered: Yes
Deposit to hold place in class (applied to tuition):
  $100, due with response to acceptance offer
Deposit refundable prior to: May 15, 2001
Estimated number of new entrants: 165 (7–10 EDP)
Starting date: Aug. 2000

TUITION AND STUDENT FEES PER YEAR FOR 1999–2000 FIRST-YEAR CLASS

Tuition
  Resident: $8,856
  Nonresident: $23,004
Student fees: $167

INFORMATION ON 1999–2000 FIRST-YEAR CLASS

Number of	*In-State*	*Out-of-State*	*Total*
Applicants	794	418	1,212
Applicants Interviewed	420	0	420
New Entrants*	165	0	165

*All took the MCAT and had baccalaureate degrees.

CHAPTER 11

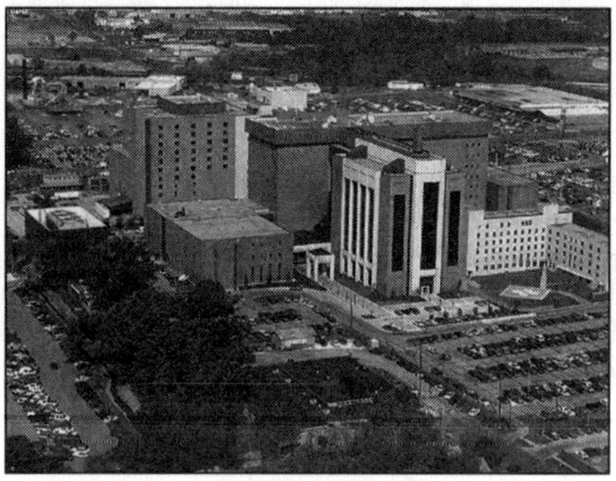

Louisiana State University School of Medicine in Shreveport

Shreveport, Louisiana

Dr. Ike Muslow, *Vice Chancellor and Interim Dean*
Dr. F. Scott Kennedy, *Assistant Dean for Student Admissions*
Sherry Gladney, *Associate Director of Student Financial Aid*

ADDRESS INQUIRIES TO:

Office of Student Admissions
Louisiana State University Health Sciences Center
School of Medicine in Shreveport
P.O. Box 33932
Shreveport, Louisiana 71130-3932
(318) 675-5190; 675-5244 (FAX)
E-mail: shvadm@lsumc.edu
Web Site: http://lib-sh.lsumc.edu/

MISSION STATEMENT

The Louisiana State University Health Sciences Center (LSUHSC) provides education, research, patient care services, and community outreach. LSU Health Sciences Center encompasses six professional schools: the School of Medicine in New Orleans, the School of Medicine in Shreveport, the School of Graduate Studies in New Orleans and Shreveport, the School of Nursing, the School of Dentistry, and the School of Allied Health Professions in New Orleans and Shreveport.

LSU Health Sciences Center educates health professionals and scientists at all levels. Its major responsibility includes the advancement and dissemination of knowledge in medicine, dentistry, nursing, allied health, public health, and basic sciences. Statewide programs of clinical and basic health science research are developed and expanded by LSU Health Sciences Center. This research results in publications, technology transfer, and related economic enhancements to meet the changing needs of the state of Louisiana and the nation.

LSU Health Sciences Center provides vital public service through direct patient care, including care of indigent patients. Health care services are provided through the LSU Clinics in New Orleans, the LSU Hospital and Clinics in Shreveport, Dental Clinics and Nursing Clinics in New Orleans, the Allied Health Professions Clinics in New Orleans and Shreveport, and numerous affiliated hospitals and clinics throughout Louisiana. LSUHSC also provides coordination and referral services, continuing education, and public information.

LSU Health Sciences Center administers the Health Care Services Division of the LSU System. This division has a dual mission: 1) to assure the availability of acute and primary health care services to the uninsured, to the underinsured, and to others with problems of access to medical care, and 2) to serve as the principal sites for the clinical education of future doctors and other health care professionals.

LSUHSC created and oversees the operation of Area Health Education Centers (AHEC's). These corporate entities, governed by boards of prominent citizens, act as liaison agencies between Louisiana's schools of health professions and Louisiana communities. AHEC programs seek to improve the number and distribution of health care providers in rural and urban underserved areas of Louisiana and support existing rural health care providers through continuing education programs.

GENERAL INFORMATION

The Louisiana State University (LSU) School of Medicine in Shreveport, a four-year school, admitted its first class in 1969; the first M.D. degrees were awarded in 1973. Teaching takes place at the school's principal teaching hospital, Louisiana State University Hospital (436 beds), and at the affiliated Shreveport Veterans Administration Hospital (450 beds). Permanent medical school facilities, consisting of a basic and clinical science building, library, and Comprehensive Care Teaching Facility, were occupied in the winter of 1975.

CURRICULUM

The curriculum is traditional in general features but not entirely classical in detail. It is flexible to permit experimentation without disruption. Contact with patients begins early, paralleling a thorough grounding in the basic medical sciences. In addition to short courses in radiology, psychiatry, biometry, and physical examination, live clinics throughout the first and second years serve to indicate application of the basic sciences in clinical medicine. A wide variety of elective instruction is available to first- and second-year students, and one-third of the senior year is elective time on campus or at other institutions. A program of comprehensive care is woven through all four years. The third and fourth years are essentially rotating clerkships in the clinical disciplines. A letter grading system is employed: A, B, C, D (barely pass), and F (fail).

REQUIREMENTS FOR ENTRANCE

The MCAT and a minimum of three years of college (at least 90 semester hours) are required. A baccalaureate degree is desirable. Required courses are:

	Sem. hrs.
Biology or zoology (with lab)	8
Inorganic chemistry (with lab)	8
Organic chemistry (with lab)	8
General physics (with lab)	8
English	6

Prospective applicants are strongly urged to take the MCAT by the spring prior to the year of application and to complete most of the required course work by the time of application. They should pursue their own particular interests in selecting college courses not required for admission; a broad educational background is desirable.

SELECTION FACTORS

Admission is based upon character, motivation, intellectual ability, and achievement as judged by recommendations of premedical advisors, personal interviews with members of the faculty at the School of Medicine, college grades, and MCAT scores. In recent years, the number of applications filed by well-qualified residents of Louisiana has been in excess of the number of places available. For this reason, places have not been offered to nonresidents. Determination of state residence is provided by LSU system regulations.

Accepted students for the 1999 entering class had the following credentials: *mean science GPA,* 3.5; *mean overall GPA,* 3.6; *sex,* 45 percent *women* (acceptance rate the same for men and women per number of applicants); *residence,* 100 percent from Louisiana; *undergraduate major,* 81 percent in the sciences and chemistry; undergraduate college, 38 schools represented.

The School of Medicine in Shreveport does not discriminate in applicant selection on the basis of race, sex, creed, national origin, age, or handicap.

FINANCIAL AID

Scholarship and long-term, low-interest loan funds are available to students with financial need. In the past, no accepted students have been unable to meet their financial needs. Scholarships and loans are available to students all four years and are based on applicants showing verified need. Certain awards are given in recognition primarily of academic accomplishment and promise. The school offers summer employment to many students but does not advise employment during school sessions, which would interfere with academic performance. Financial need has no bearing on an applicant's acceptance. Applications for financial assistance are furnished by the Financial Aid Office after students have been accepted and the class is firmly filled. Approximately 81 percent of the student body obtain financial aid in the form of loans.

INFORMATION FOR MINORITY STUDENTS

Applications from minority students are encouraged and will be given every consideration.

Public Institution

APPLICATION AND ACCEPTANCE POLICIES FOR 2001–2002 FIRST-YEAR CLASS

School participates in AMCAS. See Chapter 6.

Filing of AMCAS application
- Earliest date: June 1, 2000
- Latest date: Nov. 15, 2000

School application fee to all applicants: $50
Oldest MCAT scores considered: April 1997
Does have Early Decision Program (EDP)
- For Louisiana residents only
- EDP application period: June 1–August 1, 2000
- EDP applicants notified by: Oct. 1, 2000

Acceptance notice to regular applicants
- Earliest date: Oct. 15, 2000
- Latest date: Until class is filled

Applicant's response to acceptance offer
- Maximum time: 2 weeks

Requests for deferred entrance considered: Yes
Deposit to hold place in class (applied to tuition):
- $100, due with response to acceptance offer

Deposit refundable prior to: May 15, 2001
Estimated number of new entrants: 100 (5 EDP)
Starting date: Aug. 9, 2001

TUITION AND STUDENT FEES PER YEAR FOR 1999–2000 FIRST-YEAR CLASS

Tuition
- Resident: $8,581
- Nonresident: $22,729

Student fees: $276

INFORMATION ON 1999–2000 FIRST-YEAR CLASS

Number of	*In-State*	*Out-of-State*	*Total*
Applicants	933	0	933
Applicants Interviewed	206	0	206
New Entrants*	100	0	100

*All took the MCAT; 85% had baccalaureate degrees.

CHAPTER 11

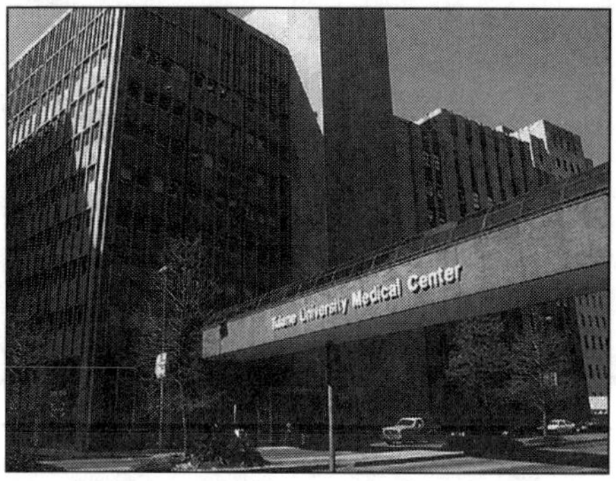

Tulane University School of Medicine

New Orleans, Louisiana

Dr. James J. Corrigan, Jr., *Dean*
Dr. Joseph C. Pisano, *Associate Dean*
Michael T. Goodman, *Director of Financial Aid*

ADDRESS INQUIRIES TO:

Office of Admissions
Tulane University School of Medicine
1430 Tulane Avenue, SL67
New Orleans, Louisiana 70112-2699
(504) 588-5187; 988-6735 (FAX)
E-mail: medsch@tmcpop.tmc.tulane.edu
Web Site: http://www.mcl.tulane.edu

GENERAL INFORMATION

Tulane University School of Medicine, a private, nonsectarian institution, was founded in 1834. Today it is one of the eleven colleges composing Tulane University and the 15th oldest medical school in the U.S. The School of Medicine is located in downtown New Orleans, a few blocks from the New Orleans Superdome and the Vieux Carré (French Quarter). While the School of Medicine has affiliation agreements with more than 10 hospitals and clinics in New Orleans and other communities, three of its principal clinical teaching facilities are immediately adjacent to the School of Medicine: Charity Hospital of New Orleans, Veterans Affairs Medical Center, and the Tulane University Center Hospital and Clinic. The School of Medicine and the Tulane University Hospital and Clinic are two components of the Tulane University Medical Center. Other components of the center include: the School of Public Health and Tropical Medicine, the J. Bennett Johnston Center for Bioenvironmental Research, the Tulane Regional Primate Research Center, and the F. Edward Hébert Center. In 1995, Tulane University and Columbia/HCA Healthcare Corporation formed a partnership that introduced to Tulane 11 centers of excellence that will serve as specialized health care education and research hubs for the region. These centers include the Tulane Hospital for Children, a center dedicated to educational research in primary care, and centers for studies in genetics, infectious diseases, neurological diseases, cardiovascular medicine, geriatrics, cancer, transplantation, women's health, and sports medicine. Through the full use of its varied resources, Tulane University School of Medicine is dedicated to conducting the highest-quality educational programs, which will result in academically and clinically prepared physicians (generalists and specialists) and biomedical scientists to satisfy regional, national, and international health needs.

CURRICULUM

The School of Medicine offers a four-year program leading to the M.D. degree. While the emphasis in the first two years is on the principles of the basic medical sciences, the goal of the first two years is helping students develop clinical problem-solving skills instead of emphasizing the transmission of facts devoid of clinical context. The program in Foundations in Medicine, which spans the first two years, is responsible for instructing students in the complex art and science of the patient-doctor interaction. This objective is accomplished through lectures, small-group discussions, clinical demonstrations, visits to community health facilities, and interactions with both real patients and individuals trained as patient instructors. The third and fourth years provide experience in clinical settings where the emphasis is on patient care and community health. Flexibility is attained throughout the four years by allowing approximately one-third of scheduled curriculum time for elective courses and selected advanced studies. Throughout all four years a number of interdisciplinary courses are offered by the combined faculties of the basic and clinical science departments. The course of study and grading methods are under review at all times by faculty and students.

Several combined-degree programs are available to medical students. Work towards a Ph.D. degree in combination with the doctorate in medicine requires concurrent enrollment in the Graduate School and the School of Medicine. Medical students may choose to concurrently enroll in the School of Public Health and Tropical Medicine to complement their doctorate in medicine with an M.P.H. degree. Students wishing to obtain the M.P.H. are encouraged to begin their studies in the School of Public Health and Tropical Medicine during the summer before their matriculation into medical school.

Tulane offers a wide variety of support systems for medical students. Such support systems include an academic year tutorial program, study and test-taking skills workshops, and review programs for the USMLE. Academic, career, and personal counseling is available for students upon request.

REQUIREMENTS FOR ENTRANCE

The MCAT and a minimum of three years of college, or 90 semester hours, are required. Four years of college and the baccalaureate degree are strongly recommended.

Applicants are strongly urged to take the MCAT in the spring of the year of application and to have their basic science requirements completed at the time of application. The required courses are:

	Sem./hrs.
Biology or zoology (with lab)	6
Inorganic chemistry (with lab)	6
Organic chemistry (with lab)	6
General physics (with lab)	6
English	6

In premedical preparation, the major program need not be in one of the science fields. Students are urged to follow their own inclinations in choosing a course of study, recognizing that a physician should have a broad educational background. Approximately one-third of the entering class each year has come from a non-science background.

SELECTION FACTORS

In evaluating applicants, the Committee on Admissions relies on such criteria as grade point averages, MCAT scores, faculty appraisals from the applicant's college, special accomplishments and talents, and the substance and level of courses taken in a particular college. While most successful applicants have attained at least a GPA of 3.5 and a composite MCAT score of 30, Tulane has not established mandatory minimal scores, as all components of the application, cognitive and noncognitive, are taken into account. Because of national priorities, most students accepted must be U.S. citizens. Personal character of the highest order is required along with strong motivation, great potential, and evidence of high-level performance. Tulane University does not discriminate on the basis of race, sex, creed, age, national origin, or handicap.

All completed applications are read in full by members of the Committee on Admissions. Selected applicants are invited for personal interviews, which are held in New Orleans on the medical school campus. Following interview sessions, the committee reviews again an applicant's record during one of its regular weekly meetings. The committee holds the authority to decide whether a candidate should be accepted, rejected, or held for further evaluation at a later date.

FINANCIAL AID

Scholarships and loans (federal, private, and Tulane programs) are available to students based on an analysis of the individual's financial needs. Additionally, each year approximately 20 students are awarded scholarships based exclusively upon academic merit. More than 85 percent of the students receive some form of financial assistance during their four years of study.

First-year students ordinarily are not encouraged to undertake employment during the session; this is also true for students in the other years if their scholastic standing would be jeopardized. A number of paid externships are available in the local hospitals, however.

INFORMATION FOR MINORITY STUDENTS

Tulane encourages qualified minority and disadvantaged students to apply. Special activities available for, but not limited to, minority students include tutorial and counseling services for students in medical school. The Committee on Admissions includes minority members, but there is no separate review for minority applicants or for any other special group.

Private Institution

APPLICATION AND ACCEPTANCE POLICIES FOR 2001–2002 FIRST-YEAR CLASS

School participates in AMCAS. See Chapter 6.

Filing of AMCAS application
Earliest date: June 1, 2000
Latest date: Dec. 15, 2000
School application fee to all applicants: $95
Oldest MCAT scores considered: 1998
Does have Early Decision Program (EDP)
EDP application period: June 1–Aug. 1, 2000
EDP applicants notified by: Oct. 1, 2000
Acceptance notice to regular applicants
Earliest date: Oct. 1, 2000
Latest date: Until class is filled
Applicant's response to acceptance offer
Maximum time: 2 weeks
Requests for deferred entrance considered: Yes
Deposit to hold place in class (applied to tuition): $500, nonrefundable
Deposit is due on: May 15, 2001
Estimated number of new entrants: 150 (10)
Starting date: Aug. 2001

TUITION AND STUDENT FEES PER YEAR FOR 1999–2000 FIRST-YEAR CLASS

Tuition: $29,145 Student fees: $1,777

INFORMATION ON 1999–2000 FIRST-YEAR CLASS

Number of	*In-State*	*Out-of-State*	*Total*
Applicants	518	7,753	8,271
Applicants Interviewed	121	787	908
New Entrants*	25	127	152

*All had baccalaureate degrees and took the MCAT.

CHAPTER 11

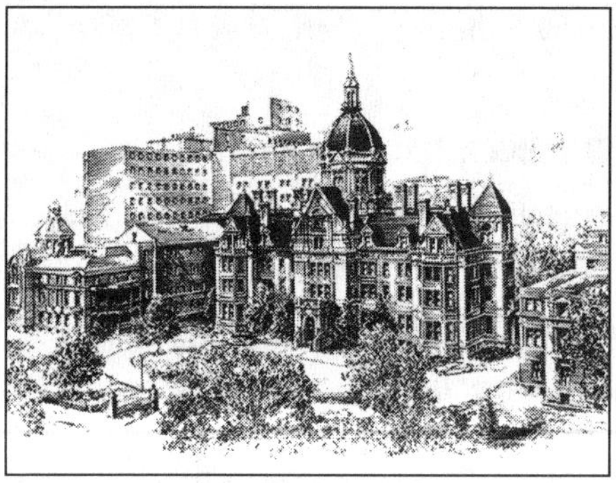

Johns Hopkins University School of Medicine

Baltimore, Maryland

Dr. Edward D. Miller, *The Baker Dean of the Medical Faculty and Chief Executive Officer, Johns Hopkins Medicine*
David M. Trabilsy, *Assistant Dean for Admissions*
Paula Abernethy, *Director of Financial Aid Services*

ADDRESS INQUIRIES TO:

Committee on Admission
Johns Hopkins University
School of Medicine
720 Rutland Avenue
Baltimore, Maryland 21205-2196
(410) 955-3182
Web Site: http://www.med.jhu.edu/admissions

MISSION STATEMENT

The Johns Hopkins University School of Medicine is dedicated to preparing students to practice compassionate medicine of the highest standards and to contributing to the advancement of medical knowledge.

GENERAL INFORMATION

Johns Hopkins University School of Medicine, founded in 1893, is a private, nondenominational institution, which fosters the training of medical practitioners, teachers, and biomedical scientists. The medical center provides: library facilities, the Reed Residence Hall, off-campus housing assistance, cafeterias, recreational sports in the Cooley Center, and performing arts programs.

Preclinical courses are given in the adjacent basic science complex. Medical care facilities such as the Johns Hopkins Hospital and the Outpatient Center provide an extensive and diverse patient base for the teaching of all clinical subjects. Students also attend educational programs conducted at community hospitals in Baltimore and pursue elective experiences at other medical schools in the United States and foreign countries.

The Ross building and other facilities house exceptional opportunities for students to engage in research. A new oncology center, dedicated to patient care and research, has recently opened. Within the Johns Hopkins Medical Institutions are the School of Hygiene and Public Health, School of Nursing, and affiliated centers such as the Kennedy Krieger Institute for children with disorders of the brain.

CURRICULUM

The Johns Hopkins curriculum provides sound foundations in basic sciences and clinical medicine while retaining the flexibility required for students to identify and to develop diverse career interests.

The M.D. program includes the integration of basic sciences and clinical experiences and the expanded use of case-based small-group learning sessions. Students have contact with clinical medicine throughout the first year by working with community physicians. The physician and society course spans the four-year program and covers topics such as ethics, finances, legal and political issues, fine arts as they relate to medicine (literature, music, art), and history of medicine.

First Year: Includes integrated coverage of introductory basic sciences, neuroscience, epidemiology, and introduction to clinical medicine.

Second Year: Study of advanced basic sciences, behavioral sciences, clinical skills, and beginning clerkships.

Third and Fourth Years: With the assistance of faculty advisors, students develop individualized programs incorporating required clerkships in major clinical areas and electives. Students may use electives for specialized clerkships, research, and public health experience.

Students interested in academic medicine can obtain combined M.D.-Ph.D. degrees by pursuing coordinated graduate studies in biochemistry and molecular biology, biological chemistry, biomedical engineering, biophysics, cell biology and anatomy, cellular and molecular medicine, epidemiology, history of medicine, human genetics, microbiology and immunology, neurosciences, pathobiology, pharmacology, and physiology. Candidates accepted for M.D.-Ph.D. studies can apply for financial support through the Medical Scientist Training Program, which provides full tuition and stipend. Students may also enroll for special studies or seek advanced degrees in any component of the Johns Hopkins University, including the M.P.H. degree at the School of Hygiene and Public Health.

The deferral plan for admitted applicants provides opportunities for delayed matriculation into the School of Medicine. Deferred admission enables students to plan and pursue alternative education, research, work experience, international fellowships, or humanitarian service, which will enhance their future careers in medicine. For more information on the deferral plan, please contact the Admissions Office.

REQUIREMENTS FOR ENTRANCE

The MCAT is required for admission. The B.A. degree or equivalent is required of all students entering the School of Medicine. Students are encouraged to complete coherent studies of sciences and liberal arts consistent with their undergraduate major. Required courses are:

	Sem. hrs.
General biology (with lab)	8
General chemistry (with lab)	8
Organic chemistry (with lab)	8
General physics (with lab)	8
Humanities and social and behavioral sciences	24
Calculus or statistics	6

Advanced placement credit is acceptable for meeting the calculus and physics requirements. A semester of biochemistry may be substituted for one semester of organic chemistry. Students are expected to be proficient in the use of computers. Required courses must be evaluated by a traditional grading system other than pass/fail grades. CLEP credit may not be used to satisfy required courses.

Johns Hopkins participates in AMCAS. Prospective applicants are advised to consult the admissions Web site or contact the Admissions Office for the latest information on admissions requirements and policies.

SELECTION FACTORS

In addition to proven academic competence, previous achievements and activities help the Committee on Admission to evaluate applicants' suitability for medicine. Students who have unusual talents, strong humanistic qualities, demonstrated leadership, and creative abilities are sought. There are no residence requirements for U.S. citizens, and applications are invited from candidates in all sections of the country. Medical students in good academic standing may apply for transfer admission. Generally there are few, if any, positions available. The Johns Hopkins University complies with federal and state law prohibiting discrimination.

FINANCIAL AID

The Johns Hopkins policy has been to keep the tuition "frozen" at the first-year amount with no increase in tuition for the second, third, and fourth years of medical school. The cost for living expenses is based on a twelve-month budget. Students are able to maintain a moderate lifestyle, because the cost of living in Baltimore is highly affordable. Financial aid in the form of federal and institutional grants and loans is awarded solely on the basis of need. Financial considerations do not influence admissions decisions. Approximately 80 percent of matriculating students receive financial assistance. Parents' financial information is required of all students requesting institutional aid. Students are awarded financial aid packages to fully meet their demonstrated financial need. Student fellowship stipends are frequently available for projects carried out in summers.

Non-U.S. citizens without permanent resident or immigrant visa status are not eligible to receive financial aid because of government restrictions on funds that support the aid program. Qualified foreign students receive final acceptance only after establishing an escrow account acceptable to the School of Medicine that is sufficient to meet all tuition, fees, and living expenses for the anticipated period of enrollment. This amount is currently $170,000.

INFORMATION FOR MINORITY STUDENTS

Johns Hopkins is committed to the enrollment and education of individuals from all disadvantaged groups. The school values having a diverse student population from all areas of the country. Hopkins has an excellent record of enrolling students from underrepresented minority groups. For information, write Dr. Roland Smoot, assistant dean for student affairs.

Private Institution

APPLICATION AND ACCEPTANCE POLICIES FOR 2001–2002 FIRST-YEAR CLASS

School participates in AMCAS. See Chapter 6.

Filing of AMCAS application
- Earliest date: June 1, 2000
- Latest date: Oct. 15, 2000

School application fee to all applicants: $60

Oldest MCAT scores considered: 1991

Does have Early Decision Program (EDP)
- EDP application period: June 1–Aug. 15, 2000
- EDP applicants notified by: Oct. 1, 2000

Acceptance notice to regular applicants
- Earliest date: Oct. 15, 2000
- Latest date: March 30, 2001

Applicant's response to acceptance offer
- Maximum time: 3 weeks

Requests for deferred entrance considered: Yes

Deposit to hold place in class: None

Estimated number of new entrants: 120 (5 EDP)

Starting date: Sept. 2001

TUITION AND STUDENT FEES PER YEAR FOR 1999–2000 FIRST-YEAR CLASS

Tuition: $25,500 Student fees: $2,628

INFORMATION ON 1999–2000 FIRST-YEAR CLASS

Number of	*In-State*	*Out-of-State*	*Total*
Applicants	290	2,713	3,003
Applicants Interviewed	67	556	623
New Entrants*	16	103	119

*All students matriculating into four-year program had baccalaureate degrees; 81% took the MCAT.

CHAPTER 11

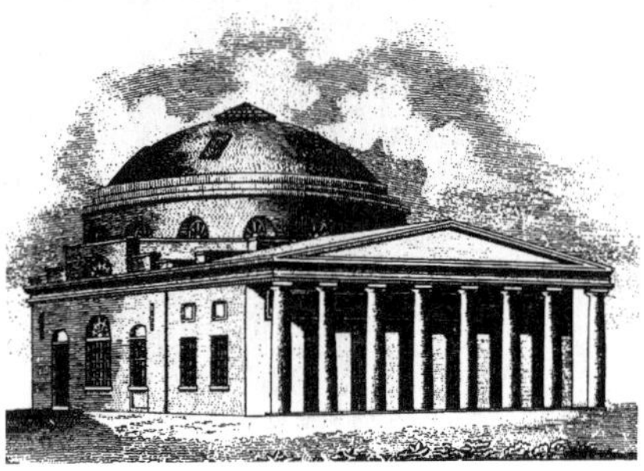

University of Maryland School of Medicine

Baltimore, Maryland

Dr. Donald E. Wilson, *Dean*
Dr. Milford M. Foxwell, Jr., *Associate Dean for Admissions*
Mary S. Vansickle, *Director of Financial Aid*

ADDRESS INQUIRIES TO:

Committee on Admissions
Room 1-005
University of Maryland
School of Medicine
655 West Baltimore Street
Baltimore, Maryland 21201
(410) 706-7478
Web Site: http://www.som1.ab.umd.edu/

MISSION STATEMENT

The University of Maryland School of Medicine is dedicated to providing excellence in biomedical education, basic and clinical research, quality patient care, and service to improve the health of the citizens of Maryland and beyond. The School is committed to the education and training of M.D., M.D.–Ph.D., graduate, physical therapy, and medical research technology students. The school will recruit and develop faculty to serve as exemplary role models for our students.

GENERAL INFORMATION

The University of Maryland School of Medicine is the fifth oldest medical college in the United States. It was organized in 1807 and chartered in 1808 under the name of the College of Medicine of Maryland; the first class was graduated in 1810. Among the first to erect its own hospital for clinical instruction in 1823, the University of Maryland established the first intramural residency for senior students.

Along with the other professional schools of the University of Maryland (dentistry, law, nursing, pharmacy, social work, and the graduate schools of basic sciences), the School of Medicine is located on the Baltimore City Campus, which is adjacent to the downtown Charles Center, Inner Harbor, Oriole Park at Camden Yards, and PSI Net Stadium.

The University of Maryland Medical System and affiliated hospitals in and around Baltimore have more than 2,300 general hospital beds for teaching purposes.

CURRICULUM

The basic sciences during the first two years of medical school will be integrated and taught as systems, using interdisciplinary teaching with both basic and clinical science faculty. Problem-based learning has been implemented throughout the basic science years. Contact hours have been reduced, with an emphasis on independent study with the availability of mentors and learning resources. A half-day course in Introduction to Clinical Practice will begin at the inception of the freshman year and will continue throughout the first two years; dedicated to the instruction of interviewing, physical examination, intimate human behavior, biomedical ethics, and the dynamics of ambulatory care. Much of this experience will be off-site in clinical settings. The clinical clerkships during the last two years of medical school will include a mandatory ambulatory month in family medicine, an emphasis on ambulatory teaching in all other disciplines, and a longitudinal half-day experience in a clinical setting in which the student will have continuity of care for patients and families.

A program offering a combined M.D.-Ph.D. is available for selected applicants. Application forms are included in the Stage II packet. After the preclinical years, M.D.-Ph.D. students perform as full-time graduate students for approximately two years, taking the required graduate courses and seminars and focusing on dissertation research. Following this period, students begin the two years of clinical clerkships, using elective time if necessary to complete Ph.D. research.

REQUIREMENTS FOR ENTRANCE

The MCAT and at least 90 semester hours of accredited arts and science college credit are required. Preference is given to applicants who will have earned a bachelor's degree. The following courses must be completed prior to matriculation:

	Sem. hrs.
Biological sciences	8
Inorganic chemistry	8
Organic chemistry	8
General physics	8
English	6

Applicants should major in the academic area of their interest. If a nonscience major is selected, sufficient science courses should be taken to acquaint the applicant with the demands of a science-oriented curriculum.

The MCAT must be taken no later than the fall test period of the year in which application is made. It is required that the MCAT be taken within four years preceding the anticipated date of matriculation.

SELECTION FACTORS

Applications are accepted from citizens and permanent residents of the United States and Canada only. All applicants from Maryland are permitted to submit a direct application (Stage II) after the AMCAS application is received. As preference is given in the selection process to residents of Maryland, nonresident applicants are sent a Stage II application only upon recommendation of the Committee on Admissions. The deadline for the Stage II application is December 1. Applications from nonresidents may be rejected on the basis of GPA and MCAT scores that appear on the AMCAS application.

Interviews are arranged for those applicants who appear to have the academic and personal qualities required for successful completion of the requirements for the practice of medicine. All interviews are conducted on campus. Applications may be rejected from both residents and nonresidents without an interview.

Selections are based on a careful appraisal of the individual's motivation for medicine, academic achievement, performance on the MCAT, letters of recommendation, extracurricular activities, community service, and interviews by faculty members.

Accepted students for the 1999 entering class had the following characteristics: *average GPA,* 3.60 (range 3.1–4.0); *MCAT average,* 10 (range 6–14); *undergraduate major,* about 70 percent science majors; *sex,* 57 percent women; *minorities,* 14 percent.

The University of Maryland School of Medicine does not discriminate on the basis of race, sex, creed, national origin, age, or handicap.

FINANCIAL AID

The school makes available financial aid in the form of scholarships and loans to those students with demonstrable financial need. The amount of the award varies according to the student's needs and the level of funding available. About 70 percent of the students receive some degree of financial aid.

INFORMATION FOR MINORITY STUDENTS

The University of Maryland School of Medicine is committed to the recruitment and retention of minority and disadvantaged students. A major focus of our recruitment effort is to provide information on admissions requirements, the admissions process, undergraduate preparation for medicine, and education opportunities including the M.D.-Ph.D. program.

All students in the above categories are encouraged to apply. The admissions procedures for minority students are the same as those for all applicants. Among the selection factors emphasized by the Admissions Committee are undergraduate or graduate GPA, MCAT scores, application essay, and personal characteristics of the applicant, including work or research experience. The interview, letters of recommendation, and the applicant's life experiences help us to evaluate the subjective qualifications.

The minority recruitment coordinator, in conjunction with other support personnel, makes a special effort to provide information relevant to minority applicants. There is no fixed quota for any special group within the applicant pool. Information may be obtained from Hermione M. Hicks, director of recruitment, Room 1-005 in the Office of Admissions.

Public Institution

APPLICATION AND ACCEPTANCE POLICIES FOR 2001–2002 FIRST-YEAR CLASS

School participates in AMCAS. See Chapter 6.

Filing of AMCAS application
- Earliest date: June 1, 2000
- Latest date: Nov. 1, 2000

School application fee after screening: $50
Oldest MCAT scores considered: 1998
Does have Early Decision Program (EDP)
- EDP application period: June 1–Aug. 1, 2000
- EDP applicants notified by: Oct. 1, 2000

Acceptance notice to regular applicants
- Earliest date: Oct. 15, 2000
- Latest date: Until class is filled

Applicant's response to acceptance offer
- Maximum time: 3 weeks

Requests for deferred entrance considered: Yes
Deposit to hold place in class: None
Estimated number of new entrants: 138 (10 EDP)
Starting date: Aug. 2001

TUITION AND STUDENT FEES PER YEAR FOR 1999–2000 FIRST-YEAR CLASS

Tuition
- Resident: $13,129
- Nonresident: $25,145

Student fees: $1,806

INFORMATION ON 1999–2000 FIRST-YEAR CLASS

Number of	*In-State*	*Out-of-State*	*Total*
Applicants	819	2,471	3,290
Applicants Interviewed	321	154	475
New Entrants*	115	23	138

*All took the MCAT and had baccalaureate degrees.

CHAPTER 11

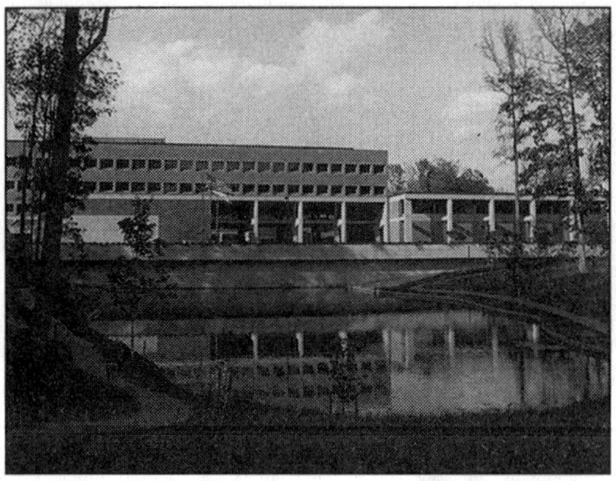

Uniformed Services University of the Health Sciences F. Edward Hébert School of Medicine

Bethesda, Maryland

Dr. Val G. Hemming, COL, USAF, MC (Ret), *Dean*
Peter J. Stavish, LTC, MS, USA (Ret), *Assistant Dean for Admissions and Academic Records*
Joan C. Stearman, *Director, Office of Admissions*

ADDRESS INQUIRIES TO:

Admissions Office, Room A-1041
Uniformed Services University
of the Health Sciences
F. Edward Hébert School of Medicine
4301 Jones Bridge Road
Bethesda, Maryland 20814-4799
(301) 295-3101; 295-3545 (FAX);
1 (800) 772-1743
Web Site: http://www.usuhs.mil

GENERAL INFORMATION

Created by public law in 1972, the Uniformed Services University of the Health Sciences (USUHS) was founded to prepare young men and women for careers as health care professionals in the uniformed services. The USUHS School of Medicine admitted its charter class in 1976. The school is located on the grounds of the Naval Hospital in Bethesda, Maryland. The school operates in close association with many federal health resources located in the greater Washington, D.C., area to provide students with a broad range of educational experiences in both the basic sciences and clinical medicine. The school's charter is to provide a comprehensive education in medicine to select individuals who demonstrate potential for, and commitment to, careers as medical officers in the uniformed services.

CURRICULUM

The school has a four-year program culminating in the doctor of medicine degree. Each of the first three academic years is 48 weeks, and the final year runs 40 weeks. Basic science instruction predominates in the initial two academic years, with the final two years being devoted to clinical education. Basic science instruction is correlated, as appropriate, both interdisciplinarily and clinically. The integration between the clinical and basic sciences is progressive and proceeds with involvement in patient care activities early in the curriculum, starting with the first semester of the freshman year. While the overall program is designed to educate students to serve as providers of primary health care, there is sufficient flexibility in the curriculum to accommodate differences in interests among students and also sufficient substances to enable graduates to pursue postgraduate activities such as research. Elective courses are offered in clinical and research facilities in this country and in areas of the world where diseases rarely seen in the United States are responsible for 80 percent of the morbidity and mortality. The curriculum also includes basic military orientation and concentration on unique aspects of military medicine. A conventional letter grading system is employed to record student progress.

REQUIREMENTS FOR ENTRANCE

Applicants must be U.S. citizens between the ages of 18 and 30 and must meet the physical and personal qualifications for a commission in the uniformed services. Applicants cannot be more than 30 years of age as of June 30 in the year of matriculation. Military applicants who have the appropriate creditable commissioned service may be considered for a waiver through age 35. The MCAT and a baccalaureate degree are required.

The following courses are required:

	Sem. hrs.
General biology (with lab)	8
General or inorganic chemistry (with lab)	8
Organic chemistry (with lab)	8
Physics (with lab)	8
Calculus	3
English	6

CLEP and advanced placement credits are acceptable for required courses. However, individuals exempted from prerequisites through these programs are required to take formal course work in the same areas at a more advanced level.

Both qualified civilians and military personnel are eligible to apply. However, individuals who are in military service or a program of study sponsored by the Armed Forces (including ROTC and the service academies) must obtain a "Letter of Approval to Apply" from their respective services before making application.

SELECTION FACTORS

The school employs a three-stage, progressive screening process for selecting entrants. The first stage consists of the submission of the standard AMCAS application form; the second, the submission of supplementary materials (a premedical committee recommendation and a personal statement describing the applicant's knowledge of and interest in a career in the service are required); and the third, personal interviews, which are conducted at the medical school campus. Advancement in the process is competitive, based on candidates' personal and intellectual characteristics. Applicants should not send transcripts, letters of recommendation, or other such materials unless specifically requested to do so by the Committee on Admissions. The Committee on Admissions does not discriminate on the basis of sex, race, religion, marital status, or national origin.

There were 2,452 applicants for the 1999 first-year class; of this total 499 were interviewed. The 165 entrants had the following credentials: *mean GPA,* 3.53; *mean MCAT,* 10.2; *mean age at time of application,* 23.5 years; *sex,* 26 percent women; *undergraduate major,* 30 percent in biology, with engineering, biochemistry, chemistry, psychology, and economics among others represented; residence, 31 percent from northern states, 26 percent from southern states, 35 percent from western states, 8 percent from central states. USUHS is a federal institution; preference is not given to in-state residents, therefore these statistics are not kept.

SERVICE BENEFITS AND MILITARY OBLIGATION

Upon entering the first-year class of the School of Medicine, the student will be commissioned and will serve on active duty in the grade of second lieutenant in either the Army or Air Force or ensign in the Navy, receiving the appropriate pay and benefits of that grade. All incoming students will be affected by the new military retirement system if not in the military prior to August 1, 1986. The time spent in medical school is not creditable toward retirement until retirement eligibility has been established.

If current promotion policies continue, the student can expect a promotion in rank to captain in the Air Force or Army or lieutenant in the Navy upon receipt of the M.D. degree. Graduates are obligated to serve on active duty as medical officers for not less than seven years as well as six years inactive ready reserve. The period of time spent in internship or residency training shall not be acceptable toward satisfying this seven-year obligation. A student who is dropped from the program for either academic deficiencies or other reasons may be required to perform active duty in an appropriate military capacity for a period equal to the time spent in the program. A disenrolled student may also be required to reimburse the government for tuition and fees. However, one year will be the minimum required active duty for persons separated from the school regardless of the time spent in the program.

INFORMATION FOR MINORITY STUDENTS

The Uniformed Services School of Medicine has an Office of Minority Affairs. The program is designed to encourage competitive minority applicants to apply. The Vice President and staff offer assistance prior to, and throughout, the application and admission processes. The application and admissions processes are the same for all students.

The Vice President and staff additionally offer encouragement and assist in offering a strong support network to minority and all students for successful matriculation. Support is also available through the Mentor Program, Women in Medicine and Science, and Student National Medical Association.

Public Institution

APPLICATION AND ACCEPTANCE POLICIES FOR 2001–2002 FIRST-YEAR CLASS

School participates in AMCAS. See Chapter 6.

Filing of AMCAS application
  Earliest date: June 1, 2000
  Latest date: Nov. 1, 2000
School application fee: None
Oldest MCAT scores considered: 1998
Does not have Early Decision Program
Acceptance notice to regular applicants
  Earliest date: Oct. 15, 2000
  Latest date: Until class is filled
Applicant's response to acceptance offer
  Maximum time: 2 weeks
Requests for deferred entrance considered: Yes
Deposit to hold place in class: None
Estimated number of new entrants: 165
Starting date: June 2001

TUITION AND STUDENT FEES PER YEAR FOR 1999–2000 FIRST-YEAR CLASS

There are no tuition or fees for attending the USUHS. Required books, equipment, and instruments are furnished without charge. Students are required to pay for housing, food, and other expenses from their annual salary, which is equivalent to the salary of a second lieutenant in the Army or Air Force, or an ensign in the Navy.

INFORMATION ON 1999–2000 FIRST-YEAR CLASS

Number of	*Total*
Applicants	2,452
Applicants Interviewed	499
New Entrants*	165

*All took the MCAT and had baccalaureate degrees.

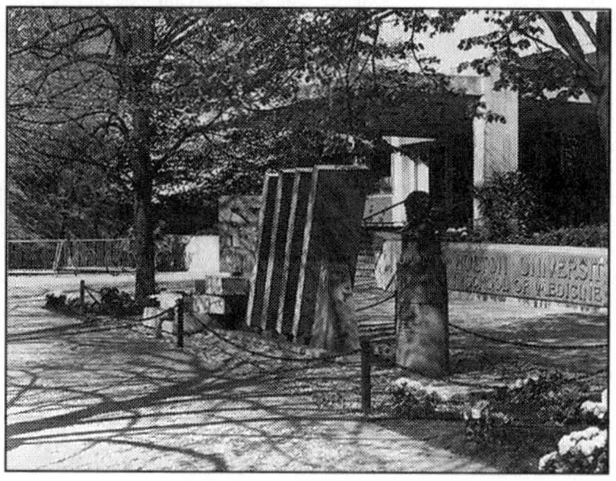

Boston University School of Medicine

Boston, Massachusetts

Dr. Aram V. Chobanian, *Dean*
Dr. John F. O'Connor, *Associate Dean for Admissions*
Charles Terrell, *Associate Dean for Financial Management*

ADDRESS INQUIRIES TO:

Admissions Office
Building L, Room 124
Boston University
School of Medicine
715 Albany Street
Boston, Massachusetts 02118
(617) 638-4630

GENERAL INFORMATION

In 1848 the New England Female Medical College was founded as the first medical college for women in the world. In 1873 the original buildings and endowment were acquired by Boston University, and the name was changed to Boston University School of Medicine. At present the School of Medicine, School of Dental Medicine, School of Public Health, Centers for Advancement in Health and Medicine, and University Hospital constitute the Boston Medical Center. All professional medical activities at Boston Medical Center are vested in the School of Medicine, and that hospital, together with 21 other health care facilities affiliated with the Medical Center, affords students varied and rich clinical experiences.

CURRICULUM

The curriculum provides the opportunity to study medicine in a flexible environment that stimulates a spirit of critical inquiry and provides sound knowledge in the biological, social, and behavioral sciences. In 1992, Integrated Problems, a course using problem-based learning, was added and the courses in introduction to clinical medicine reinforced. These courses link the discipline-specific work in basic sciences with applications in clinical medicine. They integrate longitudinally through the first two years.

During the first year, the basic medical sciences are emphasized in both departmental and interdisciplinary courses along with human development and community medicine.

The second-year program emphasizes the changes in normal structure and function that lead to disease. Major systems pathophysiology is presented in an integrated multidisciplinary format.

The third year represents the major clerkship year. In addition to the conventional clerkships in medicine, surgery, pediatrics, obstetrics, and psychiatry, a clerkship in out-patient primary care is required in either the third or fourth year.

The new curriculum includes four mandatory clerkships for the fourth year: neurology, radiology, ambulatory primary care, and home medicine. The fourth year is otherwise devoted to developing an elective program under the supervision of a faculty member. Research opportunities are available in basic science and clinical settings in an independent study program.

A dynamic generalist curriculum in the primary care disciplines of internal medicine, family practice, and pediatrics is presented throughout the four years. Faculty in nearby urban and suburban practices serve as mentors and teachers. Primary care medicine is taught in these physician's office practices, in community health centers, patients' homes, day care centers, and shelters. Experience in rural practice (in the United States and abroad) is available as electives in the fourth year.

With the approval of the promotions committee, students may complete the first-year requirements over two academic years by taking half the normal course load each year without paying any additional tuition.

In addition to the traditional M.D. degree, students may also pursue a pathway of study leading to the M.D.-Ph.D. or M.D.-M.P.H.

REQUIREMENTS FOR ENTRANCE

Applicants are required to have a baccalaureate degree from an approved college of arts and sciences. The following courses are required:

	Years
Biology (with lab)	1
Inorganic chemistry (with lab)	1
Organic chemistry (with lab)	1
Physics	1
Humanities	1
English composition or literature	1

A knowledge of a quantitation in chemistry and calculus is recommended.

Applicants are urged to acquire a broad background in the humanities and behavioral and social sciences in their college years.

All required courses must be completed before medical school work begins. If an applicant has been excused from a required college-level course, another course at the same or higher level must be substituted.

The MCAT is required. Applicants are strongly urged to take the MCAT in the spring of the year of application and to have most of their basic science requirements completed at the time of application. Applicants who have not taken the MCAT by the fall of the application year will not be considered.

SELECTION FACTORS

The Committee on Admissions chooses applicants who seem best qualified not only by scholastic record, college recommendations, and involvement in college and community activities but also by qualities of personality, character, and maturity. A personal interview is an integral part of the admissions process. Applicants who have not heard from the School of Medicine by March 1 and still wish to be considered for an interview should contact the Admissions Office. All interviews are granted at the discretion of the Committee on Admissions. The School of Medicine does not discriminate on the basis of race, sex, age, creed, or national origin.

No deferments are permitted.

If places are available, applications for transfer may be requested in January.

FINANCIAL AID

The school is committed to equal financial access for all students demonstrating need. Therefore it initiated a series of low-interest student revolving loan funds in 1975. Since that time it has tried to mitigate the cycle of mounting market-rate debt.

Student assistance is available to students in all years of the medical school curriculum; 52 percent of the student body receive institutional assistance; 90 percent receive institutional and/or outside support assistance. The school's Office of Student Financial Management administers its portfolio of 50 revolving loans, assists students in securing aid from outside sources, conducts debt management seminars and activities, conducts all required entrance and exit interviews, and provides daily student financial management information. A new series of funds, the Primary Care Pool, have been introduced to promote primary care; students are eligible if they demonstrate need and express interest. Grant aid is minimal, equaling 5 percent of student aid in full-need cases. Most assistance is based upon need. Upon acceptance, students are automatically sent a student assistance response card which generates all necessary forms and information. Financial need is not considered in the admissions process.

There are no special institutional financial funds disbursed for international students. Unless a student has an I-551 or I-151 resident alien card, federally insured loans are not available.

INFORMATION FOR MINORITY STUDENTS

Programs for the recruitment and support of minority students have been developed through the Office of Minority Affairs. One of these programs allows students to take special summer courses in anatomy, biochemistry, and knowledge acquisition skills prior to matriculation in the fall. Minority applications are processed through the regular Committee on Admissions in consultation with the Office of Minority Affairs. It is possible to have application fees defrayed.

Private Institution

APPLICATION AND ACCEPTANCE POLICIES FOR 2001–2002 FIRST-YEAR CLASS

School participates in AMCAS. See Chapter 6.

Filing of AMCAS application
Earliest date: June 1, 2000
Latest date: Nov. 15, 2000
School application fee to all applicants: $95
Oldest MCAT scores considered: 1998
Does have Early Decision Program (EDP)
EDP application period: June 1–Aug. 1, 2000
EDP applicants notified by: Oct. 1, 2000
Acceptance notice to regular applicants
Earliest date: Feb. 15, 2001
Latest date: Until class is filled
Applicant's response to acceptance offer
Maximum time: 2 weeks
Requests for deferred entrance considered: No
Deposit to hold place in class (applied to tuition): $500, due June 15, 2001; nonrefundable
Estimated number of new entrants: 150 (3 EDP)
Starting date: Aug. 2001

TUITION AND STUDENT FEES PER YEAR FOR 1999–2000 FIRST-YEAR CLASS

Tuition: $35,525 Student fees: $450

INFORMATION ON 1999–2000 FIRST-YEAR CLASS

Number of	*In-State*	*Out-of-State*	*Total*
Applicants	674	9,225	9,899
Applicants Interviewed	223	800	1,023
New Entrants*	38	112	150

*All took the MCAT; 89% had baccalaureate degrees.

CHAPTER 11

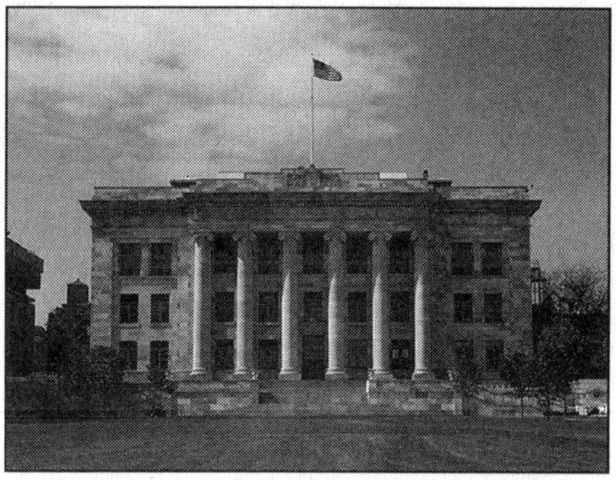

Harvard Medical School

Boston, Massachusetts

Dr. Joseph B. Martin, *Dean*
Dr. Jules L. Dienstag, *Faculty Associate Dean for Admissions; Chair, Committee on Admissions*
Theresa J. Orr, *Associate Dean for Admissions and Student Services*

ADDRESS INQUIRIES TO:

Admissions Office
Harvard Medical School
25 Shattuck Street
Boston, Massachusetts 02115-6092
(617) 432-1550; 432-3307 (FAX)
E-mail: admissions_office@hms.harvard.edu
Web Site: http://www.hms.harvard.edu

MISSION STATEMENT

Harvard Medical School is dedicated to preparing for the medicine of tomorrow. This involves taking care of patients to the best of medicine's abilities, conducting research in the sciences basic to medicine, and educating new physicians and scientists.

GENERAL INFORMATION

Harvard Medical School was established in 1782. It has occupied its present site in the Longwood Avenue Quadrangle since 1906. Adjacent are the Harvard School of Public Health, the Harvard School of Dental Medicine, and the Francis A. Countway Library. Clinical teaching is carried out in several general and specialized hospitals. These include Massachusetts General, Brigham and Women's, Children's, Beth Israel Deaconess Medical Center, Massachusetts Eye and Ear, Mount Auburn, and Cambridge hospitals. The Massachusetts Mental Health Center and the McLean Hospital are psychiatric facilities. Harvard Vanguard Medical Associates and other community-based health centers provide additional opportunities for patient care, teaching, and research. Other affiliated institutions include the West Roxbury and Brockton VA Medical Centers, the Shriners Burns Institute, and the Spaulding Rehabilitation Hospital. Vanderbilt Hall provides living facilities for single students. Apartments for married students may be found nearby.

PROGRAMS

The New Pathway Program is designed to accommodate the variety of interests, educational backgrounds, and career goals that characterize the student body. Basic science and clinical content are interwoven throughout the four years. In the first and second years, a problem-based approach that emphasizes small-group tutorials and self-directed learning is complemented by laboratories, conferences, and lectures. Students are expected to analyze problems, locate relevant material in library and computer-based resources, and develop habits of lifelong learning and independent study. Clinical clerkships and a wide variety of elective courses and research opportunities are available at Harvard Medical School, its affiliated hospitals, Harvard University, and the Massachusetts Institute of Technology (M.I.T.). One hundred thirty-five students are admitted to this program each year.

A second M.D. Pathway is the Harvard–M.I.T. Division of Health Sciences and Technology Program (HST). This program was established jointly by the faculties of these two institutions. The curriculum of this program is designed for the student with a strong interest and background in quantitative science. Courses in the first two years are taught both at Harvard Medical School and M.I.T. with faculty drawn from both institutions. The curriculum is in a semester format. HST students join students of the New Pathway Program for their clinical rotations. A thesis is required for graduation. Thirty students are admitted to this program each year.

The M.D.-Ph.D. Program exists for qualified applicants who wish to integrate medical school and intensive scientific training. Graduate study and research for the Ph.D. are pursued through one of the basic science departments or committees of the Division of Medical Sciences, other departments of the Harvard Graduate School of Arts and Sciences, or the Graduate Schools of Science and Engineering at M.I.T.

Other joint programs are offered in collaboration with the Harvard School of Public Health and the John Fitzgerald Kennedy School of Government.

ACADEMIC SOCIETIES

All students are assigned to one of five academic societies. The societies offer the perspective of smaller groupings of students and faculty who will work together during their time at Harvard Medical School. Each society has a home base in the Tosteson Medical Education Center—a state-of-the-art teaching facility.

REQUIREMENTS FOR ENTRANCE

The MCAT, at least three years of college, and a baccalaureate degree are required.

Biology—One year with laboratory experience. Courses taken should deal with the cellular and molecular aspects as well as the structure and function of living organisms.

Chemistry—Two years with laboratory experience. Full-year courses in general (inorganic) and organic chemistry meet this requirement. Other options that adequately prepare students for the study of biochemistry and molecular biology in medical school will be acceptable.
Physics—One year.
Mathematics—One year of calculus.
Expository writing—One year. May be met with writing, English, or nonscience courses that involve expository writing.
HST Program—Requirements are the same as above except that calculus through differential equations and calculus-based physics are required. A course in biochemistry is encouraged.

A variety of course formats and combinations that provide equivalent preparation will be accepted. Advanced placement credits may be used to satisfy the calculus requirement and one semester of the chemistry and physics requirements for the New Pathway program. In addition to the writing requirement, at least 16 credit hours should be completed in nonscience courses. No preference is shown toward students majoring in the sciences over students majoring in nonscience areas.

Applicants educated abroad must have completed at least one year of study in an approved college or university in the United States or Canada before applying. Foreign students who do not have a baccalaureate or advanced degree from an institution in the United States or Canada are rarely accepted for admission.

Students who have been enrolled in medical school, or who have been refused admission by us on two prior occasions are ineligible to apply.

SELECTION FACTORS

Academic excellence is expected. For the 1999 entering class, the *average GPA* was 3.8, with a range that was broader and the *average MCAT scores* were VR-10.5, PS-11.7, and BS-11.8, with a range that was in keeping with the national average. Other factors considered include the essay, out-of-classroom activities, and life experiences. Research and community work and comments contained in letters of recommendation are considered. We look for evidence of integrity, maturity, humanitarian concerns, leadership potential, and an aptitude for working with people. Interviews are scheduled selectively and are conducted on campus. Please note that secondary applications are automatically mailed to all applicants, and early application is strongly encouraged.

The Committee on Admissions welcomes applications from qualified students representing groups that historically have been underrepresented in medicine. Harvard Medical School is committed to the enrollment of a diverse body of talented students who will reflect the character of the American people whose health needs the medical profession must serve. Harvard Medical School does not discriminate on the basis of race, color, religion, sex, sexual preference, age, or handicap.

The 1999 entering class came from 54 different colleges. Forty-five percent were women and 18 percent were minorities.

Harvard Medical School does not invite applications for advanced standing because opportunities for transfer are rarely available and are limited to entry into the third-year class. Those eligible to apply are only those students who are spouses of current Harvard medical students, house officers, or faculty, and acceptance occurs infrequently.

FINANCIAL AID

All financial aid is awarded on the basis of need. A vigorous effort is made to assist accepted applicants in meeting their medical education costs through loans, medically related employment, and scholarships.

Foreign students who are not U.S. permanent residents are eligible to be considered for need-based institutional scholarships and loans; however, because such students are ineligible for federal financial aid programs, the Financial Aid Office is not able to offer them the same level of financial assistance that is available to other students. Approximately 70 percent of the student body receive financial aid.

For further information, contact the Financial Aid Office at (617) 432-1575.

Private Institution

APPLICATION AND ACCEPTANCE POLICIES FOR 2001–2002 FIRST-YEAR CLASS

School participates in AMCAS. See Chapter 6.

Filing of AMCAS application
  Earliest date: June 1, 2000
  Latest date: Oct. 15, 2000
School application fee to all applicants: $75
Oldest MCAT scores considered: 1995
Does not have Early Decision Program
Acceptance notice to regular applicants
  Earliest date: Feb. 28, 2001
  Latest date: Feb. 28, 2001
Applicant's response to acceptance offer
  Maximum time: 3 weeks
Requests for deferred entrance considered: Yes
Deposit to hold place in class: None
Estimated number of new entrants: 165
Starting date: Sept. 2001

TUITION AND STUDENT FEES PER YEAR FOR 1999–2000 FIRST-YEAR CLASS

Tuition: $27,000 Student fees: $1,676

INFORMATION ON 2000–2000 FIRST-YEAR CLASS

Number of	*In-State*	*Out-of-State*	*Total*
Applicants	439	5,578	6,017
Applicants Interviewed	92	952	1,044
New Entrants*	21	144	165

*All took the MCAT and had baccalaureate degrees.

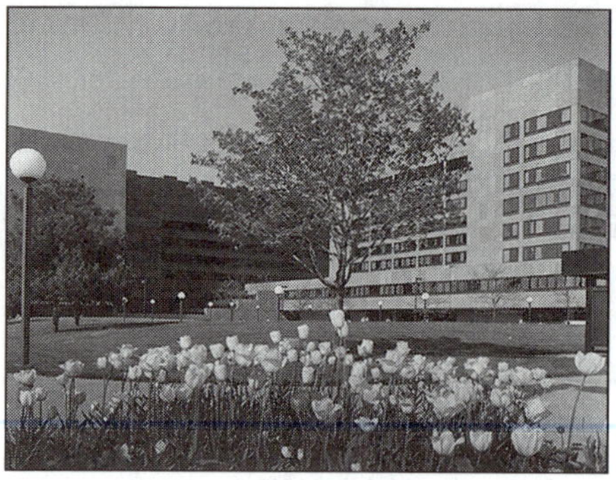

University of Massachusetts Medical School

Worcester, Massachusetts

Dr. Aaron Lazare, *Chancellor/Dean*
Dr. John Paraskos, *Associate Dean for Admissions*
Judith L. Case, *Director of Financial Aid*

ADDRESS INQUIRIES TO:

Associate Dean for Admissions
University of Massachusetts Medical School
55 Lake Avenue, North
Worcester, Massachusetts 01655
(508) 856-2323
E-mail: anne.parlante@umassmed.edu
Web Site: http://www.umassmed.edu/education/admit.cfm

GENERAL INFORMATION

Established in 1962, the University of Massachusetts Medical School accepted its first class in 1970. The school's founding mission was to provide high-quality and accessible medical education for the residents of Massachusetts. The University of Massachusetts Medical School is committed to training physicians in a wide range of medical disciplines and also emphasizes training for practice in general medicine and the primary care specialties, in the public sector and in underserved areas of Massachusetts. This mission has since been expanded to include graduate education in the biomedical sciences and nursing, graduate medical education, and continuing medical education for health professionals. The school's clinical partner is UMass Memorial Medical Center, which comprises two acute care hospitals with a total of 761 beds. Clinical education is also conducted at a number of affiliated community hospitals and health centers in the region. UMass Worcester is adjacent to the Massachusetts Biotechnology Research Park, which houses a number of UMass research programs including the Program in Molecular Medicine, the Cancer Center, and the Worcester Foundation for Biomedical Research.

CURRICULUM

The educational program stresses interdisciplinary learning and integration of the basic and clinical sciences, with special attention to clinical correlation of subject matter in the preclinical years. Emphasis in the first year is on normal structure and function, with a balance of small-group learning and large-group teaching. Through a longitudinal preceptorship program, students are provided with patient involvement beginning immediately in year one and continuing throughout the first two years. Emphasis in the second year is on the etiology of disease, pathophysiology, pharmacology, and clinical diagnosis. The two-year course on the Patient, Physician, and Society (PPS) runs throughout the preclinical program and integrates the basic sciences into medical interviewing, clinical problem solving, biomedical ethics, preventive medicine, epidemiology, and medical informatics. Led by a diversity of senior faculty, students in the PPS course learn through an interdisciplinary model and work in small groups to experience a collaborative team approach to patient care and case-based clinical problem solving.

The third and fourth years are a continuum of required clerkships and both clinical and research electives. Elements of the PPS course are revisited in the clinical years through one-week interclerkship courses, which address a broad range of important issues using an interdisciplinary approach, which combines the clinical and basic sciences. Interclerkships have addressed diverse subjects including domestic violence, environmental medicine, managed care, nutrition, and substance abuse. An International Health Program is also available for students interested in clinical and/or research experience abroad and in underserved areas of the United States. Over one-third of UMass students benefit from an international health experience. The program coordinates and oversees the placement of students in electives worldwide, and provides a learning opportunity in which students experience and understand different cultures while serving those populations most in need.

The faculty of the Medical School also encourages medical students to participate in research programs in basic and clinical science departments. A combined M.D.-Ph.D. program in basic medical sciences is also offered.

REQUIREMENTS FOR ENTRANCE

The MCAT is required and must be taken within the last three years. A baccalaureate degree is required. Required courses that must be taken within the last four years are:

	Years
Biology (with lab)	1
Inorganic chemistry (with lab)	1
Organic chemistry (with lab)	1
Physics (with lab)	1
English	1

Credit for any secondary school course may be given only if such credit appears on the college transcript. Applicants may major in the areas of either sciences or humanities, and in either case independent study is encouraged. Students able to do so are encouraged to take such courses as biochemistry, calculus, statistics, sociology, or psychology. Applicants are encouraged to complete the basic science requirements by the time of application since consideration will be delayed if required courses are in progress.

SELECTION FACTORS

Current policy limits admission to students who are Massachusetts residents. The Committee on Admissions bases its evaluation of applicants on academic ability and achievement, scores on the MCAT, and such factors as extracurricular achievement, maturity, motivation, and character as these are reflected in letters of recommendation from preprofessional advisory committees and other persons. Interviews are arranged by invitation only. Applicants are selected on the basis of their individual merits without regard to race, sex, creed, national origin, age, or disability. UMass has a set of technical standards for admission and promotion, which are available upon request. All supplementary materials must be received by December 15.

Accepted students for the class entering August 1999 had the following credentials: *science GPA,* approximately 3.6; *sex,* 55 percent women; *undergraduate major,* 60 percent in science and 40 percent in nonscience.

FINANCIAL AID

Students unable to finance their medical education should consider applying for financial aid. The Financial Aid Office sends appropriate materials and establishes individual financial aid application deadlines when applicants are accepted or placed on the alternate list. Applicants for only Federal Stafford Loans need not supply parental information on the FAFSA. Applicants for campus-based funds are required to provide complete parental financial information and signatures on both the FAFSA and the CSS Profile Form.

The financial aid application comprises the UMass Medical School Financial Aid Application, the FAFSA, the Profile Form of the College Scholarship Service, parental and student federal income tax returns and W-2 forms, and financial aid transcripts from all educational institutions previously attended.

Financial aid funds are disbursed according to institutional packaging policy established by the Student Affairs Committee. Approximately 97 percent of the student body receive some combination of scholarships, loans, and/or employment. UMass Medical School offers all students, regardless of financial need, the option of entering into a learning contract that gives students the choice of paying full tuition or deferring a portion (currently two-thirds) of tuition until after residency training. Graduates must begin payment with either money or service no later than six months after completing residency or fellowship training. Service to the Commonwealth may be provided by practicing primary care medicine anywhere in the state, practicing medical specialties in underserved areas in the state, or completing an approved activity of particular benefit to the Commonwealth. Students not able to provide service will be charged eight percent interest; interest begins accruing after completion of the medical internship. Payment may not exceed eight years.

INFORMATION FOR DISADVANTAGED STUDENTS

Please contact the associate vice chancellor of school services for additional information on programs for disadvantaged students.

Public Institution

APPLICATION AND ACCEPTANCE POLICIES FOR 2001–2002 FIRST-YEAR CLASS

School participates in AMCAS. See Chapter 6.

Filing of AMCAS application
Earliest date: June 1, 2000
Latest date: Nov. 1, 2000
School application fee to all applicants: $75
Oldest MCAT scores considered: 1998
Does have Early Decision Program (EDP)
For Massachusetts residents only
EDP application period: June 1–Aug. 1, 2000
EDP applicants notified by: Oct. 1, 2000
Acceptance notice to regular applicants
Earliest date: Oct. 15, 2000
Latest date: Varies
Applicant's response to acceptance offer
Maximum time: 2 weeks
Requests for deferred entrance considered: Yes
Deposit to hold place in class (applied to tuition): $100, due with response to acceptance offer
Deposit refundable prior to: May 15, 2001
Estimated number of new entrants: 100 (10 EDP)
Starting date: Aug. 2001

TUITION AND STUDENT FEES PER YEAR FOR 1999–2000 FIRST-YEAR CLASS

Tuition
Resident: $8,352
Nonresident: N/A

Student fees: $1,995

INFORMATION ON 1999–2000 FIRST-YEAR CLASS

Number of	*In-State*	*Out-of-State*	*Total*
Applicants	826	0	826
Applicants Interviewed	451	0	451
New Entrants*	100	0	100

*All took the MCAT and had baccalaureate degrees.

CHAPTER 11

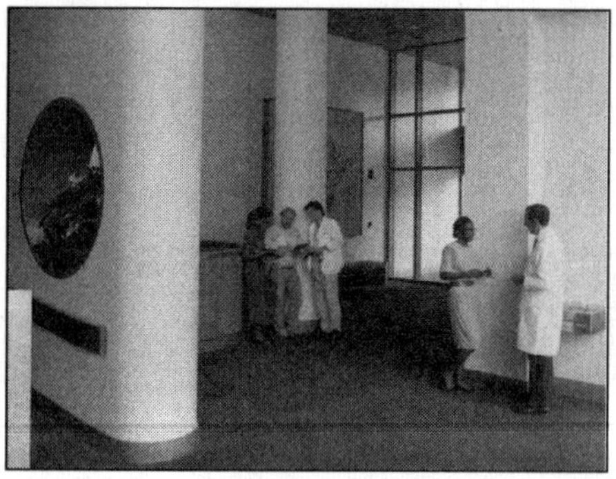

Tufts University School of Medicine

Boston, Massachusetts

Dr. John Harrington, *Dean*
Dr. Robert C. Sarno, *Dean for Admissions*
Thomas M. Slavin, *Director of Admissions*

ADDRESS INQUIRIES TO:

Office of Admissions
Tufts University
School of Medicine
136 Harrison Avenue
Boston, Massachusetts 02111
(617) 636-6571
Web Site: http://www.tufts.edu/med

GENERAL INFORMATION

Tufts University was founded in 1852 as a liberal arts college in Medford, Massachusetts, and has since grown into a modern university whose School of Medicine was established in Boston in 1893. The medical school is located within a health sciences complex, which includes the dental school, veterinary school, Sackler School of Graduate Biomedical Sciences, Sackler Center for Health Communications, Nutrition Center, and the New England Medical Center. The medical school buildings, located in the center of Boston, house the preclinical departments, research laboratories, administrative offices, seminar rooms, lecture rooms, and the library. Close association of the School of Medicine with 30-plus hospitals affords ample facilities for clinical experience.

CURRICULUM

The initial phase of the curriculum focuses on the biology of cells and their constituent molecules followed by a segment dealing with the structure and development of tissues and organs. This is followed by the functions of the organs and the organism and its environment. The biology of normal cells, tissues, and organs is presented before the students are exposed to the pathological manifestations of these components. The curriculum also includes those aspects of the nonbiological sciences that are relevant to health care delivery and patient care, such as nutrition, health care economics, family medicine, ethics, and history of medicine. The program also emphasizes problem solving and critical, analytical discussion in small groups instead of rote learning based on a large number of lectures. A strong emphasis on the use of problem-based learning, a teaching based on case studies, is an aspect of the curriculum. The cases chosen have been closely coordinated with the material from the ongoing segments of the curriculum but provide opportunities for student learning in a wide range of areas, including ethics, socioeconomics, history, culture, and the physician-patient relationship. The Preclinical Elective Program is designed to encourage students to pursue outside interests and talents as well as to foster meaningful faculty-student relationships. Students can explore opportunities in basic science, clinical medicine, or community aspects of medicine. In addition, faculty are able to work more closely with students and to serve as role models, mentors, and informal advisors.

The third year consists of rotations through the major clinical specialties and an elective period.

The fourth year consists of a minimum of eight four-week rotations. Five of these eight must be taken at Tufts-affiliated hospitals; of these, two must be ward service rotations and one must be the clinical specialties rotation. Beyond these requirements, students are free to schedule approved learning experiences as part of their elective rotations at the Tufts-associated hospitals or elsewhere in the United States or abroad.

Tufts offers a combined M.D.-M.P.H. program, leading to the awarding of both degrees in four years. The program is fully accredited by the Council on Education for Public Health and provides basic grounding in epidemiology and biostatistics, health planning and management, environmental health, and the behavioral sciences. A public health field experience and advanced course work are essential parts of the program, which is fully integrated into the medical curriculum.

Tufts, in collaboration with Northeastern and Brandeis Universities, now offers a combined M.D.-M.B.A. degree in health management. The changing nature of the nation's health care system has created a demand for physicians who are trained to plan and manage these changes in the best interests of patients, health care organizations, and the community. The curriculum is designed to provide students with a foundation in business problem-solving skills and knowledge in health care management. M.D.-M.B.A. candidates will begin their studies the summer before the start of medical school and devote the summer between the first and second years of medical school to M.B.A. courses.

Tufts also offers an M.D.-Ph.D. program.

REQUIREMENTS FOR ENTRANCE

The MCAT and a minimum of three years of college are required. College credits must include:

	Years
Biology (with lab)	1
Inorganic chemistry (with lab)	1
Organic chemistry (with lab)	1
Physics (with lab)	1

SELECTION FACTORS

The selection of candidates for admission to the first year is based not only on performance in the required premedical courses, but also on the applicant's entire academic record and extracurricular experiences. Letters of recommendation and additional information supplied by the applicant are reviewed for indications of promise and fitness for a medical career. Personal interviews are a prerequisite for admission and are granted only by invitation of the Admissions Committee.

Tufts has a strong commitment to affirmative action and seeks to provide an atmosphere of nondiscrimination for members of minority groups as well as an accessible campus and support services for persons with disabilities.

Tufts accepts transfers from other American, LCME-accredited medical schools into the second- and third-year classes in years when vacancies have been created by attrition. The number of seats available has traditionally been extremely limited. In some years, no transfer openings are available. Preference is given to American citizens and permanent residents who will receive a bachelor's degree from an American college or university prior to matriculation.

FINANCIAL AID

Up to 75 percent of students participate in the federal government's student loan programs at some time during their four years of study. Additionally, limited scholarship and loan assistance is available directly from Tufts for students who qualify on the basis of need. Approximately 33 percent of the students receive financial aid directly from Tufts at some time during their four years of study.

There are no rules prohibiting outside employment; however, first- and second-year students are urged not to seek outside work. Some opportunities for part-time employment are available in the various hospitals and in the medical school.

In situations of extreme financial need, the $95 application fee may be waived if AMCAS has first granted a similar waiver.

Private Institution

APPLICATION AND ACCEPTANCE POLICIES FOR 2001–2002 FIRST-YEAR CLASS

School participates in AMCAS. See Chapter 6.

Filing of AMCAS application
  Earliest date: June 1, 2000
  Latest date: Nov. 1, 2000
School application fee to all applicants: $95
Oldest MCAT scores considered: 1997
Does have Early Decision Program (EDP)
  EDP application period: June 1–Aug. 1, 2000
  EDP applicants notified by: Oct. 1, 2000
Acceptance notice to regular applicants
  Earliest date: Nov. 15, 2000
  Latest date: Until class is filled
Applicant's response to acceptance offer
  Maximum time: 2 weeks
Requests for deferred entrance considered: Yes
Deposit to hold place in class (applied to tuition):
  $100, due with response to acceptance offer
Deposit refundable prior to: May 15, 2001
Estimated number of new entrants: 168 (3 EDP)
Starting date: Aug. 2001

TUITION AND STUDENT FEES PER YEAR FOR 1999–2000 FIRST-YEAR CLASS

Tuition: $34,180   Student fees: $480

INFORMATION ON 1999–2000 FIRST-YEAR CLASS

Number of	*In-State*	*Out-of-State*	*Total*
Applicants	721	8,591	9,312
Applicants Interviewed	196	675	871
New Entrants*	50	118	168

*All took the MCAT and had baccalaureate degrees.

CHAPTER 11

Michigan State University College of Human Medicine

East Lansing, Michigan

Dr. William S. Abbett, *Dean*
Dr. Christine L. Shafer, *Assistant Dean for Admissions*
Dr. Wanda D. Lipscomb, *Director of Prematricular Programs*

ADDRESS INQUIRIES TO:

College of Human Medicine
Office of Admissions
A-239 Life Sciences
Michigan State University
East Lansing, Michigan 48824-1317
(517) 353-9620; 432-0021 (FAX)
E-mail: MDAdmissions@msu.edu
Web Site: http://www.chm.msu.edu/

MISSION STATEMENT

The mission of the College of Human Medicine is to educate and develop exemplary physicians who are responsive to the unmet needs of medically underserved populations in Michigan; considerate of the dignity, diversity, and values of patients; and focused in the practice and delivery of primary health care.

GENERAL INFORMATION

The College of Human Medicine (CHM) was founded in 1964 in response to Michigan's need for primary care physicians. CHM, a four-year medical school located on an active Big 10 campus, provides a small college atmosphere with an entering class of 106. The average student age is 25 (range 22–45) with men and women equally represented. Students spend the first two years at the East Lansing campus where they are taught in the classroom, laboratory, and clinical settings before moving on to one of the six community campuses for clinical training in realistic health care settings. Approximately 2,500 clinical and adjunct faculty join the more than 200 clinical and basic science faculty members in providing this unique learning environment.

CURRICULUM

The curriculum is divided into three blocks organized around a commitment to the integration of the basic biological, behavioral, and social sciences; a developmental approach to learning; early teaching of clinical skills; and clinical training utilizing a community-integrated approach.

Grading is on a modified pass/no pass system. Honors-level performance is recognized with a letter of recognition during the first two years and by a grade of "pass with honors" during the clerkship years.

Block I is a three-semester experience comprising the first year in which fundamental basic science concepts and principles are presented in a structured, discipline-based format. Basic clinical skills teaching begins, along with a mentor group experience and opportunity to participate in independent as well as supplementary learning experiences. A clinical correlations course integrates basic science information, connects these sciences to medicine, and models a team approach to the practice of medicine.

Block II is a 2½-semester experience comprising the second year in which advanced basic science concepts are organized in an integrated, problem-based format. Emphasis is on small-group instruction and problem solving. A clinical context for learning basic science concepts is also provided. Clinical skills training continues along with special topics seminars, which deal with contemporary issues in society and medicine.

Block III includes 60 weeks of required and 20 weeks of elective clerkships. Students live in Flint, Grand Rapids, Kalamazoo, Lansing, Saginaw, or the Upper Peninsula during their required clerkships. Their experiences are in a variety of hospital and ambulatory care settings. The required clerkships include a family practice/primary care clerkship with exposure to the comprehensive and continuous care of patients and families. Students have the option to complete elective clerkships in other locations including third world countries.

REQUIREMENTS FOR ENTRANCE

The MCAT and a baccalaureate degree from an accredited college or university are required. Thirteen percent of the 1999 entering class hold graduate or professional degrees.

Applicants should select the academic major that best links their interests and talents since no specific major is preferred over another. A solid background in the arts, humanities, and social sciences is recommended.

Specific course requirements with no grade less than a 2.0 are:

	Sem./Qtr. hrs.
General Biology Sequence (one lab)	8/12
General Chemistry Sequence (one lab)	8/12
Organic Chemistry Sequence (one lab)	8/12
General Physics Sequence (one lab)	8/12
English Writing (Writing in the Major)	8/12
Humanities/Social Science	8/12

Mathematics through college algebra or statistics and probability (waived with AP credit for Calculus 1, or freshman mathematics placement above college algebra) is required.

Completion of one upper-level (junior- or senior-level) biological science course from the following: biochemistry, cell biology, embryology, genetics, microbiology, molecular biology, neuroscience, or physiology, is also required.

SELECTION FACTORS

All application materials are reviewed prior to an initial decision. Approximately 900 applicants will be invited to complete the secondary application. Because MSU/CHM is a state school, approximately 80 percent of the entering class will be Michigan residents.

The college seeks to admit a class that is academically competent, reflective of both the rural and urban character of Michigan, and representative of a wide spectrum of personalities, backgrounds, and talents. Students who have the desire and aptitude to become physicians but who have experienced unequal educational opportunities because of social, cultural, or racial reasons are encouraged to apply.

From the over 3,000 applicants reviewed by the Committee on Admissions, approximately 400 applicants will be invited to Interview Day at the East Lansing campus for interviews with faculty and medical students. Selection is based on many factors, including the GPA, both year to year and cumulative; MCAT scores; fit with the school's mission; relevant community service experience; interviewers' assessments of motivation, ability to communicate, problem-solving ability, maturity, and suitability for the MSU program; state of residence; and potential to contribute to the overall quality of the entering class.

Special Programs include the Rural Physicians Program (RPP), which incorporates the successful Upper Peninsula Program that was established to meet special health care needs of patients in remote, medically underserved rural areas of Michigan through training physicians to provide on-site health care in these areas. Applicants to this program will need to complete additional essays and interviews. The Medical Scholars Program, available to high school seniors, awards a combined B.A./B.S.-M.D. degree. The Advanced Baccalaureate Learning Experience (ABLE) is designed for disadvantaged medical school applicants who have been invited to participate in a 13-month enriched academic experience that will result in regular admission if successfully completed. Opportunity exists for M.D.-Ph.D. programs as well as master's degrees in epidemiology, and ethics and humanities in the life sciences.

FINANCIAL AID

Information about specific scholarships and about financial aid can be obtained from the Office of Financial Aid, 252 Student Services Building. Ability to pay is not considered in the selection process.

INFORMATION FOR MINORITY STUDENTS

Although the College of Human Medicine does not have a separate review for minority applicants, underrepresented minority and other nontraditional students have been very competitive. The 1999 entering class had a minority enrollment of approximately 20 percent, which included African American, Mexican American, mainland Puerto Rican, and American Indian students. The college also offers a postbaccalaureate program, ABLE, for a few selected students. Questions about the prematricular programs and services afforded to minority students should be addressed to the assistant dean for admissions.

Public Institution

APPLICATION AND ACCEPTANCE POLICIES FOR 2001–2002 FIRST-YEAR CLASS

School participates in AMCAS. See Chapter 6.

Filing of AMCAS application
  Earliest date: June 1, 2000
  Latest date: Nov. 15, 2000
School application fee to all applicants: $55
Oldest MCAT scores considered: 1998
Does have Early Decision Program (EDP)
  EDP application period: June 1–Aug. 1, 2000
  EDP applicants notified by: Oct. 1, 2000
Acceptance notice to regular applicants
  Earliest date: Oct. 15, 2000
  Latest date: Varies
Applicant's response to acceptance offer
  Maximum time: 2 weeks
Requests for deferred entrance considered: Yes
Deposit to hold place in class: $55, due with response to acceptance offer
Deposit refundable prior to: May 15, 2001
Estimated number of new entrants: 106 (4 EDP)
Starting date: Aug. 2001

TUITION AND STUDENT FEES PER YEAR FOR 1999–2000 FIRST-YEAR CLASS

Tuition (3 semesters)
  Resident: $15,423
  Nonresident: $33,873

Student fees: $925

INFORMATION ON 1999–2000 FIRST-YEAR CLASS

Number of	*In-State*	*Out-of-State*	*Total*
Applicants	1,036	2,150	3,186
Applicants Interviewed	311	111	422
New Entrants*	81	24	105

*98% had baccalaureate degrees; 92% took the MCAT.

CHAPTER 11

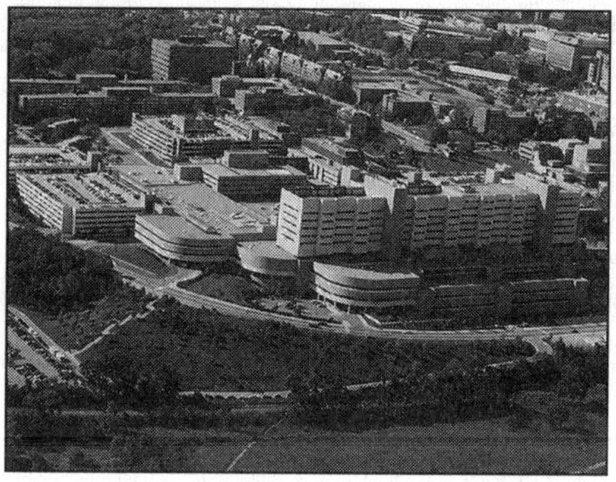

University of Michigan Medical School

Ann Arbor, Michigan

Dr. Allen S. Lichter, *Dean*
Dr. Joyce A. Wahr, *Assistant Dean of Admissions and Financial Aid*

ADDRESS INQUIRIES TO:

Admissions Office
M4130 Medical Science I Building
University of Michigan Medical School
Ann Arbor, Michigan 48109-0611
(734) 764-6317; 763-0453 (FAX)
Web Site: http://www.med.umich.edu/medschool/

MISSION STATEMENT

The University of Michigan Medical School seeks to graduate physicians who are dedicated to life-long learning. Our goals include educating individuals committed to achieving the highest standards of competency required to provide exemplary patient care. We seek to graduate culturally competent physicians who will assume leadership roles in the areas of clinical medicine, research, and teaching. Physicians who graduate from the University of Michigan will demonstrate a strong foundation in biomedical sciences; empathetic interpersonal skills; an ability to identify and reduce health risk factors; an ability to obtain and interpret relevant patient information and to make effective clinical decisions; a commitment to achieving personal and professional excellence; and the critical attributes of compassion, honesty, and integrity.

GENERAL INFORMATION

The University of Michigan Medical School was founded in 1850. This school was the first to establish a university-owned hospital. Today, the medical center occupies more than 30 buildings, the world's largest one-site complex devoted to health care, education, and research. The Health System consistently ranks as one of the top ten in the nation. Instructional sites also include nearby tertiary care hospitals and ambulatory care facilities.

CURRICULUM

The curriculum is designed to provide the integration of basic science and clinical skills necessary for all physicians. In the first year, students receive a strong foundation in the basics of biomedical science, including courses in anatomy, immunology and molecular biology, pharmacology, physiology, embryology, and human genetics. In addition, a course on Introduction to the Patient, which continues throughout year two, familiarizes the student with physical exam and patient history skills. The second-year curriculum is organized into twelve organ system and disease based sequences and is taught by interdisciplinary teams of faculty. Small group activities, pathology lab sessions, case presentations, and panel discussions are typical learning formats. The clinical years provide hands-on training in a wide variety of in- and out-patient settings, but continue didactic teaching in the form of tutorials, small group discussions, and the "Weekly Seminars in Medicine," presentations of clinical issues such as alternative medicine and cultural competency. Students rotate through the required clerkships of family medicine, internal medicine, neurology, OB/GYN, pediatrics, psychiatry, and surgery. In the fourth year, students are assigned to an eight-week subinternship in which they assume major responsibility for a patient caseload. Much of the fourth year is elective time in which the student can select clinical and research experiences of interest to them, including international rotations.

All courses in the first year are graded pass/fail. In the subsequent years, faculty assign students grades of honors, high pass, pass, or fail. Students are required to pass the USMLE, Step I, before promotion to the clinical phase in the third year, and are required to pass USMLE, Step 2, before graduation.

Opportunities exist for individual research summer programs or for special research fellowships. Students also have the option to pursue a combined M.D.–Ph.D. curriculum either as a fellow in the Medical Scientist Training Program or as a graduate student in one of the basic science departments. Another option is a combined M.D.–M.P.H. in one of the graduate programs of the School of Public Health.

Personal and academic counseling, academic enrichment programs, tutorial services, and career counseling are offered through various units of the medical school. A six-week summer prematriculation program, designed to enhance students' academic preparedness for medical school, is also offered.

REQUIREMENTS FOR ENTRANCE

The MCAT and a minimum of 90 semester hours of university work are required. Grades below C in required courses are not acceptable. The specific course requirements are:

	Sem. hrs.
Biology (with lab)	6
General/inorganic and organic chemistry (with lab)	8
Biochemistry	3
Physics (with lab)	6

English composition and literature 6
Nonscience/humanities 18

SELECTION FACTORS

The Admissions Committee is dedicated to matriculating those individuals with the skills, intelligence, and personal attributes to become leaders in medicine. Although admitted students all have demonstrated the ability to succeed academically, other attributes such as compassion, empathy, altruism, honesty, and interpersonal skills are viewed as being critical to future excellence. The Committee considers that all information pertaining to the ability, personality, and character of the applicant is relevant. Although a solid background in science is required, students with expertise in a wide variety of fields, including humanities, arts, and engineering, are encouraged to apply.

All applicants are requested to fill out a Supplemental Information form, but only about 25 percent of applicants are asked to complete the application by submitting letters of reference. The mean undergraduate GPA for admitted students has been about 3.6 for each of the past five years. Reports from college faculty, especially those who know the student best and have experience with pre-med students, are important. While only three years of undergraduate work are required, nearly all admitted students will have completed baccalaureate and more advanced degrees.

Interviews are offered to applicants based on review of submitted information and supporting documents. The interview is usually held in Ann Arbor. Applicants must have had at least one year, and preferably more, of their premedical training in the United States or Canada. International students must have a permanent resident visa in the United States. Any applicant who has been enrolled previously in a medical school in a program leading to the M.D. degree must be in good standing and eligible for re-entry to that school in order to be considered for admission to the University of Michigan Medical School. The Medical School cannot accept transfer students from other medical schools or health care programs.

FINANCIAL AID

Application for financial aid may be initiated following acceptance to the Medical School. Loan funds and some scholarships are available to assist registered students with tuition expense and a share of their living expenses. It is the goal of the Financial Aid Committee that no students should be required to interrupt their education solely for financial reasons.

INFORMATION FOR MINORITY STUDENTS

The University of Michigan is committed to training a diverse cohort of physicians who are capable of caring for an increasingly diverse patient population. The university is one of the top ten U.S. medical schools in the number of minority physicians trained. An Opportunity Award Program provides a degree of financial support for economically disadvantaged students.

Medical students of color are very active in organizations such as LANAMA (Latino/a American/Native American/ Medical Association) and BMA (Black Medical Association). We have a minority alumni group that is very supportive and involved in the lives of our minority students. Minority students are also actively involved in setting the agenda for diversity and cultural competency programs, and participate in the Health System's Multi-cultural Community Health Alliance. Minority students coming for interviews are usually hosted by current minority medical students.

Public Institution

APPLICATION AND ACCEPTANCE POLICIES FOR 2001–2002 FIRST-YEAR CLASS

School participates in AMCAS. See Chapter 6.

Filing of AMCAS application
Earliest date: June 1, 2000
Latest date: Nov. 15, 2000
School application fee to all applicants: $50
Oldest MCAT scores considered: 1997
Does not have Early Decision Program (EDP)
Acceptance notice to regular applicants
Earliest date: Oct. 15, 2000
Latest date: Until class is filled
Applicant's response to acceptance offer
Maximum time: 3 weeks
Requests for deferred entrance considered: Yes
Deposit to hold place in class: None
Estimated number of new entrants: 170
Starting date: Aug. 2001

TUITION AND STUDENT FEES PER YEAR FOR 1999–2000 FIRST-YEAR CLASS

Tuition
Resident: $18,020
Nonresident: $27,776

Student fees: $185

INFORMATION ON 1999–2000 FIRST-YEAR CLASS

Number of	*In-State*	*Out-of-State*	*Total*
Applicants	872	4,177	5,049
Applicants Interviewed	217	408	625
New Entrants*	66	75	141

*All took the MCAT and had baccalaureate degrees.

CHAPTER 11

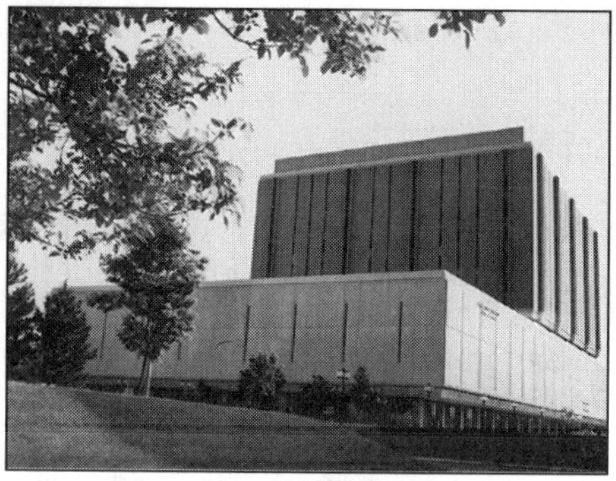

Wayne State University School of Medicine

Detroit, Michigan

Dr. John D. Crissman, *Interim Dean*
Dr. James W. Collins, *Assistant Dean for Admissions*
Kevin J. Culler, M.B.A., *Sr. Associate Director, Financial Aid*

ADDRESS INQUIRIES TO:

Assistant Dean for Admissions
Wayne State University
School of Medicine
540 East Canfield
Detroit, Michigan 48201
(313) 577-1466; 577-1330 (FAX)
Web Site: http://www.med.wayne.edu/

MISSION STATEMENT

The mission of the Wayne State University School of Medicine is to provide the Michigan community with medical and biotechnical resources, in the form of scientific knowledge and trained professionals, so as to improve the overall health of the community.

GENERAL INFORMATION

The School of Medicine, which originated in 1868, is the oldest component of Wayne State University. It is located in the 236-acre Detroit Medical Center. This center is composed of a basic science building (Scott Hall), containing modern teaching facilities for the first two years of medical school; the Shiffman Medical Library; the Lande Medical Research Building; the Elliman Clinical Research Building; C. S. Mott Building; Harper-Grace, Hutzel, and Children's hospitals; Detroit Receiving Hospital and University Health Center (an ambulatory care facility); the Rehabilitation Institute; and the Veterans Administration Hospital. The Detroit Medical Center hospitals are the major clinical teaching and treatment units of the school. In addition, the medical school is affiliated with Sinai, Saint John, William Beaumont, Oakwood, Providence, and Saint Joseph Mercy hospitals.

CURRICULUM

The curriculum is divided into four academic periods that are in sequence 9, 10, 12, and 8 months in duration. The major subjects for these respective periods are normal human biology, evidence-based medicine, public health, pathology, pharmacology, introduction to clinical medicine, clerkships, and medical electives. Year 1 is primarily disciplinary, and Year 2 is initially disciplinary progressing to an organ-systems approach. Year 3 focuses on clinical clerkships. The elective period, senior year, allows students an opportunity to define a major portion of their own academic program within a general structure under the guidance of faculty advisors.

A wide range of opportunities are offered for students to engage in research, basic and clinical, as well as graduate-degree programs (M.S. and Ph.D.) in combination with an M.D. program. Students must pass the USMLE Step 1 to be promoted into Year 3.

REQUIREMENTS FOR ENTRANCE

The MCAT is required in addition to a baccalaureate degree or its equivalent; however, the Committee on Admissions is prepared to review the records of third-year students with unusual academic attainment. The MCAT should be taken during the year of application, preferably in the spring. Required courses for medical school admission are:

	Years
General biology or zoology (with lab)	1
Inorganic chemistry (with lab)	1
Organic chemistry (with lab)	1
General physics (with lab)	1
English	1

Besides a strong preparation in the basic sciences, a broad educational background in a liberal arts-oriented program is desirable. Applicants are encouraged to select subjects that will contribute substantially to a broad cultural background.

SELECTION FACTORS

The Committee on Admissions will select those applicants who, in its judgment, will make the best students and physicians. Consideration is given to the entire record, GPA, MCAT scores, recommendations, and interview results as these reflect the applicant's personality, maturity, character, and suitability for medicine. Additionally, the committee regards as desirable certain health care experiences, such as volunteering or working in hospitals, hospices, nursing homes, or doctor's offices. The committee also values experience in biomedical laboratory research. Following an initial screening process, students with competitive applications are selected to complete a secondary application. Special encouragement is given to candidates from medically underserved areas in Michigan.

As a state-supported school, the institution must give preference to Michigan residents; however, out-of-state applicants are encouraged to apply. An applicant's residency is determined by university regulations. Students whose educational backgrounds include work outside the United States must have completed two years of course work at a U.S. or Canadian college. Interviews are required but scheduled only with those applicants who are given serious consideration. The Committee on Admissions meets on a weekly basis to evaluate candidates. Offers of acceptance will be made on four occasions during the application cycle. Students are urged to apply by November 1.

FINANCIAL AID

Scholarships, loans, and grants are awarded on the basis of academic performance, financial need, and available funding. Students may borrow through various loan programs up to the amount of total school-related costs and living expenses. Loans not based on demonstrated financial need are also available. Although the primary responsibility for financing a medical education rests with the student and the student's family, the School of Medicine will assist students with unmet need as funds are available. Short-term loans may be made for emergency purposes after registration.

Financial aid awards administered by the School of Medicine are made by the financial aid officer based on federal guidelines and those established by the Committee on Financial Aid and Scholarships, which includes student representation.

The College Work-Study Program and other medically oriented jobs are generally available to eligible students for the summer break.

Accepted students are mailed applications and updated financial aid information in February preceding matriculation. Additional information is available from the financial aid officer. Financial aid seminars are held for incoming students and their families. Financial aid appointments and information are available by calling (313) 577-1039.

INFORMATION FOR MINORITY STUDENTS

Wayne State University School of Medicine is committed to the recruitment and retention of minority and disadvantaged applicants. The school supports a one-year postbaccalaureate program for disadvantaged medical school applicants from Michigan who have been denied admission, but who appear to have the potential for academic success. The program consists of premedical science courses, academic skills training, personal adjustment counseling, and academic tutoring. Successful students are guaranteed admission to the School of Medicine. Through the minority recruitment office, the school also administers the Incoming Freshman Summer Program for minority students who are admitted to the freshman class. Additionally, college and high school premedical preparatory programs are offered. For information write Julia Simmons, director, minority recruitment and prematriculation programs.

Public Institution

APPLICATION AND ACCEPTANCE POLICIES FOR 2001–2002 FIRST-YEAR CLASS

School participates in AMCAS. See Chapter 6.

Filing of AMCAS application
- Earliest date: June 1, 2000
- Latest date: Dec. 15, 2000

School application fee after screening: $30
Oldest MCAT scores considered: 1997
Does have Early Decision Program (EDP)
- EDP application period: June 1–Aug. 1, 2000
- EDP applicants notified by: Oct. 1, 2000

Acceptance notice to regular applicants
- Earliest date: Nov. 20, 2000
- Latest date: varies

Applicant's response to acceptance offer
- Maximum time: 3 weeks

Requests for deferred entrance considered: Yes
Deposit to hold place in class (applied to tuition):
- $50, due with response to acceptance offer, nonrefundable

Estimated number of new entrants: 256 (20 EDP)
Starting date: Aug. 2001

TUITION AND STUDENT FEES PER YEAR FOR 1999–2000 FIRST-YEAR CLASS

Tuition
- Resident: $10,739
- Nonresident: $21,812

Student fees: $710

INFORMATION ON 1999–2000 FIRST-YEAR CLASS

Number of	*In-State*	*Out-of-State*	*Total*
Applicants	1,200	1,959	3,159
Applicants Interviewed	544	120	664
New Entrants*	227	26	253

*All took the MCAT and had baccalaureate degrees.

CHAPTER 11

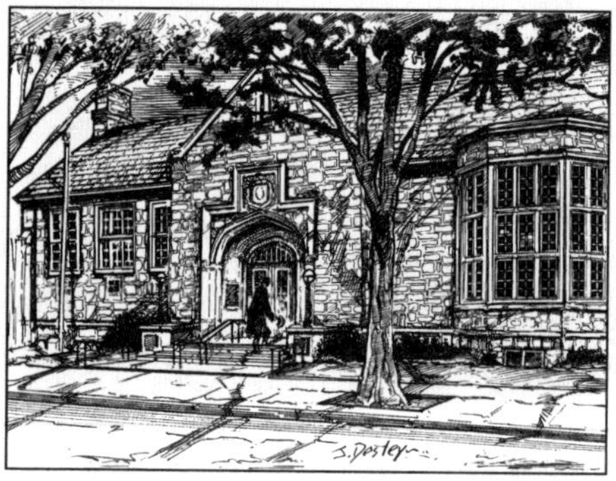

Mayo Medical School

Rochester, Minnesota

Dr. Anthony J. Windebank, *Dean*
Dr. Thomas R. Viggiano, *Associate Dean for Student Affairs*
Leibert Morris, *Assistant Dean for Student Affairs*

ADDRESS INQUIRIES TO:

Mayo Medical School
200 First Street, S.W.
Rochester, Minnesota 55905
(507) 284-3671; 284-2634 (FAX)
Web Site: http://www.mayo.edu/mms

GENERAL INFORMATION

Mayo Medical School is an integral part of Mayo Foundation and Mayo Clinic, the world's largest group practice of medicine.

Resources of MMS include a diverse patient population of more than 415,000 registrants annually, four affiliated hospitals with facilities for clinical and basic research, primary care facilities including several rural health centers, and affiliations with physicians who practice in surrounding communities and states. The faculty is drawn from the clinical and scientific staff of Mayo Clinic with locations in Rochester, Minnesota; Jacksonville, Florida; and Scottsdale, Arizona.

CURRICULUM

The curriculum is designed to emphasize the integration of basic and clinical sciences throughout all four years. Governance of the curriculum is centralized and structured around learning objectives such as the Scientific Foundations of Medical Practice; the Clinical Experiences; and the Patient, Physician, and Society. Through this mechanism, longitudinal oversight of teaching of the basic and clinical sciences can be assured and integration facilitated.

In the first year, basic sciences are taught with clinical correlation emphasizing the normal function of the cell and organ systems. Simultaneous with this learning is the introduction to clinical skills culminating in the ability to perform a history and examination on a Mayo patient by the end of the first year. Preceptor experiences throughout the first year in Continuity of Care keep the focus on the patient.

The second year is devoted to an introduction to the core clinical sciences while completing the introduction of the basic scientific underlayment of clinical practice. Emphasis here is on pathophysiology of the organ systems as students explore the use of basic clinical skills.

The third year is devoted to honing skills in all of the basic clinical clerkships, moving beyond the level of acquiring information to the level of synthesis and diagnosis. Clinical experiences at Mayo have always been both ambulatory and hospital based. Because of the small class size and more than 1,000 physician faculty, in most cases these experiences occur as one-on-one assignments with staff of the Mayo Clinic. One third of the third year is an opportunity to explore the realm of scientific investigation, as every Mayo student completes a research endeavor of his or her own choice under the mentorship of an experienced Mayo investigator. Approximately 175 Mayo scientists in 37 disciplines offer research experiences in which the students participate.

The fourth year has been carefully designed to produce students who have a well-structured completion of their undergraduate education leading to a physician who is prepared to enter any realm of medicine. Requirements include an internal medicine sub-internship and rotations in family medicine, pediatrics, and surgery. A social medicine elective to understand the role of community in the mission of medicine is also required. Integrated into the fourth-year curriculum is a three-week return to the classroom to explore issues in preventive medicine, biomedical ethics, palliative medicine, and clinical pharmacology. The remainder of the fourth year is fully elective to allow students to customize their learning to meet individual goals.

Formal evaluations are recorded as honors, high pass, pass, marginal pass, or fail, and are supplemented by narrative comments from the faculty. Individual support and tutoring are available to all students.

A combined-degree program leading to the M.D.-Ph.D. is available for six members of the entering class. This joint effort with the Mayo Graduate School allows a student to be fully prepared for clinical practice as well as have all the tools for a career in scientific research. Another program in cooperation with the Mayo Graduate School of Medicine is available for two candidates with the D.D.S. degree who are seeking an M.D. degree and certification in oral and maxillofacial surgery. Stipend support and tuition waiver are included for these programs.

All students attending Mayo Medical School are supported by scholarship funds, which significantly reduce the tuition burden. Merit scholarship renewal is dependent upon achieving a grade of pass or higher in every course, but remediation is always available. In addition to participation in federal student assistance programs, Mayo has its own loan program and need-based grant program, which are available to help offset educational expenses.

REQUIREMENTS FOR ENTRANCE

A baccalaureate degree is required, but no major field is preferred. The MCAT must have been taken within three years of application. College work must include:

	Years
Biology and/or Zoology	1
Inorganic chemistry (with lab)	1
Organic chemistry (with lab).	1
A course in Biochemistry	
Physics (with lab)	1

Mayo Medical School looks for students with excellent academic records in a breadth of educational experiences. Valued highly are the diverse talents within the class, and candidates who have a lifelong commitment to service. Experiences that demonstrate unique personal characteristics along with a commitment to medicine are evaluated in the application process. Access to a personal computer is required of all matriculants.

SELECTION FACTORS

In evaluating candidates, the entire academic record, results of the MCAT, careful reading of the candidate's personal statement, and letters of recommendation are utilized in the initial steps. A standardized telephone interview is utilized in lieu of a secondary application for those candidates who have the academic credentials. A great deal of weight is placed on the personal interview in Rochester. Evidence of integrity, adaptability, maturity, leadership, and humanitarian concern are essential. Appointment notification occurs roughly every six weeks throughout the admissions process, though appointments may be given any time up to the time classes begin in August.

Applications are accepted from all U.S. citizens and those foreign citizens possessing a permanent resident visa. Transfers to Mayo Medical School are not accepted except under very unusual circumstances.

Some characteristics of the students accepted for the 1999 entering class were: *mean GPA,* 3.80; *mean MCAT scores,* above 10 in all categories; *gender,* 60 percent women, *minorities,* 7 percent.

Mayo does not discriminate on the basis of race, sex, creed, national origin, age, or handicap in its educational programs or activities in accordance with civil rights legislation.

FINANCIAL AID

An aggressive grant and scholarship program allows every student significant financial support. Forty-five percent of entering students receive a full-tuition scholarship. A merit scholarship program reduces the cost to all other students. All scholarships are forfeited by students holding appointments at other schools after May 15. Evidence of withdrawal from other institutions must be provided by that date. Mayo provides an attractive institutional loan program. Comprehensive health care coverage is available. Further information may be obtained by telephoning the financial aid office at (507) 284-4839.

Private Institution

APPLICATION AND ACCEPTANCE POLICIES FOR 2001–2002 FIRST-YEAR CLASS

School participates in AMCAS. See Chapter 6.

Filing of AMCAS application
  Earliest date: June 1, 2000
  Latest date: Nov. 1, 2000
School application fee to all applicants: $60
Oldest MCAT scores considered: 1997
Does have Early Decision Program (EDP)
  EDP application period: June 1–Aug. 1, 2000
  EDP applicants notified by: Oct. 1, 2000
Acceptance notice to regular applicants
  Earliest date: Oct. 15, 2000
  Latest date: Until class is filled
Applicant's response to acceptance offer
  Maximum time: 2 weeks
Requests for deferred entrance considered: Yes
Deposit to hold place in class (applied to tuition):
  $100, due with response to acceptance offer
Deposit refundable prior to: May 15, 2001
Estimated number of new entrants: 42 (1 EDP)
Starting date: Aug. 2001

TUITION AND STUDENT FEES PER YEAR FOR 1999–2000 FIRST-YEAR CLASS

Tuition: $19,700*   Student fees: None

INFORMATION ON 1999–2000 FIRST-YEAR CLASS

Number of	*In-State*	*Out-of-State*	*Total*
Applicants	332	2,990	3,322
Applicants Interviewed	39	260	299
New Entrants†	15	27	42

*Mayo Scholarships and support from the state of Minnesota reduce tuition from $19,700 to $4,925 for residents of MN, AZ, and FL and $9,850 for nonresidents.

†All took the MCAT and had baccalaureate degrees.

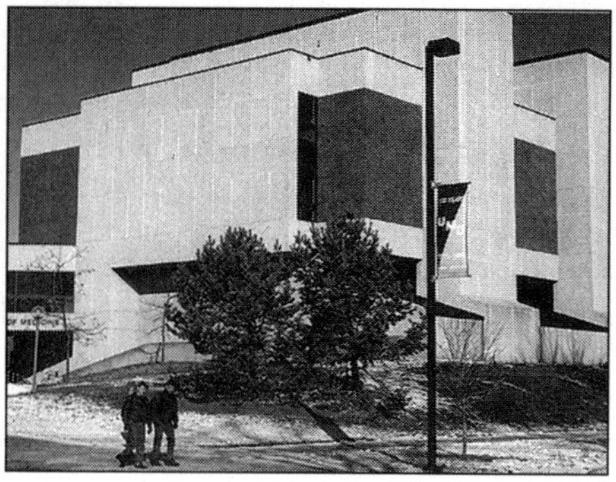

University of Minnesota—Duluth School of Medicine

Duluth, Minnesota

Dr. Richard J. Ziegler, *Dean*
Dr. Lillian Repesh, *Associate Dean for Admissions and Student Affairs*
Dina Flaherty, *Financial Aid Liaison*

ADDRESS INQUIRIES TO:

Office of Admissions, Room 180
University of Minnesota—Duluth
School of Medicine
10 University Drive
Duluth, Minnesota 55812
(218) 726-8511; 726-6235 (FAX)
E-mail: jcarls10@d.umn.edu
Web Site: http://www.d.umn.edu/medweb/admissions

GENERAL INFORMATION

The University of Minnesota—Duluth (UMD) School of Medicine admitted its first class of 24 students in September 1972 to a two-year basic medical and clinical sciences program. After these first two years, students are automatically transferred to the University of Minnesota Medical School at Minneapolis under an established, noncompetitive mechanism for completion of their training.

The UMD School of Medicine has established affiliation agreements with the St. Mary's/Duluth Clinic and Miller-Dwan medical centers and St. Luke's Hospital of Duluth. These institutions afford medical students access to health care systems that provide patients from the northern regions of Minnesota, Wisconsin, and Michigan with care for various medical problems.

The full-time teaching faculty consists of 45 basic and clinical science members. The part-time and voluntary clinical sciences faculty includes over 250 area physicians who represent all of the major medical specialties. Their close interactions with the full-time faculty in presenting the curriculum ensures a practical as well as an academic approach toward training physicians.

CURRICULUM

The two-year curriculum is designed to prepare students for future medical practice through careful and integrated instruction in basic, clinical, and behavioral sciences. Under the guidance of the volunteer clinical faculty, students have early exposure to patients, learning accurate medical history-taking and physical examination skills. Ample time is also devoted to basic science-clinical correlations allowing a student to utilize the basic sciences as they apply to clinical medicine. In addition, each student is paired with a family physician in a required preceptorship arrangement. During the first year, this entails meeting with the preceptor for at least 50 hours per year. In the second year, students spend three consecutive days three times per year with their preceptors in small towns throughout Minnesota.

REQUIREMENTS FOR ENTRANCE

The MCAT and completion of all requirements for a bachelor's degree must be completed by the time of matriculation. Applicants are strongly urged to take the MCAT in the spring of the year of application and to have their premedical course requirements completed at the time of application. The processing of an application may be delayed if MCAT scores or grades from required courses in process are not included in the original application.

Required courses are:

	Sem./Qtr.
Biochemistry	1/1
General biology (with lab)	2/2
General physics (with lab)	2/3
General/inorganic chemistry (with lab)	2/2
Organic chemistry (with lab)	2/2
English composition	2/3
Humanities	2/3
At least one course must be upper-division level.	
Behavioral sciences	2/3
At least one course must be upper-division level.	
Calculus or upper-level statistics	

Beyond these requirements, applicants are strongly encouraged to broaden their education by taking courses in non-science areas that will provide intellectual stimulation. Applicants are also encouraged to become exposed to people and their problems and to learn about the medical profession.

SELECTION FACTORS

The University of Minnesota is committed to the policy that all persons shall have equal access to its programs, facilities, and employment without regard to age, race, creed, sex, national origin, veteran's status, sexual preference, or handicap. As a state-supported school, strongest preference for selection is given to legal residents of Minnesota. Consideration will also be given to applicants from Douglas, Ashland, Bayfield, Burnett, Iron, Price, Sawyer, and Washburn

Counties of Wisconsin, and the Canadian Province of Manitoba who wish to become family practice physicians in a small-town setting. Applicants from other states, except for minorities, will not be considered for admission. Transfer requests are not considered. Applicants must be U.S. Citizens or have permanent resident status.

For each applicant, the Committee on Admissions considers the entire academic record, including trends in performance, scores from the MCAT, and responses to a questionnaire prepared by the committee. If an applicant is selected from this initial screening, the individual is then invited to the Duluth campus for interviews by two committee members. During this visit, the candidate is invited to have lunch with a current medical student. Letters of evaluation are requested of all interviewed applicants.

In keeping with the mandated goals set by the Minnesota legislature at the school's inception, the committee is seeking persons with personal and background traits that indicate a high potential for becoming a family physician in a small-town or rural setting. There is no prejudice for or against the reapplicant. If possible, reapplicants are encouraged to identify any liabilities and rectify them before reapplying through AMCAS. Individuals who are not accepted have the opportunity to review the application with an admissions officer to try to pinpoint the reasons(s) for the action. Admissions requests for advanced standing cannot be considered because of the nature of the curriculum.

The following information pertains to the 1999 entering class: *overall acceptance rate,* 83 acceptances offered to obtain a class of 52 students; mean GPA, 3.45; *mean MCAT scores, VR*-9.2, *PS*-8.8, *BS*-9.2; *sex,* 30 percent women; *residence,* 96 percent from Minnesota; *undergraduate major,* 48 percent in biology or chemistry, with the remainder from a variety of fields.

FINANCIAL AID

Financial aid is based on the demonstrated need of the student. A number of loans are available through the University Financial Aid Program, and there is limited scholarship aid. To date, no one who has been accepted has discontinued medical studies because of financial need. About 93 percent of the students are eligible for and receive financial assistance. For more information, contact financial aid liaison Dina Flaherty at (218) 726-6548.

INFORMATION FOR MINORITY STUDENTS

The school accepts the principles of affirmative action and recognizes the need to provide minority group members with the opportunity to study medicine. Academic and cultural support, particularly for American Indians, is provided through the Center for American Indian and Minority Health and through a program called Native Americans into Medicine.

Public Institution

APPLICATION AND ACCEPTANCE POLICIES FOR 2001–2002 FIRST-YEAR CLASS

School participates in AMCAS. See Chapter 6.

Filing of AMCAS application
  Earliest date: June 1, 2000
  Latest date: Nov. 15, 2000
School application fee after screening: $50
Oldest MCAT scores considered: 1997
Does have Early Decision Program (EDP)
  EDP application period: June 1–Aug. 1, 2000
  EDP applicants notified by: Oct. 1, 2000
Acceptance notice to regular applicants
  Earliest date: Oct. 15, 2000
  Latest date: Varies
Applicant's response to acceptance offer
  Maximum time: 2 weeks
Requests for deferred entrance considered: Yes
Deposit to hold place in class: None
Estimated number of new entrants: 50 (6 EDP)
Starting date: Sept. 2001

TUITION AND STUDENT FEES PER YEAR FOR 1999–2000 FIRST-YEAR CLASS

Tuition
  Resident: $13,910
  Nonresident: $25,842
Student fees: $645

INFORMATION ON 1999–2000 FIRST-YEAR CLASS

Number of	*In-State*	*Out-of-State*	*Total*
Applicants	534	297	831
Applicants Interviewed	173	18	191
New Entrants*	48	4	52

*All took the MCAT and had baccalaureate degrees.

CHAPTER 11

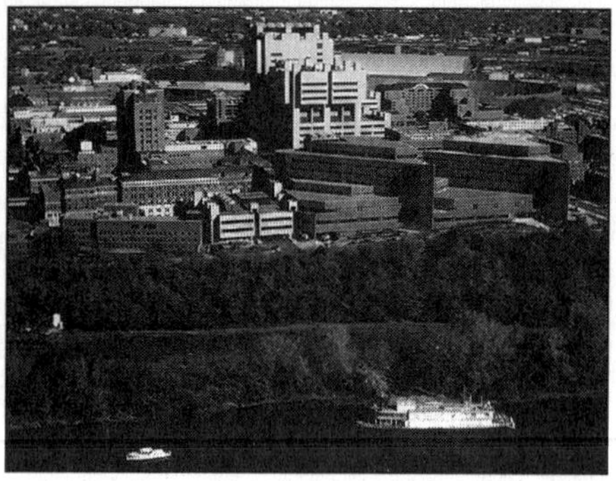

University of Minnesota Medical School—Minneapolis

Minneapolis, Minnesota

Dr. Alfred F. Michael, *Dean*
Dr. Madgetta T. Dungy, *Director of Admissions*
B. J. Gibson, *Financial Aid Officer*

ADDRESS INQUIRIES TO:

University of Minnesota Medical School
Office of Admissions
Box 293
420 Delaware Street, S.E.
Minneapolis, Minnesota 55455-0310
(612) 624-1122; 626-4200 (FAX)
E-mail: galva001@maroon.tc.umn.edu
Web Site: http://www.med.umn.edu/

MISSION STATEMENT

The mission of medical education at the University of Minnesota Medical School is to graduate physicians who serve the health needs of Minnesota, the nation, and the world through excellence in clinical medicine, research, education, and health care leadership.

GENERAL INFORMATION

Founded in 1888, the University of Minnesota Medical School is located on the Minneapolis campus of the University of Minnesota. This proximity to disciplines basic or related to medicine provides unique opportunities for interchange of information, techniques, and personnel. The Medical School is a unit of the University of Minnesota Academic Health Center and has a close working relationship with other units, including dentistry, nursing, and pharmacy. Most of the major hospitals in the Minneapolis-St. Paul area are affiliated with the Medical School, providing teaching facilities for medical students.

CURRICULUM

A major feature of the curriculum is a well-organized required course sequence in the first and second years and flexibility of the schedule in the third and fourth years. The first-year program consists of courses, which form a basis for the continued study of medicine. These include anatomy, biochemistry, histology, human genetics, human behavior, human sexuality, microbiology, neuroscience, physiology, and preventive medicine. Relevance of these areas is reinforced through weekly clinical correlations.

Clinical Medicine courses begin the first week of Year One by addressing topics in professionalism, ethical issues, cultural diversity, medical law, and environmental and occupational health. Following a "White Coat Ceremony" in January, students begin tutorials and preceptorships with community physicians where they start to acquire skills in interviewing, history taking, and physical diagnosis. Lectures and demonstrations are also given on "how to do" an interview/history taking and physical examination.

In the second year, pathology and pharmacology provide the framework for continued study of basic sciences, and pathophysiology is emphasized in organ system courses. Clinical skills are broadened through additional work in clinical medicine, in the primary care fields of medicine, pediatrics, family practice, and neurology.

The program in the third and fourth years includes 52 weeks of required externships and experiences, 24 weeks of electives, and 20 weeks of free time. Students are encouraged to undertake research and are urged to develop goals and pursue personal and special interests in medical education. A faculty advisor is selected during the second year. The advisor assumes an important role in assisting students in achieving their own special educational goals. Flexibility of scheduling in the third and fourth years provides the opportunity to pursue other clinical/academic interests.

A seven-year M.D.-Ph.D. program is offered to combine the breadth of medical education with the depth of a rigorous graduate research program for superior students seeking a career in academic medicine.

REQUIREMENTS FOR ENTRANCE

The MCAT and a bachelor's degree from an approved college or university are required. Applicants are urged to take the MCAT in the spring of the year of application and to complete all of the required science courses before taking the MCAT or making application.

Required courses are:

	Quarters
General biology or zoology (with lab)	2
General or inorganic chemistry (with lab)	2
Organic chemistry (with lab)	2
Biochemistry (with lab)	1
General physics (with lab)	3
English	3
Behavioral sciences, social sciences, or other liberal arts courses	(27 qtr. hrs.)
Upper–level statistics or calculus	

Course work in genetics, psychology, and liberal arts subjects is strongly recommended.

SELECTION FACTORS

Although scholastic aptitude is necessary in order to complete studies in medical school, neither high grades nor high MCAT scores alone or in combination are adequate to obtain admission. The Admissions Committee is looking for candidates who demonstrate the greatest promise of becoming competent physicians. Evidence of personal integrity, maturity, creativity, motivation for medicine, the ability to work cooperatively with others, and a sense of dedication in service to others are factors that will be evaluated by the committee. These qualities and attitudes will be evaluated through letters of evaluation, the scope and nature of extracurricular activities, the breadth of undergraduate education, and personal interview. The committee evaluates all aspects of the applicant's academic record, including trends in the scholastic performance.

Accepted students enter a class of 165 students, approximately 89 percent of whom are Minnesota residents. Although preference is given to legal residents of the state, applicants from other states are encouraged to apply if they can demonstrate high-level academic performance; have attained MCAT scores above the national mean; and show evidence of industriousness, creativity, and an interest in research. With a wide variety of undergraduate majors, accepted students for the 1998 entering class had the following statistics: *mean GPA*, 3.63; *mean MCAT*, 10-10-N-10; *mean age*, 23; 2 percent *minorities*; 45 percent *women* and 55 percent *men*. The University of Minnesota Medical School does not discriminate on the basis of race, gender, creed, sexual orientation, disability, or national origin.

All applications must be submitted through AMCAS. Interviews are required before an applicant is accepted. All interviews are initiated on the invitation of the Admissions Committee. Academically qualified applicants with MCAT scores and GPAs above the national mean may apply through the Early Decision Program.

Applicants not accepted in two successive years are rarely accepted on future applications unless there are significant improvements in both academic and nonacademic credentials.

Transfer students are accepted into the third year, from the two-year medical school at the University of Minnesota—Duluth. Other transfers are rarely accepted due to limits on clinical training sites.

FINANCIAL AID

Applicants for financial assistance must file the cost-free FAFSA. Long-term loans and some scholarship money are available through the Medical School Financial Aid Office for students with demonstrated financial need. Over 90 percent of the student body receives financial assistance. For additional details and assistance in financial planning, please contact the Office of Financial Aid at (612) 625-4998.

INFORMATION FOR MINORITY STUDENTS

The University of Minnesota Medical School is committed to the recruitment, enrollment, and education of students from minority groups. The medical school is committed to providing equal opportunity to students from educationally or economically disadvantaged backgrounds, those with high ability, and nonresidents. Further information may be obtained by contacting Ms. Mary Tate at (612) 6251494, the Office of Minority Affairs.

Public Institution

APPLICATION AND ACCEPTANCE POLICIES FOR 2001–2002 FIRST-YEAR CLASS

School participates in AMCAS. See Chapter 6.

Filing of AMCAS application
  Earliest date: June 1, 2000
  Latest date: Nov. 15, 2000
School application fee to all applicants (to whom supplemental materials are mailed): $50
Oldest MCAT scores considered: 1996
Does have Early Decision Program (EDP)
  EDP application period: June 1–Aug. 1, 2000
  EDP applicants notified by: Oct. 1, 2000
Acceptance notice to regular applicants
  Earliest date: Nov. 1, 2000
  Latest date: Until class is filled
Applicant's response to acceptance offer
  Maximum time: 2 weeks
Requests for deferred entrance considered: Yes
Deposit to hold place in class: None
Estimated number of new entrants: 165 (20 EDP)
Starting date: Sept. 2001

TUITION AND STUDENT FEES PER YEAR FOR 1999–2000 FIRST-YEAR CLASS

Tuition
  Resident: $17,976
  Nonresident: $33,396
Student fees: $716

INFORMATION ON 1999–2000 FIRST-YEAR CLASS

Number of	*In-State*	*Out-of-State*	*Total*
Applicants	729	1,145	1,874
Applicants Interviewed	616	112	728
New Entrants*	146	20	166

*All had baccalaureate degrees; 94% took the MCAT.

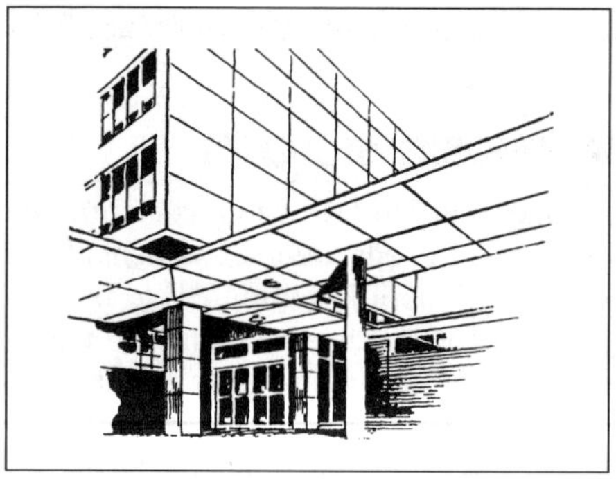

University of Mississippi School of Medicine

Jackson, Mississippi

Dr. A. Wallace Conerly, *Dean*
Dr. Steven T. Case, *Chairman, Admissions Committee*
Dr. Billy M. Bishop, *Director, Student Services and Records*

ADDRESS INQUIRIES TO:

Chairman, Admissions Committee
University of Mississippi
School of Medicine
2500 North State Street
Jackson, Mississippi 39216-4505
(601) 984-5010; 984-5008 (FAX)
Web Site: http://www.umsmed.edu

MISSION STATEMENT

The primary mission of the University of Mississippi School of Medicine is to offer an accredited program of medical education that will provide well-trained physicians and certain supporting health care professionals, in numbers consistent with the health care needs of the state, who are responsive to the health problems of the people and committed to medical education as a continuum, which must prevail throughout professional life. Related objectives are to (1) expand the body of basic and applied knowledge in biomedical sciences, (2) improve systems of health care delivery, (3) demonstrate model medical care for hospitalized and ambulatory patients, and (4) provide excellent programs of continuing education for the state's practicing physicians.

GENERAL INFORMATION

The School of Medicine, created by a special act of the Board of Trustees in June 1903, operated as a two-year school in Oxford until 1955, when it expanded to four years and moved to the University of Mississippi Medical Center in Jackson. The medical center complex includes the School of Medicine, School of Nursing, School of Health Related Professions, School of Dentistry, Graduate Programs in the Medical Sciences, and the 593-bed University Hospital. Newest campus facilities are the Guyton Research Building, the Blair E. Batson Children's Hospital, and the Norman C. Nelson Student Center. Clinical instruction is also carried out in the Veterans Administration Hospital and McBryde Rehabilitation Center for the Blind.

CURRICULUM

In the first year, the courses in anatomy, biochemistry, physiology, and psychiatry/behavioral science are reinforced with a program of clinical correlation that introduces the student to presentation of patients and clinical concepts. The second-year student has courses in biostatistics, epidemiology, genetics, microbiology, pathology, pharmacology, psychiatry/behavioral science, and the conjoint course introduction to clinical medicine. The third-year students rotate through family medicine, obstetrics-gynecology, pediatrics, psychiatry, medicine, and surgery for clinical instruction in these areas. The fourth year consists of a minimum of eight clinical clerkships (blocks), each one calendar month in length. Required blocks include core blocks in internal medicine, obstetrics-gynecology, pediatrics, and surgery. Of the required senior courses, internal medicine is largely an inpatient experience with an ambulatory component provided in medicine clinics at the Veterans Administration Medical Center or University Hospital. The required course in obstetrics-gynecology is largely ambulatory, but includes some inpatient experience in the labor and delivery suite. Of the core months required in pediatrics and surgery, one must be an inpatient clerkship. An additional ambulatory block is required. A fourth-year course in a senior seminar, which covers topics in medical ethics, medical economics and related issues, is required. The remaining months are available for elective experiences that the students select with the counsel of their advisor and the dean's office.

REQUIREMENTS FOR ENTRANCE

The MCAT and three years of college are required. Each applicant must have a minimum of 90 semester hours from an accredited college, excluding physical education, military training, and certain professional courses. However, preference is given to applicants who will have completed all requirements for a baccalaureate degree prior to matriculation.

The required courses are:

	Sem./Qtr. hrs.
General biology or zoology (with lab)	8/12
Inorganic or general chemistry (with lab)	8/12
Organic chemistry (with lab)	8/12
General physics (with lab)	8/12
Advanced science	8/12
Mathematics	6/9
English	6/9

Science courses for nonscience majors, survey courses, and CLEP credits are not acceptable for fulfilling the science requirements. Two semesters of advanced science must be taken in a senior college.

Students who qualify by placement tests for a more advanced course in mathematics must take a semester course of calculus I rather than algebra and trigonometry.

The student is advised to develop proficiency in a specific area and acquire a background in the humanities and behavioral sciences in undergraduate school.

SELECTION FACTORS

Selection of applicants is made on a competitive basis without regard to age, sex, race, creed, national origin, marital status, handicap, or veteran status. The Admissions Committee selects students who are best qualified on the basis of a demonstration of scholastic aptitude and personal achievement with due consideration of other factors. Major considerations are academic performance, MCAT results, motivation for medicine, and such personal characteristics as maturity, integrity, and stability. Additional factors are the recommendation of the premedical advisors or committee and the impression made on the personal interview. Strong preference is given to residents of Mississippi. Interviews are arranged at the discretion of the Admissions Committee.

The mean GPA for the 1999 entering class was 3.65.

Mississippi residents who are enrolled in other medical schools accredited by the Liaison Committee on Medical Education can be considered for transfer after successful completion of one or two years in another program. After completion of two years in another medical school, the transfer applicant must pass Step 1 of the United States Medical Licensure Examination before acceptance in this program.

FINANCIAL AID

Accepted students may apply for financial aid. The school participates in federal scholarship programs and federal loan programs, such as the Health Professions Student Loan Program, the Perkins Loan Program, and the Stafford Student Loan Program. Eligible students may also apply for limited scholarship funds provided by private donors. Additional financial aid is available through the American Medical Association Education and Research Foundation loan program and the Mississippi State Medical Education Scholarship Loan Program, which was established by the state legislature. In the latter program, Mississippi resident medical students who contract to practice in Mississippi may borrow up to $6,000 per school year or $24,000 in four years. Minority students are assisted by the National Medical Fellowship, Inc., program. A limited number of prizes and scholarships are awarded to outstanding students. Four dean's awards, renewable annually, are awarded each year to the freshmen with the highest academic achievement at the end of the first year. Although the study of medicine is considered a full-time occupation, students who maintain satisfactory academic standing may apply for part-time jobs in the medical center.

INFORMATION FOR MINORITY STUDENTS

The Admissions Committee recognizes the serious need for minority physicians and encourages minority students to apply for admission. Further information on the various aspects of the minority program may be obtained by writing to the director, minority student affairs.

Public Institution

APPLICATION AND ACCEPTANCE POLICIES FOR 2001–2002 FIRST-YEAR CLASS

School participates in AMCAS. See Chapter 6.

Filing of AMCAS application
  Earliest date: June 1, 2000
  Latest date: Nov. 1, 2000
School application fee: None
Oldest MCAT scores considered: 1997
Does have Early Decision Program (EDP)
  For Mississippi residents only
  EDP application period: June 1–Aug. 1, 2000
  EDP applicants notified by: Oct. 1, 2000
Acceptance notice to regular applicants
  Earliest date: Oct. 15, 2000
  Latest date: Until class is filled
Applicant's response to acceptance offer
  Maximum time: 15 days
Requests for deferred entrance considered: Yes
Deposit to hold place in class (applied to tuition):
  $50 for residents, due with response to acceptance offer
Deposit refundable prior to: May 15, 2001
Estimated number of new entrants: 100 (10 EDP)
Starting date: Aug. 2001

TUITION AND STUDENT FEES PER YEAR FOR 1999–2000 FIRST-YEAR CLASS

Tuition
  Resident: $6,838
  Nonresident: $13,198

Student fees: None

INFORMATION ON 1999–2000 FIRST-YEAR CLASS

Number of	*In-State*	*Out-of-State*	*Total*
Applicants	300	286	586
Applicants Interviewed	188	0	188
New Entrants*	100	0	100

*All took the MCAT; 98% had baccalaureate degrees.

CHAPTER 11

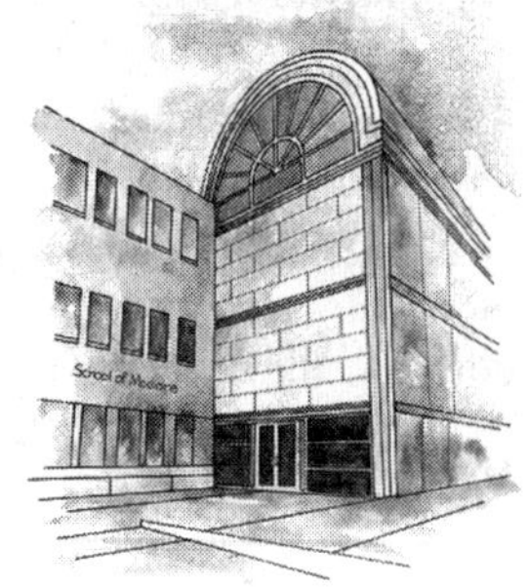

University of Missouri—Columbia School of Medicine

Columbia, Missouri

Dr. Robert J. Churchill, *Interim Dean*
Dr. Robert N. McCallum, *Assistant Dean for Student Programs*
Conway A. Jones, *Financial Aid Coordinator*

ADDRESS INQUIRIES TO:

Judy Nolke, Admissions and Recruitment Coordinator
Office of Medical Education
MA202 Medical Sciences Building
University of Missouri—Columbia
School of Medicine
One Hospital Drive
Columbia, Missouri 65212
(573) 882-2923; 884-4808 (FAX)
E-mail: nolkej@health.missouri.edu
Web Site: http://www.muhealth.org/~medicine

MISSION STATEMENT

MU's School of Medicine is committed to providing high-quality medical education and developing physicians who will meet the health-care needs of Missourians. To do so, it is committed to the following goals: *Content:* The MU School of Medicine will provide a series of learning experiences in the basic science curriculum and in the clinical clerkships to assure that graduates possess the knowledge and understanding of scientific principles and concepts essential to the practice of medicine, and master the scientific method and its application to the practice of medicine, while cultivating in them the qualities of integrity, respect, and compassion. *Application:* The MU School of Medicine will provide opportunities for students to attain skill in performance of a thorough medical history and a complete physical examination; to apply principles of diagnosis and treatment of major illnesses of patients; to incorporate the social, behavioral, and ethical aspects into their patient care; and to practice the principles of public health and preventative medicine. *Process:* The MU School of Medicine will provide an academic atmosphere emphasizing principles, independent thinking, and problem solving; a professional environment fostering and developing attitudinal and professional traits of a competent physician; and experiences for each student as a member of a health care team and a health care delivery system.

GENERAL INFORMATION

The University of Missouri-Columbia School of Medicine was established in 1872 as a two-year medical school. In 1956 the curriculum was expanded to its present four-year program. The MU Health Sciences Center includes the University Hospital, Mid-Missouri Mental Health Center, Harry S. Truman Veterans Administration Hospital, Medical Sciences Building, J. Otto Lottes Health Sciences Library, Howard A. Rusk Rehabilitation Center, Mason Institute of Opthalmology, Cosmopolitan International Diabetes Center, and Ellis Fischel Cancer Center. Students have a total of 1,000 hospital beds available for patient care. Additional local outpatient clinics and rural primary care clinics within 35 miles of Columbia are available. The School of Medicine also maintains affiliations with various other health institutions across the state.

CURRICULUM

The educational program of the School of Medicine was completely revised in 1993 to emphasize a strong foundation in the basic sciences, problem solving, clinical skills, early experiences with patients and role-model physicians, self-directed learning/lifelong learning, and the attitudes essential to competent and compassionate patient care.

Each of the first two years has four 10-week blocks with two components—Basic Science/Problem-Based Learning and Introduction to Patient Care. Bsci/PBL focuses on eight patient cases per block integrating basic sciences, clinical concepts, and psychosocial aspects of medicine. Lectures and labs correlate with the cases. Students engage in collaborative learning and problem solving as they work in groups of eight with a faculty tutor. In IPC, students develop the clinical skills and critical thinking needed for third and fourth years clinical experiences.

The third year features six eight-week required clerkships in internal medicine, surgery, psychiatry/neurology, child health, obstetrics/gynecology, and family medicine. The fourth year has three eight-week required advanced clinical selectives from a surgical area, a medical area, and one other area; eight weeks of advanced biomedical science; and 12 years of general electives. Students with an interest in rural practice may elect to take some of their third- and fourth-year clinical experiences at a rural clinical center. Students with a special interest in biomedical research follow the physician-scientist tract by engaging in guided basic science research through summer experiences, post-sophomore fellowships, and fourth-year electives and selectives which could lead to a graduate degree.

A multilevel grading system is used, with satisfactory/unsatisfactory in the first year, honors/satisfactory/unsatisfactory in the second year, and honors/letter of commendation/satisfactory/unsatisfactory in the third and fourth years.

Students must pass the USMLE Step 1 prior to their fourth year, and Step 2 to graduate.

REQUIREMENTS FOR ENTRANCE

Applicants are required to take the new MCAT (1993 or later) and to have earned a minimum of 90 semester hours (exclusive of physical education and military science) from a recognized college or university. All successful applicants will have completed a bachelor's degree. Specific courses required for admission are:

	Sem.
English composition (or writing-intensive courses)	2
College-level math or calculus	1
	Hrs.
General biology (with lab)	8
General chemistry (with lab)	8
Organic chemistry (with lab)	8
General physics (with lab)	8

Only those courses required for science majors may be used to meet these requirements, not introductory survey courses. A course in biochemistry is strongly recommended. Applicants are also strongly urged to pursue a broad-based education which includes courses in the social sciences, humanities, and oral and written communication. The entering class typically shows a wide range of undergraduate majors.

SELECTION FACTORS

The Committee on Admissions is composed of faculty members, community physicians, and medical students. Strong selection preference is given to Missouri residents.

On-campus personal interviews are required for admission. Selection for interview is based upon MCAT scores, academic performance, the AMCAS application, and letters of reference. Both academic qualifications and nonacademic attributes are important. The Committee assesses personal characteristics such as maturity, motivation, leadership, social concern, and commitment. Demographic factors may be considered.

Credentials of the members of the 1999 entering class: *mean science GPA,* 3.68; *mean GPA,* 3.74; *undergraduate major in sciences,* 78%; *sex,* 48% women; *mean MCAT,* 29.6; *Early Decision Program acceptance,* 2%; *overall acceptance rate,* 144 acceptances offered to complete a class of 96 students.

The School of Medicine participates in the Early Decision Program (EDP). Current requirements to apply are: Missouri resident with 3.75 overall GPA and MCAT sum of 30 with no individual score below 9. We accept transfer students in the third year from U.S. and/or foreign medical schools, primarily Missouri residents.

The School of Medicine does not discriminate on the basis of race, sex, creed, national origin, age, handicap, religion, or status as a Vietnam-era veteran in the admission or access to or treatment or employment in its programs and activities.

FINANCIAL AID

Students are admitted to the School of Medicine without regard to financial circumstances. After acceptance, prospective students are mailed the necessary forms to complete the financial aid process. The school participates in the federal scholarship and loan programs. The institutional scholarship program is primarily need-based. Institutional long-term loans are available to third- and fourth-year students. The school also operates an emergency short-term loan program.

INFORMATION FOR MINORITY STUDENTS

The University of Missouri is committed to the recruitment and education of minority, disadvantaged, and nontraditional applicants. The School of Medicine sponsors summer programs for minority, rural, and disadvantaged high school students interested in health care professions.

Public Institution

APPLICATION AND ACCEPTANCE POLICIES FOR 2001–2002 FIRST-YEAR CLASS

School participates in AMCAS. See Chapter 6.

Filing of AMCAS application
- Earliest date: June 1, 2000
- Latest date: Nov. 1, 2000

School application fee after screening: $50
Oldest MCAT scores considered: 1993
Does have Early Decision Program (EDP)
- For Missouri residents only
- EDP application period: June 1–Aug. 1, 2000
- EDP applicants notified by: Oct. 1, 2000

Acceptance notice to regular applicants
- Earliest date: Nov. 15, 2000
- Latest date: Varies

Applicant's response to acceptance offer
- Maximum time: 30 days

Requests for deferred entrance considered: Yes
Deposit to hold place in class (applied to tuition):
- $100, due with response to acceptance offer

Deposit refundable prior to: May 15, 2001
Estimated number of new entrants: 96 (5 EDP)
Starting date: Aug. 2001

TUITION AND STUDENT FEES PER YEAR FOR 1999–2000 FIRST-YEAR CLASS

Tuition
- Resident: $14,486
- Nonresident: $29,128

Student fees: $703

INFORMATION ON 1999–2000 FIRST-YEAR CLASS

Number of	*In-State*	*Out-of-State*	*Total*
Applicants	469	451	920
Applicants Interviewed	249	20	269
New Entrants*	94	0	94

*All had baccalaureate degrees; 73% took the MCAT.

CHAPTER 11

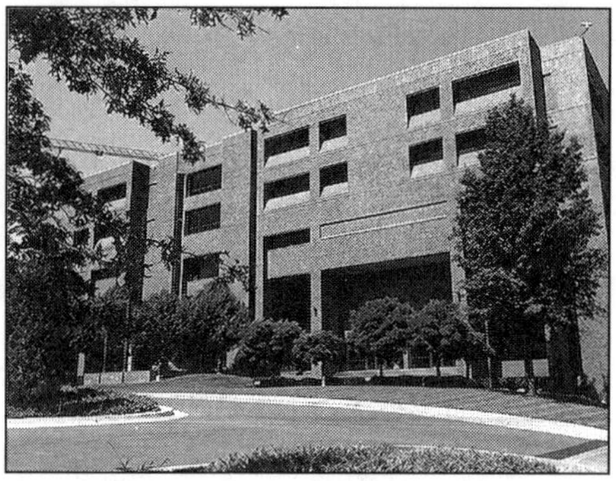

University of Missouri—Kansas City School of Medicine

Kansas City, Missouri

Dr. Michael Friedland, *Dean*
Melvin Tyler, *Director of Admissions*
Patrick McTee, *Director of Student Financial Aid*

ADDRESS INQUIRIES TO:

Council on Selection
University of Missouri—Kansas City
School of Medicine
2411 Holmes
Kansas City, Missouri 64108
(816) 235-1870; 235-5277 (FAX)
Web Site: http://research.med.umkc.edu

MISSION STATEMENT

The mission of the University of Missouri—Kansas City School of Medicine is to prepare graduates so they are able to enter and complete graduate programs in medical education, qualify for medical licensure, provide competent medical care, and have the educational background necessary for lifelong learning in order to address the health care needs of our state and nation.

GENERAL INFORMATION

The Board of Curators of the University of Missouri authorized the establishment of a medical school at the University of Missouri—Kansas City in 1969. Located on a 135-acre Hospital Hill campus, the medical school is near both the schools and colleges of the university and affiliated community hospitals.

CURRICULUM

The School of Medicine, in combination with the College of Arts and Sciences and the School of Biological Sciences, offers a year-round program leading to baccalaureate and M.D. degrees in six calendar years. The student is required to complete both degrees and has the freedom to major in any department of the School of Biological Sciences or the College of Arts and Sciences.

The program is designed primarily for high school seniors who are entering college. Students are permitted to obtain 30 semester hours of credit through the advanced placement program or the CLEP subject area examinations. To receive the baccalaureate degree, the student must complete 120 semester hours of credit.

The fundamental objective of the program is to provide students with a broad liberal arts education and to prepare physicians who are committed to providing comprehensive health care.

Under the guidance of a clinician-scholar, called a docent, small groups of first- and second-year students are introduced to medicine in several community hospitals where they can observe patients and their problems.

During the first two years of the program, the student is occupied predominantly with arts and sciences course work, with about one-fourth of the time being devoted to introduction to medicine courses. After these two years the student advances, with the approval of the Council on Evaluation, to Year 3 of the six-year program.

During the last four years of the curriculum the student, with guidance from a docent and education assistant, plans a program for meeting the curriculum requirements. Two months of Years 4 through 6 are spent with the docent unit on an inpatient internal medicine rotation. The remaining months of each year are spent in a number of other required and elective course offerings in the basic and clinical sciences and the humanities and social sciences. Students spend two academic terms in arts and sciences course work during the last four years of the program.

Basic, clinical, and behavioral science information is presented and emphasized throughout the six-year program. Thus, each student is expected to acquire a firm and broad base of information in each of these major content areas.

The academic program provides the medical student with a realistic working knowledge of community health problems and resources. The school provides an environment for learning medicine, which is enhanced by the strong student support system.

An alternative path is available for extended study.

REQUIREMENTS FOR ENTRANCE

Applicants for admission to Year 1 of the six-year baccalaureate-medical program must meet the admission requirements of both the University of Missouri—Kansas City and the School of Medicine. Applicants must graduate from an accredited U.S. high school and demonstrate the ability to perform successfully at the college level, based on a combination of high school rank and scores on the American College Test (ACT).

A student admitted to the combined program at UMKC is required to meet the following high school course requirements (one unit equals one year in class): four units of English; four units of mathematics; three units of science, including one unit of biology and one unit of chemistry; three units of social studies; one unit of fine arts; two units of a single foreign language. Applicants are strongly encouraged to pursue an extensive and challenging course of study.

Only a limited number of positions become available at the Year-3 level of the program. *Applications to the Year-3 level will be considered only from applicants who have a baccalaureate or advanced degree and are residents of Missouri or adjacent counties of Kansas.*

SELECTION FACTORS

The criteria for selection are:

1. Applicant's academic potential is judged by quality of high school courses, rank in high school class, and scores on the ACT. In the 1999–2000 entering class, the average ACT score fell at the 90th percentile, and the average rank in class was at the 95th percentile.

2. Personal qualities evaluated include maturity, leadership, stamina, reliability, motivation for medicine, range of interests, interpersonal skills, compassion, and job experience.

The Council on Selection carefully reviews all applicants to this program. Applicants who appear to be well qualified are invited for interviews at the medical school campus. If invited, the applicant is notified in writing and will be required to be present at the scheduled date and time of the interview.

Students are considered on the basis of their individual qualifications without regard to race, creed, sex, or national origin. The program does not accept transfer students.

FINANCIAL AID

There is a variety of financial assistance available to all medical students. Further information and applications for financial aid may be obtained from: Student Financial Aid Office, University of Missouri—Kansas City, 5115 Oak, Kansas City, Missouri 64110. Application should be made prior to March 15 of the year for which the student is applying.

INFORMATION FOR MINORITY STUDENTS

Information for minority students is available from Dr. Reaner Shannon, Assistant Dean for Minority Affairs, or Adela L. Fleming, Coordinator of Admissions, Council on Selection, University of Missouri–Kansas City School of Medicine.

Public Institution

APPLICATION AND ACCEPTANCE POLICIES FOR 2001–2002 FIRST-YEAR CLASS

Year 1 of six-year program.

Filing of application
  Earliest date: Aug. 1, 2000
  Latest date: Nov. 15, 2000
School application fee to all applicants: $25 (in-state)
  $50 (out-of-state)
Does not have Early Decision Program
Acceptance notice to regular applicants
  Earliest date: April 1, 2001
  Latest date: Varies
Applicant's response to acceptance offer
  Maximum time: by May 1, 2001
Requests for deferred entrance considered: No
Deposit to hold place in class (applied to tuition):
  $100, due with response to acceptance offer
  Deposit refundable prior to: May 15, 2000
Estimated number of new entrants: 100
Starting date: Aug. 2000

TUITION AND STUDENT FEES PER YEAR FOR 1999–2000 FIRST-YEAR CLASS

Tuition*
  Resident: $21,322
  Nonresident: $43,200

Student fees: $818

INFORMATION ON 1999–2000 FIRST-YEAR CLASS

Number of	*In-State*	*Out-of-State*	*Total*
Applicants	330	314	644
Applicants Interviewed	204	78	282
New Entrants	104	16	120

*These fees apply to Year 3 of the six-year program.

CHAPTER 11

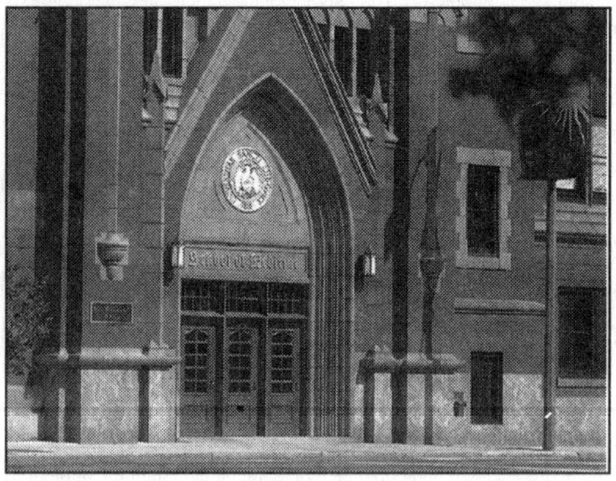

Saint Louis University School of Medicine

St. Louis, Missouri

Dr. Patricia Monteleone, *Dean*
Dr. L. James Willmore, *Associate Dean*
Mary B.W. Fenton, *Assistant Dean, Student Financial Planning*

ADDRESS INQUIRIES TO:

Nancy McPeters
Admissions Committee
Saint Louis University
School of Medicine
1402 South Grand Boulevard
St. Louis, Missouri 63104
(314) 577-8205; 577-8214 (FAX)
E-mail: medadmis@slu.edu
Web Site: http://www.slu.edu/colleges/med/

MISSION STATEMENT

Beyond the important objective of training physicians who are scholars of human biology, the School of Medicine strives to graduate physicians who manifest in their personal and professional lives a special appreciation for what may be called humanistic medicine.

We regard humanistic medicine as a constellation of ethical and professional attitudes, which affect the physician's interactions with patients, colleagues, and society. Among these attitudes are concern for the sanctity of human life; commitment to dignity and respect in the provision of medical care to all patients; devotion to social justice, especially regarding inequities in the availability of health care; humility and awareness of medicine's limitations in the care of the sick; appreciation of the role of non-medical factors in a patient's state of well-being or illness; and mature, well-balanced professional behavior that derives from comfortable relationships with members of the human family and one's Creator.

GENERAL INFORMATION

Saint Louis University is a privately endowed, coeducational institution founded by the Jesuits in 1818. The first faculty of medicine was appointed in 1836, and the school assumed its general present form in 1903. Today the Saint Louis University School of Medicine includes the University Hospital, the School of Medicine (Schwitalla Hall, Doisy Medical Research Facility, and Margaret McCormick Doisy Learning Resources Center), Firmin Desloge Towers, Bordley Pavilion, David P. Wohl Memorial Mental Health Institute, Cardinal Glennon Hospital for Children, SLU-Anheuser Busch Eye Institute, Doctors' Office Building, and the Institute of Molecular Virology. Major teaching affiliations include Forest Park Medical Center, DePaul Medical Center, St. John's Mercy Medical Center, St. Mary's Health Center, and the St. Louis Veterans Administration hospitals.

CURRICULUM

The M.D. Degree Program curriculum has undergone extensive changes in order to adapt to the needs of the evolving health care environment. All years have been subject to revision. Distinctive aspects of the program include:

1. A new Phase 1 (Year 1) that consists of a Fundamentals of Biomedical Sciences course; a Health Information Resources course to develop computer skills and proficiency in gathering information on various aspects of human disease and patient care; and a Patient, Physician, and Society course that includes units such as ethics, communication skills, and physical diagnosis.

2. Phase 2 (Year 2) will include an organ and systems approach. Phase 3 incorporates Year 3 and Year 4, with a new clerkship in Family Medicine and ample opportunities to design individualized programs including electives. Also, ambulatory care activities have been significantly expanded.

3. A Clinical Skills Center provides the latest methodology for instruction and evaluation using standardized patients and other devices to learn clinical skills, in addition to the regular training sites.

4. The opportunity to participate in a combined M.D.-Ph.D. program, in which qualified medical students undertake graduate studies leading to the Ph.D. in one of the basic science disciplines. Students interested in research may opt to receive the M.D. with Distinction in Research Award.

5. The opportunity to participate in a combined M D.-M.P.H. program.

6. The grade system consists of the following levels: Honors, Pass, and Fail.

REQUIREMENTS FOR ENTRANCE

Saint Louis University School of Medicine encourages applications from students who have demonstrated a high level of academic achievement and who manifest in their personal lives those human qualities that are required for a career of service to society. Specific academic requirements include the MCAT and a minimum of 90 semester hours (135 quarter hours) in undergraduate arts and science courses. Most accepted applicants complete a baccalaureate degree of at least 120 semester hours (180 quarter hours) from an accredited college or university. Specific course requirements are:

	Sem. hrs.
General biology or zoology (with lab)	8
Inorganic chemistry (with lab)	8
Organic chemistry (with lab)	8
Physics (with lab)	8
English	6
Other humanities and behavioral sciences	12

Biochemistry is strongly recommended.

Applicants are expected to have pursued one area of knowledge or discipline in depth. The Admissions Committee does not favor any specific major in its decisions.

SELECTION FACTORS

The selection of candidates is based upon demonstrated intellectual ability and personal qualifications, including motivation, character, emotional maturity, stability, and personality. There is no discrimination on the basis of race, color, sex, age, national origin, religion, sexual orientation, disability, or veteran status. All university policies, practices, and procedures are administered in a manner consistent with our Catholic Jesuit identity. There are no geographical restrictions or quotas for American citizens. Only U.S. citizens and full U.S. permanent residents are eligible to apply for admission. All applicants receive serious consideration, and some additional attention is given to applicants from Saint Louis University.

Students for the 1998 entering class had the following average academic credentials: *SMGPA,* 3.63; *overall GPA,* 3.68; *mean MCAT Scores, VR*-9.4, *PS*-9.9, *BS*-10.2, *WS*-Q; *sex,* 46 percent women; *residence,* 36 percent from Missouri, 29 states represented; *undergraduate major,* 54 percent in life sciences, 17 percent in chemistry.

Transfers into our School of Medicine are only possible at the beginning of the third year of studies. The only individuals who are eligible to apply for transfer are those who are currently enrolled in, and students in good standing at, other U.S. medical schools accredited by the Liaison Committee on Medical Education.

FINANCIAL AID

The Office of Student Financial Planning identifies a standard student budget and assists students in managing an aid plan to meet expenses for their directly related educational costs. Loan and scholarship aid is available and is awarded on the basis of financial need. It is absolutely necessary that an individual be "creditworthy" in order to qualify for financial assistance. Information on the financial status of parents is required of all students seeking University aid and some federal aid.

In 1998–99, 85 percent of the students received financial assistance from either school or noninstitutional sources.

Financial aid information is automatically sent upon acceptance to the School of Medicine. This information includes the need analysis document(s), descriptions of available aid sources, and the application form for financial assistance from the School of Medicine. Individuals in need of applying for financial aid may do so only after they have been accepted to the School of Medicine.

The Office of Student Financial Planning encourages financial aid applicants to contact it when questions arise regarding eligibility for aid and the financial aid process.

INFORMATION FOR MINORITY STUDENTS

The School of Medicine is committed to diversity. There is an ongoing effort to increase the number of individuals significantly underrepresented in the medical profession, in particular those of African-American descent.

The Office of Multicultural Affairs (OMA) assists students from diverse backgrounds to be successful as they progress along the educational pathway in pursuit of a career as a physician.

Private Institution

APPLICATION AND ACCEPTANCE POLICIES FOR 2001–2002 FIRST-YEAR CLASS

School participates in AMCAS. See Chapter 6.

Filing of AMCAS application
- Earliest date: June 1, 2000
- Latest date: Dec. 15, 2000

School application fee to all applicants: $100
Oldest MCAT scores considered: 1997
Does have Early Decision Program (EDP)
- EDP application period: June 1–Aug. 1, 2000
- EDP applicants notified by: Oct. 1, 2000

Acceptance notice to regular applicants
- Earliest date: Oct. 15, 2000
- Latest date: Until class is filled

Applicant's response to acceptance offer
- Maximum time: 2 weeks

Requests for deferred entrance considered: Yes
Deposit to hold place in class (applied to tuition):
- $100, due with response to acceptance offer

Deposit refundable prior to: May 15, 2001
Estimated number of new entrants: 151 (4 EDP)
Starting date: Aug. 2001

TUITION AND STUDENT FEES PER YEAR FOR 1999–2000 FIRST-YEAR CLASS

Tuition: $29,930 Student fees: $1,182

INFORMATION ON 1999–2000 FIRST-YEAR CLASS

Number of	*In-State*	*Out-of-State*	*Total*
Applicants	401	5,082	5,483
Applicants Interviewed	126	637	763
New Entrants*	51	100	151

*All took the MCAT and had baccalaureate degrees.

CHAPTER 11

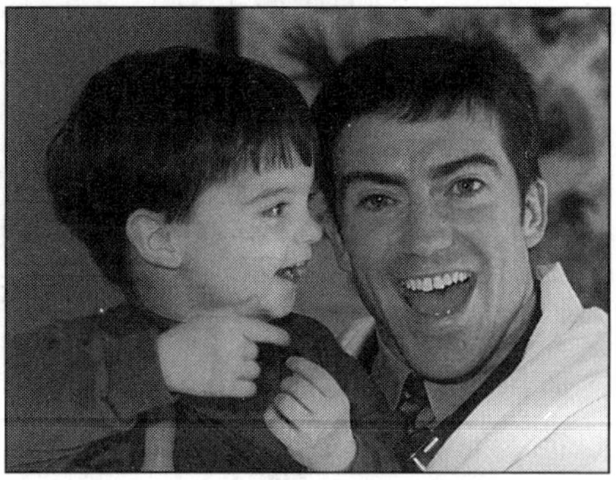

Washington University School of Medicine

St. Louis, Missouri

Dr. William A. Peck, *Dean and Vice Chancellor for Medical Affairs*
Dr. W. Edwin Dodson, *Associate Dean for Admissions*
John F. Walters, *Assistant Dean and Director of Financial Aid*

ADDRESS INQUIRIES TO:

Office of Admissions
Washington University
School of Medicine
660 South Euclid Avenue, #8107
St. Louis, Missouri 63110
(314) 362-6857; 362-4658 (FAX)
E-mail: wumscoa@msnotes.wustl.edu
Web Site: http://medschool.wustl.edu/admissions/

MISSION STATEMENT

The mission of Washington University is the promotion of learning—learning by students and by faculty. Teaching, the transmission of knowledge, is central to our mission, as is research, the creation of new knowledge. Our goals are:

- to foster excellence in our teaching, research, scholarship, and service;
- to prepare students with attitudes, skills, and habits of lifelong learning and with leadership skills, enabling them to be useful menbers of a global society; and
- to be an exemplary institution in our home community, St. Louis, as well as in the nation and the world.

GENERAL INFORMATION

Washington University School of Medicine has a rich history of success in research, education, and patient care. It pioneered bedside teaching and led in the transformation of empirical knowledge into scientific medicine. From the earliest days, there has been an understanding that "investigation and practice are one in spirit, method, and object."

Responding to a national concern for improving doctors' training, Washington University in 1891 established a medical department. By 1900, scientific progress had accelerated the reform of medical education, and the medical department assumed new importance. In 1909, Robert Brookings, successful St. Louis businessman turned philanthropist, set about transforming the medical department into a modern medical school. Today, the medical school occupies more than 4 million gross square feet of space.

Washington University School of Medicine, Barnes-Jewish, St. Louis Children's, and Barnard hospitals, and Central Institute for the Deaf compose the 230-acre Washington University Medical Center. Barnes-Jewish Hospital is a 1,442-bed teaching facility and the largest hospital in the region. St. Louis Children's Hospital is one of the top pediatric health centers in the country, providing a full range of services throughout its 200-mile service area. Barnes-Jewish and St. Louis Children's hospitals are members of BJC Health System, the largest academically linked health care system in the country.

A good doctor must be a compassionate and understanding human being as well as a good scientist. To this end, the School of Medicine has always selected applicants who, in addition to possessing keen minds, demonstrate an ability to perceive and serve their patients' interests. An education from Washington University School of Medicine provides graduates with solid opportunities for sought-after residencies and fellowships, challenging research endeavors, and rewarding medical careers.

CURRICULUM

The curriculum provides students with a stimulating education, in both the science and the art of clinical medicine. Instruction is by lecture, small-group interactive sessions with faculty, including problem-based exercises and self-directed learning using computers and other resources led by faculty facilitators. Medical humanities and ethics are integrated into the four years of medical training. Throughout the curriculum, serious consideration is given to the sociological and cultural concerns of the patients and to the necessity of adapting medical care to their needs.

Patient contact begins in the first semester of the first year. Courses address the broad issues of normal structure and function of humans with emphasis on neuroscience, cell biology, and genetics. The effect of disease on bodily structure and function characterize the second-year curriculum. Expanded clinical experience is integrated with course work in pathology, pathophysiology, and pharmacology. Core clinical clerkships occupy the entire third year with increasing emphasis on ambulatory medicine. The fourth year is a full year of electives planned and selected by the student with faculty guidance.

For students who care to participate, there are abundant opportunities to engage in basic and clinical research through summer research fellowships and research electives. A five-year M.A. and M.D. degree program is available for students desiring a full year of research training. A six-year Medical Scientist Training Program permits students seeking a career in academic medicine to obtain both M.D. and Ph.D. degrees.

A tutorial program is available to any student in the school who needs academic assistance. A pass/fail grading system is used in the first year; an honors/high pass/pass/fail grading system is used thereafter.

REQUIREMENTS FOR ENTRANCE

Accepted applicants must present evidence of superior intellectual ability and achievement, completion of at least 90 semester hours of course work in an approved college or university, satisfactory performance on the MCAT, and attributes necessary for a productive career in medicine.

Mathematics, physics, and chemistry provide the tools for modern biology, medicine, and the biological basis of patient care. Accordingly, premedical education should include a minimum of the following courses:

	Years
Biological science	1
General or inorganic chemistry	1
Organic chemistry	1
Physics	1
Mathematics (through differential and integral calculus)	1

Prerequisites are subject to waiver by the Committee on Admissions. The development of the intellectual talents of an individual often involves the in-depth pursuit of some areas of knowledge in humanities, social sciences, or natural sciences. A diversified background of cultural development is encouraged.

SELECTION FACTORS

Students are selected on the basis of character, attitude, interest, intellectual ability, motivation, maturity, and past achievement as indicated both by superior scholastic work and active participation in extracurricular activities prior to entering medical school. Washington University policies and programs are nondiscriminatory, and full consideration is given to all applicants without regard to sex, age, race, handicap, sexual preference, creed, or national or ethnic origin. Minority group students are strongly encouraged to apply.

Students in the 1999 entering class had the following credentials: *mean science GPA,* 3.80; *mean nonscience GPA,* 3.84; *mean total GPA,* 3.82; *mean MCAT scores—VR*-11.0, *PS*-12.3, *BS*-12.5; *sex,* 51 percent women; *undergraduate major,* 51 percent in biological sciences or preprofessional studies, 19 percent in chemistry or biochemistry, 10 percent in physics or engineering, 20 percent in a variety of other fields of study.

Early submission of the AMCAS application permits its prompt evaluation by the Committee on Admissions. All applicants are invited to complete their application with letters of evaluation and additional personal information. Selected applicants are invited for interview. All accepted applicants are interviewed.

FINANCIAL AID

To facilitate financial planning, tuition is set for the first year and does not increase during the four years of medical school.

The financial resources of an applicant do not enter into the admission selection process. Need-based financial aid is awarded to accepted students who document financial need. An award decision is usually made within two weeks following receipt of completed financial aid application forms. Awards consist of both scholarships and loans. Merit-based full-tuition scholarships are awarded to multiple students in each entering class and are eligible for renewal each year of study for the M.D. degree. Application to apply is by invitation of the Admissions Committee. For information contact: Committee on Student Financial Aid; 660 South Euclid Avenue, #8059; St. Louis, Missouri 63110; (314) 362-6845; 362-3045 (FAX); E-mail: money@msnotes.wustl.edu.

INFORMATION FOR MINORITY STUDENTS

The school is committed to the recruitment, enrollment, education, and graduation of an increased number of individuals from minority groups. For information contact: Will Ross, M.D.; Associate Dean for Diversity; 660 South Euclid Avenue, #8023; St. Louis, Missouri 63110; (314) 362-6854; 747-3974 (FAX); E-mail: rossw@msnotes.wustl.edu.

Private Institution

APPLICATION AND ACCEPTANCE POLICIES FOR 2001–2002 FIRST-YEAR CLASS

School participates in AMCAS. See Chapter 6.

Filing of AMCAS application
  Earliest date: June 1, 2000
  Latest date: Dec. 1, 2000
School application fee to all applicants: $50
Oldest MCAT scores considered: 1997
Does not have Early Decision Program
Acceptance notice to regular applicants
  Earliest date: Nov. 15, 2000
  Latest date: Until class is filled
Applicant's response to acceptance offer
  Maximum time: 2 weeks
Requests for deferred entrance considered: Yes
Deposit to hold place in class (applied to tuition):
  $100, due with response to acceptance offer
Deposit refundable prior to: May 15, 2001
Estimated number of new entrants: 120
Starting date: Aug. 2001

TUITION AND STUDENT FEES PER YEAR FOR 1999–2000 FIRST-YEAR CLASS

†Tuition: $31,700   Student fees: None

INFORMATION ON 1999–2000 FIRST-YEAR CLASS

Number of	*In-State*	*Out-of-State*	*Total*
Applicants	227	4,858	5,085
Applicants Interviewed	50	1,059	1,109
New Entrants*	10	111	121

*All took the MCAT and had baccalaureate degrees.

†Tuition is stabilized for four years.

CHAPTER 11

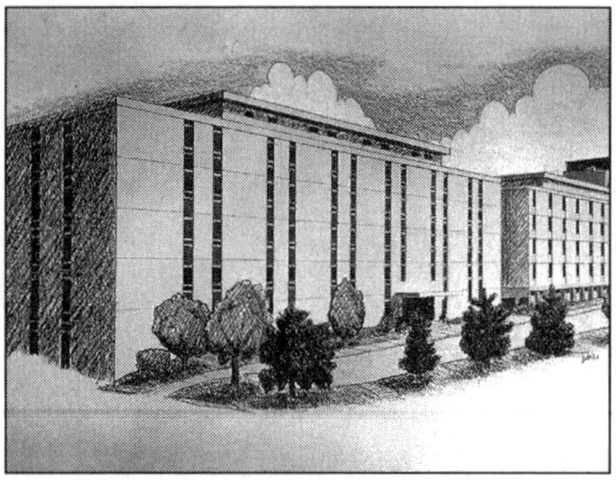

Creighton University School of Medicine

Omaha, Nebraska

Dr. M. Roy Wilson, *Dean*
Henry C. Nipper, Ph.D., *Assistant Dean for Admissions*
Tanya T. Avant, *Financial Aid Coordinator*

ADDRESS INQUIRIES TO:

Creighton University School of Medicine
Office of Admissions
2500 California Plaza
Omaha, Nebraska 68178
(402) 280-2799; 280-1241 (FAX)
E-mail: medschadm@creighton.edu
Web Site: http://medicine.creighton.edu

MISSION STATEMENT

The mission of Creighton University School of Medicine is to develop and promote an understanding of human health and the causes, treatments, and prevention of disease. To accomplish this mission in the Jesuit tradition and spirit of Creighton University, the School of Medicine will pursue the following goals: 1) create an environment in which medical and graduate students and faculty are motivated to learn, to teach, and to serve the needs of society and in which compassion, integrity, humility, and self-knowledge are united with wisdom; 2) empower future physicians with the necessary knowledge, skills, judgement, and confidence to become competent clinicians and lifelong learners; 3) promote postgraduate education of physicians so they may become excellent practitioners, teachers, and scholars instilled with a spirit of service and the highest ethical standards; 4) incorporate the concepts of disease prevention and health promotion into the art and science of medical practice; 5) motivate physicians to meet health care needs through specialty training in those disciplines where recognized shortages exist; 6) provide continuing education for health professionals so they may futher their knowledge and skills to better serve the needs of their community; and 7) promote scholarship and conduct research dedicated to improving the practice and teaching of medicine, enhancing the quality of life, and developing new knowledge.

GENERAL INFORMATION

The Creighton University School of Medicine, a Jesuit institution, was opened over 100 years ago in October 1892, 14 years after the opening of the parent university. Its plant includes four units that provide all facilities for research, basic science, and preclinical teaching. St. Joseph's Hospital, accommodating 403 patients, is the principal teaching hospital of the medical school. Clinical instruction is also carried out in the Children's Memorial, Veterans Administration, and Alegent Health System hospitals. Clinical services are also conducted at several other area hospitals. The Bio-Information Center, located on the west campus north of the hospital, contains a multimedia self-instructional component, a biomedical communication center, an educational services unit, and the traditional library facilities.

CURRICULUM

A new curriculum, designed for the twenty-first century, was introduced in the summer of 1996. The educational program has been divided into four components. Component One, Biomedical Fundamentals, serves as the foundation of the educational program followed by more complex basic science information presented in a clinically relevant context in Component Two. This component consists of a series of organ-based and disease-based courses. Component Three consists of redesigned required core clerkships emphasizing basic medical principles, primary care, and preventive medicine. Component Four provides additional responsibilities for patient care including an eight-week block of critical care medicine, a four-week surgery selective, a four-week subinternship, and twenty-four weeks of elective study. Clinical experience is a prominent part of the curriculum in all components, beginning with the physical diagnosis instruction in the first year. Students interact with standardized patients in the first year and are assigned to longitudinal clinics during the second year. The curriculum also integrates ethical and societal issues into all four components. Instructional methodology utilizes case-based small-group sessions and computer-assisted instruction in all components. A close faculty/student relationship provides for mentoring and advising of students in choosing courses that will broaden their background for a career in medicine, as well as satisfying their special interest. Competency-based evaluation is used in all components, and the students are graded on a pass/fail/honors system. Students compete against standards and not each other. Under the new curriculum, Creighton students continue to excel on USMLE Step 1.

REQUIREMENTS FOR ENTRANCE

The MCAT and three years (at least 90 semester hours) of accredited college work are mandatory. Preference is given, however, to holders of the baccalaureate degree. Applicants may take the MCAT in the fall of the year preceding their entry into medical school. All requirements for admission must be completed by June prior to entry. Course work must include:

	Sem. hrs.
General biology (with lab)	8
Inorganic chemistry (with lab)	8
Organic chemistry (with lab)	8-10
General physics (with lab)	8
English	6

Although no additional coursework is required, advanced study in human biology, including biochemistry and/or genetics, is encouraged. Applicants may pursue a baccalaureate degree with any major in science or liberal arts (except military science) appropriate to their interests. Non-science majors should elect to take advanced science study to the extent possible. Up to 27 semester hours of credit are accepted under CLEP and/or advanced placement programs.

SELECTION FACTORS

Consideration will be given to all of the qualities considered to be necessary in a physician. Intellectual ability and curiosity, emotional maturity, honesty, and proper motivation, in addition to proven scholastic ability, are of the utmost importance. A record that includes significant service to humanity and medical experience is deemed important. The preprofessional committee evaluations and letters of recommendation are equally important.

The school reserves the right to require a formal interview of every applicant selected before it finalizes the acceptance. The interview will be held on the university campus.

There are no restrictions placed on applicants because of race, religion, sex, national or ethnic origin, age, disability, or status as a disabled veteran or veteran of the Vietnam era. Candidates are not restricted by state of residence. Creighton University values diversity in its medical classes. Not only is ethnic diversity encouraged, but Creighton considers the non-traditional applicant to be a positive influence on the school and its students. Preference is given to applicants who have undertaken their preprofessional education at Creighton University. The Creighton "Guaranteed Admission Program" is in its second year. It is expected that as many as 40 to 50 seats may be awarded in this program.

Because the cumulative and science GPAs of the 115 candidates selected for the 1998 entering class were 3.73 and 3.71, respectively, it is suggested that no candidate apply whose GPA in either situation is below 3.4. Other characteristics of the 1999 entering class were: *sex*, 50 percent women; *undergraduate major*, 84 percent in science.

The AMCAS application is the principal source of information on the candidates. Additional (secondary) information is requested of all applicants upon receipt of the AMCAS form. Transfers from LCME medical schools are admitted on a space-available basis.

FINANCIAL AID

In addition to federally insured student loan programs and funds available from major foundation grants, a limited number of scholarships and fellowships are available for upperclassmen and for a few well-qualified entering students. Scholarship aid is awarded on the basis of overall qualifications and personal financial need.

Approximately 95 percent of the students receive some form of financial aid during a part or all of their four years of study. Students are discouraged from accepting outside employment because of the lack of available time during a heavy academic schedule, but spouses of students usually have no difficulty in finding employment in the Omaha metropolitan area.

INFORMATION FOR MINORITY STUDENTS

Consideration is given to applications from African American, native American, Alaskan native, native Hawaiian, Mexican American, and Puerto Rican candidates. The school application fee will be waived if AMCAS has first waived its charges. Financial aid in the form of grants and long-term loans is available on the basis of proven need.

Private Institution

APPLICATION AND ACCEPTANCE POLICIES FOR 2001–2002 FIRST-YEAR CLASS

School participates in AMCAS. See Chapter 6.

Filing of AMCAS application
  Earliest date: June 1, 2000
  Latest date: Dec. 1, 2000
School application fee to all applicants: $65
Oldest MCAT scores considered: 1998
Does have Early Decision Program
  EDP application period: June 1—Aug. 1, 2000
  EDP applicants notified by: Oct. 1, 2000
  Acceptance notice to regular applicants
  Earliest date: Oct. 15, 2000
  Latest date: Until class is filled
Applicant's response to acceptance offer
  Maximum time: 2 weeks
Requests for deferred entrance considered: Yes
Deposit to hold place in class (applied to tuition):
  $100, due with response to acceptance offer
Deposit refundable prior to: March 1, 2001
Estimated number of new entrants: 113 (15 EDP)
Starting date: Aug. 9, 2001

TUITION AND STUDENT FEES PER YEAR FOR 1999–2000 FIRST-YEAR CLASS

Tuition: $28,010 Student fees: $566

INFORMATION ON 1999–2000 FIRST-YEAR CLASS

Number of	*In-State*	*Out-of-State*	*Total*
Applicants	235	4,434	4,669
Applicants Interviewed	64	408	472
New Entrants*	13	102	115

*All took the MCAT and had baccalaureate degrees.

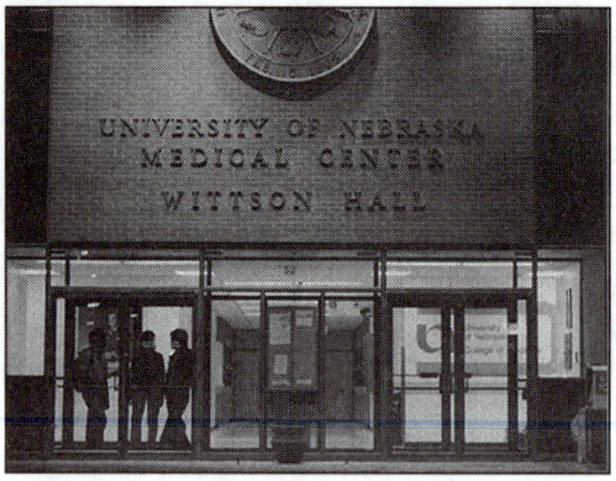

University of Nebraska College of Medicine

Omaha, Nebraska

Dean to be announced
Dr. Jeffrey W. Hill, *Associate Dean of Admissions, and Student and Multicultural Affairs*
Shirley Dohring, *Assistant Director of Financial Aid*

ADDRESS INQUIRIES TO:

Office of Academic and Student Affairs
University of Nebraska College of Medicine
986585 Nebraska Medical Center
Omaha, Nebraska 68198-6585
(402) 559-2259; 559-6840 (FAX)
Web Site: http://www.unmc.edu/UNCOM

MISSION STATEMENT

The mission of the University of Nebraska Medical Center is to improve the health of Nebraska through premier educational programs, innovative research, the highest quality patient care, and outreach to underserved populations.

GENERAL INFORMATION

Medical education has been continuous in Omaha since students first entered the Omaha Medical College in the fall of 1880. The University of Nebraska Medical Center includes colleges of dentistry, medicine, nursing, and pharmacy, a school of allied health, Nebraska Health System (University Hospital and Clarkson Hospital), University Outpatient Services, University Geriatric Center, Eppley Cancer Research Institute, and C. Louis Meyer Children's Rehabilitation Institute. These facilities are supplemented by direct teaching affiliations with the Veterans Affairs Hospital and eight private hospitals, two of which are on the medical center campus. Thus students have access to facilities with a total of approximately 2,800 teaching beds.

CURRICULUM

The goals of the College of Medicine are to provide the best possible training both in the science and art of medicine for students with the dedication and ability to become working practitioners of the healing arts. Education at the College of Medicine sets high standards for its students who, as a result, are recognized throughout the country as highly skilled practitioners with superior clinical ability. Over 85 percent of the graduates of the College of Medicine obtain one of their top three choices of residency programs nationwide. The college provides a sound basis for support of career choices in medical practice, teaching, research, or administration by stimulating students to obtain a background of basic information, a command of the language of biomedical science, a mastery of the skills necessary for clinical problem-solving, a habit of self-education, and a sympathetic understanding of the behavior of healthy and sick people. The college is particularly oriented toward training physicians to meet all the health care needs of the citizens of Nebraska.

The curriculum ensures that students develop the understanding, clinical skills, and knowledge needed for residency training and practice. The Nebraska graduate develops superior skills in problem solving and clinical reasoning, extensive knowledge of the biomedical and psychosocial sciences, and the skills needed for lifelong learning of medicine. Courses in the first two years introduce students to the basic sciences of medicine: anatomy, behavioral science, biochemistry, microbiology, pathology, pharmacology, and physiology. Here students also begin to learn clinical skills and reasoning, through preceptorships and clinical case study in small groups.

In the third and fourth years students apply their knowledge on the hospital wards and clinical offices. Under faculty guidance students develop clinical diagnostic and management skills. They learn to select clinical tests and prescribe therapies. They learn to provide comprehensive care and learn the art of medicine. During the third year, students take clinical clerkships in Family Medicine, Internal Medicine, Obstetrics and Gynecology, Pediatrics, Psychiatry, and Surgery. In the fourth year, students select from a variety of clinical and basic science experiences.

At the beginning of medical school, students work in small groups with a faculty member to solve clinical cases. This initial exercise helps develop the library and information retrieval skills they will need in their medical studies. Case study and small-group teaching emphasizing problem-based learning are becoming more prominent features of all of the basic science courses. Since 1986, simulated patients have been used to supplement the clinical experience of medical students. These trained patient simulators are used to teach and evaluate history taking and physical examination skills. All these changes are making medical education more relevant to patient care and medical practice.

REQUIREMENTS FOR ENTRANCE

The MCAT and a minimum of 90 semester hours (three years of college work) in an accredited liberal arts and sciences college are required. The completion of a college major or baccalaureate degree is strongly recommended. The undergraduate program must include:

	Sem. hrs.
Biology (with lab)	8–10
General chemistry (with lab)	8–10
Organic chemistry (with lab)	8–10
Physics (with lab)	8–10
Humanities and/or social sciences	12–16
Calculus or statistics	3
English composition or writing course	3
The following courses will also be required beginning with the 2002 entering class:	
Biochemistry	3
Genetics	3

In addition to meeting specific requirements, applicants are encouraged to adopt an educational goal that includes exploring areas of personal interest. In view of the rapidly broadening scope of medicine, a well-rounded education is considered optimum preparation. The requirements are consistent with that belief.

SELECTION FACTORS

Selection is based on a total assessment of each candidate's motivation, interests, character, demonstrated intellectual ability, previous academic record and its trends, personal interview, scores on the MCAT, and general fitness and promise for a career in medicine. Admission is based on individual qualifications without regard to age, sex, sexual preference, race, national origin, handicap, or religious or political beliefs. Academic credentials are evaluated on the basis of course level and load, involvement in cocurricular activities or employment, and other influential factors. Cutoff levels for GPAs or for scores on the MCAT are not utilized; however, applicants are reminded of the competition for entrance and are advised to be realistic. Personal attributes are assessed through letters of reference and in the interview.

Strong preference is given to residents of Nebraska, but a number of students from other states may be accepted. The University of Nebraska encourages, in particular, students from rural areas, small towns, or disadvantaged backgrounds to apply. The potential for service to underserved communities is taken into consideration during the preadmission evaluation.

Accepted students for the 1999 entering class had the following credentials: *mean* GPA, 3.70; *sex,* 43 percent women; *undergraduate major,* approximately 70 percent science majors.

FINANCIAL AID

Some scholarships are available each year. A few may be granted to entering freshmen. Several fellowships and assistantships are available to students who desire to take one or two years of graduate study or research in the basic sciences. Loan funds have been increased through efforts of physicians in Nebraska, fraternal organizations, and friends of the college. Approximately 80 percent of the students receive some financial aid.

INFORMATION FOR MINORITY STUDENTS

The University of Nebraska College of Medicine is committed to increasing the number of physicians from ethnic groups currently underrepresented in the medical profession. Applications are encouraged from resident and nonresident black Americans, American Indians, mainland Puerto Ricans, and Mexican Americans. The accomplishments of applicants will be evaluated with due consideration given to their backgrounds. Specific information is available from the Office of Student Equity and Multicultural Affairs; 984275 Nebraska Medical Center, Omaha, NE 68198-4275; (402) 559-4437.

Public Institution

APPLICATION AND ACCEPTANCE POLICIES FOR 2001–2002 FIRST-YEAR CLASS

School participates in AMCAS. See Chapter 6.

Filing of AMCAS application
Earliest date: June 1, 2000
Latest date: Nov. 1, 2000
School application fee: $25
Oldest MCAT scores considered: 1998
Does have Early Decision Program (EDP)
For Nebraska residents only.
EDP application period: June 1–Aug. 1, 2000
EDP applicants notified by: Oct. 1, 2000
Acceptance notice to regular applicants
Earliest date: December
Latest date: Until class is filled
Applicant's response to acceptance offer
Maximum time: 2 weeks
Requests for deferred entrance considered: No
Deposit to hold place in class (applied to tuition):
$100, due with response to acceptance offer
Deposit refundable prior to: May 15, 2001
Estimated number of new entrants: 120 (45 EDP)
Starting date: Aug. 2001

TUITION AND STUDENT FEES PER YEAR FOR 1999–2000 FIRST-YEAR CLASS

Tuition
Resident: $12,578
Nonresident: $24,319

Student fees: $1,225

INFORMATION ON 1999–2000 FIRST-YEAR CLASS

Number of	*In-State*	*Out-of-State*	*Total*
Applicants	313	594	907
Applicants Interviewed	282	50	332
New Entrants*	114	6	120

*97% took the MCAT; 97% had baccalaureate degrees.

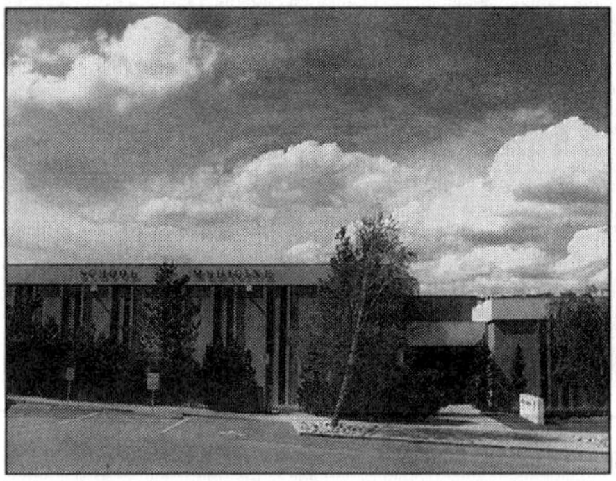

University of Nevada School of Medicine

Reno, Nevada

Dr. Robert H. Miller, *Dean*
Dr. Jerry R. May, *Associate Dean for Admissions and Student Affairs*
Peggy Dupey, *Director of Student Services*

ADDRESS INQUIRIES TO:

Office of Admissions and Student Affairs
University of Nevada
School of Medicine
Mail Stop 357
Reno, Nevada 89557
(775) 784-6063; 784-6194 (FAX)
E-mail: asa@unr.edu
Web Site: http://www.unr.edu/unr/med.html

GENERAL INFORMATION

The University of Nevada School of Medicine is a state-supported, community-based, university-integrated school which relies heavily on community physicians as teachers and community health facilities as sites for the majority of its clinical education. The school is dedicated to selecting individuals with diverse backgrounds who will learn to be compassionate and competent physicians. Students study comprehensive health care delivery considering the needs of the individual, the family, and the community.

CURRICULUM

The first two years of the program are concentrated in classrooms and laboratories on the Reno campus. The curriculum emphasizes biomedical and behavioral sciences basic to medicine. Basic science disciplines are integrated with each other and with clinical problems to promote the learning of problem-solving skills. A clinical correlation course, which explores the basics of biomedical ethics, is taught.

Early clinical training is provided for students to learn patient interviewing, doctor-patient relationship skills, and basics of physical examination and diagnosis. Throughout the first and second years, students spend time with a physician to observe medical practice in the office setting and clinic settings.

There are also opportunities to participate in basic and clinical science research throughout the curriculum. The third and fourth years emphasize a balance of ambulatory and inpatient medical education designed to better prepare students for residency in all specialties and the practice of medicine in the twenty-first century.

Individualized M.D.-Ph.D. programs are offered to students, depending upon the specific interest area.

REQUIREMENTS FOR ENTRANCE

The MCAT and a minimum of three years of college work (90 semester hours) are required. The MCAT must be taken prior to the November 1 application deadline. (It is not necessary to wait for fall MCAT scores prior to applying.) The Admissions Selection Committee strongly recommends completion of a baccalaureate degree prior to matriculation in medical school.

Applicants are encouraged to have a broad educational background and to enroll in an in-depth course curriculum that will lead to a discipline-oriented major, e.g., biology, English, psychology. However, no specific major is favored over any other. In addition to academic course work, people-oriented activities and health care exposure are important.

Course work must include:

	Sem. hrs.
Biology	12
Must include 3 sem. hrs. of upper-division credit	
Inorganic chemistry	8
Organic chemistry	8
Physics	8
Behavioral Sciences	6
Must include 3 sem. hrs. of upper-division credit	

In fulfillment of the behavioral sciences requirement, students should take courses that deal with the psychological stages of the life cycle (e.g., human growth and development, adolescence, aging, human sexuality, abnormal psychology, family dynamics, or medically oriented sociology).

Correspondence, CLEP, AP, and/or pass/fail or audit in lieu of a letter grade is not acceptable for the above required courses.

A demonstrated competency in English composition and expression is required. Generally, students are expected to satisfy the English composition requirements of their undergraduate institution. Supplementary courses strongly recommended but not required for admission include history, literature, philosophy, ethics, and computer sciences. Accepted students are responsible for completing all prerequisite course work prior to matriculation.

Early submission of the AMCAS application permits its prompt evaluation during the process. Applicants are, therefore, urged to submit their applications and supporting credentials as early as possible.

Access to a personal computer is required of all matriculants. Contact the school for minimum requirements.

SELECTION FACTORS

Candidates are evaluated on the basis of academic performance; results of the MCAT; the nature and depth of scholarly, extracurricular, and health care related activities during college years (excellence and balance of the natural sciences, social sciences, and humanities); academic letters of evaluation; and the personal interview. Select applicants are invited for interviews. Interviews are held in Reno and Las Vegas. All accepted applicants are interviewed.

A high priority is given to residents of Nevada. A small number of nonresident applicants are considered each year who have strong residential ties to Nevada (that is, parents' residence, medical catchment area) or are residents of Alaska, Idaho, Montana, or Wyoming (western rural states without medical schools). Individuals who do not meet the residential requirements should not apply.

Matriculants for the 1999 entering class had the following profile: *average science* GPA, 3.6; *accumulative* GPA, 3.7; *average MCAT scores*—VR-8.9; PS-9.4; BS-9.8; 34 percent female, *average age*, 24.

Resident and nonresident applications for the Early Decision Program (EDP) are encouraged. It is suggested that EDP applicants call for updated requirements before application. Reapplicants are not eligible for EDP.

Only those students who are currently enrolled and in good academic standing with LCME-accredited medical schools and have a strong residential tie to Nevada are considered for transfer to the second and third years. The number of positions available for transfer is strictly limited by attrition and compatibility to the school's curriculum. Only U.S. citizens are considered. Application from students attending foreign medical schools are not considered.

FINANCIAL AID

Every attempt is made to assist students and their families in meeting both their financial obligations to the School of Medicine and the student's essential personal needs. Financial status is not a determinant in selecting qualified applicants. A limited number of loans and scholarships are available to medical students on the basis of need and merit. Determination of financial aid award is made after acceptance. More than 80 percent of Nevada's medical students receive some type of financial assistance.

INFORMATION FOR MINORITY STUDENTS

The School of Medicine is committed to the recruitment, selection, and retention of individuals who are members of ethnic and racial groups traditionally underrepresented in American medicine. Residents of the state of Nevada and individuals who meet the nonresident criteria who are from minority and disadvantaged backgrounds are encouraged to apply.

The Admissions Selection Committee encourages applicants of both genders and from all socioeconomic, racial, religious, and educational backgrounds.

Public Institution

APPLICATION AND ACCEPTANCE POLICIES FOR 2001–2002 FIRST-YEAR CLASS

School participates in AMCAS. See Chapter 6.

Filing of AMCAS application
  Earliest date: June 1, 2000
  Latest date: Nov. 1, 2000
School application fee after screening: $45
Oldest MCAT scores considered: 1999
  Does have Early Decision Program (EDP)
  EDP application period: June 1–Aug. 1, 2000
  EDP applicants notified by: Oct. 1, 2000
Acceptance notice to regular applicants
  Earliest date: Jan. 15, 2001
  Latest date: Varies
Applicant's response to acceptance offer
  Maximum time: 2 weeks
Requests for deferred entrance considered: Yes
Deposit to hold place in class: None
Estimated number of new entrants: 52 (2 EDP)
Starting date: Aug. 2001

TUITION AND STUDENT FEES PER YEAR FOR 1999–2000 FIRST-YEAR CLASS

Tuition
  Resident: $7,782
  Nonresident: $22,808

Student fees: $1,918

INFORMATION ON 1999–2000 FIRST-YEAR CLASS

Number of	*In-State*	*Out-of-State*	*Total*
Applicants	201	101	302
Applicants Interviewed	130	30	160
New Entrants*	43	3	46

*All took the MCAT and had baccalaureate degrees.

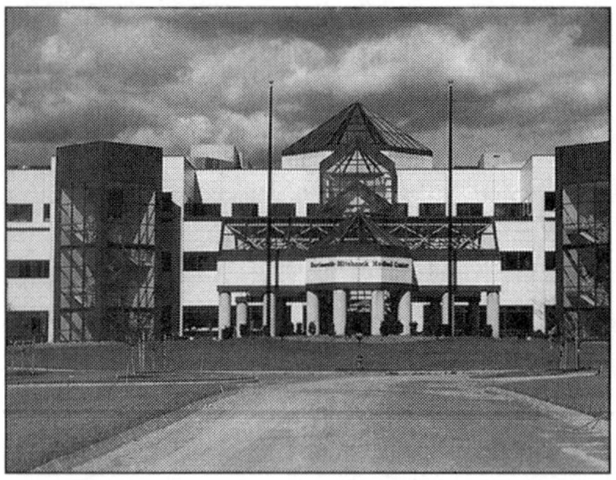

Dartmouth Medical School

Hanover, New Hampshire

Dr. John C. Baldwin, *Dean*
Andrew G. Welch, *Director of Admissions*
Nanci G. Cirone, *Director of Financial Aid*

ADDRESS INQUIRIES TO:

Admissions
Dartmouth Medical School
Office of Admissions
3 Rope Ferry Rd.
Hinman Box 7020
Hanover, New Hampshire 03755-3833
(603) 650-1505; 650-1560 (FAX)
Web Site: http://www.dartmouth.edu/dms/

MISSION STATEMENT

Dartmouth Medical School is dedicated to advancing health through the dissemination and discovery of knowledge. Our chief responsibility is to select students of exceptional character and accomplishment and prepare them to become superb and caring physicians, scientists, and teachers.

We are committed to:

- education of health professionals in an environment of discovery;
- research that advances health;
- formulation of health policies in the interest of our citizens;
- service with our partners to maintain Dartmouth-Hitchcock Medical Center as a local, regional, and national resource for health care of the highest quality.

GENERAL INFORMATION

Dartmouth Medical School, the fourth oldest medical school in the United States, is a component of the Dartmouth-Hitchcock Medical Center (DHMC), which includes the Mary Hitchcock Memorial Hospital, the Norris Cotton Cancer Center, and the White River Junction (VT) Veterans Administration Hospital. The Dartmouth-Hitchcock Clinic, headquartered at DHMC, is one of the nation's 10 largest group practices. DHMC, a state-of-the-art facility located on a 225-acre campus, serves a patient population of 1.5 million people. It includes 396 beds in two five-story in-patient towers, a diagnostic and treatment center, an ambulatory care building, the cancer center, the Borwell Research Building, and a student center. Additional clinical teaching sites include the Brattleboro Retreat (VT), the Family Medical Institute of Augusta (ME), Hartford Hospital (CT), the Tuba City Indian Health Service Hospital (AZ), and numerous primary care sites in Maine, New Hampshire, and Vermont. The C. Everett Koop Institute at Dartmouth was founded in 1992. Dr. Koop serves as the institute's senior scholar. A faculty of approximately 1,000 offers all students the opportunity for individually based instruction.

CURRICULUM

Dartmouth's "New Directions" curriculum is designed to integrate the study of basic and clinical sciences throughout medical school. The curriculum's hallmarks are longitudinal experiences in both the basic and clinical sciences, introduction to the ambulatory care setting in the earliest weeks of study, extended participation in small-group learning, close working relationships with faculty members, and increased opportunities for independent learning. The first year includes On Doctoring, a course that pairs students with faculty practitioners in local communities. Clinical training in the course alternates with biweekly, small-group tutorials on the DMS campus. A major course in the second year is the Scientific Basis of Medicine, an interdisciplinary pathophysiology course that integrates, through lectures, seminars, and problem-based learning, the basic sciences with a broad introduction to the mechanisms of disease and the principles of clinical medicine. In the third year, students begin a series of clinical clerkships in Inpatient and Outpatient Medicine, Inpatient and Outpatient Pediatrics, Inpatient OB/GYN, Surgery and Surgical Selectives, Inpatient Psychiatry, and Outpatient Family Medicine. The fourth year includes clerkships in Neurology and Women's Health plus a sub-internship and four short courses (Clinical Pharmacology; Advanced Medical Sciences; Health, Society and the Physician; and Advance Cardiac Life Support), but is largely tailored to students' individual needs and interests through substantial elective opportunities.

Entering class size at Dartmouth is 75. Most students follow the four-year curriculum at DMS and receive the M.D. degree from Dartmouth. Approximately 15 students, admitted jointly by Dartmouth and the Brown University School of Medicine, spend the first two years at Dartmouth and the last two years studying at Brown. The Brown-Dartmouth students are awarded the M.D. from Brown.

DMS offers an M.D.-Ph.D. program that provides a comprehensive academic, intellectual, and financially supportive environment enabling highly qualified students to pursue an M.D. and a Ph.D. in any of the degree-granting departments of the medical school and the college. A joint M.D.-M.B.A. program is offered through DMS and Dartmouth's Amos Tuck School of Business Administration. In addition, graduate degrees are available through Dartmouth's Center for the Evaluative Clinical Sciences.

REQUIREMENTS FOR ENTRANCE

Except in unusual circumstances, all candidates are expected to present MCAT scores. Where possible, the spring MCAT is recommended and helps the Admissions Committee to proceed expeditiously with the review of an application.

Specific courses required at college level are:

	Sem. hrs.
General biology	8
Inorganic chemistry	8
Organic chemistry	8
Physics	8
Calculus	3

Proficiency in written and oral English is required. At least three years of study at a Canadian or American college or university is required.

In general, the demonstration of excellence in an area of study is a more important criterion than the particular discipline. Hence, students are encouraged to major in the field of their special interest and, if possible, to pursue independent investigation in that field. Students majoring in nonsciences who have demonstrated ability in science are encouraged to apply.

SELECTION FACTORS

The decision of the Admissions Committee depends on appraisal of the entire application, including a thorough evaluation of personal, scholastic, and scientific qualifications. Rigid cutoff points and inflexible criteria are avoided. Dartmouth Medical School is a national institution enrolling students from across the country.

All candidates who apply to DMS through AMCAS receive a secondary application, and all applicants in the final group from which the class is chosen are interviewed in Hanover. A limited number of applicants are selected for interview and invited throughout the academic year.

It is the long-standing policy of Dartmouth Medical School to support equality of opportunity for all persons regardless of race or ethnic background, and no student shall be denied admission or financial aid or be otherwise discriminated against because of age, disability, race, creed, religion, sex, sexual orientation, or national origin.

Application for the Brown-Dartmouth program is initiated at Dartmouth. All applicants invited for interviews receive a form on which to indicate their program choices. In selecting applicants for the joint program, the admission policies and standards of both institutions are observed. Successful applicants are offered acceptance to only one program at a time. Letters of acceptance state the program to which the student has been admitted and are binding.

FINANCIAL AID

Admission decisions are made without regard to financial need. All accepted U.S. citizens and permanent residents with documented need are offered financial aid packages. Approximately 80 percent of the students receive financial aid, usually as a combination of scholarship and loan or through federally supported service programs. Scholarships and loans are awarded on the basis of need as documented on the FAFSA, the Need Access form, and the DMS financial aid application and supporting documentation (see Part 1).

Application fee waiver is granted to individuals who have received an AMCAS fee waiver. Applicants who are neither U.S. citizens nor permanent residents should be aware that financial support for foreign students is extremely limited.

INFORMATION FOR MINORITY STUDENTS

Applications from members of underrepresented minority groups are encouraged. Several members of the admissions committee are members of underrepresented minority groups. Lori Alvord, M.D., who serves as a member of the admissions committee, is Associate Dean of Student and Minority Affairs.

Private Institution

APPLICATION AND ACCEPTANCE POLICIES FOR 2001–2002 FIRST-YEAR CLASS

School participates in AMCAS. See Chapter 6.

Filing of AMCAS application
Earliest date: June 1, 2000
Latest date: Nov. 1, 2000
School application fee to all applicants: $60
Oldest MCAT scores considered: 1998
Does not have Early Decision Program
Acceptance notice to regular applicants
Earliest date: Dec. 15, 2000
Latest date: Until class is filled
Applicant's response to acceptance offer
Maximum time: 2 weeks
Requests for deferred entrance considered: Yes
Deposit to hold place in class: None
Estimated number of new entrants: 75
Starting date: Aug. 2001

TUITION AND STUDENT FEES PER YEAR FOR 1999–2000 FIRST-YEAR CLASS

Tuition: $25,800 Student fees: $1,455

INFORMATION ON 1999–2000 FIRST-YEAR CLASS

Number of	*In-State*	*Out-of-State*	*Total*
Applicants	68	6,158	6,226
Applicants Interviewed	25	613	638
New Entrants*	6	51	67†

*All had baccalaureate degrees; 96% took the MCAT.

†Plus 5 M.D.–Ph.D. candidates.

CHAPTER 11

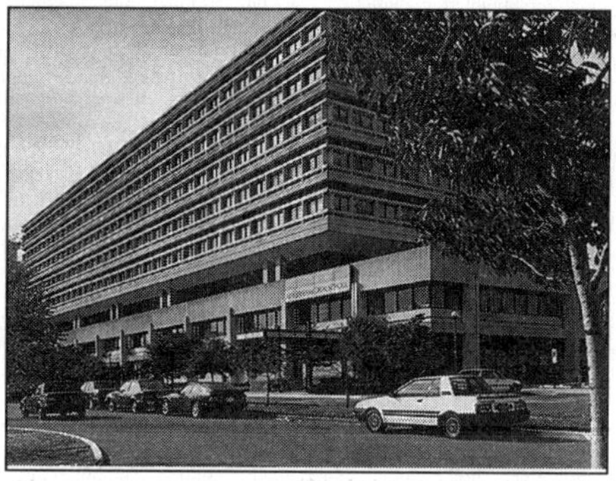

UMDNJ—New Jersey Medical School

Newark, New Jersey

Dr. Ruy V. Lourenço, *Dean*
Dr. George F. Heinrich, *Assistant Dean for Admissions*
Michael Katz, *Director of Financial Aid*

ADDRESS INQUIRIES TO:

Director of Admissions
UMDNJ—New Jersey Medical School
185 South Orange Avenue
Newark, New Jersey 07103
(973) 972-4631; 972-7986 (FAX)
E-mail: njmsadmiss@umdnj.edu
Web Site: http://www.umdnj.edu/njmsweb

MISSION STATEMENT

The University of Medicine and Dentistry of New Jersey (UMDNJ), the state's university of the health sciences, is the "largest free-standing health sciences university in the United States." It has four main academic health center campuses in Newark, Camden, New Brunswick/Piscataway, and Stratford and also at educational and health care institutions in communities throughout the state.

UMDNJ is dedicated to the pursuit of excellence in:

- the undergraduate, graduate, postgraduate, and continuing education of health professionals and scientists;
- the conduct of basic biomedical, psychosocial, clinical, and public health research;
- health promotion, disease prevention, and the delivery of health care; and
- service to our communities and the entire state.

UMDNJ seeks to advance the health sciences; to prepare future health professionals for leadership roles; to respond to academic, health personnel, and service delivery needs, while recognizing the diversity of our constituencies; to provide educational opportunities to New Jerseyans; and to improve the health and quality of life of the citizens of New Jersey and society at large.

GENERAL INFORMATION

The New Jersey Medical School of the University of Medicine and Dentistry of New Jersey (UMDNJ-NJMS) moved into facilities situated in Newark in 1977. A $350 million complex contains the teaching-research Biomedical Science Building, a hospital, an ambulatory care center, a library, a dental school, and a community mental health center.

Major clinical instruction is carried out at University Hospital, Hackensack University Medical Center, Veteran's Affairs Medical Center in East Orange, Morristown Memorial Hospital, and Kessler Institute for Rehabilitation.

CURRICULUM

During the first two years, a thorough coverage of the basic medical sciences is implemented through a hybrid curriculum with departmental and integrated interdepartmental studies. A first-year course, The Art of Medicine, utilizes office–based preceptorships along with small group problem-based learning. Part of the second year is devoted to an introduction to the clinical sciences, during which the student receives instruction in history-taking, physical diagnosis, and pathophysiology. In addition, courses in preventive medicine and community health, behavorial science, and psychiatry are offered. The third year is spent in rotations through core clinical departments. This is a closely supervised, hands-on, comprehensive learning experience in which the student acquires the basic knowledge and techniques of clinical medicine. Instruction is carried out mainly in small groups and is individualized. The fourth year is devoted to advanced required work and elective programs. The required courses are emergency medicine, neurology, surgical subspecialties, physical medicine and rehabilitation, and an acting internship, all of which bring together the ethical, legal, and social factors that are part of total patient care. Sixteen weeks of electives are available.

An ongoing curriculum renewal process is aimed at achieving an organ-system approach in the preclinical years and strengthening clinical and professional skills in the clinical years.

REQUIREMENTS FOR ENTRANCE

The MCAT and a minimum of three years of college (90 credit hours) are required. Three-year applicants with good credentials are encouraged to apply.

The minimum requirements are:

	Sem. hrs.
Biology or zoology (with lab)	8
Course work must be exclusive of botany and invertebrate zoology.	
Organic chemistry (with lab)	8
Other chemistry (with lab)	8
Inorganic, physical, analytical chemistry or biochemistry will satisfy the requirement.	
General physics (with lab)	8
English	6

A course in mathematics is recommended but not required.

Specific requirements may be waived or imposed at the discretion of the Admissions Committee in any individual case.

The Admissions Committee urges all candidates to prepare themselves further by completing courses in social or cultural fields and generally broadening their academic backgrounds. Candidates who are not premedical or science majors are given equal consideration if they have demonstrated academic excellence in the course requirements listed above.

New Jersey Medical School offers a limited number of Academic Excellence Scholarships for entering first-year students.

Available combined degree programs are: M.D.-Ph.D., M.D.-J.D., M.D.-M.P.H., and M.D.-M.B.A.

SELECTION FACTORS

Students are selected on the basis of scholastic achievement, fitness, and aptitude for the study of medicine, and other personal qualifications. Since success in medicine depends on a number of related factors in a student's development, of which scholastic accomplishments are only a part, the Admissions Committee also gives consideration to the use of language, special aptitudes, mechanical skill, stamina, perseverance, and motivation.

New Jersey Medical School applies no GPA or MCAT cutoff levels in its selection process. It must be remembered, however, that competition is very keen, and applicants who are high in all determinable categories often receive the highest priority for acceptance. There are no restrictions as to race, creed, sex, national origin, age, or handicap.

Accepted students in the 1999 entering class had the following profile: *average* GPA, 3.49; *gender,* 47 percent women; *residence,* 11 nonresidents; *minorities,* 28 students.

Applications from nonresidents are accepted.

The UMDNJ policy is that no program or activity administered by the University shall exclude from participation, admission, treatment or employment, or deny benefits to, or subject to discrimination any qualified individual solely by reason of his or her disability.

FINANCIAL AID

No questions of financial need are involved in the selection of students. All students who are accepted and wish to matriculate are advised to contact the financial aid officer immediately to discuss aid and fill out all necessary forms. All aid is given on the basis of financial need as assessed by an outside source. The needs analysis is usually adjusted upward to reflect costs in the northeastern United States. Approximately 70 percent of the students receive some form of financial aid. The Financial Aid Office extends itself to help all students in financial need.

INFORMATION FOR MINORITY STUDENTS

NJMS has a long-standing strong commitment to the recruitment of minority applicants. A special summer program is open to economically and educationally disadvantaged students who have been accepted, as well as to others in various stages of their undergraduate careers. Information is available from Lonnie Wright, Director of the Students for Medicine and Dentistry Program, at (973) 972-5433 or James Foster, Assistant Dean for Student Affairs, at (973) 972-5431.

SPECIAL RECOGNITION

NJMS is proud to have received the 1994 Outstanding Community Service Award by the AAMC. This award acknowledges the extensive community service programs developed by NJMS.

Public Institution

APPLICATION AND ACCEPTANCE POLICIES FOR 2000–2001 FIRST-YEAR CLASS

School participates in AMCAS. See Chapter 6.

Filing of AMCAS application
- Earliest date: June 1, 2000
- Latest date: Dec. 1, 2000

School application fee to all applicants: $75
Will accept MCAT scores from any year
Does have Early Decision Program (EDP)
- For exceptional New Jersey residents only
- EDP application period: June 1–Aug. 1, 2000
- EDP applicants notified by: Oct. 1, 2000

Acceptance notice to regular applicants
- Earliest date: Oct. 15, 2000
- Latest date: Until class is filled

Applicant's response to acceptance offer
- Maximum time: 2 weeks

Requests for deferred entrance considered: Yes
Deposit to hold place in class (applied to tuition):
- $100, due with response to acceptance offer

Deposit refundable prior to: May 15, 2001
Estimated number of new entrants: 170 (3 EDP)
Starting date: Aug. 2001

TUITION AND STUDENT FEES PER YEAR FOR 1999–2000 FIRST-YEAR CLASS

Tuition
- Resident: $16,052
- Nonresident: $25,119

Student fees: $1,122

INFORMATION ON 1999–2000 FIRST-YEAR CLASS

Number of	*In-State*	*Out-of-State*	*Total*
Applicants	1,023	1,721	2,744
Applicants Interviewed	589	154	743
New Entrants*	159	11	170

*All took the MCAT; 89% had baccalaureate degrees.

CHAPTER 11

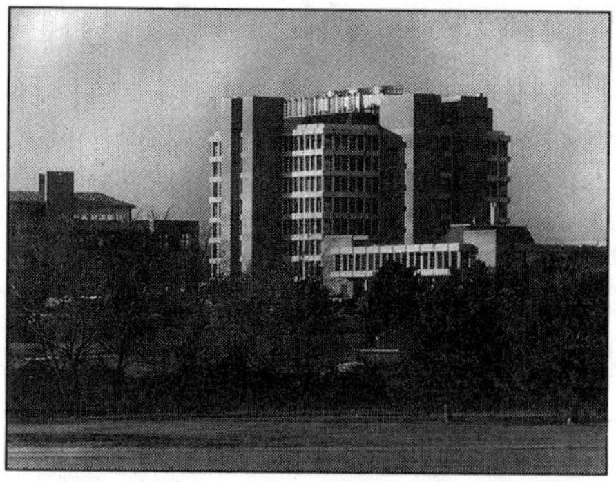

University of Medicine and Dentistry of New Jersey Robert Wood Johnson Medical School

Piscataway, New Jersey

Dr. Harold L. Paz, *Dean*
Dr. David Seiden, *Associate Dean for Admissions and Student Affairs*
Paul D. Koch, *Associate Director of Financial Aid*

ADDRESS INQUIRIES TO:

Office of Admissions
UMDNJ—Robert Wood Johnson Medical School
675 Hoes Lane
Piscataway, New Jersey 08854-5635
(732) 235-4576; 235-5078 (FAX)
Web Site: http://www2.umdnj.edu/rwjms.html

GENERAL INFORMATION

Robert Wood Johnson Medical School, formerly known as Rutgers Medical School, was named after the former president and chairman of the board of Johnson & Johnson Company and the benefactor of the Robert Wood Johnson Foundation.

The Basic Science Building is located adjacent to the science campus of Rutgers University. University Behavorial Healthcare, which houses the Department of Psychiatry, adjoins the building. Facilities shared with Rutgers University include the Library of Science and Medicine, the Center for Advanced Biotechnology and Medicine, and the Environmental and Occupational Health Science Institute.

Robert Wood Johnson University Hospital is the core teaching hospital in New Brunswick. Cooper Hospital/University Medical Center is the core teaching hospital in Camden. These two centers, supplemented by affiliations with community hospitals in central New Jersey, provide the Medical School with a full complement of diverse clinical training facilities.

The Medical School has a division at Camden. Separate applications are not required. All students receive their basic education at the Piscataway campus. Students who matriculate in the Camden program receive their clinical education at the Camden campus.

CURRICULUM

The curriculum is newly revised. It provides for an early introduction to patient care, an integration of clinical skills into the preclinical curriculum, and the opportunity for self-directed learning within the context of a rigorous basic science education during the first two years. Multiple learning modalities are used including lectures, laboratory exercises, small-group discussions, and computer-assisted instruction. During the first two years, in addition to the traditional basic sciences, there are courses in ethics, introduction to the patient, case-based learning, clinical prevention, clinical pathophysiology, human genetics, and community and environmental medicine, among others. The third-year curriculum consists of an introduction to the clinical experience followed by six eight-week clerkships in medicine, surgery, family medicine, psychiatry, obstetrics-gynecology, and pediatrics. There is also a formative clinical skills assessment at the beginning of the third year, with a summative clinical skills assessment at the end of the year. The fourth-year curriculum includes an advanced clerkship in ambulatory medicine, an advanced clerkship in surgery, neurology, a subinternship, and a minimum of 16 weeks of electives. Grades are reported as honors, high pass, pass, low pass, and fail. Students must pass USMLE Step 1 prior to completing the third year and must pass USMLE Step 2 prior to graduation.

In conjunction with the School of Public Health, a combined M.D.-M.P.H. program is available. Combined M.D.-Ph.D. programs are available in the medical school and in conjunction with Rutgers University. Financial support that includes both tuition remission and stipends is available throughout the seven-year program. A new combined M.D.-J.D. program, in conjunction with Rutgers Law School; a combined M.D.-M.S. in Jurisprudence, in conjunction with Seton Hall Law School; a combined M.D.-M.S. in Medical Informatics, in conjunction with the New Jersey Institute of Technology; and a combined M.D.-M.B.A. in conjunction with Rutgers School of Management are also available.

REQUIREMENTS FOR ENTRANCE

The MCAT and a minimum of three years of college consisting of 90 semester hours of college work (exclusive of military and physical education) are required. The MCAT must be taken within the four years preceding application and no later than the fall of the year of application. The following undergraduate courses are required:

	Semesters
Biology or zoology (with lab)	2
Inorganic chemistry (with lab)	2
Organic chemistry (with lab)	2
Physics (with lab)	2
College mathematics	1
English	2

Must include one semester of a college writing course. College-approved "writing intensive courses" may substitute for English.

Robert Wood Johnson Medical School places high value on a balanced undergraduate education. While this balance will vary with the background and interests of the individual, it is expected that applicants will have exposed themselves to course work in the humanities, the behavioral sciences, and liberal arts as well as the premedical sciences. In addition, applicants may be asked to demonstrate competence in written English.

Students capable of superior performance in any academic field, whether in the sciences or humanities, should feel free to pursue their intellectual interests in depth, provided only that they can do well in the required courses mentioned above. The Admissions Committee may waive or impose specific requirements at its discretion. Applicants must be U.S. citizens or permanent residents to be eligible for admission.

SELECTION FACTORS

Preference for admission is given to bona fide residents of New Jersey. While no set number exists, the school accepts some students from outside New Jersey. Competition in this category is keen.

Admission is determined on the basis of academic achievement in a balanced undergraduate education, results of the MCAT, preprofessional committee evaluations, other recommendations, character, motivation, and personal interview. Applications from qualified members of racial minority groups are encouraged. Interviews are arranged by invitation.

Accepted students for the 1999 entering class had a *mean GPA* of 3.59 (10 percentile-3.24, 90 percentile-3.91). Women represented 44 percent of the class.

FINANCIAL AID

Accepted students who believe they will need financial aid are encouraged to request information and application forms from the Financial Aid Office. About 80 percent of the student body received some sort of financial assistance during the 1998–99 academic year. Financial aid is awarded on the basis of evaluated need computed by an approved needs analysis method. All awards consist of a package of loans and grants when funds are available. Funds have been allocated for freshman scholarships, which are renewable annually.

INFORMATION FOR MINORITY STUDENTS

UMDNJ—Robert Wood Johnson Medical School is committed to the education and training of minority physicians. Applications from both in-state and out-of-state candidates are welcome, and ample financial aid assistance is offered. Numerous support services are available, including a preenrollment summer program for accepted students. A summer Biomedical Careers Program for undergraduates interested in health care careers is also offered. Further information is available from Betty Treadwell-Oglesby.

Public Institution

APPLICATION AND ACCEPTANCE POLICIES FOR 2001–2002 FIRST-YEAR CLASS

School participates in AMCAS. See Chapter 6.

Filing of AMCAS application
- Earliest date: June 1, 2000
- Latest date: Dec. 1, 2000

School application fee to all applicants: $75
Oldest MCAT scores considered: 1996
Does have Early Decision Program (EDP)
- EDP application period: June 1–Aug. 1, 2000
- EDP applicants notified by: Oct. 1, 2000

Acceptance notice to regular applicants
- Earliest date: Nov. 15, 2000
- Latest date: Until class is filled

Applicant's response to acceptance offer
- Maximum time: 2 weeks

Requests for deferred entrance considered: Yes
Deposit to hold place in class (applied to tuition):
- $50, due with response to acceptance offer

Deposit refundable prior to: May 15, 2001
Estimated number of new entrants: 142 (5 EDP)
Starting date: Aug. 2001

TUITION AND STUDENT FEES PER YEAR FOR 1999–2000 FIRST-YEAR CLASS

Tuition
- Resident: $16,052
- Nonresident: $25,119

Student fees: $1,187

INFORMATION ON 1999–2000 FIRST-YEAR CLASS

Number of	*In-State*	*Out-of-State*	*Total*
Applicants	1,044	1,427	2,471
Applicants Interviewed	548	161	709
New Entrants*	124	19	143

*All took the MCAT and had baccalaureate degrees.

CHAPTER 11

University of New Mexico School of Medicine

Albuquerque, New Mexico

Dr. Paul B. Roth, *Dean*
Dr. Roger J. Radloff, *Interim Assistant Dean for Admissions*

ADDRESS INQUIRIES TO:

Office of Admissions and Student Affairs
University of New Mexico
School of Medicine
Basic Medical Sciences Building, Room 107
Albuquerque, New Mexico 87131-5166
(505) 272-4766; 272-8239 (FAX)
Web Site: http://hsc.unm.edu/som/admiss

MISSION STATEMENT

The mission of the University of New Mexico School of Medicine is to educate physicians, scientists, and allied health professionals through the transmission of biomedical knowledge acquired from research and patient care. The school is dedicated to the creation, evaluation, transmission, and application of biomedical knowledge to be applied directly for the improvement of the health of the public. Our primary focus is on the unique health needs of New Mexico's culturally and ethnically diverse populations. The environment in which we work recognizes and respects all who make up the community and those we serve.

GENERAL INFORMATION

The establishment of a school of the basic medical sciences was authorized by the regents and the faculty of the University of New Mexico (UNM) in 1961. The first entering class of 24 students was enrolled in September 1964, and progress to the full four-year program was approved by the New Mexico State Legislature in 1966.

The medical school facilities are located on the north campus of the university and include a basic medical sciences building, biomedical research facility, medical center library, UNM Mental Health Center, UNM Children's Psychiatric Hospital, family practice center, Center for Non-Invasive Diagnosis, and an international cancer center. The 421-bed University of New Mexico Hospital serves as the major teaching hospital of the medical school, with additional teaching at the 257-bed Regional Federal Medical Center in Albuquerque. The faculty numbers 623, with 540 full-time appointments.

The School of Medicine is a professional and graduate school of the university. In addition to providing education in the basic and clinical sciences for the doctor of medicine degree, opportunities are available for work leading to a doctor of philosophy degree. Medical education at the resident and postgraduate levels is offered through the university's teaching hospitals.

CURRICULUM

The University of New Mexico School of Medicine implemented a new curriculum in the fall of 1993, which incorporated aspects of its prior educational innovations from the Conventional Curriculum Track, Primary Care Curriculum, and Health of the Public Program.

The goals of the new curriculum are to graduate physicians who: are excited and enthusiastic about learning; have assumed a major responsibility for their continued learning; have the ability to define problems, formulate questions, and carry out scholarly inquiry; are skilled in self and peer assessment; have a broad perspective on the importance of human biology, behavior, environment, culture and social setting, in the health of individuals and of populations.

Educational innovations include the following: the integration of the basic and clinical sciences throughout undergraduate medical education, early clinical skills training and community-based learning, the incorporation of a population and behavioral perspective into the clinical years, and peer teaching and computer-assisted instruction.

Student assessment will value mastery of knowledge, writing skills, critical appraisal, interpersonal and clinical skills, teaching ability, and peer and self-assessment. Assessment will be competency-based and cumulative.

REQUIREMENTS FOR ENTRANCE

The MCAT and three years of college are required. A college program leading to the bachelor's degree from an accredited college of arts and sciences is ordinarily recommended.

Minimum course requirements are:

	Sem. hrs.
General biology (with lab)	8
General or inorganic chemistry (with lab)	8
Organic chemistry (with lab)	8
General physics	6
Biochemistry	3

The following courses are strongly recommended: calculus, anatomy, physiology, microbiology, and Spanish.

SELECTION FACTORS

All applicants for first-year positions must apply through AMCAS. All New Mexico applicants will be sent additional application materials upon receipt of their application from AMCAS. Nonregional applicants, including WICHE and former New Mexico residents, must apply through the Early Decision Program to receive any consideration for admission. Those who pass an initial screening process will be sent full application materials and invited for interviews.

Selection is based upon scholastic achievement, performance on the MCAT, personal interviews with members of the Admissions Committee, and recommendations of a college professional advisory committee. The University of New Mexico is committed to providing equal educational and employment opportunities regardless of sex, marital or parental status, race, religion, age, or physical handicap. Preference is given to residents of New Mexico and next to applicants who are residents of western states that participate in the WICHE program.

To guide applicants in considering application to the School of Medicine, the following information is provided on the 1999 applicant pool: 1,080 total applicants, 98 accepted, 73 matriculated; 329 New Mexico applicants, 96 accepted, 71 matriculated; 22 WICHE applicants, 1 accepted, 1 matriculated; 729 nonregional applicants, 1 accepted, 1 matriculated. Some characteristics of the 1999 entering class were *average GPA*, 3.62 (96 percent above 3.0); *average MCAT* 9.2; sex, 53 percent *women*; *ethnic minorities*, 33 percent. All students offered acceptance were interviewed at this school.

TRANSFER

Applications for transfer into Phase II (years 3 and 4) will be considered from New Mexico and WICHE residents in Liaison Committee on Medical Education approved four-year U.S. medical and American Osteopathic Association approved osteopathic schools. New Mexico and WICHE residents in approved World Health Organization foreign schools who have completed the equivalent of the first two years of basic science course work will also be considered for transfer. Applicants will be accepted on a space-available basis, and all acceptances will be contingent upon passing the USMLE, Step 1. Criteria for acceptance will be based on medical school academic performance, residency considerations, and a compelling need to transfer to this school.

FINANCIAL AID

The school makes available financial aid in the form of loans and scholarships to those students with demonstrated financial need. The amount of award varies according to the student's need and the level of funding available. A short-term, no-interest loan fund is available to all students in need of immediate financial help. The Student Affairs Office assists all students in locating necessary funds to support their medical education.

INFORMATION FOR MINORITY STUDENTS

The School of Medicine is committed to the recruitment, selection, and retention of qualified Black and Hispanic residents of New Mexico and American Indian residents of New Mexico and the Navajo Nation. The Office of Cultural and Ethnic Programs, directed by Dr. Roberto Gomez, offers several programs to support the above commitment. Additional information may be obtained by contacting the Office of Cultural and Ethnic Programs at (505) 272-2728.

Public Institution

APPLICATION AND ACCEPTANCE POLICIES FOR 2001–2002 FIRST-YEAR CLASS

School participates in AMCAS. See Chapter 6.

Filing of AMCAS application
Earliest date: June 1, 2000
Latest date: Nov. 15, 2000
School application fee after screening: $50
Oldest MCAT scores considered: 1991
Does have Early Decision Program
Nonresidents must apply through EDP
EDP application period: June 1–Aug. 1, 2000
EDP applicants notified by: Oct. 1, 2000
Acceptance notice to regular applicants
Earliest date: March 15, 2001
Latest date: Varies
Applicant's response to acceptance offer
Maximum time: 4 weeks
Requests for deferred entrance considered: Yes
Deposit to hold place in class: None
Estimated number of new entrants: 73 (30 EDP)
Starting date: Aug. 2001

TUITION AND STUDENT FEES PER YEAR FOR 1999–2000 FIRST-YEAR CLASS

Tuition
Resident: $7,126
Nonresident: $20,429

Student fees: $1,270

INFORMATION ON 1999–2000 FIRST-YEAR CLASS

Number of	*In-State*	*Out-of-State*	*Total*
Applicants	329	751	1,080
Applicants Interviewed	311	4	315
New Entrants*	71	2	73

*All took the MCAT and had baccalaureate degrees.

CHAPTER 11

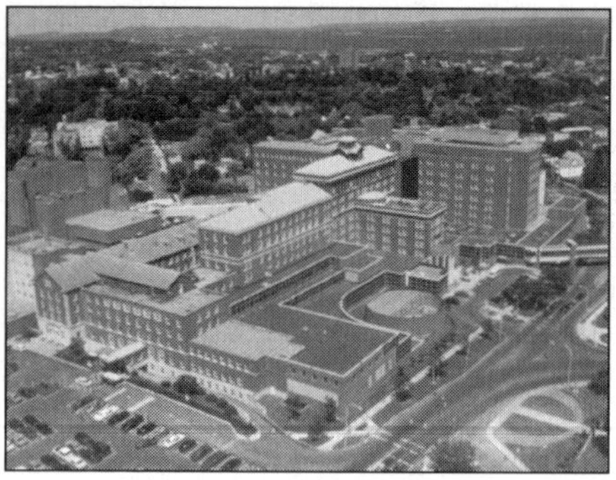

Albany Medical College

Albany, New York

Dr. James Mandell, *Dean*
Sara J. Kremer, *Assistant Dean of Admissions and Records*
Tor Shekerjian, *Assistant Dean of Academic and Student Services*

ADDRESS INQUIRIES TO:

Office of Admissions, Mail Code 3
Albany Medical College
47 New Scotland Avenue
Albany, New York 12208
(518) 262-5521; 262-5887 (FAX)
Web Site: http://www.amc.edu

MISSION STATEMENT

The goal of the admissions process is to recruit, select, and enroll a class of students who have the potential to develop into excellent physicians. Excellence is broadly defined as pertaining to a range of competencies that will enable physicians to meet the needs of the "total patient" and to contribute in constructive and important ways to the profession of medicine and health care systems.

Therefore, we seek students who are academically qualified and exhibit high moral character, demonstrate the potential for professional growth and development, and can make significant and unique contributions to the Albany Medical College community and to medical science and clinical practice. Accordingly, the ideal candidate for admission will hold clear promise of developing competencies in all dimensions of patient care, including scientific, technical, psychosocial, interpersonal, and ethical.

GENERAL INFORMATION

Founded in 1839, the Albany Medical College is one of the oldest medical schools in the country. The college is coeducational, nondenominational, and privately supported.

The college buildings and those of the 650-bed Albany Medical Center Hospital are physically joined in one large complex that comprises Albany Medical Center. The hospital is both a community hospital for people of the immediate area and a tertiary diagnostic and treatment center for over two million residents of eastern New York and western New England. Additional clinical facilities are provided by the Albany Veterans Administration Medical Center, the Capital District Psychiatric Center, and other affiliated hospitals located nearby.

CURRICULUM

The Albany Medical College implemented a new curriculum in 1993. Basic and clinical sciences are integrated into themes (primarily organ systems) stressing normal function in Year 1 and pathological function in Year 2. All four years of school offer three themes that include clinical skills, ethical and health systems issues, and evidence-based medicine. In every theme, students receive exposure to clinical presentations. These begin with the development of patient interviewing skills at the start of Year 1, and by year's end have included clinical exposure in the ICU, the neonatal units, and the cardiac operating rooms. First-year students spend an afternoon in a nursing home learning to interview the elderly. Basic science seminars reinforce the importance of the basic sciences in years 3 and 4. Emphasis is placed on primary care throughout the four years, with an increased emphasis on care in ambulatory settings in the clinical rotations of Year 3. Year 4 emphasizes specialty care in some required rotations. Elective rotations are available in Year 4 at Albany Medical Center Hospital, other affiliated hospitals, and at other institutions in the United States and abroad. Senior students may plan programs with their advisors that provide opportunities to explore career possibilities.

SPECIAL PROGRAMS

The Albany Medical College provides various pathways for admission including several combined-degree programs offered conjointly with Rensselaer Polytechnic Institute, Union College, and Siena College. Information on these programs is included in Chapter 10.

REQUIREMENTS FOR ENTRANCE

Applicants for admission must have completed at least three years of study at an accredited college preferably in the United States or Canada. Most students admitted, however, will have earned the bachelor's degree.

Minimal course requirements for admission are:

	Sem./Qtr. hrs.
Biology or zoology (with lab)	6/9
Inorganic chemistry (with lab)	6/9
Organic chemistry (with lab)	6/9
General physics (with lab)	6/9

Proficiency in oral and written English is required.

When achievement in the required science courses is less than optimum, the desirability of augmenting the minimum requirements with additional experience in the fields of chemistry, embryology, genetics, and mathematics should be considered. On the other hand, ideally a physician's education should also rest on a base of general knowledge that includes a broad liberal arts education. Accordingly, students who have majored in the arts or humanities are considered on an equal basis with those who have majored in the sciences, provided that these students have demonstrated good capability in the required science studies.

The MCAT is also required and must be taken no later than the fall one year prior to the intended date of matriculation.

SELECTION FACTORS

In selecting students, emphasis is placed upon integrity, character, academic achievement, motivation, emotional stability, and social and intellectual suitability. The Albany Medical College is committed to the belief that educational opportunities should be available to all eligible persons without regard to race, creed, age, sex, religion, marital status, handicap, or national origin. Admission is not restricted to New York State residents. Although preference is usually given to U.S. citizens, the committee will from time to time admit outstanding applicants who are citizens of other countries.

For the 1999 entering class, all matriculants had a *mean cumulative GPA* of 3.4.

All applications are reviewed in the order in which they are received and are given equal consideration. Applications are individually reviewed by admissions committee members, who are looking for qualities other than, and in addition to, the MCAT scores and GPA. Invitations for interview are made at the discretion of the Committee and all interviews are conducted on campus. Preapplication inquiries or questions from applicants concerning the status of their applications are welcome at any time.

A transfer admission program is no longer offered.

FINANCIAL AID

The college attempts to assist all students by locating and awarding scholarship and loan assistance, as well as through guidance in employment. Eighty-four percent of the student body receive some scholarship and/or loan assistance. An announcement regarding applying for financial assistance is distributed to all students by December 15 for the following academic year. Awards of scholarship and loan assistance begin in April by the Financial Aid office. Scholarships are awarded until the funds are depleted. Additional or new requests for financial assistance in the form of loans are accepted throughout the year. In the Albany Medical Center there are opportunities for part-time employment for students through a federally funded work-study program. International students, who are not U.S. citizens or eligible non-citizens, must make their own financial arrangements to attend the school.

INFORMATION FOR MINORITY STUDENTS

The Office of Minority Affairs is actively involved in the recruitment and retention of qualified minority applicants. We also host a high school program for promising junior high and high school students.

Because of our firm commitment to educating and graduating minority students, guidance is offered to minority students from the application stage forward. The Minority Affairs Director is available for counseling and assistance at any time. Our Admissions Committee is sensitized to important factors in the selection of minority students. Albany Medical College has graduated an impressive number of minority students who are practicing in a wide variety of specialties across the nation.

Albany Medical College maintains a Minority Scholarship fund and an endowed scholarship fund. Minority students who meet the eligibility criteria are awarded grants from this fund. There are a limited number of institution and donated scholarships available.

This office also coordinates academic, social, and cultural support services for minority students. More information may be obtained by contacting the Office of Minority Affairs: telephone (518) 262-5824.

Private Institution

APPLICATION AND ACCEPTANCE POLICIES FOR 2001–2002 FIRST-YEAR CLASS

School participates in AMCAS. See Chapter 6.

Filing of AMCAS application
  Earliest date: June 1, 2000
  Latest date: Nov. 15, 2000
School application fee to all applicants: $75
Oldest MCAT scores considered: 1996
Does not have Early Decision Program
Acceptance notice to regular applicants
  Earliest date: Oct. 15, 2000
  Latest date: Until class is filled
Applicant's response to acceptance offer
  Maximum time: 2 weeks
Requests for deferred entrance considered: Yes
Deposit to hold place in class (applied to tuition):
  $100, due with response to acceptance offer
Deposit refundable prior to: May 15, 2001
Estimated number of new entrants: 128
Starting date: Aug. 2001

TUITION AND STUDENT FEES PER YEAR FOR 1999–2000 FIRST-YEAR CLASS

Tuition: $30,797 Student fees: None

INFORMATION ON 1999–2000 FIRST-YEAR CLASS

Number of	*In-State*	*Out-of-State*	*Total*
Applicants	1,666	5,364	7,030
Applicants Interviewed	182	453	635
New Entrants*			
(Regular Program)	21	64	85
(Special Programs and deferred)	22	17	39

*69% took the MCAT; 76% had baccalaureate degrees.

(NOTE: Students applying through AMCAS must take the MCAT; those matriculating through Albany's accelerated program have not earned their baccalaureate degree and are not required to take the MCAT prior to enrolling.)

CHAPTER 11

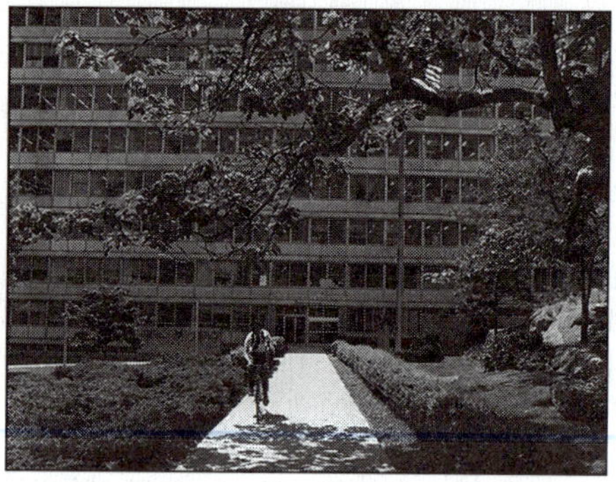

Albert Einstein College of Medicine of Yeshiva University

Bronx, New York

Dr. Dominick P. Purpura, *Dean*
Noreen Kerrigan, *Assistant Dean for Student Admissions*
Lloyd Greenberg, *Financial Aid Officer*

ADDRESS INQUIRIES TO:

Office of Admissions
Albert Einstein College of Medicine
of Yeshiva University
Jack and Pearl Resnick Campus
1300 Morris Park Avenue
Bronx, New York 10461
(718) 430-2106; 430-8825 (FAX)
E-mail: admissions@aecom.yu.edu
Web Site: http://www.aecom.yu.edu

MISSION STATEMENT

To conduct educational programs of the highest quality in the biomedical and clinical sciences. To conduct fundamental biomedical and clinical research related to health and disease and health policy. To maintain excellent patient care in association with the education and training of medical students and postgraduate physicians. To conduct collaborative educational, research, and training programs with affiliated institutions. To provide, sustain, and improve health care in our community. To encourage widespread participation in the evolution of public policy in biomedical science, education, and health care.

GENERAL INFORMATION

The Albert Einstein College of Medicine is a privately endowed, coeducational, and nondenominational institution situated on a 17-acre site in a residential area of the northeast Bronx. Clinical education takes place in affiliated acute care hospitals, long-term care and skilled nursing facilities, hospices, and neighborhood health centers that serve the health care needs of a very diverse population of patients in the boroughs of the Bronx, Queens, and Manhattan. These institutions include Jacobi Medical Center, which is a municipal hospital, and four private voluntary hospitals—Beth Israel Medical Center, Montefiore Medical Center, Bronx Lebanon Hospital Center, and Long Island Jewish Medical Center. In addition to these clinical sites, there are extensive facilities devoted to biomedical research and teaching.

Apartments for students are located on and close to the campus, and a recreational sports center with a swimming pool is located on the grounds of the main apartment building complex.

CURRICULUM

Students in the first two years participate in an innovative interdisciplinary series of biomedical science courses in which there are abundant opportunities for self-directed learning and application of basic science knowledge to clinical problems. Two new interdisciplinary courses are Molecular and Cellular Foundations of Medicine and Nervous System and Human Behavior, both of which exemplify our attempts to integrate basic science disciplines with each other and with the clinical sciences. Running parallel to the biomedical science courses is the Introduction to Clinical Medicine program in which students encounter patients in various hospital and non-hospital settings, learn and practice the basic skills of communication and the clinical examination, and discuss psychosociocultural and ethical aspects of the doctor-patient relationship in small-group conferences. A one-year period of clerkship rotations in the third year enables students to acquire clinical skills and knowledge while working with patients at various health care sites in inpatient and outpatient settings. The senior year provides extensive experience in ambulatory care as well as additional responsibilities for the care of hospitalized patients during a subinternship. Special senior elective opportunities include overseas exchange programs, international health fellowships, and a research program that leads to the M.D. degree with distinction in the student's research discipline. Evaluation of performance is on a pass/fail basis in Year 1, supplemented by honors in Year 2 and further supplemented by detailed narrative reports in clinical courses.

A fully funded M.D.-Ph.D. program is offered to students in the first year; several students may also be selected at the end of the second year. It is a requirement that all students pursue an in-depth study of an area of interest and prepare a written, referenced report of scholarly substance prior to graduation. A generalist mentorship program has been established to meet the particular needs of students with career interests in generalist disciplines.

Tutoring in most basic science courses is available, and individual counseling is provided to students in need of long-term assistance to assure retention.

REQUIREMENTS FOR ENTRANCE

The MCAT and a minimum of three years of full-time undergraduate study are required; four years are preferred. The minimum course requirements are:

	Sem. hrs.
Biology (with lab)	8
General chemistry (with lab)	8
Organic chemistry (with lab)	8
Physics (with lab)	8
College mathematics (May include statistics and computer science)	6
English	6

The undergraduate major is not an important selection factor, and the scholarly pursuit of a broad liberal arts education, including the study of humanities and social sciences, is strongly recommended.

Applicants should provide evidence of participation in intra- or extramural activities that serve to enhance one's communication and interpersonal skills. Such activities may include tutoring, counseling, and community service, as well as experience in the health care system.

SELECTION FACTORS

Students are carefully selected on the basis of academic performance, letters of recommendation, MCAT scores, potential for professional achievement, and motivation and evidence of other personal qualities deemed essential for the study and practice of medicine. Letters of recommendation from commercial educational consultants will not be considered. Applicants are considered without regard to race, age, sex, religion, national origin, state of residence, or physical handicap. Students who do not gain admission are discouraged from reapplying the subsequent year or until such time as they can present new data to warrant a more favorable decision.

Foreign nationals may apply for admission; however, because they are ineligible for federal loan programs, it is their responsibility to secure private funding for tuition. The 1999 entering class represented 22 states, 75 undergraduate colleges, and is 54 percent female; 45 percent of the entering class had a total undergraduate GPA of at least 3.70; the range, however, is broad. Receipt of the application will be acknowledged, and the applicant will be requested to submit letters of recommendation and the college application fee. A decision regarding a formal interview is made upon receipt of all supporting documents. Interviews are required of all applicants under serious consideration.

FINANCIAL AID

Every attempt is made to assist students and their families in meeting both their financial obligations to the college and the student's essential personal needs. Financial status is not a determinant in selecting among qualified applicants. Awards and loans from the college are available after all other means of financial assistance have been exhausted. Financial aid applications are available only after acceptance. Advice on financial assistance and applications is available from the Student Finance Office. About 50 percent of the students receive institutional loans and/or scholarships, and about 75 percent of them qualify for outside loans and/or grants.

The application fee may be waived upon written request from the financial aid officer of the undergraduate college. It may be waived also upon a written request from the applicant after a fee waiver from AMCAS has been granted.

INFORMATION FOR MINORITY STUDENTS

The College of Medicine is actively seeking and welcomes applications from minority students. The college's Office of Minority Student Affairs provides abundant opportunities for medical students to participate in special programs for high school and college students.

Private Institution

APPLICATION AND ACCEPTANCE POLICIES FOR 2001–2002 FIRST-YEAR CLASS

School participates in AMCAS. See Chapter 6.

Filing of AMCAS application
  Earliest date: June 1, 2000
  Latest date: Nov. 1, 2000
School application fee to all applicants: $85
Oldest MCAT scores considered: 1997
Does have Early Decision Program (EDP)
  EDP application period: June 1–Aug. 1, 2000
  EDP applicants notified by: Oct. 1, 2000
Acceptance notice to regular applicants
  Earliest date: Jan. 15, 2001
  Latest date: Until class is filled
Applicant's response to acceptance offer
  Maximum time: 2 weeks until May 1, 2001
    1 week thereafter
Requests for deferred entrance considered: Yes
Deposit to hold place in class (applied to tuition):
  $100, due with response to acceptance offer
Deposit refundable prior to: June 1, 2001
Estimated number of new entrants: 180 (Varies EDP)
Starting date: Aug. 2001

TUITION AND STUDENT FEES PER YEAR FOR 1999–2000 FIRST-YEAR CLASS

Tuition: $28,650 Student fees: $1,700

INFORMATION ON 1999–2000 FIRST-YEAR CLASS

Number of	*In-State*	*Out-of-State*	*Total*
Applicants	1,671	5,371	7,042
Applicants Interviewed	482	1,025	1,507
New Entrants*	80	101	181

*All took the MCAT and had baccalaureate degrees.

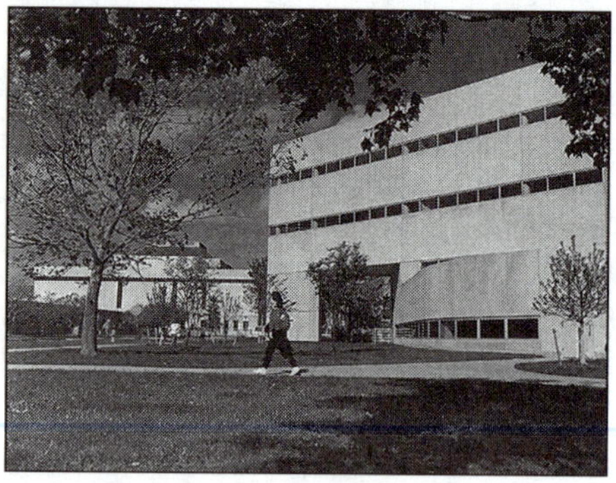

University at Buffalo School of Medicine and Biomedical Sciences

Buffalo, New York

Dr. John R.Wright, *Dean*
Dr. Thomas J. Guttuso, *Assistant Dean, Admissions*
Elias G. Eldayrie, *Director, Student Finances and Records*

ADDRESS INQUIRIES TO:

Office of Medical Admissions
University at Buffalo
45 Biomedical Education Building
Buffalo, New York 14214-3013
(716) 829-3466; 829-3849 (FAX)
E-mail: jjrosso@acsu.buffalo.edu
Web Site: http://www.smbs.buffalo.edu/ome

MISSION STATEMENT

- To provide well-trained physicians and other health care professionals who will attend to the health needs of citizens.
- To offer a source of continuing education to the community of health care providers, and
- To provide a center of research and scholarship that will advance and promote health-related services.

As a public institution, the mission places particular emphasis on diversity, inclusion, and the special needs of New York State such as generalist education, minority recruitment and retention, and the underserved urban and rural health populations.

GENERAL INFORMATION

The School of Medicine was founded by Millard Fillmore and a group of physicians in 1846. It was a privately supported school until the University of Buffalo joined the State University of New York (SUNY) system in 1962. The University at Buffalo has the most comprehensive campus in the SUNY system and was honored in 1989 with election to the Association of American Universities. The preclinical campus and library are located on the Main Street Campus at the northeastern corner of the city. The clinical education program is conducted in cooperation with nine area hospitals.

CURRICULUM

The curriculum is designed to emphasize the relevance of medical education to the practice of medicine, demonstrate the relevance of basic science to clinical practice, introduce patient contact and patient-centered learning in the first year of medical school, and increase the experience in ambulatory care in the clinical years. Innovative new courses, including Introduction to Clinical Medicine and Interdisciplinary Medicine, will be taught throughout the first two years and are designed to prepare students in the knowledge, skills, and attitudes required to successfully enter the clinical clerkships in the third year and provide the foundation for their medical careers. Ethics, the doctor-patient relationship, principles of health promotion, disease prevention, and promotion of self-learning and inquiry are emphasized, in addition to extensive education in the skills basic to medical practice and patient care. All students must pass Step I of the USMLE within three attempts before being allowed to matriculate in the clinical years. The clinical years include required clerkships in internal medicine, surgery, pediatrics, obstetrics and gynecology, psychiatry, neurology, family medicine, primary ambulatory care, and surgical specialties. There is ample free time in the senior year for electives here or away. UB's goal is to prepare its graduates to enter and complete graduate education, qualify for licensure, provide excellence in medical care, and have the educational background for continued learning.

REQUIREMENTS FOR ENTRANCE

The MCAT is required and should be taken no later than the fall of the year preceding admission. A bachelor's degree from an approved college or university is desired. The following minimal premedical course requirements must be completed prior to enrollment:

	Semesters
Biology (with lab)	2
With not more than one semester of botany.	
General Chemistry (with lab)	2
Organic Chemistry (with lab)	2
General physics	2
English	2

The choice of undergraduate concentration is optional. The prerequisites for admission reflect the need for a basic preparation in the sciences and are meant to encourage the student to develop a foundation in the social sciences and the humanities.

The Medical Scientist Training Program (MSTP) is a seven- to eight-year program designed for preparation for careers in biomedical sciences and combines the training for both the M.D. and Ph.D. degrees. Interested applicants should request an application from the MSTP Office, University at Buffalo, 143 Cary Hall, Buffalo, NY 14214; (716) 829-3236.

EARLY ASSURANCE PROGRAM

Undergraduate sophomores can apply to this program if they have demonstrated a high level of academic competence by attaining around a 3.5 GPA in science and nonscience courses and have completed at least half of the premedical course requirements. Minorities with a competitive record are especially encouraged to apply. Application deadline is February 1, 2001. Submission of SAT scores is required. Accepted candidates are not required to take the MCAT, are encouraged to pursue their intellectual interests in their remaining college years, and will commence their medical education in August 2003. Approximately 30 are accepted each year.

SELECTION FACTORS

The Admissions Committee seeks to identify and select students who display favorable qualities deemed important for the pursuit of a career in medicine. In making its assessments and determinations, the committee relies on information contained in the application and in documents submitted in support of the applicant. Based on careful screening, applicants are invited to appear for an interview. Reapplications are treated no differently than initial applications. Rejected applicants should seek the advice and counsel of their premedical advisor.

Students are accepted without regard to race, sex, creed, national origin, age, or handicap. All applicants will receive the *Essential Functions of the Medical School Curriculum* including technical standards with our secondary application. Preference is given to qualified residents of New York State. Out-of-state applicants should consider this carefully before applying. Applications are not accepted from foreign nationals. All applicants must have completed at least two full years or 60 credit hours of higher education in the United States or Canada. The present freshman class has an average GPA of 3.60 and an average MCAT of 9.5 with a composition of 55 percent female and 9 percent minority. Transfer students are accepted into the third year only. Transfers from American and foreign schools are considered only under conditions of hardship.

FINANCIAL AID

The FAFSA should be received at the Federal Student Aid Office (see Part 1) by May 15, 2001, for all students applying to the 2001 entering class. Forms received after the deadline are subject to funds available. Requests for financial aid are considered after admission, and awards are made based on the student's need as estimated by the university's Office of Financial Aid. In most financial aid requests, parental income information is required regardless of dependency status. All financial aid is need based. A limited number of scholarships based on academic merit and financial need are provided each year.

INFORMATION FOR MINORITY STUDENTS

A Summer Enrichment and Support Program is available to facilitate students' retention in medical school. The enrichment program, designed for first-year educationally and socioeconomically disadvantaged students admitted to SUNY-Buffalo, offers histology, a preceptorship program, and learning skills development. The program begins June 1 and runs through July. Tutorial and counseling services are offered during the summer and throughout the academic year. The School of Medicine has a strong retention program; however, each student must meet the academic standards established by the faculty.

Public Institution

APPLICATION AND ACCEPTANCE POLICIES FOR 2001–2002 FIRST-YEAR CLASS

School participates in AMCAS. See Chapter 6.

Filing of AMCAS application
- Earliest date: June 1, 2000
- Latest date: Nov. 1, 2000

School application fee to all applicants: $65
Oldest MCAT scores considered: 1997
Does have Early Decision Program (EDP)
- EDP application period: June 1–Aug. 1, 2000
- EDP applicants notified by: Oct. 1, 2000

Acceptance notice to regular applicants
- Earliest date: Oct. 15, 2000
- Latest date: Until class is filled

Applicant's response to acceptance offer
- Maximum time: 2 weeks

Requests for deferred entrance considered: Yes
Deposit to hold place in class (applied to tuition):
- $100, due with response to acceptance offer

Deposit refundable prior to: May 1, 2001
Estimated number of new entrants: 135 (10 EDP)
Starting date: Aug. 2001

TUITION AND STUDENT FEES PER YEAR FOR 1999–2000 FIRST-YEAR CLASS

Tuition
- Resident: $10,840
- Nonresident: $21,940

Student fees: $950

INFORMATION ON 1999–2000 FIRST-YEAR CLASS

Number of	*In-State*	*Out-of-State*	*Total*
Applicants	1,780	377	2,157
Applicants Interviewed	464	21	485
New Entrants*	136	2	138

*All took the MCAT and had baccalaureate degrees. This does not include EAP.

CHAPTER 11

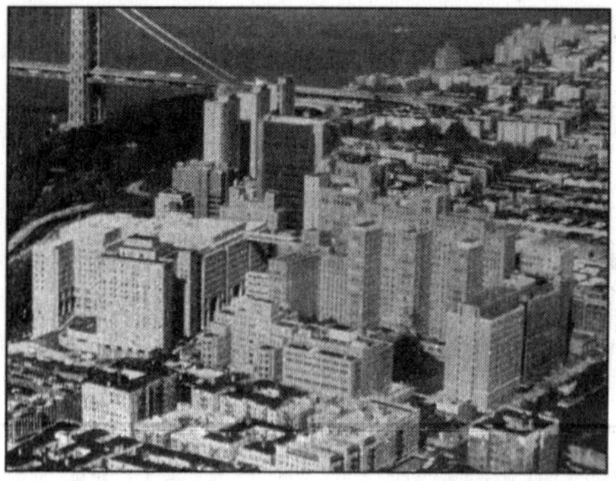

Columbia University College of Physicians and Surgeons

New York, New York

Dr. Thomas Q. Morris, *Interim Dean*
Dr. Andrew G. Frantz, *Associate Dean for Admissions*
Ellen Spilker, *Director, Office of Student Affairs (Financial Aid)*

ADDRESS INQUIRIES TO:

Columbia University
College of Physicians and Surgeons
Admissions Office, Room 1-416
630 West 168th Street
New York, New York 10032
(212) 305-3595
Web Site: http://www.columbia.edu/dept/ps/

GENERAL INFORMATION

The College of Physicians and Surgeons originated in 1767 as the Medical Faculty of King's (later Columbia) College and was the first school to award an earned doctor of medicine degree in the American colonies. The college is now a part of the Columbia-Presbyterian Medical Center. Clinical teaching is provided at the Medical Center; Roosevelt-St. Luke's Hospital Center and Harlem Hospital Center in Manhattan; Bassett Hospital in Cooperstown, New York; and Overlook Hospital in New Jersey.

University housing is available for unmarried and married students.

CURRICULUM

Our curriculum aims to prepare students with a solid foundation in basic sciences, as well as in the art and practice of clinical medicine that will equip them for a wide range of careers. Recent revision of our curriculum has been carried out to develop an interdisciplinary and integrative approach to the basic science subjects taught in the first two years, and which intertwines basic science and clinical education throughout the four years. Teaching in small groups is emphasized. Patient contact begins in the first year and is maintained throughout the year by means of selective clinical courses in which students participate with physicians in a variety of settings involving community clinics and doctors' offices. Clinical correlation with basic sciences is emphasized, and, in the second year, all topics in pathophysiology are studied by means of case-based histories led by preceptors in small-discussion groups. In addition to the evaluation of scientific data, the program is designed to inculcate the school's attitudes about patient care, which include the attitude that the patient is not simply a disease entity and is being improperly cared for if treated as such. The concept of the patient as a whole person is fostered by means of a variety of teaching experiences, including an interdisciplinary course in the first year entitled Introduction to Clinical Practice. Ethical problems as well as topics in health care are discussed in this course, which continues in the second year. Student participation in research is encouraged, and many opportunities for laboratory and clinical clinical research under faculty guidance are available. These take place principally during the summer between the first and second years, as well as in the fourth year.

In early July after the second year, students begin a full year of clerkships in which they participate in all of the clinical services. From July after the third year until graduation, the student follows an individually selected program of studies. A great variety of elective courses are offered, including research electives and opportunities for study abroad. Courses also may be taken in other branches of the university. In cooperation with 14 of the university's departments and programs, an M.D.-Ph.D. program is offered for which a maximum of eight openings are usually available annually.

An M.D.-M.P.H. program also is offered in conjunction with our School of Public Health.

Courses are graded on the basis of honors, pass, and fail.

REQUIREMENTS FOR ENTRANCE

The MCAT and a minimum of three years of full-time study in an accredited college are required; four years are recommended. The undergraduate program must include the following courses:

	Years
Biology	1
Mammalian biology preferred.	
General chemistry	1
Organic chemistry	1
Physics	1
English	1

Applicants who have more than one of the required courses to complete are at a disadvantage in the competition for admission.

Admission is possible for all qualified applicants regardless of sex, race, age, religion, national origin, or handicap.

The area of undergraduate concentration is not an important selection factor.

SELECTION FACTORS

Admission is offered to those applicants who have given evidence that they are qualified to complete all of the curriculum requirements of the college and have shown the greatest promise that they are likely to graduate as ethical, compassionate, and competent physicians. Competence implies, in part, mastery of the scientific basis of medicine. Competence also requires mastery of the art of medicine for which certain personal qualities and attitudes are essential. These qualities and attitudes are evaluated by several means: the tenor of letters of recommendation, the nature of extracurricular and summer activities (assuming choice was not restricted by financial need), the breadth of the undergraduate education, and the personal interview.

Each year, some applicants are accepted who display extraordinary promise with regard to either the science or art of medicine, even though they do not meet, in optimal measure, all of the criteria described above.

FINANCIAL AID

Financial aid is based solely on need and consists of scholarship awards and long-term loans. Accepted applicants, along with their parents, complete a financial aid questionnaire if aid is to be requested. An appropriately sized combination of scholarship money and loans is awarded in accordance with guidelines provided by the Financial Aid Office. Financial aid resources are equally available to the four classes.

The college cannot promise to meet fully the financial needs of students, although it makes every effort to do so. Its resources provide aid for a substantial segment of the student body, however. About 68 percent of the students currently receive financial aid.

INFORMATION FOR MINORITY STUDENTS

The college has a strong commitment to increase the numbers of medical students from minority groups. There are relatively large numbers of minority faculty members and a highly diverse student body. Applications from minority students are welcomed. Additional information can be sought from Gerald E. Thomson, M.D., senior associate dean, Office of Minority Affairs, (212) 305-4158.

Private Institution

APPLICATION AND ACCEPTANCE POLICIES FOR 2001–2002 FIRST-YEAR CLASS

Filing of application
  Earliest date: June 1, 2000
  Latest date: Oct. 15, 2000
School application fee to all applicants: $75
Oldest MCAT scores considered: 1997
Does not have Early Decision Program
Acceptance notice to regular applicants
  Earliest date: Feb. 1, 2001
  Latest date: Varies
Applicant's response to acceptance offer
  Maximum time: 3 weeks
Requests for deferred entrance considered: Yes
Deposit to hold place in class: None
Estimated number of new entrants: 150
Starting date: Aug. 2001

TUITION AND STUDENT FEES PER YEAR FOR 1999–2000 FIRST-YEAR CLASS

Tuition: $29,548   Student fees: $1,723

INFORMATION ON 1999–2000 FIRST-YEAR CLASS

Number of	*In-State*	*Out-of-State*	*Total*
Applicants	697	2,600	3,297
Applicants Interviewed	306	1,032	1,338
New Entrants*	43	109	152

*All took the MCAT and had baccalaureate degrees.

CHAPTER 11

Mount Sinai School of Medicine of New York University

New York, New York

Dr. Arthur Rubenstein, *Dean*
Dr. Richard D. Kayne, *Associate Dean for Admissions*
Glenda Palmer, *Director of Student Financial Services*

ADDRESS INQUIRIES TO:

Office of Admissions
Mount Sinai School of Medicine
Annenberg Building, Room 5-04
One Gustave L. Levy Place-Box 1002
New York, New York 10029-6574
(212) 241-6696; 828-4135 (FAX)
Web Site: http://www.mssm.edu
E-mail: admissions@mssm.edu

GENERAL INFORMATION

Mount Sinai School of Medicine is privately endowed, coeducational, and nondenominational. Developed from the 140-year tradition of patient care, professional education, and research of the Mount Sinai Hospital, it enrolled its first students in 1968 and is officially affiliated with New York University.

The campus's 22 buildings include a hospital, numerous research and service laboratories, teaching facilities, the Postgraduate School of Medicine, and the Graduate School of Biological Sciences.

The Mount Sinai Hospital, a 1,300-bed facility with a clinical research center, constitutes the basic resource for clinical training. Additional clinical training sites in our health system extend throughout New York City, New Jersey, Westchester County, and Long Island. They include municipal hospitals, a Veteran's Affairs Medical Center, and private community hospitals, as well as private practitioners' offices.

CURRICULUM

Mount Sinai School of Medicine has completely revised its curriculum to give our graduates a core knowledge of the biological basis of human function in health and disease, skills in critical thinking, dedication to lifelong learning, professional and humanistic attitudes, a scientific approach to medicine, and an appreciation of their obligation to society and the community in which they live. Our curriculum emphasizes the interdisciplinary nature of the various basic sciences, clinical sciences, as well as the interface between the two. A variety of pedagogic methods are used including lecture, small group seminars, and problem-based learning. Courses are graded pass/fail during the first two years, honors/pass/fail in the last two.

Student–patient interactions begin in the first month of school with Introduction to Clinical Medicine and continue throughout. In addition to three introductory courses: Student Well Being, Introduction to Emergency Medicine, and Ethics; the first year focuses on an integrated approach to the study of Molecules and Cells, Structure and Function, and Pathogenesis and Host Defense Mechanisms. A case-based sequence is used to provide clinical relevance for the basic science that is being learned. Case-based Integration and Intro to Clinical Medicine continue during the second year, along with a focus on Epidemiology and Biostatistics. These are accompanied by a year-long study of mechanisms of Disease and Pharmacology.

Clinical rotations include new and innovative clerkships which combine the disciplines of Medicine and Geriatrics, and Pediatrics and Obstetrics/Gynecology. An integrated seminar series spans the entire third year.

The fourth year provides the student an increasing degree of patient care responsibility, and allows for extended electives. An Emergency Medicine rotation and a subinternship in Medicine or Pediatrics immerses students in the care of the acutely ill patient. A Clinical Translational Fellowship combines the clinical practice of medicine with the relevant basis science. Our year-end Post-match Integrated Selective focuses on mastering the skills that are necessary to ensure a productive and educational internship experience.

One of our unique educational resources is the Morchand Center for Clinical Competence, the first media training facility of its kind in New York. Here, with the aid of state-of-the-art audiovisual systems and standardized patients, students develop the interpersonal communication, history taking, and physical exam skills essential to a successful physician-patient relationship.

The Medical Scientist Training Program (MSTP) was developed for students interested in a career in medical research and academic medicine. This M.D.-Ph.D. program is funded by a training grant from the NIH as well as by other extramural and intramural awards. Students may apply for the combined program at the time of application for admission or during the second year of medical school.

A master of science degree in community medicine is available, and is designed to produce a new generation of leaders in preventive medicine while providing advanced training in the population-based medical sciences.

REQUIREMENTS FOR ENTRANCE

A minimum of three years of college and the MCAT are required. Most students admitted have earned the bachelor's degree. The prospective student should have basic knowledge of the biological and physical sciences and mathematics, plus an appreciation of the social forces influencing man. Students majoring in nonscience disciplines who meet all admission requirements will be given consideration on an equal basis with those having specific scientific backgrounds.

Admission requirements include accredited college work in the following subjects:

	Years
Biology	1
Inorganic chemistry	1
Organic chemistry	1
Physics	1
Mathematics	1
English	1

Biology and Chemistry courses must be accompanied by laboratory experience. Courses in Statistics or Computer Science may fulfill the Mathematics requirements.

SELECTION FACTORS

The school is keenly interested in a total appraisal of a student's potential for a career in medicine. Excellence in scholarship, personal maturity, integrity, intellectual creativity, and motivation for medicine are important factors. A personal interview is required, and all interviews are conducted at Mount Sinai. The interview is given considerable weight; premedical advisory committee letters of recommendation and MCAT scores are criteria for evaluation. All applicants, regardless of race, sex, color, creed, age, national origin, handicap, veteran status, marital status, or sexual orientation, are given serious and thorough consideration by the Admissions Committee. Transfer students are not accepted.

Accepted students for the 1999 entering class had the following characteristics: *mean GPA,* 3.64; *mean MCAT,* 10.63; *sex,* 49 percent women. Distribution of undergraduate major reflects the distribution in the applicant pool.

FINANCIAL AID

It is the policy of the school to provide as much financial assistance as possible to students who require such assistance in order to maintain attendance. Students who are accepted for admission are provided financial assistance applications on which they may document their request for financial aid. Applications are treated confidentially, and awards are made by a faculty committee on financial aid. Each applicant is considered on an individual basis so that the greatest support for the most needy students can be distributed.

Financial aid may be offered in the form of a scholarship, a loan, or both, in accordance with the requirements of the individual situation and the availability of funds in the various categories. Over 75 percent of the students receive financial assistance; 70 percent receive direct institutional support. Students who are not citizens or permanent residents of the United States are not eligible for financial assistance.

INFORMATION FOR MINORITY APPLICANTS

Strongly motivated students from minority backgrounds are actively sought and encouraged to apply. A pre-entrance summer enrichment program is available for students who are accepted to the freshman class. Tutorial assistance is available for all students.

The school's Office of Multicultural and Community Affairs serves to support its commitment to cultural and ethnic diversity within the school. This office provides leadership and coordination for minority affairs activities, multicultural diversity program activities, and a variety of enrichment programs. In addition, this office assists in providing advisory and career counseling services for all students.

Private Institution

APPLICATION AND ACCEPTANCE POLICIES FOR 2001–2002 FIRST-YEAR CLASS

School participates in AMCAS. See Chapter 6.

Filing of AMCAS application
  Earliest date: June 1, 2000
  Latest date: Nov. 1, 2000
School application fee to all applicants: $100
Oldest MCAT scores considered: 1997
Does have Early Decision Program (EDP)
  EDP application period: June 1–Aug. 1, 2000
  EDP applicants notified by: Oct. 1, 2000
Acceptance notice to regular applicants
  Earliest date: Nov. 15, 2000
  Latest date: Varies
Applicant's response to acceptance offer
  Maximum time: 2 weeks
Requests for deferred entrance considered: Yes
Deposit to hold place in class: None
Estimated number of new entrants: 105 (1 EDP)
Starting date: Aug. 2001

TUITION AND STUDENT FEES PER YEAR FOR 1999–2000 FIRST-YEAR CLASS

Tuition: $22,750   Student fees: $1,675

INFORMATION ON 1999–2000 FIRST-YEAR CLASS

Number of	*In-State*	*Out-of-State*	*Total*
Applicants	1,350	3,856	5,206
Applicants Interviewed	319	518	837
New Entrants	59	46	105

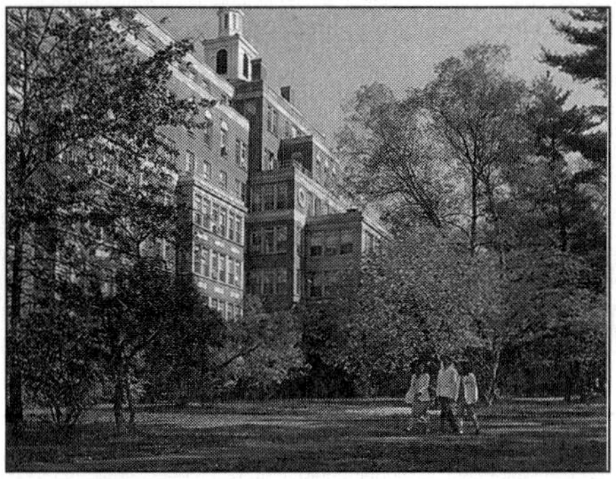

New York Medical College

Valhalla, New York

Dr. Ralph A. O'Connell, *Provost and Dean; School of Medicine*
Dr. Fern R. Juster, *Associate Dean and Chair, Committee on Admissions*
Anthony M. Sozzo, *Associate Dean and Director of Student Financial Planning*

ADDRESS INQUIRIES TO:

Office of Admissions
Sunshine Cottage
New York Medical College
Valhalla, New York 10595
(914) 594-4507; 594-4976 (FAX)
Web Site: http://www.nymc.edu

GENERAL INFORMATION

Founded in 1860, New York Medical College is a private university comprising a medical school and two graduate schools in health sciences and basic medical sciences. As a health sciences university in the Catholic tradition, the college's mission emphasizes a special responsibility to the underserved. Located on a suburban campus in Westchester County, 25 miles from New York City, the college is home base for students in the first two years. The school is affiliated with more than 20 hospitals in the New York City metropolitan area, from which students select the sites for clinical clerkships in years three and four. These affiliations include urban medical centers, small suburban hospitals, and technologically advanced, regional tertiary care facilities. This vast network endows the university with diverse resources for teaching, learning, research, and patient-care activities.

CURRICULUM

Though centered on the basic sciences, the curriculum of the first two years maintains a consistent clinical focus. The program was revised and expanded to bring clinical relevance and small-group teaching into all courses. The core of the first-year curriculum—anatomy, histology, biochemistry, physiology, neural science, and behavioral science—is supplemented by clinical case correlations and courses in epidemiology and biostatistics. All first-year students have regular patient contact working in the office of a primary care physician. This one-on-one placement affords both clinical exposure and an individualized mentor relationship.

The redesigned second-year curriculum, with its strong focus on pathology/pathophysiology, emphasizes small-group discussion, problem-based learning, and self-study. Clinical skills training, pharmacology, and medical microbiology prepare students for full entry into the clerkship experience of the next two years.

The third year runs for a full calendar year. Students complete clerkships in seven disciplines—medicine, neurology, obstetrics and gynecology, pediatrics, psychiatry, surgery, and family medicine. Because of the medical school's unique location just outside New York City, students can choose from demographically and clinically diverse settings which extend from the city to suburban and rural Hudson Valley sites. About half the third-year class moves into New York City for their clinical years, and many live in college-owned housing in Manhattan.

The fourth year comprises required clinical rotations taken at affiliated hospitals and electives at medical institutions across the country and around the world. Approximately 15 percent of the fourth-year students take international electives each year.

Special programs are available through the college's two graduate schools. Medical students can simultaneously pursue an M.P.H. degree through the Graduate School of Health Sciences. The dual degree can be finished within the four years of medical school or can be extended to five years. Similarly, the Graduate School of Basic Medical Sciences affords the opportunity for joint M.D.–Ph.D. degrees, which typically require six to seven years to complete. These programs do not have a separate application process; applicants apply first to the School of Medicine.

Anticipating the need for more generalist physicians, a decade ago the college began offering medical students primary care training and mentors. This initiative continues today and includes the following programs:

Introduction to Primary Care—This innovative program, begun in 1988, places all first-year students in the offices of generalist faculty. Students work closely with a physician preceptor, examining patients and focusing on issues such as health maintenance, ethics, and cultural perspectives of health care.

Family Medicine Clerkship—This third-year clerkship allows students to work directly with primary care physicians in outpatient settings that stress continuity, preventive medicine, and the integration of the behavioral sciences in clinical medicine.

Six-Year Program—This program allows students to condense into six years the four years of medical school and three years of residency in internal medicine, by overlapping the last year of medical school with the first year of residency. Loans for the fourth year of medical school are forgiven for those who practice primary care for three years after completing the program.

REQUIREMENTS FOR ENTRANCE

It is strongly recommended that the applicant complete undergraduate work leading to a baccalaureate degree from an accredited college of arts and sciences in the United States or Canada. All courses offered in satisfaction of the requirements for admission must be taken in or accepted as transfer credit by an accredited college in the United States or Canada and must be acceptable to that institution toward a baccalaureate degree in general arts or sciences. The Committee on Admissions has no preference for a major field of undergraduate study, but any college work submitted must include the specified credits below.

	Sem. hrs.
Biology (with lab)	8
Inorganic chemistry (with lab)	8
Organic chemistry (with lab)	8
Physics (with lab)	8
English	6

All candidates are required to take the MCAT.

SELECTION FACTORS

The Committee on Admissions selects students after carefully considering all those factors of intellect, character, and personality that point toward their ability to become informed and caring physicians. This basic platform must include a history of academic excellence. Although the majority of students have had undergraduate majors in the sciences, it is not at all a requirement or a factor in selection. We welcome applicants with a broad education in the humanities who have completed their premed requirements in a postbaccalaureate program.

In addition to purely academic factors, we look for students who show clear evidence through their activities of strong motivation toward medicine and a sense of dedication to the service of others. Personal qualities of character and personality are evaluated from letters of recommendation, from the personal statement, and from the interview. New York Medical College does not deny admission to any applicant on the basis of race, gender, religion, national origin, age, or handicap.

Secondary applications are mailed to all applicants upon receipt of the AMCAS application. After the completed secondary application and all letters of recommendation have been processed, the applicant's file is reviewed for consideration. Interviews are by invitation and are conducted on campus. We generally interview from October through April and decisions are made on a rolling basis.

In the most recent entering first-year class, the class of 2002, students had the following credentials: *mean GPA 3.5; mean total MCAT; 31; mean age, 23; gender, 47* percent women.

FINANCIAL AID

Approximately 85 percent of the student body receives some financial assistance. Financial aid is awarded on the basis of need; limited grants and scholarships are also available. The college provides services including debt management and loan counseling. Students are discouraged from seeking outside employment during the academic year. All accepted students will receive an informational financial aid packet. For further information call the Office of Student Financial Planning at (914) 594-4491.

INFORMATION FOR MINORITY STUDENTS

Strongly motivated students from educationally deprived and minority groups are actively sought and encouraged to apply. The Office of Minority Affairs is responsible for developing and implementing special programs to enhance educational opportunities, recruit, and retain minority students for careers in medicine. This office also coordinates academic and social support services, individual career counseling, mentoring, and scholarships. For further information, call the Office of Minority Affairs at (914) 594-3014.

Private Institution

APPLICATION AND ACCEPTANCE POLICIES FOR 2001–2002 FIRST-YEAR CLASS

School participates in AMCAS. See Chapter 6.

Filing of AMCAS application
Earliest date: June 1, 2000
Latest date: Dec. 1, 2000
School application fee to all applicants: $100
Oldest MCAT scores considered: 1997
Does have Early Decision Program (EDP)
EDP application period: June 1–Aug. 1, 2000
EDP applicants notified by: Oct. 1, 2000
Acceptance notice to regular applicants
Earliest date: Oct. 15, 2000
Latest date: Until class is filled
Applicant's response to acceptance offer
Maximum time: 2 weeks
Requests for deferred entrance considered: Yes
Deposit to hold place in class (applied to tuition):
$100, due May 15, 2001
Deposit refundable prior to: May 15, 2001
Estimated number of new entrants: 185 (10 EDP)
Starting date: Aug. 2001

TUITION AND STUDENT FEES PER YEAR FOR 1999–2000 FIRST-YEAR CLASS

Tuition: $29,150 Student fees: $620

INFORMATION ON 1999–2000 FIRST-YEAR CLASS

Number of	*In-State*	*Out-of-State*	*Total*
Applicants	1,830	7,521	9,351
Applicants Interviewed	424	993	1,417
New Entrants*	64	120	184

*All took the MCAT and had baccalaureate degrees.

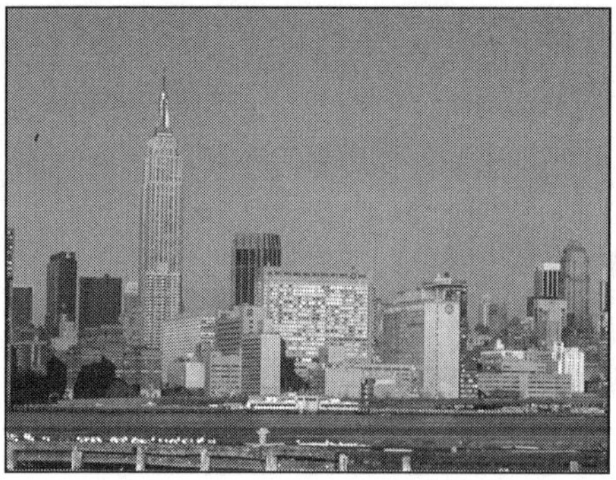

New York University School of Medicine

New York, New York

Dr. Robert M. Glickman, *Dean*
Raymond J. Brienza, *Assistant Dean for Admissions and Director of Financial Aid*

ADDRESS INQUIRIES TO:

Office of Admissions
New York University
School of Medicine
P.O. Box 1924
New York, New York 10016
(212) 263-5290
Web Site: http://www.med.nyu.edu

GENERAL INFORMATION

The New York University School of Medicine was founded in 1841 when it admitted a class of 239 students to a four-month course of lectures conducted by six professors on the faculty. The medical school is a constituent of New York University (NYU), one of the oldest and largest private universities in the United States.

CURRICULUM

Several changes in the curriculum have been implemented in the past few years. These innovations are designed to promote independent learning through an increase of small-group seminars, problem-solving exercises, and computer-assisted instruction. Study of the basic sciences provides students with the essential facts, concepts, and skills necessary to understand the scientific principles upon which clinical medicine is based. The basic science program is enriched by the honors program, the Hippocrates project, and opportunities for independent study research. Study of the clinical sciences, which begins in the third year, promotes excellence in clinical and decision-making skills. Flexibility in the scheduling of required clerkships and electives throughout the third and fourth years permits students to design a course of study specific to their educational and career goals. A rich ambulatory care experience provides students with an understanding of the physician-patient relationship and underscores issues of disease prevention.

REQUIREMENTS FOR ENTRANCE

The requirements for admission are as follows: the MCAT; a minimum of three years of college work; and the following courses plus an acceptable concentration in any of these fields, or in any other field, at the college level:

	Sem. hrs.
Biology (with lab)	6
Inorganic chemistry (with lab)	6
Organic chemistry (with lab)	6
General physics (with lab)	6
English	6

Biochemistry is strongly recommended for all students.

Genetics and a course in embryology or developmental biology are recommended for students who select extra work in biology and have all options open to them as far as their college is concerned.

It is strongly recommended that candidates complete their college work for the baccalaureate degree.

Applicants should take the MCAT in the spring of the year in which they are applying to medical school to achieve an earlier processing of their applications in the fall. In no case should the MCAT be taken later than August of the application year.

SELECTION FACTORS

The selection process involves judging the applicant from several viewpoints, among them the following: excellence in course work at the college level; evaluation of the student by college instructors, premedical committees, and other similar mechanisms provided by the colleges; an interview at NYU; and the results of the MCAT. The Committee on Admissions does not computerize the candidate's profile in terms of MCAT scores and GPAs because qualitative considerations, such as college evaluation and interview impression, are also given great weight in the final evaluation. The Committee on Admissions does lend some weight to trends in the student's college progress. Students who may, for one reason or another, get off to a slow start in college and then show that they are capable of honors work in later years are given sympathetic consideration. The medical school's student body is drawn mainly from the eastern seaboard—a reflection of the composition of the applicant pool. Applications from outside the region are welcome. NYU is a private institution and has no geographical or other quotas. It should be noted, however, that foreign nationals who do not hold a permanent resident visa have only a slight chance of being admitted.

Women have constituted from 42 to 46 percent of recent entering classes. The acceptance rates for men and women are approximately the same.

Only those students who on the basis of application data appear to merit serious consideration for admission are interviewed.

FINANCIAL AID

The Financial Aid Office reviews all applications for financial assistance. The school's resources are drawn from scholarships and loan programs. Enrolled students and those students accepted for admission to the school are eligible to file applications for assistance. The School of Medicine participates in the Primary Care Loan and the Perkins Loan Program, which provide low-interest support for deserving students. Federal Stafford loans are also available through the New York Higher Education Assistance Corporation. New York State Tuition Assistance Program Awards are available to many residents of New York who are degree candidates.

INFORMATION FOR MINORITY STUDENTS

Minorities are welcomed into the school. Every effort is made in the case of all candidates, including minorities, to reach some determination on motivation, character, and capacities of the candidate, regardless of such standard measures as test scores and college performance. Considerable reliance is placed on the evaluation of students by their college teachers. This is particularly important in terms of the candidate's motivation under adverse circumstances. It is possible to have application fees waived in cases of demonstrated need.

Private Institution

APPLICATION AND ACCEPTANCE POLICIES FOR 2001–2002 FIRST-YEAR CLASS

Filing of application
  Earliest date: Aug. 14, 2000
  Latest date: Nov. 17, 2000
School application fee to all applicants: $75
Oldest MCAT scores considered: 1997
Does not have Early Decision Program
Acceptance notice to regular applicants
  Earliest date: Dec. 18, 2000
  Latest date: Until class is filled
Applicant's response to acceptance offer
  Maximum time: 2 weeks
Requests for deferred entrance considered: Yes
Deposit to hold place in class (applied to tuition):
  $100, due with response to acceptance offer
Deposit refundable prior to: May 1, 2001
Estimated number of new entrants: 160
Starting date: Aug. 2001

TUITION AND STUDENT FEES PER YEAR FOR 1999–2000 FIRST-YEAR CLASS

Tuition: $23,285 Student fees: $4,320

INFORMATION ON 1999–2000 FIRST-YEAR CLASS

Number of	*In-State*	*Out-of-State*	*Total*
Applicants	*	*	3,647
Applicants Interviewed	*	*	971
New Entrants†	80	80	160

*Information not available.

†All took the MCAT and had baccalaureate degrees.

CHAPTER 11

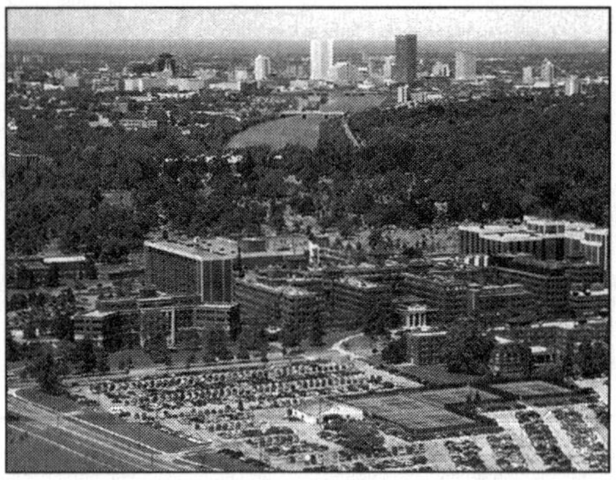

University of Rochester School of Medicine and Dentistry

Rochester, New York

Dr. Lowell A. Goldsmith, *Dean*
Dr. John T. Hansen, *Associate Dean for Admissions*
Patricia Samuelson, *Director of Admissions*

ADDRESS INQUIRIES TO:

Director of Admissions
University of Rochester
School of Medicine and Dentistry
Medical Center Box 601A
Rochester, New York 14642
(716) 275-4539; 756-5479 (FAX)
E-mail: mdadmish@urmc.rochester.edu
Web Site: http://www.urmc.rochester.edu/smd/admiss

MISSION STATEMENT

As the home of the biopsychosocial model, Rochester offers a student-centered educational program that prepares physicians for the twenty-first century. Our curriculum fosters knowledge, skills, attitudes, and behaviors of the physician/scientist/humanist by combining cutting-edge, evidence-based medical science with the relationship-centered art that is medicine's distinctive trademark.

GENERAL INFORMATION

The School of Medicine and Dentistry was established in 1920 as an academic division of the University of Rochester, a privately endowed institution founded in 1850. The university was one of the first to combine a medical school and a teaching hospital within the same facility. The original medical center has been greatly expanded to include a new medical education wing, new research facilities and clinical centers, the new Strong Memorial Hospital, and a recently completed Ambulatory Care Center. Clinical teaching also is conducted at five affiliated hospitals within the community. Opportunities for independent work include summer and full-year fellowships and a wide selection of elective offerings.

CURRICULUM

Rochester's Double Helix Curriculum represents a major revision, beginning with the entering class of 1999, that captures the integrated strands of basic science and clinical medicine as they are woven throughout the four-year curriculum. The focus of our educational program is not merely the transfer of information but the transformation of the learner in a culture providing that ingenious combination of support and challenge, which leads to education. Every course is interdisciplinary and, unlike most medical schools, clinical skills training from day one leads not to shadowing or preceptor experiences but to the start of real clinical work as part of the health care team.

Students' actual clinical cases drive the learning of science, and students return to increasingly advanced basic science in the second, third, and fourth years through an integrated series of problem-based learning (PBL) exercises. Multidisciplinary PBL cases are used in all courses with usually three PBL tutorials per week and an average of no more than ten lecture hours per week. Clinical exposure begins during the first week of school with an introduction to clinical medicine in the fall semester and the start of the ambulatory care experience beginning during the first spring semester. This experience, unlike any other in the country, includes all the ambulatory components of family medicine, pediatrics, internal medicine, women's health, psychiatry, and ambulatory surgery, and is completed by the end of the second year.

Years 2, 3, and 4 conclude with case seminars that present basic and clinical science with increasing levels of depth each year. Inpatient clerkships are completed by December of the fourth year and focus on acute care experiences in adult medicine, women's and children's health, mind/brain/behavior, and urgent/emergent care.

A formal tutoring system and assistance programs are available to all students with special academic needs.

A rich and diverse menu of opportunities is available to students, including a strong M.D.-Ph.D. program and a yearlong research fellowship program, reflecting the institution's commitment to research and the preparation of medical scientists and academicians. Master's programs are offered in public health, environmental medicine, industrial hygiene, and business. Opportunities to participate in volunteer service to the Rochester community and to experience medicine through our international medicine program reflect the school's commitment to providing the broadest possible educational experience.

REQUIREMENTS FOR ENTRANCE

All entering students have completed the baccalaureate degree. Rochester belongs to AMCAS and requires the MCAT examination.

Satisfactory completion of the following premedical course work is required:

	Sem. Hr.
Biology (with lab)	6-8

General or inorganic chemistry 6-8
Organic chemistry 6-8
One semester of biochemistry may be substituted for a semester of organic chemistry. Within the two-year chemistry sequence, one year of laboratory is required.
Physics (with lab) 6-8
Expository Writing 6-8
May be met with writing, English, or nonscience courses that involve expository writing
Humanities and/or social or behavioral sciences 12-16

The requirements above are designed with the expectation that students will enter with a liberal and diversified education. Courses in calculus and statistics, biochemistry, and experience in research, clinical practice, public health, or health policy issues are strongly recommended.

Advanced placement (AP) credit may not be used to satisfy the biology, English, or nonscience requirements. AP credit may substitute for one semester of general chemistry and/or one semester of physics only.

SELECTION FACTORS

Evaluation of applicants includes a careful examination of the entire academic record, letters of recommendation, and the candidate's personal statement. Candidates who show particular promise of achievement are invited for interviews.

Demonstrated excellence in a demanding academic program, including a high level of achievement in the natural sciences, is an absolute requirement for acceptance. Evidence of intrinsic intellectual drive and curiosity is highly valued since the program at Rochester emphasizes independent opportunities for individual students. Particular attention is given to achievements that demonstrate breadth and commitment. The school is characterized by an atmosphere in which students and faculty work closely together towards the attainment of knowledge and understanding and in which patients are treated with compassion and sensitivity. Students are sought who will contribute to this climate for learning.

Selections are made without regard to gender, sexual orientation, race, religion, national origin, age, or handicap. State residency is not a factor in selection. Transfer applicants are rarely accepted.

All applicants must have completed at least two years of undergraduate college study in the United States, including all premedical requirements. International students, unless they are Rochester graduates, are not considered.

Applicants who have not been accepted may reapply in a subsequent year, but applicants who twice have been unsuccessful in gaining admission are discouraged from reapplying.

The 1999 entering class came from 20 different states and attended over 50 different colleges and universities. The *mean age* of the class was 24 years (range 21–31), 46 percent were women, and 9 percent minorities. The *mean GPA* was 3.61, and the *average MCAT scores* were VR-10.5, PS-10.9, and BS-11.0.

FINANCIAL AID

The medical school offers scholarships and long-term loans to those students who demonstrate financial need. Decisions concerning admission are made independently of financial circumstances.

In 1999–2000, 85 percent of the enrolled students received financial assistance from either school or noninstitutional sources. Entering students applying for institutional financial aid are required to provide a FAFSA, an additional more detailed financial statement including parent information, and the School of Medicine's financial aid application.

INFORMATION FOR MINORITY STUDENTS

The Office of Ethnic and Multicultural Affairs represents a serious commitment on the part of the University of Rochester School of Medicine and Dentistry to meet the urgent need for minority physicians in all aspects of the medical profession. An active recruitment program seeks applicants for both the M.D. and M.D.-Ph.D. programs.

Private Institution

APPLICATION AND ACCEPTANCE POLICIES FOR 2001–2002 FIRST-YEAR CLASS

Filing of application
Earliest date: June 1, 2000
Latest date: Oct. 15, 2000
School application fee to all applicants: $75
Oldest MCAT scores considered: 1997
Does not have Early Decision Program
Acceptance notice to regular applicants
Earliest date: Nov. 1, 2000
Latest date: Until class is filled
Applicant's response to acceptance offer
Maximum time: 2 weeks
Requests for deferred entrance considered: Yes
Deposit to hold place in class (applied to tuition): $100, due with response to acceptance offer
Deposit refundable prior to: May 15, 2001
Estimated number of new entrants: 100
Starting date: Aug. 2001

TUITION AND STUDENT FEES PER YEAR FOR 1999–2001 FIRST-YEAR CLASS

Tuition: $26,900 Student fees: $1,568

INFORMATION ON 1999–2000 FIRST-YEAR CLASS

Number of	*In-State*	*Out-of-State*	*Total*
Applicants	1,403	4,439	5,842
Applicants Interviewed	218	432	650
New Entrants*	43	57	100

*All had baccalaureate degrees; 86% took the MCAT.

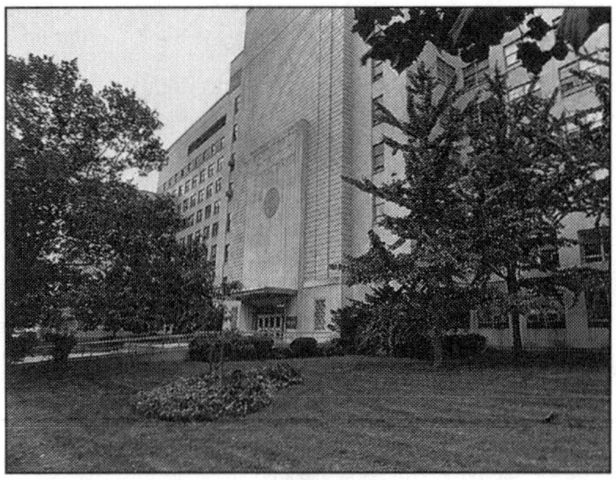

State University of New York Downstate Medical Center College of Medicine

Brooklyn, New York

Dr. Eugene B. Feigelson, *Dean*
Thomas Lo, *Director of Admissions*
Julia B. Clayton, *Director of Financial Aid*

ADDRESS INQUIRIES TO:

Director of Admissions
State University of New York
Health Science Center at Brooklyn
450 Clarkson Avenue-Box 60M
Brooklyn, New York 11203
(718) 270-2446; 270-7592 (FAX)
E-mail: admissions@netmail.hscbklyn.edu
Web Site: http://www.hscbklyn.edu

MISSION STATEMENT

Our primary mission is to make high quality education available to New York's next generation of health professionals. Integral to our concept of professional education are both a commitment to confront the health problems of urban communities and a responsibility to advance the state of knowledge and practice in the health disciplines through basic and applied clinical research.

GENERAL INFORMATION

The College of Medicine of the State University of New York Downstate Medical Center College of Medicine traces its roots to the founding in 1860 of the Long Island College Hospital, the first hospital-based medical school in the country. In 1950, the College of Medicine joined the State University of New York system and developed into a major center for health sciences. The University Hospital, a 376-bed teaching hospital, opened in 1966. In addition to its own hospital, the Health Science Center uses several major affiliated community hospitals in the clinical years. In 1992, the campus' new Health Science Education Building opened. It houses state-of-the-art classrooms, laboratories, a 500-seat auditorium, and the Medical Research Library of Brooklyn.

CURRICULUM

In preparing physicians to practice in the future health care system, the medical education process is under constant evaluation. The curriculum at the Downstate Medical Center at Brooklyn has undergone a total revision and the main goals are: to improve the integration of basic and clinical science throughout the four years of medical school; to provide earlier exposure to patient care by introducing a weekly clinical experience in the first and second years of medical school; to provide for a more small-group, self-directed and case-based learning; and to foster lifelong learning skills through the introduction of new applications of information science, outcome studies, and evidence-based medicine. An organ system approach is followed, with first-year topic areas such as genes to cells, skin and connective tissue, musculoskeletal, lymphoid/head and neck, cardiovascular, respiratory, gastrointestinal/nutrition, urinary, endocrine/reproduction, and neuroscience. Each course and clerkship has been or is under revision in view of current trends. The emphasis is on the development of clinical reasoning and problem-solving skills. During the first year, attention is focused on the basic components of human biology and behavior, as well as on the essential aspects of physician-patient relationship. The second year begins the study of human disease, its diagnosis, prevention, and treatment. All students are required to sit for Step 1 of the USMLE at the end of their second year. The third year is currently devoted to clerkships in six disciplines of medicine but will also undergo a revision, as will the fourth-year curriculum.

All courses are graded fail, conditional, pass, high pass, and honors.

The College of Medicine and the School of Graduate Studies sponsor a combined M.D.-Ph.D. program designed for students who are interested in academic medicine involving a combination of research, teaching, and clinical activities.

A B.A.-M.D. Honors program is offered in conjunction with Brooklyn College of the City University of New York. Information on special admission and matriculation criteria is available from the Office of Admissions at Brooklyn College. Early Assurance Programs are offered in Queens College and Staten Island College.

REQUIREMENTS FOR ENTRANCE

Applicants must have taken the new MCAT and completed a minimum of 90 semester credits of undergraduate work at an accredited college. Courses required for admission are:

	Semester Credits
General biology (with lab)	8
Inorganic chemistry (with lab)	8
Organic chemistry (with lab)	8
General physics (with lab)	8
English	6

If freshman English is exempted, a more advanced course is required.

The remainder of the courses should be in the liberal arts curriculum and credited toward a bachelor's degree. At least one year of college mathematics, one of an advanced scientific subject, and a course in biochemistry are recommended. Students educated abroad must complete a minimum of one year of full-time college study in an accredited college or university in the United States or Canada.

Applicants are urged to take the MCAT in the spring of the year of application and to have completed the premedical requirements at the time of application.

SELECTION FACTORS

The Committee on Admissions considers the total qualifications of each applicant without regard to sex, sexual orientation, race, color, creed, religion, national origin, age, or disability. Women and members of minority groups are encouraged to apply. Decisions are based on a number of factors, including prior academic performance; completion of required courses; the potential for academic success including performance on the MCAT; communication skills, character, personal skills; demonstrated commitment to community-social service outreach activities; and motivation for medicine. Preference is given to qualified New York State residents. Reapplicants adhere to the same procedures, policies, and deadlines as first-time applicants.

Secondary applications and an informational brochure are sent to all applicants who apply to our school. Applications are screened once all of the required information has been submitted (AMCAS application, secondary application, MCAT scores, and recommendations).

The 1999 entering class attended 72 different colleges and universities. It was 48.1 percent women and 11 percent minorities; age ranged from 20 to 38, with the mean on matriculation being 24.1. The *mean GPA* was 3.56; *MCAT scores* averaged verbal reasoning, 8.9; physical sciences, 10.1; biological sciences, 10.3. These numbers, however, represent a range of scores, and each applicant is considered individually on more than quantitative variables.

Admission to advanced standing is limited to U.S. citizens or permanent residents who are matriculated, in good standing, and in attendance as second-year medical students in an LCME college of medicine in the United States. Applications are accepted to the third-year class, and admissions preference is given to New York State residents.

FINANCIAL AID

The college is committed to help students meet their educational expenses through various types of financial assistance. Aid is granted on the basis of need (determined in accordance with federal regulations), and for some scholarships, on academic achievement. The major portion of our assistance is derived from federal and state allocations: grants, scholarships, loans and/or college work study. Loans are the most common form of assistance. Financial aid application materials are sent to all accepted applicants, and students' financial aid needs are reviewed annually.

INFORMATION FOR MINORITY STUDENTS

The SUNY Downstate Medical Center maintains a tradition of commitment to the enrollment of historically underrepresented groups. The Office of Minority Affairs directs several programs targeted to furnish information and support to students from minority backgrounds. Operation Success is an eight-week elective summer enrichment program designed to provide first-year minority students with a head start on the first-semester medical curriculum. Entering minority students are matched with a faculty mentor. The Daniel Hale Williams Society, the primary voice of minority students on campus, provides peer support.

Public Institution

APPLICATION AND ACCEPTANCE POLICIES FOR 2001–2002 FIRST-YEAR CLASS

School participates in AMCAS. See Chapter 6.

Filing of AMCAS application
Earliest date: June 1, 2000
Latest date: Dec. 15, 2000
School application fee to all applicants: $65
Oldest MCAT scores considered: 1998
Does have Early Decision Program (EDP)
For New York State residents only
EDP application period: June 1–Aug. 1, 2000
EDP applicants notified by: Oct. 1, 2000
Acceptance notice to regular applicants
Earliest date: Oct. 15, 2000
Latest date: Until class is filled
Applicant's response to acceptance offer
Maximum time: 2 weeks
Requests for deferred entrance considered: Yes
Deposit to hold place in class (applied to tuition): $100, due with response to acceptance offer; refundable upon written request prior to May 15, 2001
Estimated number of new entrants: 180 (20 EDP)
Starting date: Aug. 2001

TUITION AND STUDENT FEES PER YEAR FOR 1999–2000 FIRST-YEAR CLASS

Tuition
Resident: $10,840
Nonresident: $21,940
Student fees: $1,010

INFORMATION ON 1999–2000 FIRST-YEAR CLASS

Number of	*In-State*	*Out-of-State*	*Total*
Applicants	2,115	981	3,096
Applicants Interviewed	639	26	665
New Entrants*	184	5	189

*All had baccalaureate degrees; 89% took the MCAT.

CHAPTER 11

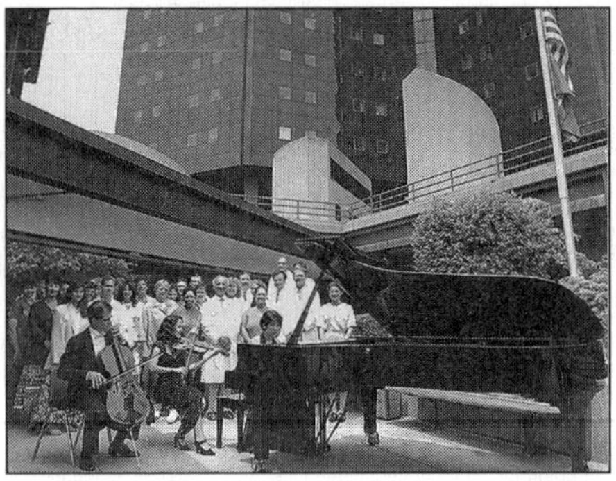

SUNY at Stony Brook School of Medicine Health Sciences Center

Stony Brook, New York

Dr. Norman H. Edelman, *Vice President, Health Sciences Center and Dean, School of Medicine*
Dr. Jack Fuhrer, *Associate Dean for Admissions*
Dr. Aldustus E. Jordan, *Associate Dean for Minority and Student Affairs*

ADDRESS INQUIRIES TO:

Committee on Admissions
Level 4 Health Sciences Center
SUNY Stony Brook
School of Medicine
Stony Brook, New York 11794-8434
(631) 444-2113; 444-6032 (FAX)
E-mail: admissions@dean.som.sunysb.edu
Web Site: http://www.hsc.sunysb.edu/som/

MISSION STATEMENT

The mission of the School of Medicine is to improve the quality of health care available to the citizens of New York and the nation by demonstrating national leadership in education, research, patient care, and community service.

To this end, the School of Medicine aims to achieve excellence in the preparation of students for careers in medical practice or research through its curriculum, and through activities that are designed to provide students with the skills that are appropriate for success in all fields of medicine.

GENERAL INFORMATION

SUNY Stony Brook School of Medicine accepted its first class in 1971. It is part of the SUNY-Stony Brook Health Sciences Center, which includes the 540-bed University Hospital.

CURRICULUM

The curriculum of the School of Medicine is designed to provide the opportunity for extensive training in the basic medical sciences and teaching in the clinical disciplines of medicine. The curriculum requires the acquisition and utilization of a variety of skills in basic and clinical sciences. The faculty has determined that a successful candidate for the M.D. degree must pass each unit of curriculum and that waiver of units of curriculum is offered only to those who because of prior experience are able to place out through examination. The grading system is honors/pass/fail.

The first year of the curriculum consists of integrated instruction in the basic sciences and introductions to clinical skills, human behavior, nutrition, and preventive medicine. The second-year curriculum includes microbiology, pharmacology, and an interdisciplinary course in pathophysiology of the different organ systems. In both the first and second years, students participate in the introduction to clinical medicine and medicine in contemporary society courses.

In the third year, students move to a series of clinical clerkships in medicine, surgery, pediatrics, obstetrics and gynecology, psychiatry, and family medicine, where opportunities for problem solving and patient responsibility are presented. Additional experiences are provided in radiology and emergency medicine. Clinical teaching in the introduction to clinical medicine course, in the systems program, and in the clinical clerkships takes place at the University Hospital and various clinical facilities affiliated with the School of Medicine. The clerkship program is followed by selectives and electives in the fourth year. The curriculum emphasizes social issues in medicine and bioethics at each level of medical training.

In addition, four-year programs leading to the M.D. with recognition in research, M.D. with recognition in humanities, and a six- to eight-year federally funded MSTP (M.D.-Ph.D. program) are available.

REQUIREMENTS FOR ENTRANCE

In anticipation that both the spring and fall administrations of the MCAT will be offered in the state of New York and that official test scores will be forwarded to New York schools, candidates for admission to the 2001 entering class are required to take the MCAT no later than fall 2000 and have official scores sent to Stony Brook. Because of the rigorous competition, candidates are advised to submit applications early in the application period. All applications must be submitted through AMCAS. Prospective applicants should be aware that those who successfully applied to us in the past represent an exceptional, able, and diverse group.

Specific minimum course requirements are:

	Years
Biology (with lab)	1
Inorganic chemistry (with lab)	1
Organic chemistry (with lab)	1
Physics (with lab)	1
English	1

This minimum of preparation should be completed prior to filing the application. The Committee on Admissions makes a careful examination of the candidate's preparation and promise for creative work in medicine, regardless of the area of concentration prior to medical school. A basic course in biochemistry is very helpful in preparing students for the first year of medical school; however, it is neither a requirement nor a criterion for admission. It is expected that each student admitted will be capable of completing the full curriculum of required courses and electives under the established policies.

SELECTION FACTORS

Grades, MCAT scores, letters of evaluation, and extracurricular and work experiences are carefully examined. Motivational and personal characteristics as indicated in the application, letters of evaluation, and a personal interview are also a major part of the admissions assessment. There is no discrimination in the admissions review and selection process on the basis of sex, race, religion, national origin, age, marital status, or handicap.

Students learn from each other as well as from their teachers, their textbooks, and their patients; therefore, the school attempts to acquire a class representative of a variety of backgrounds and academic interests. Indeed, given the demands on physicians in the twenty-first century, breadth of individual background is particularly important. SUNY-Stony Brook hopes to attract a significant representation of groups that have historically been underrepresented in medicine. Applicants from foreign schools must have completed at least one year in an American college or university. Residents of New York constitute the majority of the applicants and entrants; and applications from out-of-state candidates are not encouraged unless the application is being made to the joint M.D.-Ph.D. (MSTP) program.

Required supporting documentation includes official transcripts of all college work and a letter of official evaluation from the applicant's premedical advisor (or, when no advisor exists at the applicant's college, from two instructors, one of whom must be from science field). If there are other individuals who also may be in a position to provide important information, the school would be happy to receive letters from them. Personal interviews will be arranged at the initiative of the school for candidates who appear to be serious contenders for admission.

The 1999 entering class was 49 percent *women*, 29 percent *Asian/Pacific Islander*, and 6 percent *minority students*. The *mean GPA* of this class was 3.55; *MCAT scores averaged* verbal reasoning, 10; physical sciences, 11; writing sample, P; and biological sciences, 11. It must be emphasized, however, that these numbers represent a range of scores, and that Stony Brook does not utilize a "cut-off" in grades or MCATs in making admissions decisions.

The school is committed to giving all applicants the individualized attention that they merit.

FINANCIAL AID

SUNY Stony Brook participates in all financial aid programs available at the medical schools of the SUNY system. Financial aid and counseling are available through the Office of Student Affairs, as is assistance in securing housing and in meeting other personal needs. On-campus housing is available. Students are advised to have transportation available because there is no public transportation to the outlying clinical facilities.

The secondary application fee of $75 will be waived for those who forward a copy of the AMCAS fee waiver. Other students who believe they are eligible for a fee waiver must present supporting documentation from the financial aid advisor at their institution.

INFORMATION FOR MINORITY STUDENTS

SUNY Stony Brook encourages applications from minority students, and the school makes a detailed review of these applications.

Public Institution

APPLICATION AND ACCEPTANCE POLICIES FOR 2001–2002 FIRST-YEAR CLASS

School participates in AMCAS. See Chapter 6.

Filing of AMCAS application
- Earliest date: June 1, 2000
- Latest date: Nov. 15, 2000

School application fee to all applicants: $75
Oldest MCAT scores considered: 1996
Does have Early Decision Program (EDP)
- EDP application period: June 1–Aug. 1, 2000
- EDP applicants notified by: Oct. 1, 2000

Acceptance notice to regular applicants
- Earliest date: Oct. 15, 2000
- Latest date: Until class is filled

Applicant's response to acceptance offer
- Maximum time: 15 days, unless otherwise specified

Requests for deferred entrance considered: Yes
Deposit to hold place in class: $100, (applied to tuition), due with response to acceptance offer
Deposit refundable prior to: May 15, 2001
Estimated number of new entrants: 100 (5 EDP)
Starting date: Aug. 2001

TUITION AND STUDENT FEES PER YEAR FOR 1999–2000 FIRST-YEAR CLASS

Tuition
- Resident: $10,840
- Nonresident: $21,940

Student fees: $250

INFORMATION ON 1999–2000 FIRST-YEAR CLASS

Number of	*In-State*	*Out-of-State*	*Total*
Applicants	2,175	1,110	3,285
Applicants Interviewed	595	8	603
New Entrants*	100	0	100

*All took the MCAT and had baccalaureate degrees.

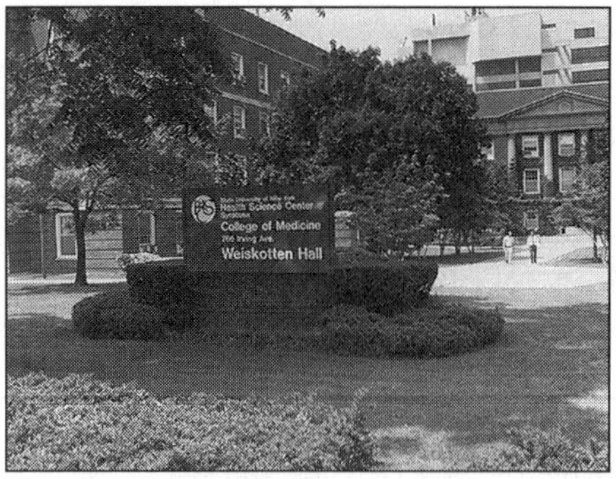

State University of New York Upstate Medical University College of Medicine

Syracuse, New York

Dr. Gregory Eastwood, *Dean, College of Medicine*
Ronald Wolk, *Associate Dean, Student Affairs*
Irvin Bodofsky, *Director of Financial Aid*

ADDRESS INQUIRIES TO:

Admissions Committee
State University of New York
Upstate Medical University
College of Medicine
155 Elizabeth Blackwell Street
Syracuse, New York 13210
(315) 464-4570; 464-8867 (FAX)

MISSION STATEMENT

The central mission of the SUNY Upstate Medical University is the education of professionals in health care and biomedical research. Excellence in patient care and the generation of new knowledge including understanding of disease, technology, and therapy are intrinsic to this mission. To this end, Upstate Medical University clinical faculty members and health care professionals commit themselves not only to their educational activities but also to patient care, demonstrating, in both areas, excellence and compassion. Similarly, a large segment of the faculty and staff must engage in research, both basic and applied, to acquire and generate new knowledge and technologies in the effort to promote health and provide a stimulating environment for the training of future scientists. In pursuing its mission, the Upstate Medical University provides its family of faculty, staff, students, and volunteers an environment of mutual trust and respect with opportunities to grow personally and professionally and to make a positive difference in the lives of others.

GENERAL INFORMATION

Upstate Medical University was established in 1834 as the Geneva Medical College. The college joined Syracuse University in 1872 and was transferred to the State University of New York (SUNY) in 1950 as the Upstate Medical Center. Since 1986, the university has been known as the SUNY Health Science Center at Syracuse. In 1999, our name was changed to SUNY Upstate Medical University to best reflect our academic mission in medical care and research, nursing, health professional training, and graduate education.

CURRICULUM

The medical education program is designed in three phases. During the first phase, students directly explore the normal structure, function, and systemic processes of the human body. In the second phase, students develop an understanding of the nature and progression of disease, the interaction and response of the human host to microorganisms, the principles of human behavior, pharmacology, and patient and population-based prevention. Interviewing and counseling skills, physical diagnosis, ethics, law, and economic issues also are addressed throughout the second phase. During the third phase, the students apply the principles of basic science to clinical problem-solving. Clinical clerkships in pediatrics, neurosciences, family medicine, medicine, surgery, obstetrics-gynecology, psychiatry, and radiology constitute the core of this phase. Clerkships in subspecialty services are required for all students. Thereafter, each student has the opportunity to attain individual educational objectives during 22–24 weeks of available elective time.

The clinical campus at Binghamton provides a core curriculum with programs in internal medicine, growth and development, perinatology, child and adolescent health, geriatrics, ambulatory surgery, neuropsychiatry, and primary care. A community orientation fosters a close working relationship between the campus and practicing physicians and other health care professionals.

A medical student research track is available, as are other research opportunities. Students who wish to develop skills in research may elect a special course of study. After selecting a project advisor, these students spend the first two summers as well as elective time on an independent research project.

Early assurance and deferred matriculation programs are available for qualified candidates. The M.D.-Ph.D. program is designed for those interested in investigating fundamental and applied issues of human health and disease. The central goal is to emphasize the best training in contemporary science in combination with the most practical experience in patient care. The Rural Medical Education program places students in rural communities for nine consecutive months of clinical and didactic education, including a community project.

An extended program under which the first two academic phases are spread over three years is available upon request and approval.

A modified pass/fail grading system is used; however, students may earn honors for outstanding performance in their courses.

REQUIREMENTS FOR ENTRANCE

Admissions preference is given to New York State residents. However, out-of-state applicants are admitted each year.

Applications are accepted from U.S. citizens and from permanent residents who have completed at least three years of college study (90 semester hours) in the United States or Canada in an accredited institution of higher education. International applicants and individuals from foreign schools must complete at least two years of study, which include all course requirements, in an accredited American or Canadian college or university prior to application and demonstrate competency in English composition and expression. Preference is also given to those applicants who have completed the courses required for admission at the time of application. Reapplicants are discouraged unless their qualifications have significantly improved.

The MCAT and satisfactory completion of the following courses are required:

	Sem. hrs.
Chemistry	8–12
Inorganic (with lab)	6–8
Organic (with lab)	6–8
Biology or zoology (with lab)	6–8
Physics (with lab)	6–8
English	6

Choice of major should be determined by the student's chief interests. Achieving excellence in the basic sciences is essential; however, academic work in the humanities and social sciences is equally important, as are meaningful experiences in relating to people.

SELECTION FACTORS

The Admissions Committee endeavors to take into consideration as much information as possible that delineates an applicant's total qualifications for the study and practice of medicine, without regard to race, creed, religion, national origin, age, sex, marital status, or degree of physical handicap. Several application forms are used in the medical school admission process. Each form collects information appropriate to the program an applicant may be seeking. Preadmission inquiries, which relate to gender, age, ethnicity, veteran status, or other characteristics, are collected for statistical purposes only. This information has no bearing on the selection process or final decisions regarding admission to the college.

Major factors in selection of applicants include: review of college records, which include scholastic aptitude and science aptitude; MCAT scores; letters of recommendation from premedical advisory committees; communication skills; character; motivation; and an evaluation of the personal interview.

FINANCIAL AID

Accepted applicants are eligible to apply for financial aid to the Office of Admissions and Student Affairs. Financial need is determined by the ACT needs analysis system (see Part 1). The Financial Aids Committee generally makes awards in July. The major portion of financial aid for each student is in loans. Scholarships are not readily available except for those state residents who qualify for the Tuition Assistance Program Awards.

INFORMATION FOR MINORITY STUDENTS

The SUNY Upstate Medical University is committed to making student enrollment reflective of the diverse population in New York state. Minorities and disadvantaged students are actively sought. A matriculation summer program and an extended curriculum are available. Premed counseling, application fee waivers, and off-campus interview programs are available. Program descriptions and further information can be obtained from either the Admissions Office or the Office of Multicultural Resources.

Public Institution

APPLICATION AND ACCEPTANCE POLICIES FOR 2001–2002 FIRST-YEAR CLASS

School participates in AMCAS. See Chapter 6.

Filing of AMCAS application
  Earliest date: June 1, 2000
  Latest date: Nov. 1, 2000
School application fee to all applicants: $100
Oldest MCAT scores considered: 1997
Does have Early Decision Program (EDP)
  EDP application period: June 1–Aug. 1, 2000
  EDP applicants notified by: Oct. 1, 2000
Acceptance notice to regular applicants
  Earliest date: Oct. 15, 2000
  Latest date: Varies
Applicant's response to acceptance offer
  Maximum time: 2 weeks
Requests for deferred entrance considered: Yes
Deposit to hold place in class: None
Estimated number of new entrants: 150 (5 EDP)
Starting date: Aug. 2000

TUITION AND STUDENT FEES PER YEAR FOR 1999–2000 FIRST-YEAR CLASS

Tuition
  Resident: $10,840
  Nonresident: $21,940
Student fees: $410

INFORMATION ON 1999–2000 FIRST-YEAR CLASS

Number of	*In-State*	*Out-of-State*	*Total*
Applicants	2,173	745	2,918
Applicants Interviewed	582	44	626
New Entrants*	148	5	153

*All had baccalaureate degrees and took the MCAT.

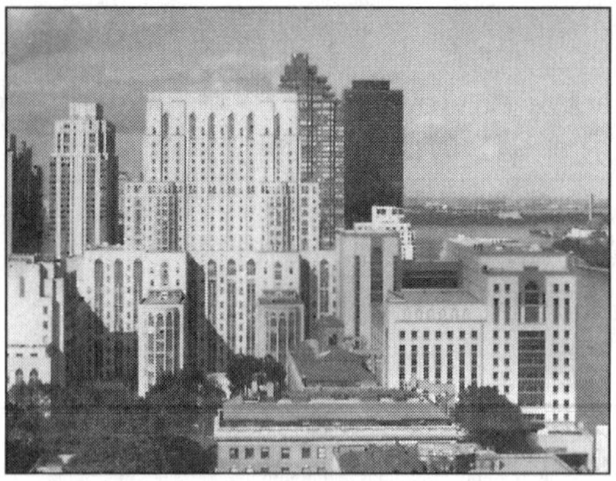

Weill Medical College of Cornell University

New York, New York

Dr. Antonio M. Gotto, *Dean*
Dr. Charles L. Bardes, *Associate Dean and Chairman, Committee on Admissions*
Joan M. May, *Assistant Dean for Financial Aid*

ADDRESS INQUIRIES TO:

Office of Admissions
Weill Medical College of Cornell University
445 East 69th Street
New York, New York 10021
(212) 746-1067; 746-8052 (FAX)
Web Site: http://www.med.cornell.edu

GENERAL INFORMATION

Cornell University Medical College was established in 1898. In 1998, the name was changed to the Weill Medical College of Cornell University. Although the university is situated in Ithaca, the Medical College was opened in New York City to take advantage of the facilities of a large urban area. Clinical instruction is carried on in the New York–Presbyterian Hospital; Memorial Sloan-Kettering Cancer Center; the Hospital for Special Surgery; the New York Hospital Medical Center of Queens; the New York Methodist Hospital; Flushing Hospital Medical Center in Queens; the New York Community Hospital; St. Barnabas Hospital; Lincoln Medical and Mental Health Center; Wyckoff Heights Medical Center in Brooklyn; the Burke Rehabilitation Hospital in White Plains, New York; United Hospital Medical Center in Port Chester, New York; and the Cayuga Medical Center in Ithaca, New York.

CURRICULUM

Medical education at Cornell aims to develop individuals who not only recognize and are dedicated to the highest quality patient care, but also understand their responsibility for contributions through continuing personal scholarship. Many Cornell alumni pursue academic and research careers in addition to the clinical practice of medicine. The education process at Cornell has undergone a recent revision with the major goals of integrating the teaching of the basic and clinical sciences throughout the four years of study and emphasizing problem-solving in the context of scientific inquiry and clinical care.

Core basic science materials are presented during Years 1 and 2, and advanced basic science courses are offered during Years 3 and 4. Learning during the first two years occurs in the setting of problem-based tutorials, small-group conferences, laboratories, lectures, and a journal club. Information is presented in a series of highly integrated, multi-disciplinary block courses: Molecules to Cells, Genes and Development, Human Structure and Function, Host Defenses, Brain and Mind, and Basis of Disease.

Clinical instruction begins in Year 1 with a full day-a-week course, Medicine, Patients, and Society I, during which the student acquires early clinical skills in an ambulatory setting and studies the doctor-patient relationship and socioeconomic, behavioral, and public health issues. This course continues as Medicine, Patients, and Society II in Year 2 with the student gaining experience in the physical examination of patients and clinical problem solving and medical ethics. In Year 3, the focus of Medicine, Patients, and Society III is on student experience with patients, clinical dilemmas, and multiculturalism. Clinical clerkships begin during the later third of Year 2 and include a new primary care clerkship, which, in conjunction with the Medicine, Patients, and Society sequence, constitutes the central features of the primary care curriculum. The clinical clerkships include rotations in medicine, neurology, obstetrics and gynecology, pediatrics, psychiatry, and surgery. Year 4 provides the major time block for clinical electives. Performance is graded by an honors/pass/fail system during the basic science curriculum and an honors/high pass/pass/fail system during the core curriculum.

For students interested in teaching and research careers in the medical sciences, Cornell offers a fully funded Tri-Institutional M.D.-Ph.D. Program, which is coordinated with the Cornell University Graduate School of Medical Sciences, Memorial Sloan-Kettering Cancer Center, and Rockefeller University. Applicants interested in applying to this program should contact the Tri-Institutional M.D.-Ph.D. Program, 1300 York Avenue, Room D-115, or telephone (212) 746-6023. The deadline to apply is October 15.

REQUIREMENTS FOR ENTRANCE

A minimum of three years in an accredited college and the MCAT are required; most students have completed four years of undergraduate work and hold a baccalaureate degree. The Committee on Admissions considers a strong foundation in the sciences a fundamental requirement but does not wish to establish rigid guidelines for admission. Therefore, Cornell requires satisfactory completion of at least 24 semester hours in science courses including biology or zoology, general chemistry, organic chemistry, and physics. In addition, six semester hours are required in English literature or composition. For non-science majors, at least two terms of biology beyond the introductory course are suggested. Cornell regards a broad liberal arts education as fundamental for the making of a good physician. The Committee on Admissions will review and evaluate achievement in the humanities and social sciences.

SELECTION FACTORS

Students are selected for their leadership potential in various areas of medicine. There is an attempt to select the best qualified students from various academic, geographic, and social backgrounds. Maturity, stability, motivation, academic achievement, and other qualities are evaluated. Recent preparation for the study of medicine, particularly in the sciences, is preferred.

The 1999 entering class had the following characteristics: 55 percent, *women; mean science GPA* 3.66; *average MCAT scores,* VR-10.3 , PS-11.4, BS-11.3; 18 percent, *minority students*; 70 percent, *sciences majors.*

Cornell's policy actively supports equality of education and employment opportunity and is committed to the maintenance of affirmative action programs, which will assure the continuation of such equality of opportunity.

Students who are unsuccessful in gaining acceptance to Cornell are rarely successful on reapplication unless there has been substantial improvement in their qualifications.

FINANCIAL AID

Admissions decisions are made without regard to financial need. Every effort is made to assist students to finance their medical education without incurring unreasonable debt. Substantial institutional grants and subsidized loans are available and are allocated according to need after an analysis of student and family resources. Fifty percent of the students receive Medical College support, and 80 percent receive grants or loans from some source. Since subsidized housing is available for all students at the Medical College and cars are not necessary, living costs and transportation expenses are reasonable. Support for community service, summer research, and international electives is available for all students. The application fee will be waived if it represents a hardship to the applicant.

Unfortunately, students who are not citizens or permanent residents of the United States are not eligible for Medical College financial aid, institutional grants, or loans. Any non-U.S. citizen or permanent resident who is accepted for admission to Cornell will be expected to comply with one of the two requirements listed below on or before July 1 of the year of matriculation.

1. The accepted student must deposit in an escrow account (to be established under terms acceptable to the Medical College) funds sufficient to meet tuition charges for the total period of enrollment.
2. The accepted student must pre-pay his or her four years of tuition by multiplying the current tuition at the time of matriculation by four.

Details of the agreements and/or requirements listed above are available in the Office of Admissions. *In all cases, students are responsible for any and all fees and other expenses.*

INFORMATION FOR MINORITY STUDENTS

The Medical College makes a nationwide effort to enroll qualified minority group students, and we have one of the best records in minority recruitment and retention among private U.S. medical schools.

Cornell conducts a research fellowship program for about 25 minority group premedical students during the summer between their junior and senior college years. The program consists of research activities with faculty members of the medical center and brief course work in cardiovascular physiology, which provides a preview of the basic science years of medical school. The participants are housed in the medical students' residence.

Private Institution

APPLICATION AND ACCEPTANCE POLICIES FOR 2001–2002 FIRST-YEAR CLASS

School participates in AMCAS. See Chapter 6.

Filing of AMCAS application
  Earliest date: June 1, 2000
  Latest date: Oct. 15, 2000
School application fee to all applicants: $75
Oldest MCAT scores considered: 1997
Does have Early Decision Program (EDP)
  EDP application period: June 1–Aug. 1, 2000
  EDP applicants notified by: Oct. 1, 2000
Acceptance notice to regular applicants
  Earliest date: Oct. 15, 2000
  Latest date: Until class is filled
Applicant's response to acceptance offer
  Maximum time: 2 weeks
Requests for deferred entrance considered: Yes
Deposit to hold place in class (applied to tuition):
  $100, due May 15, 2001
Deposit refundable prior to: June 1, 2001
Estimated number of new entrants: 101 (2 EDP)
Starting date: Aug. 2001

TUITION AND STUDENT FEES PER YEAR FOR 1999–2000 FIRST-YEAR CLASS

Tuition: $27,000 Student fees: $640

INFORMATION ON 1999–2000 FIRST-YEAR CLASS

Number of	*In-State*	*Out-of-State*	*Total*
Applicants	1,401	5,379	6,780
Applicants Interviewed	300	797	1,097
New Entrants*	45	56	101

*All took the MCAT and had baccalaureate degrees.

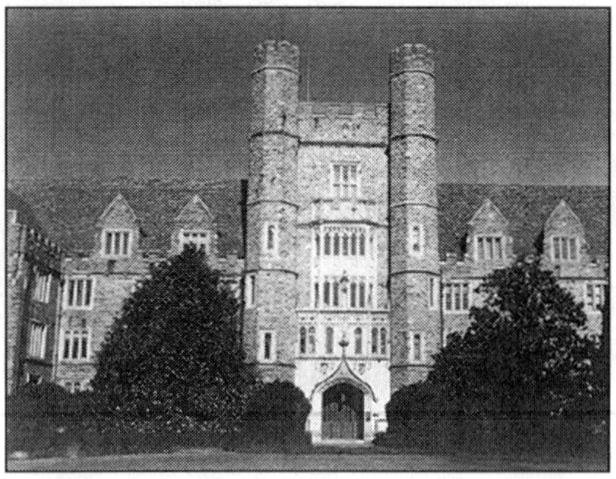

Duke University School of Medicine

Durham, North Carolina

Dr. Russel E. Kaufman, *Vice Dean for Education*
Dr. Brenda E. Armstrong, *Associate Dean and Director of Admissions*
Stacey R. McCorison, *Director of Financial Aid*

ADDRESS INQUIRIES TO:

Committee on Admissions
Duke University
School of Medicine
Duke University Medical Center
P.O. Box 3710
Durham, North Carolina 27710
(919) 684-2985; 684-8893 (FAX)
Web Site: http://www.mc.duke.edu/depts/som

GENERAL INFORMATION

The Duke University Medical Center is located on the campus of Duke University in Durham, North Carolina. A hospital was opened for patients in July 1930, and the first medical students were admitted in October of that year. The first doctor of medicine degrees were conferred in June 1932. Duke Hospital (1,000 beds) is supplemented by the Durham Veterans Administration Hospital (489 beds) for clinical teaching.

CURRICULUM

The curriculum has been designed to provide the flexibility to encompass the rapid expansion of medical knowledge as well as the broad range of individual student interests and talents. First-year students receive instruction in the basic science principles of modern medicine. A two-year introduction to clinical medicine complements instruction in each of the first two years of the medical school curriculum. The second year is the clinical clerkship year. The third and fourth years are elective; and with the guidance of an advisory dean and several senior faculty advisors, students design their programs to include half basic science and half clinical course work. In the third year each student may participate in a mentored research project enabling them to learn basic principles of research and to critically evaluate the research of others. Having completed the required courses in the first and second years, students may explore relevant areas of basic science in more depth and complement their first-year acquisition of science knowledge. Students who elect dual-degree programs (M.D.-M.P.H., M.D.-M.P.P., M.D.-M.B.A., M.D.-J.D., and M.D./M.A.-Ph.D. in medical history) begin their respective curricula during the third year. In the fourth year, clinical courses may be elected to enhance general medical education in more depth and breadth. Students graduate prepared to pursue careers in community practice, academic medicine, or public health and to contribute expertise in health policy and medical ethics issues.

The Medical Scientist Training Program is designed to provide both the M.D. and Ph.D. degrees over a six- to seven-year period of study. The first two years are spent in the medical school program, followed by a three- to four-year period of graduate study. Upon completion of the Ph.D. degree, the last year is spent in the clinical sciences. It is expected that candidates for this combined degree plan to have careers in academic medicine.

REQUIREMENTS FOR ENTRANCE

The MCAT and three years of college are required. The spring MCAT is preferred and advantageous. A minimum of 90 semester hours of approved college credit is also required. Prerequisite courses must be taken within seven years before application. Course work must include:

	Years
Biology	1
Inorganic chemistry	1
Organic chemistry	1
General physics	1
Calculus	1
English	1

An introductory course in biochemistry is suggested during the senior year.

Premedical students should be aware of the importance of a well-rounded general education as preparation for the study of medicine and not limit themselves to scientific courses. The Committee on Admissions places more importance on the way applicants handle their undergraduate work than on the subject matter taken.

SELECTION FACTORS

The selection of students is based upon the quality rather than the quantity of preparation and upon demonstrated evidence of personal attributes of intelligence, character, and general fitness for the study and practice of medicine. In considering an applicant, many sources of information may be consulted: curricular and extracurricular college record; fitness as reflected by carefully prepared, confidential appraisals by teachers who know the individual well; MCAT scores; and the applicant's showing in the interview that is held with members of the Committee on Admissions or one of its regional representatives.

Accepted students for the 1999 entering class had high GPAs and MCAT scores. Special consideration is given to residents of North Carolina. There were 45 women in the 1999 entering class. The Committee on Admissions does not discriminate on the basis of race, sex, sexual preference, creed, age, handicap, or national origin.

FINANCIAL AID

The Office of Financial Aid asks that students who wish to be considered for institutional funds complete the *Need Access* diskette and the federal government's Free Application for Federal Student Aid (FAFSA). These may be obtained via Internet or the Office of Financial Aid. Students seeking to apply for only Federal Stafford Loans need to complete the FAFSA. We urge that students complete and submit the applications as soon as possible. Accepted students will receive an award notice once we have received the FAFSA and the *Need Access* computations.

Students applying for institutional funds who demonstrate need as determined by both the FAFSA and the *Need Access* analysis will receive approximately 40 percent Stafford and/or Duke loan and 60 percent institutional grant. While more than 80 percent of currently enrolled medical students receive some type of scholarship, grant, or loan, the financial circumstance has no bearing on the admissions process.

Eight Nanaline H. Duke Scholarships in the amount of current tuition are awarded each year by the Dean to academically excellent first-year students. Seven Dean's Tuition Scholarships in the amount of current tuition are awarded each year by the Dean to academically excellent under-represented minority students.

Financially needy, disadvantaged, and minority students selected for the North Carolina Board of Governors Medical Scholarship will receive full tuition, fees, and a stipend.

Students who enter the Medical Scientist Training Program receive full tuition, fees, and a stipend.

INFORMATION FOR MINORITY STUDENTS

An aggressive effort to identify and recruit talented minority students is in place, supported by significant minority house staff and faculty numbers, and has resulted in the consistent enrollment of significant numbers of minorities to the School of Medicine. Minority medical students have access to a dean/faculty/student group that supports freshman students and meets regularly to discuss common issues pertinent to minority student experience. These efforts are supplemented by departmental and medical school-wide programs to address cross-cultural issues in medicine.

Private Institution

APPLICATION AND ACCEPTANCE POLICIES FOR 2001–2002 FIRST-YEAR CLASS

School participates in AMCAS. See Chapter 6.

Filing of AMCAS application
  Earliest date: June 1, 2000
  Latest date: Nov. 1, 2000
School application fee to all applicants: $65
Oldest MCAT scores considered: 1997
Does not have Early Decision Program
Acceptance notice to regular applicants
  Earliest date: Feb. 28, 2000
  Latest date: Until class is filled
Applicant's response to acceptance offer
  Maximum time: 3 weeks
Requests for deferred entrance considered: Yes
Deposit to hold place in class (applied to tuition):
  $100, due May 15, 2001; nonrefundable
Estimated number of new entrants: 100
Starting date: Aug. 2001

TUITION AND STUDENT FEES PER YEAR FOR 1999–2000 FIRST-YEAR CLASS

Tuition: $26,700 Student fees: $2,600

INFORMATION ON 1999–2000 FIRST-YEAR CLASS

Number of	*In-State*	*Out-of-State*	*Total*
Applicants	369	5,296	5,665
Applicants Interviewed	*	*	1,240
New Entrants†	17	83	100

*Data not available.

†All took the MCAT and had baccalaureate degrees.

CHAPTER 11

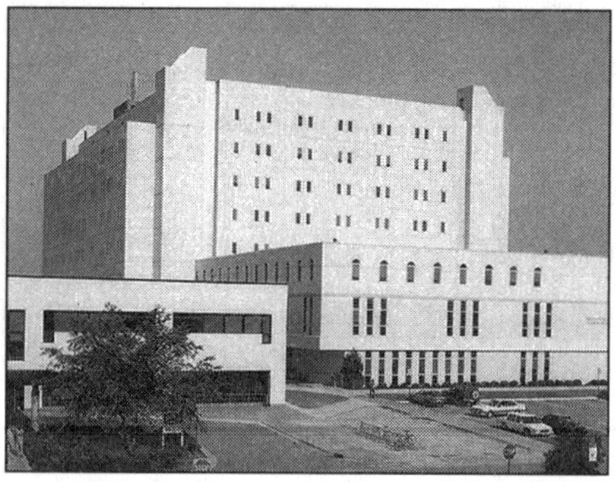

The Brody School of Medicine at East Carolina University

Greenville, North Carolina

Dr. James A. Hallock, *Vice Chancellor for Health Sciences and Dean*
Dr. James G. Peden, Jr., *Associate Dean for Admissions*
Vicki Ogden, *Director of Financial Aid and Student Services*

ADDRESS INQUIRIES TO:

Associate Dean
Office of Admissions
The Brody School of Medicine
at East Carolina University
Greenville, North Carolina 27858-4354
(252) 816-2202
Web Site: http://www.med.ecu.edu/htdocs/admiss/som.htm

MISSION STATEMENT

Simply stated, our goal at the Brody School of Medicine at East Carolina University is to provide students with the knowledge and clinical experience needed to attain successful careers in medicine. Our mission is threefold: educating primary care physicians, making medical care more readily available to the people of eastern North Carolina, and providing opportunities for disadvantaged students. Among the most important elements making up the educational approach at the School of Medicine are the relatively small class sizes, a highly competent and concerned faculty, and exceptional facilities.

GENERAL INFORMATION

In 1972 East Carolina University enrolled students in the First-Year Program in Medical Education. The Board of Governors of the University of North Carolina system and the General Assembly of North Carolina authorized East Carolina University to expand the First-Year Program and establish a degree-granting School of Medicine. The School of Medicine enrolled the first class of students in August 1977.

The school's educational facilities are located on the 100-acre Health Sciences Center campus. Preclinical instruction is offered in the nine-story Brody Medical Sciences Building, which is contiguous to the Pitt County Memorial Hospital. Comprehensive clinical instruction is offered in the hospital (731 beds). Other clinical settings, either adjacent to or near the Health Sciences Center, include the Leo W. Jenkins Cancer Center, Child Development Evaluation Clinic, Mental Health Center, Alcoholic Rehabilitation Center, Rehabilitation Center, Area Health Education Center, and the Intensive/Intermediate Care Neonatal Unit.

Our Generalist Physician Program was designed to amplify and complement activities to meet the school's major mission of educating primary care physicians. The generalist program extends across the entire four-year curriculum and involves intensive contact with community physicians. Emphasis is placed on meeting the primary health care needs of those in rural and underserved areas. All students interested in primary care careers are given the opportunity to develop long-term mentor relationships with community-based family physicians, general pediatricians, and general internists.

CURRICULUM

The first year of the four-year curriculum is devoted to the study of the anatomy and functions of the body through courses in gross and microscopic anatomy, biochemistry, physiology, microbiology/immunology, and genetics. Correlative clinical lectures in these as well as courses in psychosocial basis of medical practice, ethical and social issues in medicine, and clinical skills I are presented. A primary care preceptorship is mandatory.

The second-year curriculum is directed toward clinical medicine. Courses include clinical skills II, pathogenic microbiology, pharmacology, pathology, and introduction to medicine. Also included in the second-year curriculum are courses in psychiatry, psychopathology and human sexuality, life-style abuse, ethical and social issues in medicine, and a primary care preceptorship.

The third year is composed of six required clerkships: 8 weeks each in family medicine, internal medicine, obstetrics and gynecology, pediatrics, psychiatry, and surgery. At least 12 weeks of ambulatory care are included in the third year.

The fourth year is composed of 36 weeks of clinical and basic science electives, which must include blocks in primary care, medicine, and surgery. Students select an individualized curriculum after consulting with faculty advisors.

Student performance is evaluated by letter grade, and promotion to the next year's class is recommended to the dean by the Promotions Committee of the respective year.

A combined M.D.-M.B.A. program is available to students. Coursework in the School of Business is completed in 12 months, usually taken between the second and third years of the medical curriculum. Both the M.D. and M.B.A. degrees are awarded after five years of study.

REQUIREMENTS FOR ENTRANCE

The MCAT and a minimum equivalent of three undergraduate years of preparation are required. Minimum course work requirements are:

	Semester Hours
General biology or zoology (with lab)	8
Inorganic chemistry (with lab)	8
Organic chemistry (with lab)	8
Physics (with lab)	8
English	6

Additional courses in the humanities and social sciences and a second year of English are recommended.

SELECTION FACTORS

Factors considered in the selection process encompass the social, personal, and intellectual development of each applicant. All available application data are evaluated: MCAT scores; academic performance; comments contained in letters of reference/recommendation; and the results of two personal interviews, conducted only at the medical school campus, with two members of the Admissions Committee.

The Brody School of Medicine at East Carolina University seeks competent students of diverse personalities and backgrounds, and all applicants are evaluated without regard to race, religion, sex, age, national origin, or handicap. Very strong preference is given to qualified residents of North Carolina.

Characteristics of the 1999 entering class of 72 students were: *mean GPA,* 3.5; *sex,* 33 women; *minorities,* 26 students. *MCAT scores* (mean and ranges): *VR*-8.8 (4–13); *PS*-8.7 (5–13); *WS*-O (K–S); *BS*-9.0 (6–13).

Qualified North Carolina residents from schools with similar medical curriculae may be considered for transfer into the second- or third-year classes. Advanced standing positions are dependent on the very limited number of seats that become available through attrition. Interested students should send letters describing their circumstances to the Office of Admissions for further information.

FINANCIAL AID

Resources are available for loans and scholarships. The Financial Aid Office will make every effort to provide information and financial aid to those students who demonstrate need for financial assistance in order to meet the costs of their educational and living obligations. Awards are based on need as determined by confidential information supplied by the student. Merit awards are available.

Part-time employment is not permitted during the first two years and may be undertaken during the last two years only by permission of the dean. Sixty-five percent of the student body receive some financial assistance.

INFORMATION FOR MINORITY STUDENTS

Those members of minority groups holding residence in North Carolina are encouraged to apply. Minority representation on the Admissions Committee is significant, and the Academic Support and Counseling Center offers a wide range

Public Institution

APPLICATION AND ACCEPTANCE POLICIES FOR 2001–2002 FIRST-YEAR CLASS

School participates in AMCAS. See Chapter 6.

Filing of AMCAS application
  Earliest date: June 1, 2000
  Latest date: Nov. 15, 2000
School application after screening: $50*
Oldest MCAT scores considered: 1998
Does have Early Decision Program (EDP)
  For North Carolina residents only
  EDP application period: June 1–Aug. 1, 2000
  EDP applicants notified by: Oct. 1, 2000
Acceptance notice to regular applicants
  Earliest date: Oct. 15, 2000
  Latest date: Class matriculation date
Applicant's response to acceptance offer
  Maximum time: 3 weeks
Requests for deferred entrance considered: No
Deposit to hold place in class (applied to tuition):
  $100, due with response to acceptance offer
Deposit refundable prior to: May 15, 2001
Estimated number of new entrants: 72 (9 EDP)
Starting date: Aug. 2001

TUITION AND STUDENT FEES PER YEAR FOR 1999–2000 FIRST-YEAR CLASS

Tuition
  Resident: $2,280
  Nonresident: $21,962

Student fees: $1,006

INFORMATION ON 1999–2000 FIRST-YEAR CLASS

Number of	*In-State*	*Out-of-State*	*Total*
Applicants	755	692	1,447
Applicants Interviewed	503	0	503
New Entrants†	72	0	72

*Subject to approval by UNC Board of Governors.
†All took the MCAT; all had baccalaureate degrees.

CHAPTER 11

University of North Carolina at Chapel Hill School of Medicine

Chapel Hill, North Carolina

Dr. Jeffrey L. Houpt, *Dean and Vice Chancellor for Medical Affairs*
Dr. Axalla J. Hoole, *Associate Dean for Admissions*
Sheila M. Graham, *Financial Aid Officer*

ADDRESS INQUIRIES TO:

Admissions Office
CB# 7000 121 MacNider Hall
University of North Carolina at Chapel Hill
School of Medicine
Chapel Hill, North Carolina 27599-7000
(919) 962-8331; 966-9930 (FAX)
E-mail: admissions@med.unc.edu
Web Site: http://www.med.unc.edu/

MISSION STATEMENT

The University of North Carolina School of Medicine prepares students for the broad range of professional activities open to physicians. Graduates of the UNC School of Medicine become practitioners in the community, formulate health policy at the highest state and national levels, and make seminal contributions in research, both at the bench and in the clinic.

GENERAL INFORMATION

The School of Medicine of the University of North Carolina (UNC) at Chapel Hill was established in 1879 and expanded to a four-year school in 1952. Schools of dentistry, nursing, pharmacy, and public health are adjacent to the medical school on the university campus. Physical facilities include modern classrooms, multidisciplinary student laboratories, and a health sciences library with 290,000 print volumes, 8,900 audiovisual and micro-computer software programs, 36,000 microform pieces, and current subscriptions to 4,590 periodicals. The University of North Carolina Hospitals, the Biological Sciences Center, and the Cancer Research Center are major on-campus teaching resources. Area Health Education Centers throughout the state provide clinical experience in community settings. Additional information, including the entire content of the current catalog, is available on-line at <http://www.med.unc.edu>.

CURRICULUM

The curriculum emphasizes the application of biomedical science to the solution of clinical problems. Clinical experience is included in each of the first two years. Required clinical clerkships make up the third year. The fourth year consists primarily of clinical electives including two required rotations in community primary care settings. Students may participate in original or ongoing individualized research projects under faculty direction at any time during the course of their studies. Programs leading to M.D.-Ph.D. or M.D.-M.P.H. degrees are offered. The honors/pass/fail grading system is used.

REQUIREMENTS FOR ENTRANCE

Requirements for admission are under review and are subject to change. At this time a minimum of 96 semester hours of accredited college work and the MCAT are required. The test must be taken no later than the August prior to the intended August date of admission. Scores from an MCAT administered more than five years before the projected date of matriculation are not accepted.

Students are encouraged to pursue one or more scholarly interests in depth during the undergraduate years, but course work must demonstrate proficiency in the natural sciences. Course work in the humanities and social sciences, as well as advanced work in the sciences and mathematics, is valued. Proficiency in the use of the English language is essential. Specific course work must include:

	Suggested Sem. hrs.
English	6
Biology (including at least one course with lab). It is strongly suggested that students take at least one course in cell and molecular biology	8
General and Organic Chemistry (with labs)	16
Physics (with labs)	8

SELECTION FACTORS

The Committee on Admissions evaluates the qualifications of all applicants to select those with the greatest potential for accomplishment in one of the many careers open to medical graduates. Preference is given to North Carolina residents. The University of North Carolina does not discriminate on the basis of race, national origin, religion, sex, age, or handicap.

The AMCAS application is used for initial screening. Qualified North Carolina applicants and selected nonresidents are sent a supplementary application. Following receipt of a supplementary application, applicants are invited for an interview. In making its final selections from the group of qualified in-state applicants, the committee considers evidence of each candidate's motivation, maturity, leadership, integrity, and a variety of other personal qualifications and accomplishments in addition to the scholastic record. All information available about each applicant is considered without assigning priority to any single factor. No special admission tracks or quotas are applied among in-state applicants. The undergraduate major is not an important consideration, but excellence in the chosen field is expected. Previously rejected applicants are considered without prejudice, but re-applications are compared to those previously submitted to assess changes in the applicants qualifications.

FINANCIAL AID

Grants and low-interest, long-term loans are available to students with financial need, determined through an evaluation of the total resources available to the student. Awards are based on information obtained from the Free Application for Federal Student Aid (FAFSA) submitted by the student. At last calculation, 85 percent of the student body apply for aid from funds for which eligibility is certified by the university. Financial need will not adversely affect a student's chances of admission, and no student, once admitted, should have to leave for personal financial need. Part-time employment is discouraged. A few scholarships are awarded for academic achievement and promise; there is no separate application for these.

Economically or environmentally disadvantaged students admitted to the School of Medicine are eligible for nomination to the Board of Governors' Medical Scholars Program. Those students who are selected receive annual stipends of $5,000 plus tuition and fees. Recipients must be residents of North Carolina who demonstrate exceptional financial need and are enrolled in one of the schools of medicine on a full-time basis.

For additional information, contact the Student Aid Section at (919) 962-6118.

INFORMATION FOR DISADVANTAGED STUDENTS

Disadvantaged students are urged to apply, and there is an active recruitment program for minority students. The Medical Education Development Program is available to premedical disadvantaged students to acquaint them with the medical school curriculum and faculty and to assist them with learning skills development for medical school.

The Office of Student Affairs provides academic counseling after admission. Academic assistance is provided through tutorial programs, the Learning and Assessment Laboratory, and other resources within the university. Faculty members are available to assist students, and students are encouraged to see them for specific curricular problems. For students who have significant problems mastering the curriculum, a reduction in courses can be considered. A review program during the summer is provided for students with limited academic deficiencies. Students are reexamined at the end of the review period and promoted upon successfully passing the reexamination.

Public Institution

APPLICATION AND ACCEPTANCE POLICIES FOR 2001–2002 FIRST-YEAR CLASS

School participates in AMCAS. See Chapter 6.

Filing of AMCAS application
  Earliest date: June 1, 2000
  Latest date: Nov. 15, 2000
School application fee after screening: $60
Oldest MCAT scores considered: 1995
Does have Early Decision Program (EDP)
  EDP application period: June 1–Aug. 1, 2000
  EDP applicants notified by: Oct. 1, 2000
Acceptance notice to regular applicants
  Earliest date: Oct. 15, 2000
  Latest date: Until class is filled
Applicant's response to acceptance offer
  Maximum time: 3 weeks
Requests for deferred entrance considered: Yes
Deposit to hold place in class (applied to tuition):
  $100, due with response to acceptance offer
Deposit refundable prior to: May 15, 2001
Estimated number of new entrants: 160 (10 EDP)
Starting date: Aug. 2001

TUITION AND STUDENT FEES PER YEAR FOR 1999–2000 FIRST-YEAR CLASS

Tuition
  Resident: $2,552
  Nonresident: $23,444

Student fees: $801

INFORMATION ON 1999–2000 FIRST-YEAR CLASS

Number of	*In-State*	*Out-of-State*	*Total*
Applicants	818	2,138	2,956
Applicants Interviewed	457	78	535
New Entrants*	140	20	160

*All took the MCAT and had baccalaureate degrees.

CHAPTER 11

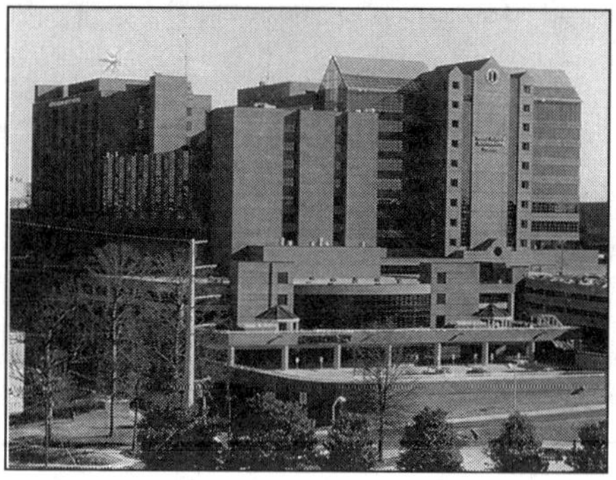

Wake Forest University School of Medicine

Winston-Salem, North Carolina

Dr. James N. Thompson, *Vice President and Dean*
Dr. Lewis H. Nelson, III, *Associate Dean for Student Services and Admissions*
Melissa Stevens, *Financial Aid Director*

ADDRESS INQUIRIES TO:

Office of Medical School Admissions
Wake Forest University School of Medicine
Medical Center Boulevard
Winston-Salem, North Carolina 27157-1090
(336) 716-4264; 716-5807 (FAX)
E-mail: medadmit@wfubmc.edu
Web Site: http://www.wfubmc.edu/education/admissions/

GENERAL INFORMATION

The School of Medicine was established in 1902 at Wake Forest, North Carolina, and of the existing 166 medical schools, it was one of 11 that required college preparation. Patient care, research, education, and community service remain the fourfold mission of the school as part of the Wake Forest University Baptist Medical Center. The name of the medical school has changed from Bowman Gray School of Medicine to Wake Forest University School of Medicine, the Bowman Gray Campus.

The main teaching hospital of the medical school is the 880-bed North Carolina Baptist Hospitals, Inc. Affiliated institutions include the 896-bed Forsyth Memorial Hospital, Reynolds Health Center, and Northwest Area Health Education Center.

CURRICULUM

The curriculum is organized to meet the seven stated goals of the undergraduate medical education program: self-directed learning and life-long learning skills, core biomedical science knowledge, clinical skills, problem solving/clinical reasoning skills, interviewing and communication skills, information management skills, and professional attitudes and behavior.

A new curriculum, Prescription for Excellence: A Physician's Pathway to Lifelong Learning, was implemented in 1998. This curriculum was founded upon the following ten principles: 1) Leadership; 2) Life-long learning; 3) Exploration and Discovery; 4) Practice of Medicine; 5) Professional Attitudes and Behaviors; 6) Health Promotion and Disease Prevention; 7) Teaching-Learning Process; 8) Admissions Process; 9) Student Evaluation; and 10) Faculty Development and Recognition.

Students study the basic and clinical sciences in an integrated fashion throughout the four-year curriculum utilizing a variety of educational methods including small-group problem-based learning. Early community-based clinical experience, as well as a focus on population health are hallmarks of the curriculum. Professionalism issues are addressed longitudinally across the curriculum in formats designed to provide students with a clear understanding of the role and responsibilities of physicians within society. Information technology has been integrated into the curriculum to a considerable degree, and all incoming students are provided with an IBM ThinkPad laptop computer.

Pharmacology, pathology, microbiology, and radiology topics are integrated with clinical topics within the organ system-based topics in the Systems Pathophysiology 1 course. Evidence-based decision making is the focus of the second-year clinical decision-making course. Issues related to the practice of medicine are discussed within, Medicine as a Profession (MAAP). Students continue their development of clinical skills during the second year within the Foundations of Clinical Medicine (FCM) course. The third phase consists of required clerkships in medicine, surgery and anesthesiology, pediatrics, psychiatry, obstetrics and gynecology, family medicine, neurology/rehabilitation medicine, and women's health. The fourth phase consists of 11 four-week rotations: two advanced in-patient management clerkships, intensive care and emergency medicine. The remainder are electives. The fifth phase completes the fourth year with a return to basic science within a clinical context. Performance is evaluated on a zero-to-four scale across the four-year curriculum.

EARLY ASSURANCE PROGRAM (EAP)

Well-qualified college students, who are residents of North Carolina, upon completion of the sophomore year, may apply for acceptance to the class entering two years later. Eligibility requires a GPA of 3.5, a science GPA of 3.5, and completion of half of the required prerequisites. The MCAT will not be required.

A student applies early in the junior year through the AMCAS process (November 1 deadline), asking consideration for the EAP. The applicant must agree to complete requisite courses, to continue academic excellence, to demonstrate high ethical conduct, and not to apply to any other medical school. Non-acceptance by the EAP does not influence future applications. The EAP should not be confused with the Early Decision Program.

JOINT-DEGREE PROGRAMS

The Wake Forest University School of Medicine offers two five-year joint-degree programs and the M.D.-Ph.D. The

M.D.–M.B.A. program is offered in conjunction with the Babcock Graduate School of Management, and the M.D.-Ph.D. is offered in conjunction with the Graduate School of Wake Forest University. The five-year M.D.-Master of Arts in Intercultural Studies is offered in conjunction with the Southeastern Theological Seminary.

The M.D.-M.B.A. program responds to the growing need for professionals who are trained in both medicine and management. The M.D.-Masters of Arts in Intercultural Studies is designed for students with an interest in medical missions. The M.D.-Ph.D. program is expected to be completed within seven years. All joint degrees require completion of all requirements of both programs before degrees are awarded.

Applicants for the joint-degree programs must be accepted via a separate admissions process to the business and graduate schools. The Babcock School of Management requires applicants to take the GMAT; the Graduate School accepts the MCAT.

REQUIREMENTS FOR ENTRANCE

The MCAT is required except for EAP. The minimum requirement for admission is 90 semester hours of college work, although most candidates benefit from a well-rounded four-year college curriculum. Required courses should be completed by the time of application. Generally, prerequisites are:

	Sem. hrs.
General biology	8
General or inorganic chemistry	8
Organic chemistry	8
General physics	8

SELECTION FACTORS

Candidates are selected on the basis of the quality of their academic records, MCAT scores, and general qualifications. Although North Carolina residents compose the majority of the class (50 to 60 percent), nonresidents are given equal and careful consideration. There are no restrictions because of race, creed, sex, religion, age, physical disadvantages, marital status, or national origin.

The Committee on Admissions (COA) will evaluate each application. Applicants whose performance suggests they would have difficulty in handling the curriculum are notified. All other applicants are sent a supplemental application. Applicants who have completed files are considered for local interviews at the discretion of the COA. No regional interviews are conducted.

The School of Medicine may be able to accept an application for transfer from a student who is currently enrolled, and in good standing, in a medical school accredited by the Liaison Committee on Medical Education and who meets the prerequisite requirements.

Characteristics of the 1998 entering class are students from 23 states and 54 colleges and universities; *gender*, 49 percent women; *acceptance rate,* 8 percent of all applicants were interviewed and 43 percent of those interviewed offered acceptance for 108 places.

FINANCIAL AID

Loans and scholarships are awarded to qualified applicants on the basis of financial need and academic standing. Applicants must complete required application forms prior to the April 1 deadline. Students receive a significant amount of their funding from federal student loan programs. Eighty percent of the student body receive financial assistance. Students should not work part-time because of the demands of the study of medicine.

INFORMATION FOR MINORITY STUDENTS

The Office of Minority Affairs actively recruits minority students and has developed summer enrichment, academic reinforcement, tutorial, and counseling services for enrolled students. Address inquiries to the Office of Minority Affairs.

Private Institution

APPLICATION AND ACCEPTANCE POLICIES FOR 2001–2002 FIRST-YEAR CLASS

School participates in AMCAS. See Chapter 6.

Filing of AMCAS application
Earliest date: June 1, 2000
Latest date: Nov. 1, 2000
School application fee after screening: $55
Oldest MCAT scores considered: 1997
Does have Early Decision Program (EDP)
EDP application period: June 1–Aug. 1, 2000
EDP applicants notified by: Oct. 1, 2000
Acceptance notice to regular applicants
Earliest date: Nov. 1, 2000
Latest date: Until class is filled
Applicant's response to acceptance offer
Maximum time: 2 weeks
Requests for deferred entrance considered: Yes
Deposit to hold place in class (applied to tuition): $100, due with response to acceptance offer
Deposit refundable prior to: May 15, 2001
Estimated number of new entrants: 108 (2 EDP)
Starting date: Aug. 2001

TUITION AND STUDENT FEES PER YEAR FOR 1999–2000 FIRST-YEAR CLASS

Tuition: $27,500 Student fees: None

INFORMATION ON 1999–2000 FIRST-YEAR CLASS

Number of	*In-State*	*Out-of-State*	*Total*
Applicants	672	4,726	5,398
Applicants Interviewed	258	238	496
New Entrants*	67	41	108

*99% had baccalaureate degrees; 97% took the MCAT.

CHAPTER 11

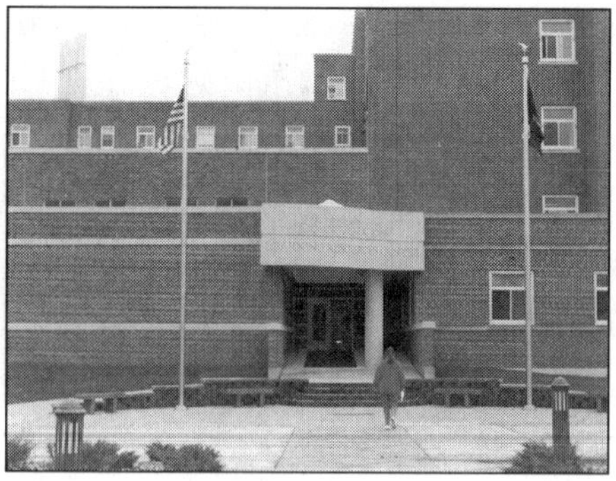

University of North Dakota School of Medicine and Health Sciences

Grand Forks, North Dakota

Dr. H. David Wilson, *Dean*
Judy L. DeMers, *Associate Dean, Student Affairs and Admissions*
Sandra K. Elshaug, *Financial Aid Administrator*

ADDRESS INQUIRIES TO:

Secretary, Committee on Admissions
University of North Dakota
School of Medicine and Health Sciences
501 North Columbia Road, Box 9037
Grand Forks, North Dakota 58202-9037
(701) 777-4221; 777-4942 (FAX)
E-mail: jdheit@medicine.nodak.edu
Web Site: http://www.medicine.nodak.edu/

MISSION STATEMENT

The mission of the University of North Dakota School of Medicine and Health Sciences is to educate and prepare physicians, medical scientists, and other health professionals for service to North Dakota and the nation, and to advance medical and biomedical knowledge through research.

GENERAL INFORMATION

The School of Medicine was established in 1905 as a basic science school offering the first two years of medical education. In 1973, legislative action created an expanded curriculum with the third year at the University of Minnesota or Mayo medical schools and the fourth year of elective clerkships on community campuses in North Dakota. In 1981, the legislature approved a full four-year medical school program within the state of North Dakota. The School of Medicine is university based but utilizes community physicians, clinics, and hospitals for the last two years of clinical education.

CURRICULUM

The School of Medicine emphasizes the training of primary care physicians. The freshman and sophomore years are spent at the University of North Dakota (UND) in Grand Forks. Beginning with the 1998-99 academic year, the school initiated a new curriculum, utilizing a "patient-centered learning" (PCL) approach. The number of traditional lecture hours is reduced significantly and greater emphasis is placed on small-group teaching and learning, active student participation, and early clinical experience. The curriculum is integrated across disciplines and consists of four 10-week blocks of instruction during each of the first and second years. Students are assigned to either the Bismarck or Fargo campuses for the third year and to one of four clinical campuses for the fourth year. A student also may participate in the ROME (Rural Opportunities in Medical Education) program during the third year, completing eight months of clinical experience in a rural community. A two-year curricular continuum offers a comprehensive, integrated, practice-based learning experience, which emphasizes continuity of care and provides a rural building block for all students. Comprehensive and continuing assessment of student learning is stressed throughout the four years of medical education.

The School of Medicine offers accredited undergraduate degrees in the allied health fields of clinical laboratory science, cytotechnology, occupational therapy, and sports medicine. A physician assistant program also is offered on a non-degree basis. Graduate degrees in anatomy, biochemistry, clinical laboratory science, microbiology, physical therapy, physiology, and pharmacology also are offered. Information on these programs may be obtained from the UND undergraduate and graduate catalogs.

A student, additionally, may apply for a combined M.D.-Ph.D. program once accepted for admission to the School of Medicine.

The school utilizes a grading system of satisfactory-unsatisfactory.

REQUIREMENTS FOR ENTRANCE

The MCAT and the equivalent of three academic years or a minimum of 90 semester hours from an approved college are required for admission. Preference is given to applicants who will have completed an undergraduate degree and who are broadly educated in the sciences and the humanities.

Course work must include the following:

	Sem. hrs.
General biology or zoology	8
Inorganic and qualitative chemistry	8
Organic chemistry*	8
General physics	8
College algebra	3
Psychology or sociology	3
English composition and literature	6

*A semester or quarter of biochemistry may be substituted for the final semester/quarter of organic chemistry.

It also is highly recommended that students be computer literate.

SELECTION FACTORS

A student should have maintained a GPA of 3.0 or better (A=4.0) to be considered for admission. Selection is based upon the scholastic record, letters of recommendation, MCAT scores, and a personal interview. Interviews are conducted only at the medical school.

In addition to high academic achievement, selection is based on a number of factors, including the demonstration of such qualities as motivation and commitment to a medical career, empathy, compassion in interpersonal relationships, and problem solving.

Qualified North Dakota residents are given preference in admission. Almost all accepted students in recent classes have been residents of North Dakota. The only exceptions for non-North Dakota residents include a limited number of Minnesota residents or admission through either the Indians into Medicine (INMED) Program or through WICHE participation. Only persons who are U.S. citizens or legal permanent residents of the United States are eligible for consideration for admission. Women are considered on the same basis as men.

The School of Medicine participates in the Professional Students Exchange Program administered by WICHE, under which legal residents of western states without a medical school may receive preference in admission. Certified WICHE students pay resident tuition. To be certified as eligible for this program, students must write to the WICHE certifying officer in their state of legal residence for the program application form. The number of students to be supported in each state in the field of medicine depends upon state appropriations. Addresses of state certifying officers are available from the Office of Student Affairs at the UND School of Medicine and Health Sciences or from WICHE (see Part 1).

The School of Medicine and Health Sciences does not utilize AMCAS. Once applications are received, they are ranked based on a combination of state residency, grade-point average, and MCAT scores. The top ranking candidates are automatically invited to interview. The records of all other candidates are reviewed by the Admissions Committee. A majority vote is required to issue an invitation to interview. The School of Medicine is unable to accept transfer students from other medical schools.

The fall 1999 entering class had the following profile: *GPA mean*: overall undergraduate, 3.54; science, 3.50; *GPA range*: overall undergraduate, 2.55–3.98; science, 2.50–4.00. *The mean MCAT scores were as follows*: VR-9.07; PS-8.48; BS-9.16. *The range of the MCAT variables* was 12 to 6. The MCAT writing score ranged from R to S with a median score of O. *Gender*, 51 percent female; *minorities*, 9 students (16.1 percent) from minority groups; 6 of which were INMED students.

It is the policy of the University of North Dakota that there shall be no discrimination against persons because of race, religion, age, creed, color, sex, disability, sexual orientation, national origin, marital status, veterans' status, or political belief or affiliation, and that equal opportunity and access to facilities be available to all.

FINANCIAL AID

The financial resources of applicants are not considered in the selection process. Immediately after acceptance into the School of Medicine, the applicant is sent all available financial aid information and may make application for financial aid.

The awarding of financial aid is based on documented need. Loans and a limited number of scholarships and prizes are available. Some awards and scholarships are based on scholarship as well as need. Approximately 85 percent of the students receive some form of financial aid. Students are discouraged from working. The financial aid office may be reached at (701) 777-2849.

INFORMATION FOR MINORITY STUDENTS

The INMED Program is a minority recruitment program for American Indian students. Up to seven qualified Native American students are admitted yearly through this program. State residency is not a consideration for admission through the INMED Program, but applicants must be enrolled in a federally recognized tribe.

Public Institution

APPLICATION AND ACCEPTANCE POLICIES FOR 2001–2002 FIRST-YEAR CLASS

Earliest date: July 1, 2000
Latest date: Nov. 1, 2000
School application fee to all applicants: $35
Oldest MCAT scores considered: Fall 1997
Does not have Early Decision Program
Acceptance notice to regular applicants
  Earliest date: Dec. 15, 2000
  Latest date: Until class is filled
Applicant's response to acceptance offer
  Maximum time: 4 weeks
Requests for deferred entrance considered: Yes
Deposit to hold place in class (applied to tuition):
  $75, due with response to acceptance offer
Deposit refundable prior to: May 15, 2001
Estimated number of new entrants: 57
Starting date: Aug. 2001

TUITION AND STUDENT FEES PER YEAR FOR 1999–2000 FIRST-YEAR CLASS

Tuition
  Resident: $10,956
  Nonresident: $29,250

Student fees: $801

INFORMATION ON 1999–2000 FIRST-YEAR CLASS

Number of	*In-State*	*Out-of-State*	*Total*
Applicants	140	147	287
Applicants Interviewed	101	54	155
New Entrants*	42	14†	56

*All took the MCAT and had baccalaureate degrees.
†Includes INMED, MN, and WICHE applicants.

CHAPTER 11

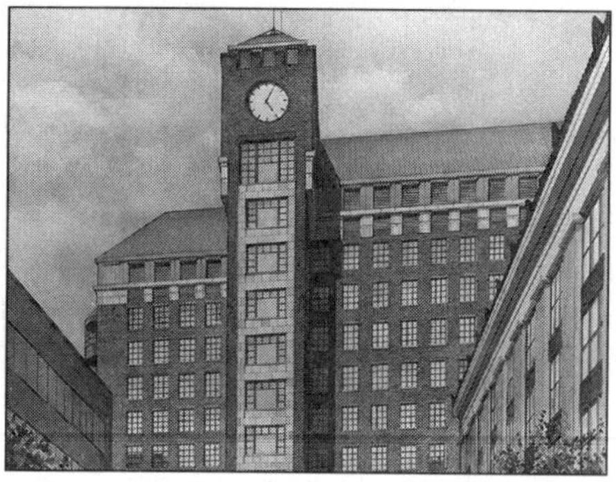

Case Western Reserve University School of Medicine

Cleveland, Ohio

Dr. Nathan A. Berger, *Dean, and Vice President for Medical Affairs*
Dr. Albert C. Kirby, *Associate Dean for Admissions and Student Affairs*
Wanda L. Rollins, *Director, Financial Aid*

ADDRESS INQUIRIES TO:

Associate Dean for Admissions and Student Affairs
Case Western Reserve University
School of Medicine
10900 Euclid Avenue
Cleveland, Ohio 44106-4920
(216) 368-3450; 368-6011 (FAX)
Web Site: http://mediswww.cwru.edu

GENERAL INFORMATION

The School of Medicine is located on the campus of Case Western Reserve University (CWRU), an independent and privately supported institution. Case Western Reserve is a comprehensive university with colleges of applied social sciences, dentistry, engineering, law, liberal arts, management, medicine, nursing, and a graduate school. The Ph.D. is available in 43 programs and the master's in 49. The university is one of over 90 cultural, educational, health, and service institutions in University Circle, a park-like area of 600 acres located five miles east of downtown Cleveland. Affiliated teaching hospitals are University Hospitals of Cleveland, MetroHealth Medical Center, and Veterans Affairs Cleveland Medical Center, all in Cleveland and the Henry Ford Health System in Detroit, Michigan.

CURRICULUM

The School of Medicine offers an environment in which students are encouraged to take initiative and responsibility in self-education. This atmosphere is fostered by early exposure to patient care responsibilities, a significant commitment to elective time, problem-based learning, and an evaluation system, which minimizes competition. Graduates will have a solid foundation in the basic and clinical sciences, expertise in areas of special interest, the ability to integrate science and humanistic values across disciplines, be responsive to patients and communities, recognize the role of the physician in the distribution of resources, and take initiative in their chosen fields.

Integrated teaching of the basic sciences by multidisciplinary faculty teams focusing on the organ systems of the body occupies much of the first two years. Case-oriented problem solving is featured as part of mastering the basic sciences.

Clinical education is introduced early in the first year with each student being responsible for a patient in the family care clinic. Required third-year clerkships are in family medicine, internal medicine, neurosciences, obstetrics-gynecology, pediatrics, psychiatry, and surgery and must be taken in our affiliated hospitals.

In order to develop expertise in areas of the student's own interest, the curriculum features significant time for electives in the pre-clinical years and the fourth year is available for clinical and basic science electives. Fourth-year electives may be taken at other teaching institutions. The Office of International Health provides opportunities for fourth-year students to study outside the United States.

The Primary Care Track is designed to stimulate careers in the primary care specialties (family medicine, internal medicine, and pediatrics) by providing early mentoring with primary care physicians and a summer research project relating to health care delivery. A unique, year-long, integrated primary care clerkship is available in the third year in place of the traditional rotations to students selecting the Primary Care Track.

CWRU School of Medicine, through its affiliated hospitals, offers accelerated residency programs in family medicine and general internal medicine in which the fourth year of medical school and the first year of residency are combined.

Students must pass USMLE Step 1 to be promoted to the third year and pass USMLE Step 2 in order to qualify for graduation.

Joint-degree programs are available with the Schools of Management and Law and the basic science departments of the School of Medicine, all of which offer the Ph.D. Several special Master's programs are available including Anatomy and Biomedical Ethics. An M.D.-Ph.D. program is available in Health Services Research. A Medical Scientist Training Program (combined M.D.-Ph.D.) is available. Students interested in these degrees must apply independently to these schools or programs and the School of Medicine and must satisfy all admissions requirements of both.

REQUIREMENTS FOR ENTRANCE

Only three years of college are required, but in practice, few students without the baccalaureate degree have ever been admitted. All candidates are expected to take the MCAT. The quality of work done is much more important than the field in which the student has majored. Specific requirements are minimal and include:

Biology: A one-year course in modern biology that emphasizes biochemical and quantitative concepts. Courses in anatomy, botany, ecology, and taxonomy will not fulfill this requirement.

Chemistry: Two years of chemistry including organic. Courses with an organic/biological chemistry content are acceptable.

Physics: A one-year course in introductory physics.

Demonstration of writing skills: This can be met by a course in freshman expository writing; however, other courses with significant writing content are acceptable.

SELECTION FACTORS

The Admissions Committee selects students without regard to age, national origin, race, religion, sex, or sexual orientation. With respect to disability, technical standards for admission are available upon request. The School of Medicine deliberately seeks a diverse student body. Over 20 states of residence and 70 to 80 undergraduate colleges are represented in a typical entering class.

While the Committee does not rely on grades and MCAT scores alone in the selection process, all students have demonstrated exceptional academic strength. Completed secondary applications are reviewed with great attention given to the candidate's written statements and letters of recommendation in the decision to invite an applicant for an interview.

Some characteristics of the 1999 entering class include: 40 percent women; 14 percent *minority students*; 10 percent over age 28; 60 percent legal residents of Ohio; undergraduate major, 65 percent in the sciences. The *average GPA* was 3.6 and the *average MCAT* was 10.7.

CWRU School of Medicine rarely accepts transfer students and then only from LCME-accredited schools and when the transfer will alleviate an extreme hardship situation. Students wishing to transfer must submit their requests in writing.

FINANCIAL AID

Financial aid is based on demonstrated need of the student. All applicants for aid must submit data for an analysis of need by NEED ACCESS. This requires complete disclosure of resources available to the student from all sources. Students are also required to submit income and asset information from parents. Approximately 75 percent of the students receive financial aid. Applications for financial aid are sent to accepted students in January with awards being made by May 15. Funds from the University are limited, consequently students have to rely on other sources of support including the Stafford Student Loan Program and alternative loan programs. Aid available from CWRU is a combination of loan and scholarship with the proportion of each being dependent upon total need.

Up to 15 merit scholarships can be awarded each year to students displaying outstanding personal and academic achievement.

INFORMATION FOR MINORITY STUDENTS

The Office of Minority Programs and the Office of Student Services offer a wide variety of academic and personal support programs for all minority students. These include special speakers, mentoring with minority faculty, a tutoring program, and counseling.

Two summer programs are sponsored for minority college students interested in careers in medicine. The Health Career Enhancement Program is a rigorous six-week enrichment program for highly motivated and capable students. Review of the sciences and MCAT preparation are major components. Part of the program includes medical apprenticeships with working physicians. A research program is also available for minority students interested in careers in biomedical research.

There is an active Student National Medical Association chapter, which sponsors many activities including tutoring and community projects. The Latino Organization of Medical Students is especially interested in health care in Cleveland's Latino community.

More information, including applications for the summer program, may be obtained from the Office of Minority Programs at the address at the top of this entry or call (216) 368-2212.

Private Institution

APPLICATION AND ACCEPTANCE POLICIES FOR 2001–2002 FIRST-YEAR CLASS

School participates in AMCAS. See Chapter 6.

Filing of AMCAS application
- Earliest date: June 1, 2000
- Latest date: Nov. 1, 2000

School application fee after screening: $60

Oldest MCAT scores considered: 1997

Does have Early Decision Program (EDP)
- EDP application period: June 1–Aug. 1, 2000
- EDP applicants notified by: Oct. 1, 2000

Acceptance notice to regular applicants
- Earliest date: Oct. 15, 2000
- Latest date: Until class is filled

Applicant's response to acceptance offer
- Maximum time: 4 weeks

Requests for deferred entrance considered: Yes

Deposit to hold place in class: None

Estimated number of new entrants: 145 (10 EDP)

Starting date: Aug. 2001

TUITION AND STUDENT FEES PER YEAR FOR 1999–2000 FIRST-YEAR CLASS

Tuition: $30,600 Student fees: $904

INFORMATION ON 1999–2000 FIRST-YEAR CLASS

Number of	*In-State*	*Out-of-State*	*Total*
Applicants	955	5,540	6,495
Applicants Interviewed	324	498	822
New Entrants*	78	67	145

*All had baccalaureate degrees; 97% took the MCAT.

CHAPTER 11

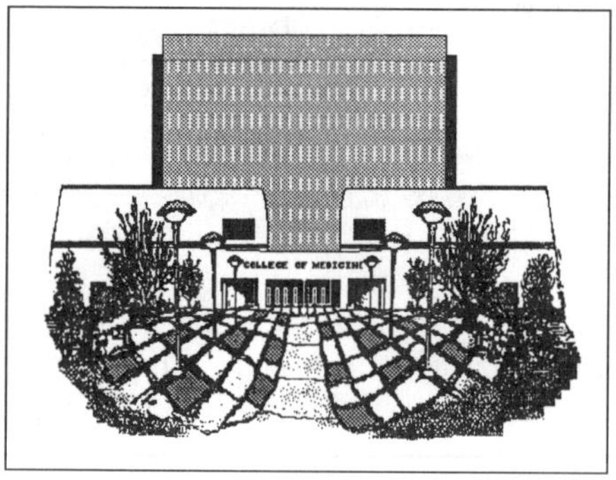

University of Cincinnati College of Medicine

Cincinnati, Ohio

Dr. John J. Hutton, *Dean*
Dr. J. Robert Suriano, *Associate Dean for Student Affairs/Admissions*
Clarice P. Fooks, *Assistant Dean for Admissions*

ADDRESS INQUIRIES TO:

Office of Student Affairs/Admissions
University of Cincinnati
College of Medicine
P.O. Box 670552
Cincinnati, Ohio 45267-0552
(513) 558-7314; 558-1165 (FAX)
Web Site: http://www.med.uc.edu/

MISSION STATEMENT

The University of Cincinnati College of Medicine envisions medical education as an integrated, systematic, and student-centered learning process rooted in the principles of both population-based and patient-centered medical care. As graduates, each student will possess an excellent conceptual knowledge base, critical lifelong learning and thinking skills, outstanding interpersonal and clinical abilities, and an understanding of and commitment to the physician's role and responsibility in society.

GENERAL INFORMATION

The College of Medicine provides both outstanding research facilities and superb clinical and teaching experiences. Graduates, ranked highly competitive by national residency program directors, choose careers in a broad range of specialty areas. Approximately 63 percent of the 1999 graduating class chose a residency program likely to lead to a primary care career (family medicine, internal medicine, obstetrics/gynecology, and pediatrics).

Research opportunities for students are extensive. Nationally, the College of Medicine and Children's Hospital Medical Center are ranked in the top 25 percent among all public medical schools in National Institutes of Health research funding, and ranked among the top third in outside research funding.

CURRICULUM

The focus of the first year is on the normal structure, function, and development of the human body using an integrated systems approach to basic and clinical science topics. It includes an introduction to doctor/patient relationships and physical diagnosis skills. The second year continues the integrated systems approach focusing on the disease processes, prevention, and the further development of physical diagnosis skills.

Third-year clerkships include 8-week rotations each in internal medicine, obstetrics-gynecology, pediatrics, and surgery; a 6-week rotation in psychiatry; a 4-week rotation in family medicine, a 2-week rotation in radiology; and 4 weeks of electives.

The fourth-year requirements are an 8-week acting internship in internal medicine, a 4-week clinical neuroscience selective; and 24 weeks of electives, which must include a 4-week internal medicine elective, a 4-week outpatient elective, and a 4-week Area Health Education Center (AHEC) elective in an underserved rural or urban community in Ohio. Portions of the elective time may be taken at other U.S. medical centers or abroad.

Evaluation of students is by an honors, high pass, pass, remediate, and fail grading system. Students are required to take and pass Step 1 and Step 2 of the USMLE examinations. All students are required to pass Step 1 prior to promotion into Year 3.

SUMMER PREMATRICULATION PROGRAM

A Summer Prematriculation Program (SPP) is offered to any accepted student. The program provides exposure to actual first year lectures, labs, course-related discussion groups, and tests. There are also sessions on study strategies, test taking skills, stress management, and leadership skills.

REQUIREMENTS FOR ENTRANCE

Applicants must complete a minimum of 90 semester hours at a U.S. accredited, four-year, degree-granting institution of higher education. Students who have attended an undergraduate college outside of the United States should have a graduate degree or a minimum of 20 hours of science course work in a U.S. accredited, four-year, degree-granting institution of higher education.

Students currently in a professional school or a degree-granting graduate program must complete all degree requirements and show documentation of graduation or completion of requirements *prior to matriculation.*

A baccalaureate degree is encouraged but not required. MCAT scores received within the past three years are required.

All majors are valued. Students are expected to engage in a rigorous academic program that enables them to understand the basic principles of the sciences fundamental to medicine and to appreciate the psychosocial nature of man. *All* applicants are expected to have the knowledge usually obtained in one-year courses in biology, general chemistry, organic chemistry, physics, and mathematics. In addition, the undergraduate program should provide an understanding of the basic social, cultural, and behavioral factors that influence individuals, families, and communities. Regardless of the area of concentration, the applicant should have acquired effective learning, communication, and problem-solving skills. A knowledge of the basic principles of statistics and computer literacy are strongly recommended.

As a state-supported university, priority will be given to Ohio residents.

All applicants must meet the College of Medicine Admissions and Graduation Standards (technical standards) with or without reasonable accommodations.

SELECTION FACTORS

Upon review of academic information including MCAT scores, applicants will be selected to receive a Secondary Application. All interviews are generated by the Admissions Committee. Approximately 650 candidates will be invited to interview each year. The interview day will include: one interview, lunch, a presentation on the curriculum, financial aid, and a tour.

Notification of final decisions will be made on or near the 15th of each month. Prior to January, acceptances may be sent on a weekly basis.

Offers of acceptance are based upon the overall evaluation of academic and personal qualities. Postbaccalaureate and graduate course work will be considered. Personal characteristics include demonstrated motivation, maturity, coping skills, leadership abilities, interpersonal skills, sensitivity and tolerance toward others, and critical-thinking skills. Students are admitted on the basis of individual qualifications, regardless of age, sex, sexual orientation, race, color, national origin, or physical or mental disabilities.

FINANCIAL AID

The college provides students with information about options for funding a medical education and counseling to help them make sound financial decisions. Over 80 percent of enrolled students receive some type of financial assistance. A financial aid packet is mailed to accepted applicants in February. Students who wish to be considered for need-based funds administered by the college must submit the Need Access diskette.

The current level of indebtedness for graduates is below the national mean for all medical students. For further information, please contact the Financial Aid Office at (513) 558-6797.

INFORMATION FOR MINORITY AND NONTRADITIONAL STUDENTS

Members of minority groups and nontraditional students are encouraged to apply. The College provides a strong supportive environment for all students and welcomes diversity in each entering class. The College also sponsors several summer programs for high school and college students. Please write or call for additional information.

PHYSICIAN SCIENTIST TRAINING PROGRAM

The Physician Scientist Training Program (PSTP) of the College is a rigorous and prestigious integrated program that leads to the M.D.-Ph.D. combined degree. PSTP students are provided full financial support, including stipend ($16,000 in 1999), tuition and health insurance. For more detailed information, visit the PSTP web site at http://www.med.uc.edu/pstp.

Public Institution

APPLICATION AND ACCEPTANCE POLICIES FOR 2001–2002 FIRST-YEAR CLASS

School participates in AMCAS. See Chapter 6.

Filing of AMCAS application
- Earliest date: June 1, 2000
- Latest date: Nov. 15, 2000

School application fee to all applicants: $25
Oldest MCAT scores considered: 1998
Does have Early Decision Program (EDP)
- EDP application period: June 1–Aug. 1, 2000
- EDP applicants notified by: Oct. 1, 2000

Acceptance notice to regular applicants
- Earliest date: Oct. 15, 2000
- Latest date: Until class is filled

Applicant's response to acceptance offer
- Maximum time: 2 weeks

Requests for deferred entrance considered: Yes
Deposit to hold place in class: None
Estimated number of new entrants: 160
Starting date: Aug. 2001

TUITION AND STUDENT FEES PER YEAR FOR 1999–2000 FIRST-YEAR CLASS

Tuition
- Resident: $12,612
- Nonresident: $22,545

Student fees: $561

INFORMATION ON 1999–2000 FIRST-YEAR CLASS

Number of	*In-State*	*Out-of-State*	*Total*
Applicants	1,203	2,497	3,700
Applicants Interviewed	500	168	668
New Entrants*	133	26	159

*All took the MCAT and had baccalaureate degrees.

CHAPTER 11

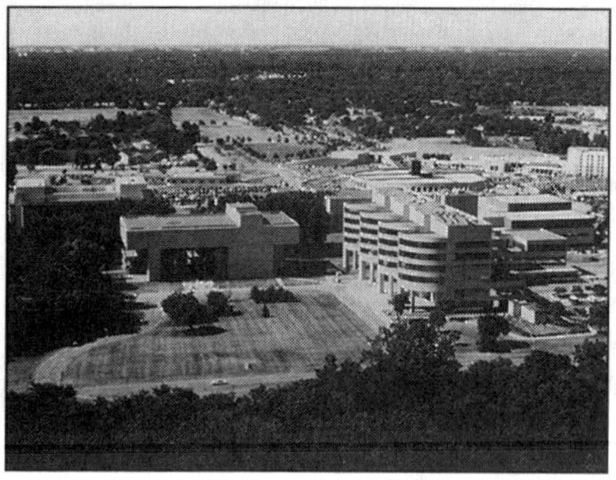

Medical College of Ohio

Toledo, Ohio

Dr. Amira F. Gohara, *Vice President for Academic Affairs and Dean, School of Medicine*
Dr. Mary Ann Myers, *Associate Dean for Admissions*
Dr. Robert A. Burns, *Assistant Dean for Admissions*

ADDRESS INQUIRIES TO:

Admissions Office
School of Medicine
3045 Arlington Avenue
Toledo, Ohio 43614
(419) 383-4229; 383-4005 (FAX)
Web Site: http://www.mco.edu

GENERAL INFORMATION

The Medical College of Ohio graduated its first students in June 1972. The institutional mission statement focuses on the creation and maintenance of an academic environment that attracts the most highly qualified faculty and fosters the pursuit of excellence in health education, research, and service. The academic medical center is located on 475 acres in a residential/commercial area of south Toledo. The center has almost 400 faculty members and 1,100 volunteer faculty members. The faculty is dedicated to establishing a learning atmosphere through balanced teaching, research, and patient care.

The Medical College of Ohio has five endowed chairs and conducts biomedical research in many areas, including genetics of hypertension, autoregulation of blood pressure, genetics of carcinogenesis, mechanism of fungi formation, role of immunophilius in steroid action carcinogenesis, and environmental microbiology.

In this medical school setting, the entering student is considered a graduate scholar by faculty members at all levels of seniority. The Medical College of Ohio seeks students who can grow intellectually and personally in this academic atmosphere.

CURRICULUM

The curriculum of the Medical College of Ohio is composed of an integrated basic science/clinical science four-year approach to medical education with emphasis on clinically oriented objectives and problem-based learning. The first year is devoted to integrated blocks of cellular and molecular biology, growth and development, human structure and neuroscience, and behavioral science. Each of these sections will have a corresponding integrated clinical applied component. Also included will be Introduction to Primary Care (IPC), which runs concurrently throughout the first two years. The basic and clinical sciences are more intently brought together by the Pathophysiology course, which acts as a conduit between the basic sciences and the IPC experience.

The second year is composed of immunity and infection, an integrated systems course involving pathology, pharmacology, and physiology. Each section will have an appropriate integrated clinical component. There is continuation of IPC and pathophysiology. During the first two years, approximately 45 percent of the student's time will be spent in a non-lecture format with emphasis placed on small-group interaction. Students will be required to pass Step 1 of the USMLE and Step 2 for graduation.

The last two years of the curriculum are devoted to mandatory clerkships in internal medicine, surgery, pediatrics, obstetrics and gynecology, psychiatry, and family practice; neurology; and electives. All students are required to rotate through a clinical Area Health Education Center (AHEC) comprising 10 percent of their total clerkship time. Most components of the curriculum are evaluated on an honors, high pass, pass, fail system. The Medical College of Ohio also has an M.D.-Ph.D. and M.D.-M.S. program. Additionally, there is a FLEX program, which is a five-year curriculum for disadvantaged students.

During the clinical phase, each student is exposed to one or two months of internal medicine in generalist settings. One of these months is spent in an area health education center so that the student will see health care delivery in a rural setting. Additionally there is a four week exposure to family medicine.

Our third- and fourth-year students are also offered a separate two-year clinical track at the Henry Ford Health System, which is designed to attract those students with a long term interest in the practice of primary care medicine in a managed care environment. This is a competitive program, and 10 students are selected for this unique educational opportunity.

The Medical College of Ohio School of Medicine offers a substantial amount of required generalist physician educational experiences and a wide variety of electives to enhance experiences in the specialist areas, which provide our students with a well-rounded basic medical education.

REQUIREMENTS FOR ENTRANCE

The MCAT is required. A baccalaureate degree is required.

Students must plan their educational sequence with due appreciation for the biologically oriented, psychologically sensitive task that they are undertaking for their life's work. The minimal premedical course requirements are:

	Years
Biology	1
Inorganic chemistry	1
Organic chemistry	1
Physics	1
College mathematics	1
College English	1

Additional upper-level biology courses are recommended.

A comprehensive command and understanding of the English language are essential.

Beyond these requirements, concentration in humanities, sciences, or other areas is viewed with equal favor. Close attention will be paid to the general scope of the applicant's academic background and to whether or not there is an adequate general understanding of the physical, biological, chemical, and social sciences and some reasonable sensitivity to the humanities.

SELECTION FACTORS

In selecting applicants, the Medical College of Ohio looks more for evidence of general competence and capability than for specific areas of study. Students are admitted on the basis of individual qualifications, regardless of sex, religion, race, age, or handicap.

Students in the 1998 entering class had the following credentials: *mean science GPA,* 3.47; *mean total GPA,* 3.51; *mean MCAT scores, VR*-9.19, *PS*-9.47, *BS*-9.77; *sex,* 37 percent women; *minorities,* 8 percent; *undergraduate major,* 86 percent in science. Interviews are by invitation only. Reapplicants are not penalized. Preference is given to Ohio residents.

FINANCIAL AID

Financial aid is awarded on the basis of demonstrated financial need according to federal methodology. Applicants for financial aid must file the FAFSA. Several scholarships are available on a competitive basis. These scholarships are funded by the Office of the Dean, the MCO Foundation, and the Associated Physicians of MCO. Approximately 50 students are employed during the academic year in the Federal Work-Study Program. Summer employment opportunities also exist with the Summer Research Program, the Community Health Project, and the Preceptorships in Family Practice Program.

INFORMATION FOR MINORITY STUDENTS

The Medical College of Ohio is committed to increasing opportunities for individuals from traditionally underrepresented groups, as well as those from economically disadvantaged backgrounds. The Office of Multicultural Affairs works in cooperation with the Admissions Committee, the Office of Student Affairs, and all other campus departments in the recruitment, selection, and retention of qualified students. For more information write, Dr. Barry Richardson, assistant vice president for multicultural affairs.

Public Institution

APPLICATION AND ACCEPTANCE POLICIES FOR 2001–2002 FIRST-YEAR CLASS

School participates in AMCAS. See Chapter 6.

Filing of AMCAS application
- Earliest date: June 1, 2000
- Latest date: Nov. 1, 2000

School application fee after screening: $30
Oldest MCAT scores considered: 1998
Does have Early Decision Program (EDP)
- For Ohio residents only
- EDP application period: June 1–Aug. 1, 2000
- EDP applicants notified by: Oct. 1, 2000

Acceptance notice to regular applicants
- Earliest date: Oct. 15, 2000
- Latest date: Until class is filled

Applicant's response to acceptance offer
- Maximum time: 2 weeks

Requests for deferred entrance considered: Yes
Deposit to hold place in class: None
Estimated number of new entrants: 140 (10 EDP)
Starting date: Aug. 2001

TUITION AND STUDENT FEES PER YEAR FOR 1999–2000 FIRST-YEAR CLASS

Tuition
- Resident: $11,854
- Nonresident: $25,898

Student fees: $1,916

INFORMATION ON 1999–2000 FIRST-YEAR CLASS

Number of	*In-State*	*Out-of-State*	*Total*
Applicants	1,109	2,003	3,112
Applicants Interviewed	434	107	541
New Entrants*	127	13	140

*All had baccalaureate degrees; 46% took the MCAT.

CHAPTER 11

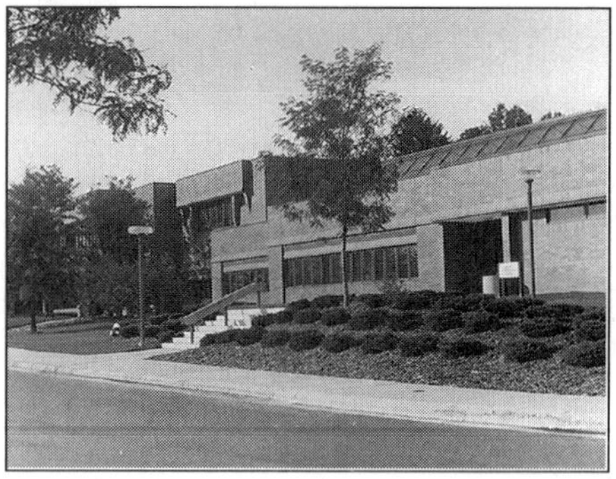

Northeastern Ohio Universities College of Medicine

Rootstown, Ohio

Dr. Robert S. Blacklow, *President and Dean*
Dr. Bonnie Jones, *Associate Dean for Admissions and Institutional Research*
R. Stephen Manuel, *Director of Admissions*

ADDRESS INQUIRIES TO:

Office of Admissions
Northeastern Ohio Universities
College of Medicine
P.O. Box 95
Rootstown, Ohio 44272-0095
(330) 325-6270; 325-8372 (FAX); 1(800) 686-2511
E-mail: admission@neoucom.edu
Web Site: http://www.neoucom.edu

MISSION STATEMENT

The mission of the Northeastern Ohio Universities College of Medicine (NEOUCOM) is to graduate qualified physicians oriented to the practice of medicine at the community level, with an emphasis on primary care: family medicine, internal medicine, pediatrics, and obstetrics/gynecology.

GENERAL INFORMATION

NEOUCOM is a publicly supported medical school consisting of a basic medical sciences campus in Rootstown, three major public universities, and 16 community hospitals with over 6,500 teaching beds in the greater Akron, Canton, and Youngstown areas. The faculty numbers over 1,500.

CURRICULUM

NEOUCOM offers primarily a combined B.S.-M.D. degree curriculum for honors-level high school graduates who have not begun college study and, supplementarily, a four-year program leading to the M.D. degree. NEOUCOM also conducts an Advanced Standing admission program for students seeking transfer from U.S. and/or foreign medical schools.

B.S.-M.D. degree students spend their first two or three years at either the University of Akron, Kent State University, or Youngstown State University studying the sciences, mathematics, and the humanities while in the process of completing most or all of the required courses for the baccalaureate degree.

NEOUCOM's education of physicians is oriented to the practice of medicine at the community level. The freshman medical student concentrates on the basic medical sciences during the nine months spent on the Rootstown campus. During the freshman and sophomore years, students enroll in introduction to clinical medicine at the ambulatory care teaching centers of the major associated teaching hospitals. They continue their clinical education through the core clerkships (internal medicine, surgery, pediatrics, psychiatry, obstetrics-gynecology, and family medicine) and a primary care preceptorship during the junior year at hospitals on the Akron, Canton, or Youngstown clinical campuses. There is an expanding problem-based learning (PBL) program across the first two years of the curriculum, both as a stand-alone course and within core clerkships. The senior medical year includes electives and specially designed selectives in the medical humanities as well as a community health clerkship. All students are required to pass Step 1 and Step 2 of the USMLE.

REQUIREMENTS FOR ENTRANCE

Admission to the combined B.S.-M.D. degree program is restricted to students who have taken no college course work following high school graduation. Applicants should take the full science-oriented college preparatory sequence which their high school offers. The American College Test (ACT) or Scholastic Aptitude Test (SAT) must be taken, and the application deadline is December 15 of the year preceding anticipated entrance. Applications may be requested after September 1. Each year 105 students are chosen for the B.S.-M.D. degree program.

Persons who have completed the equivalent of at least three years of undergraduate study may be admitted to the M.D. degree program. These applicants are required to have completed at least one year each of university-level organic chemistry and physics. All students seeking direct entry into the M.D. degree program are required to take the MCAT no later than the fall prior to the year of anticipated enrollment. The number of spaces available for M.D. degree program candidates varies with the amount of attrition from Year 2 or Year 3 of the B.S.-M.D. degree program. If an applicant (for the 4-year M.D. program) possessing the equivalent of three years of study shows unusual promise, is considered and subsequently accepted, NEOUCOM requires the student to complete the baccalaureate degree before the M.D. degree will be granted.

SELECTION FACTORS

Applicants must demonstrate strong academic preparation as measured by GPAs and entrance examination scores. In addition, they must show appropriate personal characteristics and motivation for the practice of medicine. Selection interviews are by invitation only.

Admissions preference is given to Ohio residents. Typically, no more than 10 percent are non-Ohio residents.

Applicants to the M.D. degree program who meet NEOUCOM's minimum academic criteria and who have taken the required course work are sent a supplementary application. Only those who complete supplementary applications are given full consideration by the Admissions Committee. Early submission of application materials is strongly encouraged, particularly through the Early Decision program if the applicant is competitive.

NEOUCOM does not discriminate on the basis of race, sex, creed, national origin, age, or handicap.

FINANCIAL AID

Campus-based financial aid is awarded on the basis of demonstrated need. In general, students apply for this aid by completing the FAFSA application (see Part 1) and the NEOUCOM financial aid application, and by submitting copies of federal income tax forms and financial aid transcripts. The awards are made through the Student Aid and Awards Committee after a thorough analysis of the student's financial situation.

Long-term federal educational loans are a major part of the aid program. A limited number of need-based scholarships of $1,000 each are available, as well as other limited scholarship funds for disadvantaged and/or medical minority students. About 80 percent of enrolled students receive some form of financial aid. Financial need is not a factor in admissions considerations.

INFORMATION FOR MINORITY STUDENTS

It is one of the goals of the Admissions Committee to seek out, recruit, and support qualified nontraditional applicants (members of medically underrepresented racial minorities and disadvantaged rural students). Students interested in further information should contact admissions or Dr. Kenneth Durgans, assistant to the president for minority affairs and affirmative action.

Public Institution

APPLICATION AND ACCEPTANCE POLICIES FOR 2001–2002 FIRST-YEAR CLASS

School participates in AMCAS. See Chapter 6.

Filing of AMCAS application
  Earliest date: June 1, 2000
  Latest date: Nov. 1, 2000
School application fee after screening: $30
Oldest MCAT scores considered: 1998
Does have Early Decision Program (EDP)
  EDP application period: June 1–Aug. 1, 2000
  EDP applicants notified by: Oct. 1, 2000
Acceptance notice to regular applicants
  Earliest date: Oct. 15, 2000
  Latest date: Until class is filled
Applicant's response to acceptance offer
  Maximum time: 2 weeks
Requests for deferred entrance considered: No
Deposit to hold place in class: None
Estimated number of new entrants: 20 (5 EDP)
Starting date: Aug. 2001

TUITION AND STUDENT FEES PER YEAR FOR 1999–2000 FIRST-YEAR CLASS

Tuition
  Resident: $11,919
  Nonresident: $23,838

Student fees: $564

INFORMATION ON 1999–2000 FIRST-YEAR CLASS

Number of	*In-State*	*Out-of-State*	*Total*
Applicants	703	293	996
Applicants Interviewed	94	6	100
New Entrants*	23	2	25

NOTE: Figures do not include combined B.S.-M.D. degree program students.

*All took the MCAT and had baccalaureate degrees.

CHAPTER 11

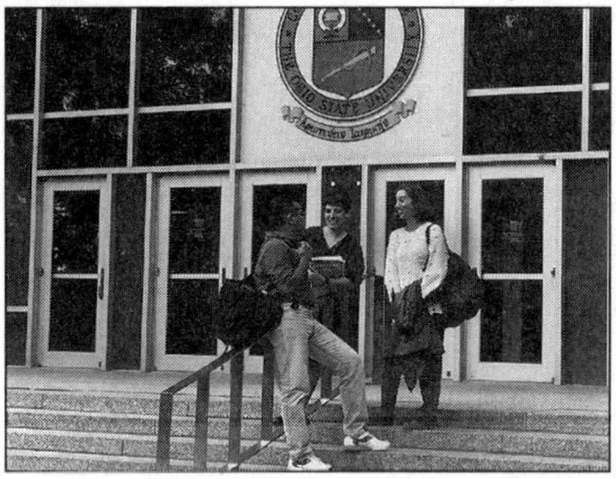

Ohio State University College of Medicine and Public Health

Columbus, Ohio

Dr. Daniel D. Sedmak, *Interim Dean*
Dr. Mark Notestine, *Assistant Dean, Admissions*
Marla Nawrocki, *Financial Aid Coordinator*

ADDRESS INQUIRIES TO:

Admissions Committee
270-A Meiling Hall
Ohio State University
College of Medicine and Public Health
370 West Ninth Avenue
Columbus, Ohio 43210-1238
(614) 292-7137; 292-1544 (FAX)
E-mail: admiss-med@osu.edu
Web Site: http://www.med.ohio-state.edu

GENERAL INFORMATION

Established in 1914, the Ohio State University College of Medicine blends traditional medical education, innovative learning opportunities, and a strong reputation in the preparation of students for primary care and specialized residencies. As part of one of the largest public universities in the country, the College of Medicine provides an environment that encourages the research interests of students. Strong emphasis is placed on medical humanities and a biopsychosocial approach to patient care.

The College of Medicine is on the south edge of the main university campus, located in metropolitan Columbus. Medical center facilities include university hospitals, the Arthur G. James Cancer Hospital and Richard J. Solove Research Institute, and a network of outpatient facilities and affiliated small-town and rural hospitals and clinics. In addition, students can spend part of their clinical clerkships in other Columbus hospitals and at the Cleveland Clinic Foundation.

CURRICULUM

Following an intensive initial 12-week course in anatomy, there are three different pre-clinical tracks for the first two years: a traditional lecture-discussion pathway; an independent study pathway; and a problem-based learning pathway. In all three pathways, the curriculum is interdisciplinary, using an organ systems approach, with an emphasis on providing a clinical context for learning.

The lecture-discussion pathway focuses on large-group presentations accompanied by tutorials and laboratories for selected topics. Lectures are held in the mornings, with afternoons used for tutorials and study.

In the independent study pathway (ISP) students use highly structured objectives, resource guides, and computer-based materials to read, review, and learn on their own. They proceed through the curriculum at their own pace within certain time limits. Faculty are available to coach students through difficult concepts and materials. Students who are successful in their first year in the ISP can request to spend their second year in the ISP at the Cleveland Clinic Foundation. It is possible to complete the independent study pathway program over a three-year period, an option that may interest non-traditional students with family obligations.

The problem-based learning pathway emphasizes student-centered, self-directed learning. Groups of seven students meet with a faculty facilitator two to three times per week. Students review cases and identify learning issues or areas they need to study. Students then work independently on learning issues before the next meeting, at which time the new information is discussed and refined.

All first-year students spend Wednesday in a medical humanities and behavioral sciences course. Some of the major components include the doctor-patient relationship, the physician's role in society, health care delivery, human development, human sexuality, and bioethics. Alternative medicine and the health care needs and issues of special populations are also presented and discussed. Emphasis is placed on small-group learning and discussion, including opportunities for electives on special topics. The first year also includes a longitudinal experience with a primary care physician in an outpatient setting.

During the second year, in addition to their science study, students take a physical examination course that includes preceptorships in both in-patient and out-patient settings. A more in-depth study of health care delivery systems, issues, and public health is also part of the second year.

The third year includes foundation clerkships in family medicine, general internal medicine, internal medicine, obstetrics and gynecology, pediatrics, psychiatry, and surgery. The fourth-year requirements include neuroscience and the differentiation of care selectives. The selectives are a series of four clerkships, each of which focuses on the care of patients at various stages of illness and wellness: the undifferentiated patient; the differentiated ambulatory patient; the patient with chronic care needs; and the acutely ill patient (subinternship). With the exception of the subinternship, all required clerkships include ambulatory experiences, with some done entirely in outpatient settings. Three electives and a month of vacation are also part of the fourth year.

The M.D.-Ph.D. Medical Scientist program, M.D.-M.P.H., and M.D.-M.H.A. programs are also available.

REQUIREMENTS FOR ENTRANCE

The MCAT and a bachelor's degree or certified eligibility for a degree in absentia are required. No specific undergraduate curriculum or major is required or preferred. A medical school candidate should follow an undergraduate program that is as broad and comprehensive as possible in order to prepare best for a career in a people-oriented profession in a changing society. Candidates are urged to take advantage of the undergraduate opportunity to study history, art, literature, creative writing, philosophy, social sciences, and communications skills.

The minimum course requirements are:

	Years
Biology	1
Inorganic chemistry (with lab)	1
Organic chemistry (with lab)	1
General physics	1

Waiver of any requirement must be approved by the Admissions Committee.

SELECTION FACTORS

First consideration is given to applicants who are Ohio residents and whose academic record and MCAT scores predict a high degree of academic accomplishment in medical school.

Successful candidates have had the following general profile of characteristics: *GPA,* 3.59 (95 percent over 3.0); *MCAT* subscore average, above 10; *residence,* about 80 percent from Ohio.

Applicants who have received and returned completed Secondary Applications are carefully reviewed by the staff and faculty of the Admissions Committee. All completed applications are given thorough review to be certain that excellent candidates who do not fit the general profile are not overlooked.

Additional factors that lend significant weight in further consideration are undergraduate academic recommendations and personal information in the application itself. Further consideration by way of interview is by invitation; interviews are held on the campus. Nonacademic accomplishments and evidence of suitability for the study of medicine are carefully considered and account for a significant range in grades, MCAT scores, and other parameters of the admitted class.

FINANCIAL AID

Scholarships and loans are awarded on the basis of need. All accepted candidates are mailed financial aid materials prior to entering to be considered with students already in school. Financial need is not a deterrent to acceptance, and no students are lost through inability to find sufficient resources for continuing their education.

Roessler Foundation Student Research Scholarships provide stipends for many students doing part-time and full-time research during their medical school career.

INFORMATION FOR DISADVANTAGED STUDENTS

Students whose previous educational and economic deprivation warrant special consideration are carefully evaluated and are offered special help in the acquisition of additional resources. Special programs, such as the MedPath Medical Careers Pathway, are provided to enhance students' educational development.

The Medpath Medical Careers Pathway is a five-quarter postbaccalaureate program aimed at developing the academic knowledge-base and skills of students prior to their entrance into medical school.

Public Institution

APPLICATION AND ACCEPTANCE POLICIES FOR 2001–2002 FIRST-YEAR CLASS

School participates in AMCAS. See Chapter 6.

Filing of AMCAS application
  Earliest date: June 1, 2000
  Latest date: Nov. 1, 2000
School application fee after screening: $30 ($40 for international applicants)
Oldest MCAT scores considered: 1998
Does have Early Decision Program (EDP)
  EDP application period: June 1–Aug. 1, 2000
  EDP applicants notified by: Oct. 1, 2000
Acceptance notice to regular applicants
  Earliest date: Oct. 15, 2000
  Latest date: Varies
Applicant's response to acceptance offer
  Maximum time: 2 weeks
Requests for deferred entrance considered: Yes
Deposit to hold place in class: $25, due May 15, 2001
Estimated number of new entrants: 210 (15 EDP)
Starting date: Aug. 2001

TUITION AND STUDENT FEES PER YEAR FOR 1999–2000 FIRST-YEAR CLASS

Tuition
  Resident: $12,771
  Nonresident: $33,786
Student fees: $594

INFORMATION ON 1999–2000 FIRST-YEAR CLASS

Number of	*In-State*	*Out-of-State*	*Total*
Applicants	1,204	2,104	3,308
Applicants Interviewed	454	232	686
New Entrants*	174	36	210

*All took the MCAT and had baccalaureate degrees.

CHAPTER 11

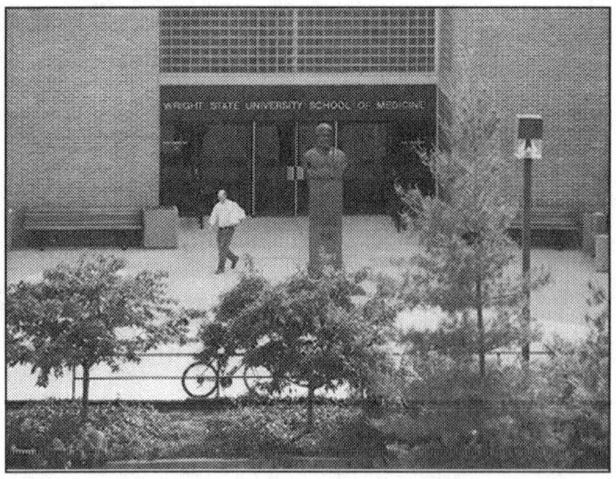

Wright State University School of Medicine

Dayton, Ohio

Dr. Howard Part, *Dean*
Dr. Paul G. Carlson, *Associate Dean for Student Affairs/Admissions*
Gwen Sloas, *Director of Financial Aid*

ADDRESS INQUIRIES TO:

Office of Student Affairs/Admissions
Wright State University
School of Medicine
P.O. Box 1751
Dayton, Ohio 45401-1751
(937) 775-2934; 775-3322 (FAX)
E-mail: som_saa@desire.wright.edu
Web Site: http://www.med.wright.edu/

MISSION STATEMENT

The mission of the school is to provide for the general professional education of students with an emphasis on primary care preparation in an environment that advances medical knowledge and is responsive to lifelong learning, research, and the community we serve. These goals and objectives are achieved through an educational program with the following core components:

- opportunities to learn in clinical settings beginning in the first quarter;
- integration of basic and clinical science knowledge throughout a four-year curriculum;
- instruction in community-based, in-patient, and out patient settings;
- utilization of diverse learning strategies and training methods;
- interaction with faculty in an atmosphere that fosters teamwork, camaraderie, and collegiality; and
- diversity in the student body and patient population, reflecting many ethnic, racial, social, age, lifestyle, and gender differences.

GENERAL INFORMATION

The Wright State University School of Medicine was established in 1973 and enrolled its first class of students in 1976. It is located on the university campus in Fairborn, a suburb of Dayton. Clinical facilities associated with the medical school include seven major teaching hospitals with 3,823 patient beds. These hospitals emphasize and provide experience with modern scientific technology. A faculty of over 1,000 provides students with the opportunity for individualized attention. The school has a strong interest in preparing students for careers in primary care as family practitioners, general internists, and general pediatricians. The educational program emphasizes early patient exposure, humanistic and compassionate care, outpatient experiences, health promotion and disease prevention, the provision of care to underserved populations, and cultural diversity.

CURRICULUM

The primary goal of the educational program is to educate students to provide comprehensive care to patients and their families. During the first two years, students are taught in an interdisciplinary fashion using large-group lectures, small-group discussions, computer-based instruction, and case-based/problem-based learning. The curriculum introduces students to normal structure and functioning in an integrated fashion. Instruction progresses through various organizational levels from molecular to organ. The basic principles and mechanisms of disease are taught in the first year.

Throughout the first two years, the curriculum integrates the behavioral sciences, humanities, wellness, and disease prevention. Regular didactic instruction by clinical faculty is provided. Students are taught medical history taking and physical examination skills, evaluation of patients' concerns, and are provided with an understanding of catastrophic illnesses. Students meet regularly with preceptors to develop clinical skills. To provide additional opportunities for clinical exposure and enrichment, clinically based electives are offered as immersion experiences between academic periods in the first two years.

In the third year, students are exposed to the basic disciplines of medicine through six clerkship rotations. Primary care clerkships are offered as part of a block rotation to coordinate instruction among the three disciplines. The fourth year includes clerkship rotations, time for board study, and junior internships, and students may choose from over 140 elective offerings.

REQUIREMENTS FOR ENTRANCE

The MCAT and three years (90 semester hours or 135 quarter hours) of collegiate preparation in an approved college or university in the United States or Canada are required. Applicants must be U.S. citizens or possess a permanent resident visa. Applicants are expected to present the equivalent of the usual premedical preparation. Course work must include:

	Years
Biology	1
Chemistry	2
Must include organic chemistry.	
Physics	1
College mathematics	1
English	1

Courses in calculus and biochemistry are strongly recommended. The Admissions Committee is interested in students with broad education in the humanities, biological, and social sciences. Each applicant's credentials for admission will be individually reviewed and evaluated. The MCAT should be taken in the spring of the year in which the application is filed and no more than three years prior to making application. Only those MCAT scores available at the time of review will be considered by the Admissions Committee.

A minimum MCAT score or GPA is not required by the Admissions Committee.

SELECTION FACTORS

It is the philosophy of the School of Medicine to seek a student body of diverse social, ethnic, and educational backgrounds. Women, minority students, and applicants from rural Ohio are particularly encouraged to apply. However, applicants are admitted solely on the basis of individual qualifications without regard to race, religion, gender, sexual orientation, disability, veteran status, national origin, age, or ancestry. Dedication to human concerns, compassion, intellectual capacity, and personal maturity in the applicant are of greater importance to the Admissions Committee than specific areas of preprofessional preparation. The Admissions Committee, which is broadly based, also seeks positive evidence of motivation, altruism, selflessness, and human empathy in the prospective medical student. The committee carefully reviews the completed application, the academic record, MCAT performance, letters of recommendation, and the results of a personal interview (by invitation only) in making its final selection. Ohio residents are given preference, but some nonresidents are accepted.

Upon receipt of the AMCAS application, all applicants will be invited to submit a supplementary application and letters of evaluation. After review of all submitted material, applicants are selected for interviews.

FINANCIAL AID

Financial aid in the form of scholarships, grants, loans, and various work opportunities is available to assist students in financial need. The Office of Student Affairs/Admissions offers financial counseling services and assists students in obtaining needed support. An emergency loan fund for students in good academic standing is also available through this office. The financial status of applicants has no effect whatever on their acceptance to the School of Medicine.

INFORMATION FOR MINORITY STUDENTS

The Wright State University School of Medicine and its faculty have a stated policy of providing educational opportunities to disadvantaged and minority applicants. The school is in the top 15 percent of the U.S. medical schools in the enrollment of students from minority groups. Special support services that meet the needs of minority students include a prematriculation program, a mentoring program in which students are paired with minority physicians in the community, a big brother/big sister program, tutoring, board preparation courses, and assistance in development of skills in critical thinking and learning. The admissions process gives careful consideration to minority applicants. Both resident and nonresident minority students are strongly encouraged to apply.

Public Institution

APPLICATION AND ACCEPTANCE POLICIES FOR 2001–2002 FIRST-YEAR CLASS

School participates in AMCAS. See Chapter 6.

Filing of AMCAS application
- Earliest date: June 1, 2000
- Latest date: Dec. 15, 2000

School application fee to all applicants: $30
Oldest MCAT scores considered: 1997
Does have Early Decision Program (EDP)
- EDP is for residents of Ohio only.
- EDP application period: June 1–Aug. 1, 2000
- EDP applicants notified by: Oct. 1, 2000

Acceptance notice to regular applicants
- Earliest date: Oct. 15, 2000
- Latest date: Until class is filled

Applicant's response to acceptance offer
- Maximum time: 3 weeks

Requests for deferred entrance considered: Yes
Deposit to hold place in class: None
Estimated number of new entrants: 90 (5 EDP)
Starting date: Aug. 2000

TUITION AND STUDENT FEES PER YEAR FOR 1999–2000 FIRST-YEAR CLASS

Tuition
- Resident: $10,842
- Nonresident: $15,348

Student fees: $662

INFORMATION ON 1999–2000 FIRST-YEAR CLASS

Number of	*In-State*	*Out-of-State*	*Total*
Applicants	1,089	1,963	3,052
Applicants Interviewed	316	82	398
New Entrants*	80	10	90

*All took the MCAT and had baccalaureate degrees.

CHAPTER 11

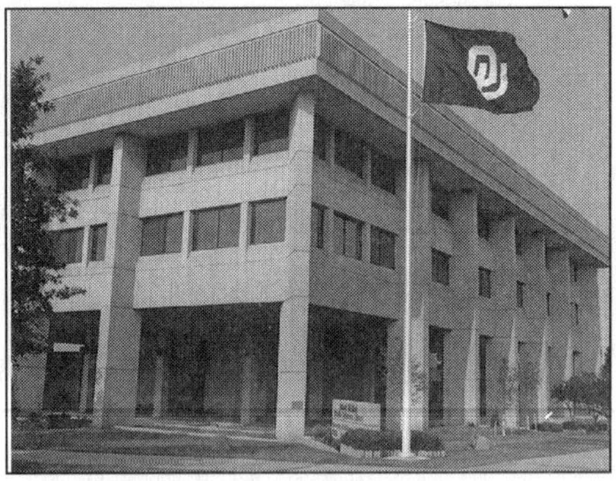

University of Oklahoma College of Medicine

Oklahoma City, Oklahoma

Dr. Nancy K. Hall, *Associate Dean of Admissions and Medical Education*
Dotty Shaw Killam, *Director of Admissions*
Martha Starling, *Director, Financial Aid*

ADDRESS INQUIRIES TO:

Dotty Shaw Killam
University of Oklahoma
College of Medicine
P.O. Box 26901
Oklahoma City, Oklahoma 73190
(405) 271-2331; 271-3032 (FAX)
E-mail: Dotty-Shaw@ouhsc.edu
Web Site: http://www.ouhsc.edu

MISSION STATEMENT

The Mission of the University of Oklahoma is to provide the best possible educational experience for our students through excellence in teaching, research and creative activity, and service to the state and society.

New structures, new facilities, and new technology—plus an internationally prominent faculty—will undoubtedly make the University of Oklahoma Health Sciences Center and the O.U. College of Medicine one of the next century's regional leaders in education, research, and patient care. OUHSC is ideally positioned to meet the demands of a rapidly changing health care system and to provide a model environment for medical education.

GENERAL INFORMATION

The University of Oklahoma College of Medicine offers students a quality education with added advantages. Access to modern patient care facilities and an aggressive research program are provided at a reasonable cost with a proven record of first-choice residency placement.

Students gain experience in a variety of settings. The college is part of a modern health sciences complex that serves as the state's principal education and research facility for physicians, dentists, nurses, biomedical scientists, pharmacists, public health administrators, and a wide range of allied health professionals.

Seven colleges—medicine, dentistry, nursing, pharmacy, public health, allied health, and the graduate college—educate more than 3,000 graduate and undergraduate students through programs offering degrees at several levels from baccalaureate through doctorate. The College of Medicine offers programs in Oklahoma City and Tulsa. The Health Sciences Center in Oklahoma City is part of a 200-acre complex of 17 public and private institutions known as the Oklahoma Health Center.

CURRICULUM

The four-year curriculum consists of two years of study in the basic sciences and two in the clinical sciences. Letter grades are awarded for all course work on a course-hour basis rather than a credit-hour basis. The first two years are complemented by a Web-based on-line curriculum. All students are required to have a computer.

There are 17 required courses in the basic science portion of the curriculum. They account for 1,973 hours of instruction or 35 percent of the total. First-year courses provide a strong basic science foundation, and second-year classes form a bridge leading directly into the clinical portion of the curriculum. A significant feature of this portion of the curriculum is early exposure to patients through the continuum courses: principles of clinical medicine I and II. The bioethical and legal issues in medicine courses are also offered.

The clinical program provides training at two sites. "The Tulsa Option" offers third- and fourth-year students the opportunity to complete their clinical training in the setting of a community-based educational program. Approximately 25 percent of the class will complete their education in several community hospitals in the Tulsa area. The clinical curriculum consists of 3,654 hours of instruction representing 65 percent of the total curriculum. A unique feature of the fourth year is a required rural preceptorship experience under the guidance of a physician in an Oklahoma community of less than 10,000 people.

Dual-degree programs are offered by the College of Medicine with full funding in place for the M.D.–Ph.D. program.

REQUIREMENTS FOR ENTRANCE

The MCAT is required and should be taken the year in which the application is filed. Applicants who have completed only 90 semester hours of college work may be considered; however, the college discourages such applications except from students who have demonstrated personal and intellectual maturity.

The following courses are required:

	Semesters
General zoology or general biology (with lab)	1
Cell biology, embryology, histology, genetics,	

or comparative vertebrate anatomy	1
Inorganic (general) chemistry	2
Organic chemistry	2
General physics	2
English	3
Psychology, sociology, anthropology, philosophy, humanities, or foreign language (any combination)	3

Additional course work in the social sciences is suggested.

Pass/fail grading, advanced placement, and CLEP courses are accepted. It is required that higher courses be taken for a grade.

No particular major is given preference; however, the applicant must provide evidence of their capability of understanding and utilizing scientific methods.

The University of Oklahoma has an October 15 deadline for applications to be submitted to AMCAS. A request for supplemental information is sent upon notification from AMCAS of a candidate's interest. The supplemental information consists of a filing fee, a premedical advisory committee letter of recommendation, plus an additional faculty recommendation, or three faculty letters. Applicants must have a complete file by November 1.

SELECTION FACTORS

Acceptance into the College of Medicine is based on GPA, MCAT scores, letters of evaluation from faculty and premedical committees, and personal interviews conducted on campus by members of the Admissions Board. Emphasis is placed on noncognitive evaluations, including health care experience, commitment, maturity, leadership, community service, and altruism. Nonresidents can represent 15 percent of the student body.

In the 1999 entering class there were 62 women, the *mean GPA* of the class was 3.59, and the *MCAT average* was 9.51.

The University of Oklahoma College of Medicine does not discriminate on the basis of race, sex, creed, national origin, age, or handicap.

FINANCIAL AID

The College of Medicine offers a number of financial assistance opportunities in addition to the federally sponsored programs. The most prominent scholarships are the Regents' Scholarship Fee Waiver, the Oklahoma Rural Medical Education Loan Scholarship Fund designed for residents wishing to practice in rural communities, and the Oklahoma Tuition Aid Grant. The loan funds established by the Shepherd Foundation, Inc., and the Lew Wentz Foundation, along with over 20 other scholarships, also aid many students annually. Additional support for minority students is available through the State Regents for Higher Education, the Ungerman Trust, and the Belknap, Culpeper, Maurer, and Reid-Winnie scholarships.

About 94 percent of all students receive some form of assistance through the Office of Financial Aid.

INFORMATION FOR MINORITY STUDENTS

The University of Oklahoma has a strong commitment to identify, recruit, and educate qualified minorities (African Americans, Native Americans, and all Hispanics). Applications are strongly encouraged from these ethnic groups as well as from any candidate with a disadvantaged background. Special consideration is given to each application.

A federally funded Native American Center of Excellence Consortium has been established in the colleges of dentistry and medicine to recruit more Native Americans into the colleges, to develop curriculum components related to Native American health issues, to recruit Native American faculty, and to stimulate research activities related to Native American health issues.

Public Institution

APPLICATION AND ACCEPTANCE POLICIES FOR 2001–2002 FIRST-YEAR CLASS

School participates in AMCAS. See Chapter 6.

Filing of AMCAS application
- Earliest date: June 1, 2000
- Latest date: Oct. 15, 2000

School application fee to all applicants: $50
Oldest MCAT scores considered: 1997
Does have Early Decision Program (EDP)
Acceptance notice to regular applicants
- Earliest date: Dec. 1, 2000
- Latest date: Until class is filled

Applicant's response to acceptance offer
- Maximum time: 2 weeks

Requests for deferred entrance considered: No
Deposit to hold place in class (applied to tuition): $100, due with response to acceptance offer
Deposit refundable prior to: May 15, 2001
Estimated number of new entrants: 150
Starting date: Aug. 2001

TUITION AND STUDENT FEES PER YEAR FOR 1999–2000 FIRST-YEAR CLASS

Tuition
- Resident: $9,552
- Nonresident: $23,606

Student fees: $629

INFORMATION ON 1999–2000 FIRST-YEAR CLASS

Number of	*In-State*	*Out-of-State*	*Total*
Applicants	314	707	1,021
Applicants Interviewed	229	35	264
New Entrants*	139	11	150

*All took the MCAT; 95% had baccalaureate degrees.

CHAPTER 11

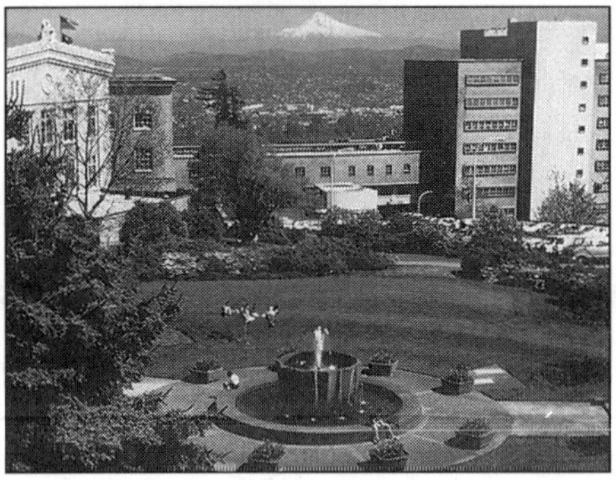

Oregon Health Sciences University School of Medicine

Portland, Oregon

Dr. Edward Keenan, *Associate Dean, Medical Education*
Vicki Fields, *Administrative Director, Education and Student Affairs*
Debbie Melton, *Admissions Officer*

ADDRESS INQUIRIES TO:

Office of Education and Student Affairs, L102
Oregon Health Sciences University
3181 S.W. Sam Jackson Park Road
Portland, Oregon 97201-3098
(503) 494-2998; 494-3400 (FAX)
Web Site: http://www.ohsu.edu/som-Dean/admit.html

GENERAL INFORMATION

The University of Oregon Medical School was established by charter from the Board of Regents of the University of Oregon in 1887. The name was changed in November 1974 when the School of Medicine and the schools of nursing and dentistry reorganized under the University of Oregon Health Sciences Center; in 1981 it was renamed Oregon Health Sciences University (OHSU). The OHSU occupies a 101-acre site in Sam Jackson Park overlooking the city but within one and a half miles of the business center. Campus physical facilities include basic science, research, and laboratory buildings; two hospital units with a licensed capacity of 509 beds; an outpatient clinic; Crippled Children's Division; Child Development and Rehabilitation Center; a hearing and speech center; a library and auditorium; and a student activities building. The School of Medicine is affiliated with the 563-bed Veterans Administration Hospital. A residence hall is provided on the campus, and apartment rentals are available in the area.

The School of Medicine provides educational programs for medical students, nurses, graduate students in basic medical sciences, and residents and interns as well as programs for radiologic technologists, medical technologists, and dietitians. An extensive postgraduate program exists.

CURRICULUM

The first two years of the curriculum are primarily devoted to the sciences basic to medicine, focusing initially on the normal structure and function of the human body and continuing with the study of the pathological basis of disease and its treatment. Principles of Clinical Medicine is presented concurrently during the first and second years to develop fundamental knowledge and skills in patient interviewing and physical diagnosis. The socioeconomic, behavioral, and population health issues are also introduced during this period. Clinical clerkship experiences undertaken at University Hospital and Clinics as well as affiliate hospitals in the Portland area constitute the third and fourth years of the curriculum. During the clinical phase of the curriculum, a six-week community health experience is required and opportunities to pursue elective courses in clinical and basic sciences.

The M.D.-Ph.D. Combined Degree Program in the School of Medicine at the Oregon Health Sciences University (OHSU) provides an opportunity for students to experience rewards of research and graduate study, while at the same time pursuing a medical education. The School of Medicine and its affiliated units have vigorous research and training programs funded by grants exceeding $100 million annually. Ph.D. degrees may be obtained in the following basic science departments: Behavioral Neuroscience, Biochemistry and Molecular Biology, Cell and Developmental Biology, Molecular and Medical Genetics, Molecular Microbiology and Immunology, and Physiology and Pharmacology, as well as in the Neuroscience program. Research training is also available through the School of Medicine in the Vollum Institute for Advanced Biomedical Research, the Center for Research on Occupational and Environmental Toxicology, the Veterans Affairs Medical Center, the Oregon Regional Primate Research Center, the Shriners Hospital for Crippled Children, and the Neurological Sciences Institute.

The combined degree program is designed for superior students with a strong basic science background. Successful applicants must show evidence of potential for excellent performance in both the M.D. and Ph.D. programs and of a firm commitment and potential for a career in academic medicine. Prior research experience is advantageous. Funding, including tuition waivers and stipend support, is provided for up to four students per year.

The Oregon Health Sciences University M.D.-M.P.H. Combined Degree Program offered by the Department of Public Health and Preventive Medicine provides an opportunity for medical students to obtain a professional degree in public health at the same time as pursuing a medical education. The Master of Public Health Epidemiology and Biostatistics track at OHSU is open to medical school applicants who wish to pursue this joint degree program.

Although the Master of Public Health Program at OHSU is part of a consortium, only the Epidemiology and Biostatistics track at OHSU is available for students in the M.D.-M.P.H. Combined Degree Program.

Admission into the M.D.-M.P.H. Combined Degree Program for medical students is designed for superior students who show evidence of potential for excellent performance in both the M.D. and M.P.H. programs and a firm commitment and potential for a career in which the population-based clinical practice model would be particularly useful.

REQUIREMENTS FOR ENTRANCE

To receive serious consideration by the Admissions Committee, all applicants must meet the following requirements.

A bachelor of arts or bachelor of science degree, or its equivalent, from an accredited college or university is required prior to matriculation to medical school. No particular major is preferred, but a broad educational background is encouraged.

The following are prescribed as the minimum acceptable college-level courses for admission. Note: One academic year is equivalent to two semesters or three quarters.

Chemistry—two academic years of chemistry (with lab) to include general chemistry (with lab) and organic chemistry (with lab). An introductory course in biochemistry is advantageous. Courses in advanced chemistry are recommended for applicants considering special medical programs with emphasis in the basic sciences (e.g., M.D.-Ph.D. Combined-Degree Program).

Biology—one academic year of general biology. A course in basic genetics is advantageous. Advanced courses in molecular biology are recommended for applicants considering the M.D.-Ph.D. Program.

Physics—one academic year of general physics (with lab).

College mathematics—one college level math course (semester/quarter) such as algebra, calculus, etc.

Humanities, Social Sciences, and English—one academic year of humanities, one academic year of social sciences, and one academic year of English to include at least one course in composition.

MCAT test scores from 1998 or later will be accepted.

SELECTION FACTORS

In evaluating candidates, attention is given to the entire academic record, the results of the MCAT, college recommendations by the premedical committee or individuals of the college faculty, and personal interviews with representatives of the Admissions Committee. Preference is given to residents of Oregon, ethnic minorities, WICHE certified residents from Montana and Wyoming, M.D.-Ph.D. and M.D.-M.P.H. candidates, and applicants with superior achievements in academics and related experiences. All applicants must have citizenship or resident alien status with a green card indicating they are a permanent resident of the United States. Each applicant is considered on the basis of qualifications without regard to race, creed, age, disability, marital status, national origin, or sex.

The *mean GPA* was 3.6 for the 1999 entering class.

FINANCIAL AID

About 90 scholarships of approximately $500 to $3,000 each are available.

Loan funds have been established to help worthy students in need of financial aid. Both short-term and long-term loans are available at reasonable interest rates.

INFORMATION FOR MINORITY STUDENTS

The School of Medicine is committed to the recruitment, selection, and retention of qualified minorities. The Admissions Committee encourages applicants of both genders and from all socioeconomic, racial, religious, and educational backgrounds. More information may be obtained by contacting the Office of Multicultural Affairs at (503) 494-7574.

Public Institution

APPLICATION AND ACCEPTANCE POLICIES FOR 2001–2002 FIRST-YEAR CLASS

School participates in AMCAS. See Chapter 6.

Filing of AMCAS application
  Earliest date: June 1, 2000
  Latest date: Oct. 15, 2000
School application fee after preliminary screening: $60
Oldest MCAT scores considered: 1998
Does not have Early Decision Program
Acceptance notice to regular applicants
  Earliest date: Nov. 1, 2000
  Latest date: Until class is filled
Applicant's response to acceptance offer
  Maximum time: 2 weeks
Requests for deferred entrance considered: No
Deposit to hold place in class: None
Estimated number of new entrants: 96
Starting date: Aug. 29, 2001

TUITION AND STUDENT FEES PER YEAR FOR 1999–2000 FIRST-YEAR CLASS

Tuition
  Resident: $14,688
  Nonresident: $30,960

Student fees: $1,950

INFORMATION ON 1999–2000 FIRST-YEAR CLASS

Number of	*In-State*	*Out-of-State*	*Total*
Applicants	283	2,169	2,452
Applicants Interviewed	141	124	265
New Entrants*	76	20	96

*All took the MCAT and had baccalaureate degrees.

CHAPTER 11

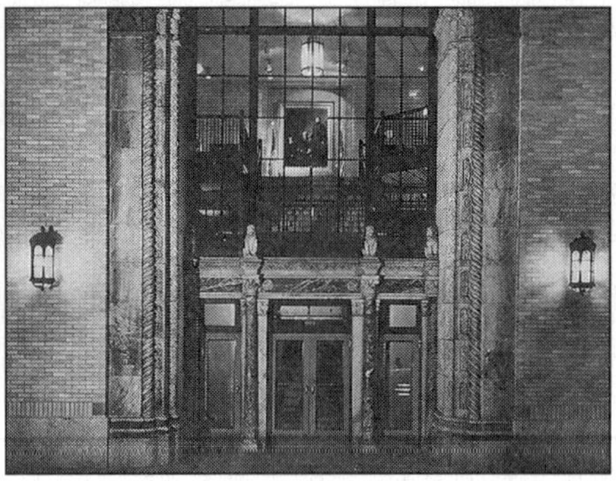

Jefferson Medical College of Thomas Jefferson University

Philadelphia, Pennsylvania

Dr. Joseph S. Gonnella, *Senior Vice President and Dean*
Dr. Clara Callahan, *Associate Dean and Director of Admissions*
Dr. Raelynn Cooter, *Director of Student Financial Aid*

ADDRESS INQUIRIES TO:

Associate Dean for Admissions
Jefferson Medical College
of Thomas Jefferson University
1015 Walnut Street, Suite 110
Philadelphia, Pennsylvania 19107-5099
(215) 955-6983; 955-5151 (FAX)
E-mail: jmc.admissions@mail.tju.edu
Web site: http://www.tju.edu/

GENERAL INFORMATION

As one of the oldest institutions of higher education in the nation, Thomas Jefferson University has, since its founding as the Jefferson Medical College in 1824, emphasized the attainment of clinical excellence in its educational programs. A recent significant expansion of the research programs has created a better balanced institutional mission and has enhanced the clinical instruction at Thomas Jefferson University Hospital and 15 affiliated federal and community hospitals.

CURRICULUM

The goals of the curriculum at Jefferson Medical College are to provide learning experiences that will enable students to acquire basic knowledge and skills as well as to develop the proper habits and attitudes needed by all physicians. The curriculum also allows students to pursue some of their special interests early in their medical training.

The first two years of instruction will encompass both a departmental and systems approach. The first-year curriculum includes anatomy, biochemistry and molecular biology, ethics, nutrition, biostatistics, histology, physiology, neuroscience, life cycle, genetics, and introduction to clinical medicine. The curriculum in the second year includes microbiology and immunology, pathology, pharmacology, introduction to clinical medicine, and medicine and society.

The clinical program consists of two 42-week phases. Phase I covers required clerkships, including family medicine, general surgery, internal medicine, pediatrics, psychiatry, and obstetrics and gynecology. Advanced basic science, rehabilitation medicine, the medical and surgical subspecialties and inpatient and outpatient subinternships in medicine or surgery are usually included in the second clinical phase. Courses in the basic sciences are given numerical grades.

Jefferson Medical College and the Pennsylvania State University select highly qualified high school seniors to earn both the B.S. and M.D. degrees in six years. The Medical Scholars Program involving the University of Delaware and Jefferson Medical College allows highly qualified students a coordinated program of education for the baccalaureate and medical degrees. The Physician Shortage Area Program serves to recruit selected students who agree to practice family medicine in physician shortage areas (especially in rural communities of Pennsylvania). Residents of the state of Delaware are admitted to Jefferson Medical College through a program involving the Delaware Institute of Medical Education and Research. There are M.D.-Ph.D. programs for students interested in research and academic medicine, as well as an M.D.-M.B.A. and M.D.-M.H.A. progam. Opportunities in basic science research and in clinical research are also available to students.

REQUIREMENTS FOR ENTRANCE

A minimum of three years (90 semester hours or equivalent) in an accredited college or university, a personal on-site interview (by invitation), and the MCAT are required. A baccalaureate degree is preferred. It is recommended that, regardless of major, each student acquire a baccalaureate education, which includes broad study in the natural and social sciences and in the humanities. The undergraduate program should include a strong preparation in the sciences and mathematics basic to medical school studies. Courses taken to meet the basic requirements should be rigorous and, in general, comparable to courses accepted for concentration in these disciplines.

Course work must include:

	Years
General biology (with lab)	1
Inorganic chemistry (with lab)	1
Organic chemistry (with lab)	1
General physics (with lab)	1

In individual cases, specific requirements may be modified at the discretion of the admissions committee.

Students are encouraged to take additional upper-level science courses out of interest or to fulfill requirements of their major.

If advanced placement credits in required subjects are submitted, additional courses in similar subjects are encouraged.

All academic requirements must be completed prior to the date of matriculation.

Students are advised to take the MCAT in the spring prior to the year of application.

SELECTION FACTORS

Jefferson, in accordance with local, state, and federal law, is committed to providing equal educational and employment opportunities for all persons, without regard to race, color, national and ethnic origin, religion, sexual orientation, age, handicap, or veteran's status. Jefferson complies with all relevant ordinances and state and federal statutes in the administration of its educational and employment policies and is an affirmative action employer. The selection of students is made after careful consideration of many factors, including the college attended, the academic record, the letters of recommendation, the MCAT scores, and the interview results of the Committee on Admissions and their opinion of the applicant's personal qualities, motivation, interpersonal skills, and achievement in nonacademic areas. Jefferson Medical College traditionally has given special consideration to offspring of alumni and faculty, minority applicants, applicants to Jefferson's special programs and, in the past, residents of Pennsylvania. Foreign applicants must have a degree from an accredited U.S. or Canadian college or university.

The 223 members of the 1999 entering class came from 91 different undergraduate schools, 22 different states, Canada, and Puerto Rico. A profile of the matriculated students includes the following: *mean science GPA*, 3.5; *mean MCAT score,* 10; *sex,* 46 percent women; *mean age,* 23.5 (range 19–44).

Each year several applicants are accepted who display extraordinary personal qualities and promise in regard to medicine, even though they do not meet all of the criteria described above.

FINANCIAL AID

Financial aid awards are based on need determined by a confidential analysis of information that is provided by the student and the student's family to the designated needs analysis service. If need is established, the student is directed to obtain a federally subsidized Stafford loan. If need exists beyond this program, Jefferson will try to meet a portion of this need from loan and grant funds. Applications for financial aid are available after December 18 from the Office of Student Financial Aid. Completed financial aid applications for the next academic year must be submitted before April 1 or within two weeks of the date of acceptance. Seventy-two percent of the 1998 entering class received financial assistance.

INFORMATION FOR MINORITY STUDENTS

Applications from qualified members of racial minority groups are encouraged.

Private Institution

APPLICATION AND ACCEPTANCE POLICIES FOR 2001–2002 FIRST-YEAR CLASS

School participates in AMCAS. See Chapter 6.

Filing of AMCAS application
  Earliest date: June 1, 2000
  Latest date: Nov. 15, 2000
School application fee to all applicants: $65
Oldest MCAT scores considered: 1997
Does have Early Decision Program (EDP)
  EDP application period: June 1–Aug. 1, 2000
  EDP applicants notified by: Oct. 1, 2000
Acceptance notice to regular applicants
  Earliest date: Oct. 15, 2000
  Latest date: Until class is filled
Applicant's response to acceptance offer
  Maximum time: 2 weeks
Requests for deferred entrance considered: Yes
Deposit to hold place in class (applied to tuition):
  $100, due on May 15, 2001
Deposit refundable prior to: May 15, 2001
Estimated number of new entrants: 223 (20 EDP)
Starting date: Aug. 2001

TUITION AND STUDENT FEES PER YEAR FOR 1999–2000 FIRST-YEAR CLASS

Tuition: $28,376 Student fees: None

INFORMATION ON 1999–2000 FIRST-YEAR CLASS

Number of	*In-State*	*Out-of-State*	*Total*
Applicants	1,043	7,129	8,172
Applicants Interviewed	330	463	793
New Entrants*	88	135	223

*All took the MCAT; 92% had baccalaureate degrees; 8% were in the B.S.-M.D. program.

CHAPTER 11

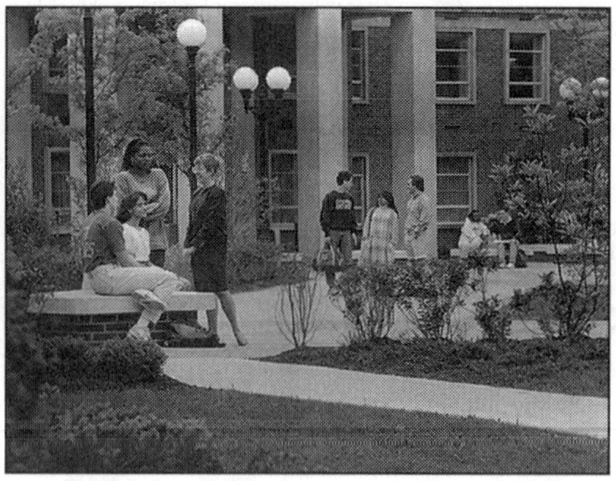

MCP Hahnemann University School of Medicine

Philadelphia, Pennsylvania

Dr. Warren E. Ross, *Interim Dean*
Kelli Kennedy, *Director of Admissions*
Cynthia A. DeLone, *Associate Director for Student Financial Aid*

ADDRESS INQUIRIES TO:

Admissions Office
MCP Hahnemann University School of Medicine
2900 Queen Lane
Philadelphia, Pennsylvania 19129
(215) 991-8202; 843-1766 (FAX)
E-mail: MCPHU.MedAdmissions@drexel.edu
Web Site: www.mcphu.edu

GENERAL INFORMATION

The Medical College of Pennsylvania (MCP) was founded in 1850 as the first medical school in the nation for women. Coeducational since 1969, the college continues to live up to its rich history, actively seeking students with diverse backgrounds and experiences. Hahnemann University, a private nondenominational institution, was founded in 1848. These two institutions have come together as part of MCP Hahnemann University, melding their rich histories and many resources to provide diversity, strength, and excellence in medical education. The medical school has a supportive environment that fosters a spirit of teamwork and personal interaction. It draws on its strengths as the academic medical anchor in a multihospital system.

MCP Hahnemann University School of Medicine is managed by Drexel University. Medical students have the opportunity for clinical training in the extensive, integrated network of hospitals of the Tenet system and at a large number of affiliated hospitals and clinics. In 1992 the School of Medicine opened a new education and research facility on a 15-acre site. This facility is the home of the first and second years of medical education.

CURRICULUM

MCP Hahnemann medical students are trained to consider each patient's case and needs in a comprehensive, integrated manner, taking into account many more factors than the presenting physiological condition. Because of this tradition, the school is dedicated to preparing "physician healers," doctors who practice the art, as well as the science and skill, of medicine.

Recognizing that different students have different ways of learning, MCP Hahnemann offers a choice between two innovative academic curricula for their first two years of study. Interdisciplinary Foundations of Medicine (IFM) integrates basic-science courses and presents them through clinical symptom-based modules. IFM is faculty-driven; students learn in lectures, labs, and small groups. The Program for Integrated Learning (PIL), a problem-based curriculum, is student-driven, supervised and facilitated by faculty. Students learn in small groups, labs, and resource sessions by focusing on case studies.

Both options focus on professional medical education, preparing students to pursue careers in either a generalist or a specialty discipline. Both stress problem solving, lifelong learning skills, and the coordinated training of basic science with clinical medicine. Both curricula also include the introduction of clinical skills training very early in the first year.

The basic clinical clerkships are offered in the third year and include experiences in all major disciplines of medical practice. The pathway program in the fourth year includes a balance of four week-long required and elective clinical experiences arranged by students with the pathway advisors to be consistent with general medical training and the student's ultimate career goals.

MCP Hahnemann University School of Medicine has joint accelerated, early assurance and post-baccalaureate programs with several colleges and universities. Combined M.D.-M.P.H., M.D.-M.B.A., and M.D.-Ph.D. programs are available for qualified students.

REQUIREMENTS FOR ENTRANCE

The MCAT and a minimum of 90 semester hours from an accredited college are required. The baccalaureate degree is highly desirable. To expedite the processing of applications, the MCAT and the required course work should be completed prior to the time of application.

The required courses are:

	Semesters
Chemistry (with lab)	2
Organic chemistry (with lab)	2
Biology (with lab)	2
Physics (with lab)	2
English	2

Biochemistry should not be counted in this total but may be taken in addition. A course in molecular and cell biology is recommended.

SELECTION FACTORS

In accord with the historical commitment of this institution, applications from women, students brought up in small towns or rural areas, those who come from Pennsylvania, students interested in a career as a generalist physician, and minorities are particularly encouraged.

Matriculated students had an average GPA of 3.35 and MCAT scores at or above the 75th percentile level. In addition to academic criteria, the interviews, which are conducted by a faculty member and a current student, are used in selecting our students.

Administrative regulations relative to the application of Public Law 93-380 (Family Educational Rights and Privacy Act) shall govern.

The medical school reserves the right to change, without notice, degree requirements, curriculum, courses, teaching personnel, rules, regulations, tuition, fees, and any other information published herein.

The medical school actively supports equality of educational opportunity. The school does not discriminate on the basis of race, color, national origin, gender, sexual preference, age, religion, creed, or handicap in admission or access to, or treatment or employment in, its programs or faculties activities. The compliance coordinator in the Office of Student Affairs is the senior associate dean.

All students must be able to meet the essential functions of the medical school.

STUDENT FINANCIAL AID

In addition to the Federal Stafford Student Loan Program, the Primary Care Loan Program, other federally funded aid programs, and assistance in obtaining money from foundation sources, the Office of University Student Financial Affairs has at its disposal limited private grant and loan funds. A College Work-Study Program for qualified students is also available. Money allocated by the school is awarded on the basis of financial need and merit. Information and applications are available from the Office of University Student Financial Affairs. Please review our Web site for more information: www.mcphu.edu/medsfa/index.html.

INFORMATION FOR MINORITY STUDENTS

Applications are actively encouraged from students of minority and disadvantaged backgrounds.

Private Institution

APPLICATION AND ACCEPTANCE POLICIES FOR 2001–2002 FIRST-YEAR CLASS

School participates in AMCAS. See Chapter 6.

Filing of AMCAS application
  Earliest date: June 1, 2000
  Latest date: Dec. 1, 2000
School application fee to all applicants: $65
Oldest MCAT scores considered: 1998
Does have Early Decision Program (EDP)
  EDP application period: June 1–Aug. 1, 2000
  EDP applicants notified by: Oct. 1, 2000
Acceptance notice to regular applicants
  Earliest date: Oct. 15, 2000
  Latest date: Until class is filled
Applicant's response to acceptance offer
  Maximum time: 15 days
Requests for deferred entrance considered: Yes
Deposit to hold place in class (applied to tuition):
  $100, due with response to acceptance offer
Deposit refundable prior to: May 15, 2001
Estimated number of new entrants: 220 (15 EDP)
Starting date: Aug. 2001

TUITION AND STUDENT FEES PER YEAR FOR 1999–2000 FIRST-YEAR CLASS

Tuition: $27,000 Student fees: $560

INFORMATION ON 1999–2000 FIRST-YEAR CLASS

Number of	*In-State*	*Out-of-State*	*Total*
Applicants	976	6,575	7,551
Applicants Interviewed	378	690	1,068
New Entrants*	106	129	235

*All took the MCAT; 98% had baccalaureate degrees.

CHAPTER 11

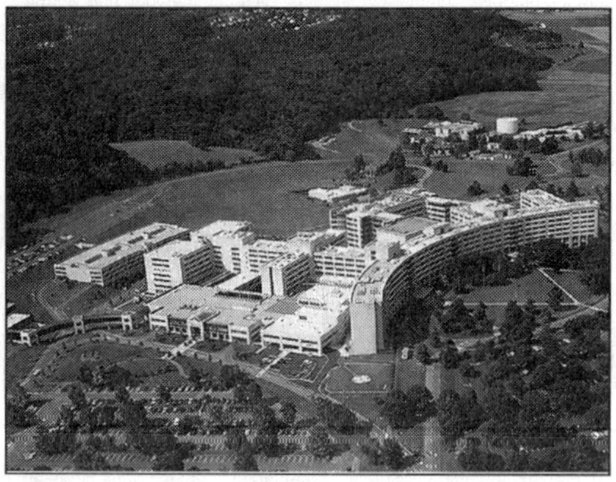

Pennsylvania State University College of Medicine

Hershey, Pennsylvania

Dr. C. McCollister Evarts, *Senior Vice President for Health Affairs and Dean*
Dr. Dwight Davis, *Associate Dean for Admissions and Student Affairs*
Jill B. Wagner, *Admissions Representative*

ADDRESS INQUIRIES TO:

Office of Student Affairs
Pennsylvania State University
College of Medicine
500 University Drive H060
Hershey, Pennsylvania 17033
(717) 531-8755; 531-6225 (FAX)
E-mail: student_affairs_SCR@psghs.edu
Web Site: http://www.collmed.psu.edu

MISSION STATEMENT

The Pennsylvania State University College of Medicine is strongly committed to the education and training of medical students, basic science graduate students, medical residents, sub-specialty fellows, other students in health-related professions, and practicing health professionals.

We seek to enroll exceptional students from all regions of the United States and to provide them with an education based on present and national health care needs. Students will be exposed to a medical environment of active basic science and clinical research where patient medical care is provided in a humanistic fashion.

Our objective is to provide a full range of patient care services, which extend from prevention of illness and maintenance of health through primary care to highly sophisticated tertiary care.

We strive to be a national leader in pursuing scientific investigation and developing programs to advance medical and scientific knowledge.

GENERAL INFORMATION

In 1963, the M.S. Hershey Foundation offered $50 million to the Pennsylvania State University to establish a medical school in Hershey. With this grant and $21.3 million from the U.S. Public Health Service, the University built a medical school, teaching hospital, and research center. Penn State's Milton S. Hershey Medical Center opened its doors to the first class of students in 1967 and became the first College of Medicine in the nation to establish a Department of Humanities, introducing humanistic disciplines into the required medical curriculum. It also was the first to start an independent Department of Family and Community Medicine. From its beginning, medical education and patient care have been guided by the institution's commitment to provide humane, compassionate, and expert care, emphasizing individual dignity.

In July 1997, two premier health institutions, the clinical enterprises of the Milton S. Hershey Medical Center and the Geisinger Health System merged to form the Penn State Geisinger Health System. This physician-led, non-profit health organization creates the only health system of its type that includes both a college of medicine and a health maintenance organization, the Penn State Geisinger Health Plan. The Penn State Geisinger system spans 40 contiguous counties in Pennsylvania, and includes a quaternary and tertiary care hospital, a community hospital, and more than 75 group practice sites.

The 550-acre medical campus is located in the rolling hills of southeastern Pennsylvania approximately eight miles from the state capital, Harrisburg. The main facility houses the College of Medicine and the Biomedical Research Building, which remain part of Penn State University; and the 504-bed Milton S. Hershey Medical Center, including the Children's Hospital, Rehabilitation Hospital and Center for Emergency Medical Services, which are part of the Penn State Geisinger Health System. The Medical Center serves as the Level 1 Regional Adult and Pediatric Trauma Center for South Central Pennsylvania.

Surrounding the main facility are the outpatient physicians center, a magnetic resonance imaging (MRI) building, a heliport for LIFE LION, the health system's aeromedical service, an animal research farm, the Penn State Center for Sports Medicine, the University fitness center, student apartments, a child care center, and outdoor recreational facilities.

CURRICULUM

In recent years the practice of medicine has undergone major changes. Many of these changes are part of a transformation that will significantly alter the way health care is organized and delivered well into the next century. Therefore, the curriculum is learner-centered and has been designed to prepare our students for the challenges of a restructured medical environment and for work in a more integrated health care system.

A single integrated curriculum for Years 1 and 2 has been developed, which combines elements of traditional medical teaching and problem-based learning. The first-year curriculum and courses are interdisciplinary rather than departmental or discipline based, combine case-based, student-centered learning with strategic lectures, laboratories, and small-group discussions. A parallel course during Years 1 and 2 entitled Physicians, Patients, and Society provides students with a core background in the important areas of humanistic medicine, psychosocial aspects of illness, epidemiology, medical ethics, and the physician-patient relationship. The second-year curriculum is more heavily oriented to case-based learning in an organ-system approach to human health, pathophysiology, and disease.

Years 3 and 4 are considered a single academic unit with Year 3 having a sequence of required core clinical clerkships in internal medicine, general surgery, pediatrics, obstetrics and gynecology, psychiatry, family and community medicine, and primary care supplemented by two selectives. Year 4 consists of a minimum of four elective rotations and four required advanced experiences, including acting internships in a medical and a surgical discipline, a primary care area, and the humanities. The College of Medicine offers a wide variety of both clinical and research electives. Students may select outpatient clinical rotations at the teaching hospitals or in university-affiliated physician offices located in a variety of rural and metropolitan communities across Pennsylvania. In addition, there are many opportunities for clinical experiences in other regions of the country and abroad.

All students must complete a medical student research project and pass USMLE Steps 1 and 2 to earn the M.D. degree.

There is an honors, high pass, pass, and fail grading system in all four years.

REQUIREMENTS FOR ENTRANCE

The MCAT and three years of college are required for admission. The baccalaureate degree is highly desirable.

The following subjects are considered by the Medical Student Selection Committee to be required:

	Years
Biology	1
Inorganic chemistry	1
Organic chemistry	1
Physics	1
Mathematics	1
Humanities	1/2
Behavioral Science	1/2

Other recommended courses are calculus, statistics, psychology, sociology, radiobiology, genetics, and anthropology.

Students should be exposed to a broad background in the humanities and social sciences. Studies that develop verbal competence and enlarge perspectives and capacities for critical, historical, and moral judgments are especially encouraged.

Students are urged to take the MCAT in the spring of the year they expect to apply. Taking the MCAT in the fall will delay consideration of the application. It is recommended that basic science courses be completed before applying.

SELECTION FACTORS

Applicants must show evidence of superior undergraduate achievement and outstanding personal characteristics. Each application is considered individually; a decision is reached after thorough evaluation of the applicant's academic record, letters of assessment, MCAT scores, and personal interview. Since the practice of medicine requires a lifelong devotion to self-education, emphasis is placed on the excellence of the individual scholar no matter what the student's previous area of study.

Applicants admitted to the College of Medicine have a *mean GPA* of 3.62 and *mean MCAT scores* of 10.

FINANCIAL AID

All financial aid is granted to students on the basis of need as determined by a federally approved needs analysis document. Approximately 85 percent of the student body receive financial assistance from some source. All funds disbursed by the school, including Federal Work-Study Program funds, are described in detail in the school catalog. Specific inquiries should be addressed to the Office of Student Affairs.

INFORMATION FOR MINORITY STUDENTS

Applications from minority group students are encouraged. Faculty members, with student support, are active in the recruitment of minority students.

Private Institution

APPLICATION AND ACCEPTANCE POLICIES FOR 2001–2002 FIRST-YEAR CLASS

School participates in AMCAS. See Chapter 6.

Filing of AMCAS application
- Earliest date: June 1, 2000
- Latest date: Nov. 15, 2000

School application fee to all applicants: $40

Deadline of completed secondary application: Jan. 15, 2001

Oldest MCAT scores considered: 1998

Does have Early Decision Program (EDP)
- EDP application period: June 1–Aug. 1, 2000
- EDP applicants notified by: Oct. 1, 2000

Acceptance notice to regular applicants
- Earliest date: Oct. 15, 2000
- Latest date: Until class is filled

Applicant's response to acceptance offer
- Maximum time: 2 weeks

Requests for deferred entrance considered: Yes

Deposit to hold place in class (applied to tuition): $100, due May 15, 2001

Deposit refundable prior to: May 15, 2001

Estimated number of new entrants: 110 (2 EDP)

Starting date: Aug. 13, 2001

TUITION AND STUDENT FEES PER YEAR FOR 1999–2000 FIRST-YEAR CLASS

Tuition
- Resident: $17,176
- Nonresident: $25,208

Student fees: $35

INFORMATION ON 1999–2000 FIRST-YEAR CLASS

Number of	*In-State*	*Out-of-State*	*Total*
Applicants	1,023	5,359	6,382
Applicants Interviewed	251	414	665
New Entrants*	53	53	106

*All took the MCAT and had baccalaureate degrees.

CHAPTER 11

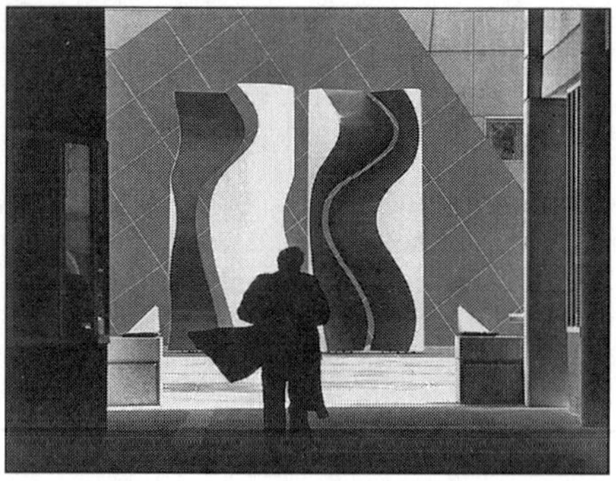

University of Pennsylvania School of Medicine

Philadelphia, Pennsylvania

Dr. William N. Kelley, *CEO and Dean*
Dr. Gail Morrison, *Vice Dean for Education*
Gaye W. Sheffler, *Director of Admissions and Financial Aid*

ADDRESS INQUIRIES TO:

Director of Admissions and Financial Aid
Edward J. Stemmler Hall, Suite 100
University of Pennsylvania
School of Medicine
Philadelphia, Pennsylvania 19104-6056
(215) 898-8001; 573-6645 (FAX)
Web Site: http://www.med.upenn.edu/admiss

GENERAL INFORMATION

The School of Medicine, the first in the United States, was founded in 1765 and is a private, nondenominational school located on the urban campus of the University of Pennsylvania.

As part of the one university concept, medical students participate throughout their enrollment as members of the university as well as the School of Medicine community. In their clinical years, medical students receive their education mostly in the Hospital of the University of Pennsylvania and the Children's Hospital of Philadelphia, the Veterans Administration of Philadelphia hospitals, Presbyterian Medical Center of Philadelphia, Pennsylvania Hospital, and Phoenixville Hospital. Student housing, both on and off campus, is plentiful.

CURRICULUM

To prepare students with diverse talents and interests for a range of career paths, the objective of Curriculum 2000™ is to facilitate the development of skills, competencies, and professional attitudes, which will help all students, as future physicians, master the challenges that they will face in an ever-changing practice environment. Across the five modules of the curriculum, concepts in basic science and clinical medicine are integrated in order to emphasize the intrinsic inextricability of these disciplines. Professional attitudes and communication abilities are fostered and invaluable skills for lifelong learning are developed.

Module 1: Core Principles. The first four months of Year 1 provide the student with fundamental concepts in basic science that underlie the biomedical basis of disease.

Module 2: Integrative Systems and Diseases. The latter six months of Year 1 and the first four months of Year 2 are organized along five organ system blocks each of which, through the integration of anatomy, histology, physiology, pathophysiology, pathology, microbiology, and pharmacology, provides the student with an all-encompassing picture of each organ system in normal and abnormal states. To acquaint students with fundamental concepts in pathology, which will be expanded upon during the organ system blocks, Module 2 begins with a transitional block.

Concurrent with Modules 1 and 2 is Module 3: The Art and Practice of Medicine. Module 3 facilitates development of competencies and attitudes in history-taking, physical exam administration, differential diagnosis, clinical epidemiology, managed care policies and practices, ethics, and professionalism and humanism. Mini-courses comprising Module 3 are coordinated with subject matter addressed in Modules 1 and 2 expanding upon and providing clinical relevance to basic science concepts. A component of Module 3 is open time for students to explore individual interests through elective course work in other schools of the university as well as projects in the community.

Module 4: Core Clinical Clerkships. One year of required clinical experiences, begins January of Year 2. While primary emphasis is upon the development of clinical skills, re-emphasis of basic science concepts and formal attention to professionalism, humanism, and ethics are ensured through symposia and interdisciplinary problem-based learning sessions based upon cases of clinical significance. The curricula of all required clerkships include ambulatory and inpatient experiences.

The final 16 months of Curriculum 2000™ are occupied by Module 5: Electives, Selectives, and Scholarly Pursuit. Students are encouraged to explore individual interests and to prepare for future career paths. Required experiences include advanced clinical electives, "Frontiers in Medical Science" mini-courses and a "scholarly pursuit" of at least three months in length.

Many opportunities exist for students of the School of Medicine to become involved in both basic science and clinical research, to study medicine through international exchange programs, and to participate in study and special projects through other schools of the university. Long-term opportunities are available through dual-degree programs. Students interested in pursuing careers in academic medicine or research and possessing strong science backgrounds and research experience may apply to the M.D.-Ph.D. program while students who are interested in careers that include responsibilities as community leaders may augment their qualifications through combined-degree programs offering graduate degrees in business/health care economics, government administration, clinical epidemiology, and education.

REQUIREMENTS FOR ENTRANCE

The MCAT and a baccalaureate degree from an accredited U.S. college or university are required. Students with degrees from foreign institutions must have completed one year of course work in the sciences in a U.S. college or university.

Students are encouraged to obtain a broad education in the liberal arts while undertaking rigorous preparation in the sciences. Science courses should include laboratory experience, which enables students to become active participants in problem solving.

Because the content of courses varies among different educational institutions, the School of Medicine does not have specific course requirements. Students are expected to acquire appropriate competence in English and communication, biology, chemistry, physics, and mathematics. The school has developed general outlines of the requisite knowledge and skills in these disciplines.

In addition, students should carry out additional work in accordance with their own interests and curiosity. They should attempt to develop, through their formal course work and other educational experiences, an appreciation of the basic social, cultural, and behavioral factors that influence both individuals and communities in their approach to health and disease.

SELECTION FACTORS

The School of Medicine will emphasize those qualities of motivation, intellect, and character essential to the physician. Consideration also will be given to special features of background and experience, which may contribute to a candidate's potential for a medical career. Applicants should give evidence of their capacity to deal effectively with other people, organize their own activities, set priorities, accept responsibility, and function under stress.

While the Committee on Admissions has no preference regarding the area of concentration, applicants are expected to have approached their chosen field in scholarly fashion and to have demonstrated excellence in whatever courses of study they have pursued.

In evaluating candidates, the Committee on Admissions reviews the academic record, recommendations from college premedical committees, scores on the MCAT, quality of and commitment to extracurricular activities, and strength of personal qualifications. Interviews are required for admission and are arranged by invitation of the Committee on Admissions. Applicants from all sections of the country are invited to apply, although some preference is given to Pennsylvania residents.

In recent years, applicants granted admission have had a *mean GPA* of 3.78 and *mean MCAT scores* of 11.4.

The class entering in September 1999 was composed of 46 percent *women;* 19 percent *Pennsylvania residents;* 37 percent *nonwhite ethnic groups,* of which 13 percent are underrepresented *minorities;* and 25 percent *nonscience majors.*

The University of Pennsylvania does not discriminate on the basis of race, sex, sexual preference, age, religion, national or ethnic origin, or physical handicap. There is no transfer admissions program.

FINANCIAL AID

Grant and loan assistance is available for students who qualify on the basis of need and who are U.S. citizens or permanent residents. Over 75 percent of the student body receive loans, and approximately one-third of the students receive school scholarship and loan funds. The ability of students to pay for their medical education does not affect the decision on their applications for admission.

INFORMATION FOR MINORITY STUDENTS

Detailed information and statistics on minority applicants, acceptances, and enrollment are available in the *Information for Minority Applicants* brochure, which can be obtained by writing to the Office of Minority Affairs, Suite 100, Stemmler Hall.

Private Institution

APPLICATION AND ACCEPTANCE POLICIES FOR 2001–2002 FIRST-YEAR CLASS

School participates in AMCAS. See Chapter 6.

Filing of AMCAS application
- Earliest date: June 1, 2000
- Latest date: Nov. 1, 2000

School application fee to all applicants: $65
Oldest MCAT scores considered: 1991
Does not have Early Decision Program
Acceptance notice to regular applicants
- Earliest date: March 1, 2001
- Latest date: Until class is filled

Applicant's response to acceptance offer
- Maximum time: 2 weeks

Requests for deferred entrance considered: Yes
Deposit to hold place in class (applied to tuition):
- $100, due on May 15, 2001

Deposit refundable prior to: May 15, 2001
Estimated number of new entrants: 145
Starting date: Aug. 8, 2001

TUITION AND STUDENT FEES PER YEAR FOR 1999–2000 FIRST-YEAR CLASS

Tuition: $29,670 Student fees: $1,780

INFORMATION ON 1999–2000 FIRST-YEAR CLASS

Number of	*In-State*	*Out-of-State*	*Total*
Applicants	774	5,843	6,617
Applicants Interviewed	130	816	946
New Entrants*	28	116	144

*All took the MCAT and had baccalaureate degrees.

University of Pittsburgh
School of Medicine

University of Pittsburgh School of Medicine

Pittsburgh, Pennsylvania

Dr. Arthur S. Levine, *Senior Vice Chancellor for Health Sciences and Dean, School of Medicine*
Dr. Edward I. Curtiss, *Associate Dean of Admissions*
Linda A. Berardi-Demo, *Director of Admissions*

ADDRESS INQUIRIES TO:

Office of Admissions
518 Scaife Hall
University of Pittsburgh
School of Medicine
Pittsburgh, Pennsylvania 15261
(412) 648-9891; 648-8768 (FAX)
E-mail: admissions@fsl.dean-med.pitt.edu
Web Site: http://www.dean_med.pitt.edu

MISSION STATEMENT

The principal goal of the University of Pittsburgh School of Medicine remains the education of scholarly physicians. This goal is to be achieved by emphasizing the centrality of the patient as the focus of health care, by providing a firm understanding of the sciences basic to medicine, and by fostering the application of principles of biomedical problem solving to the care of patients. We feel that students must develop an understanding of ethical principles in medicine and share in the application of these principles to specific problems. Development, early in the student's career, of habits of self-education by methods that include problem-based and self-directed learning, communication skills, and computer-assisted education is critical to the learning process, which must occur throughout the professional life of a physician.

GENERAL INFORMATION

The Western Pennsylvania Medical College, chartered in 1886, became associated with the University of Pittsburgh in 1908. The School of Medicine is located in the Oakland district of Pittsburgh in the Alan Magee Scaife Hall of the Health Professions.

The University of Pittsburgh Medical Center includes UPMC Presbyterian and UPMC Shadyside, large tertiary care hospitals; specialty hospitals, including Western Psychiatric Institute and Clinic, Eye & Ear, Magee-Women's Hospital, and UPMC Rehabilitation Hospital; and nine community hospitals throughout the region. The University of Pittsburgh Medical Center coordinates its activities with other university-affiliated hospitals and facilities, including Children's Hospital of Pittsburgh and the Veterans Affairs Medical Centers.

CURRICULUM

The School of Medicine has initiated extensive curricular revisions that were implemented in the fall of 1992. The goal-oriented, integrated, and centrally governed new curriculum emphasizes general principles and encourages student self-learning based on actual clinical cases. In the first two years, the curriculum employs a multidisciplinary approach organized by organ systems (such as the heart, lungs, and kidneys) rather than by individual disciplines (e.g., physiology and biochemistry). It emphasizes problem-solving skills and learning in smaller groups. The curriculum mainstreams social, cultural, and ethical issues and introduces the student to clinical medicine during the first year. The final several weeks of the second year are devoted to an Integrated Case Studies course. This course emphasizes data acquisition, problem solving, and communication skills. It is intended to help the student actively review the material presented during the first two years and serves as a bridge to the patient-care responsibilities assumed in the third-year clinical clerkships. In the third year of medical school, all students have required rotations in family medicine, internal medicine, obstetrics-gynecology, pediatrics, psychiatry, surgery, as well as ambulatory subspecialties. Some students rotate through anesthesia during the third year, while others take it during the fourth year. All fourth-year students rotate through both neurology and diagnostic imaging clerkships. Some students have one elective scheduled during the third year, and all students have extensive elective time during the fourth year.

In addition to the curricular offerings, there are opportunities for students to interact with community physicians through the Western Pennsylvania Health Preceptorship Program.

An honors/pass/fail system is used for grading.

The M.D.-Ph.D. Program of the University of Pittsburgh and Carnegie Mellon University offers exceptionally talented students the opportunity to undertake a physician-scientist training program tailored to their specific research interests. Over a period of seven or eight years, these individuals meet the degree requirements of both a graduate school and the medical school. Information may be obtained from the M.D.-Ph.D. office in 526 Scaife Hall. The telephone number is (412) 648-2324.

The School of Medicine offers two other combined-degree programs where the course of study is five years—M.D-M.P.H. and M.D-M.A. in Ethics.

REQUIREMENTS FOR ENTRANCE

The faculty of the School of Medicine consider currently enrolled students and graduates of accredited collegiate institutions for admission. Only under exceptional circumstances are students accepted to the School of Medicine with fewer than 120 hours of undergraduate work or without an undergraduate degree. The MCAT is required.

Specific minimum admission requirements include:

	Years
Biology, exclusive of botany (with lab)	1
General or inorganic chemistry (with lab)	1
Organic chemistry (with lab)	1
Physics (with lab)	1
English	1

English courses must engender effective writing skills as well as familiarity with the great works of literature. A strong background in mathematics is highly recommended. Studies in social and behavioral sciences and humanities are strongly encouraged.

Acceptance of course requirements taken at foreign universities is determined on an individual basis at the discretion of the dean of admissions.

Applicants should have completed most premedical requirements to receive serious consideration. All requirements must be met prior to matriculation.

Students whose applications have been refused by us in three prior submissions will not be considered.

SELECTION FACTORS

Applicants are chosen on the basis of intellect, integrity, maturity, and the ability to interact sensitively with people. In the competitive evaluation of applicants, consideration is given to the past academic record and MCAT scores; evaluations of college preprofessional committees; letters of recommendation, preferably from faculty members with whom the student has interacted in scholarly pursuits; extracurricular activities; and personal interviews. No one is accepted without an interview. Interviews are conducted only at the medical school campus. All applicants are considered without regard to race, color, religion, ethnicity, national origin, age, sex, sexual orientation, marital, veteran, or handicap status. Foreign nationals must have permanent resident visas and have completed at least one full year of undergraduate education in the United States, preferably the premedical requirements. Some preference is given to Pennsylvania residents since the university is a state-related school. For the entering class of 1999, matriculated students had an *average science GPA* of 3.66 and a *mean MCAT* of 10.5.

The School of Medicine is committed to increasing the number of minority students (African American, Mexican American, Mainland Puerto Rican, and Native American) in medicine, and thus actively recruits and strongly encourages applications from minority students. The school hosts premedical summer enrichment programs, as well as a prematriculation program for admitted students. Following admission, a broad range of support services are available to ensure retention. Specific information on the services provided to minority applicants can be obtained by contacting the Office of Student Affairs/Minority Programs at (412) 648-8987.

FINANCIAL AID

All loans and scholarships are awarded on the basis of financial need as documented by the FAFSA. Students demonstrating financial need are expected to obtain the first $8,500 from the Federal Stafford Student Loan.

Private Institution

APPLICATION AND ACCEPTANCE POLICIES FOR 2000–2001 FIRST-YEAR CLASS

School participates in AMCAS. See Chapter 6.

Filing of AMCAS application
  Earliest date: June 1, 2000
  Latest date: Dec. 1, 2000
School application fee to all applicants: $60
Oldest MCAT scores considered: 1997
Does have Early Decision Program (EDP)
  EDP application period: June 1–Aug. 1, 2000
  EDP applicants notified by: Oct. 1, 2000
Acceptance notice to regular applicants
  Earliest date: Feb. 21, 2001
  Latest date: Until class is filled
Applicant's response to acceptance offer
  Maximum time: 2 weeks
Requests for deferred entrance considered: Yes
  Deposit to hold place in class: $100, (which must reach our office between May 16–23, 2001).
Estimated number of new entrants: 146 (2 EDP)
Starting date: Aug. 2001

TUITION AND STUDENT FEES PER YEAR FOR 1998–99 FIRST-YEAR CLASS

Tuition
  Resident: $21,354
  Nonresident: $28,832

Student fees: $1,726

INFORMATION ON 1998–99 FIRST-YEAR CLASS

Number of	*In-State*	*Out-of-State*	*Total*
Applicants	900	3,717	4,617
Applicants Interviewed	266	783	1,048
New Entrants*	71	72	143

*All took the MCAT and had baccalaureate degrees.

CHAPTER 11

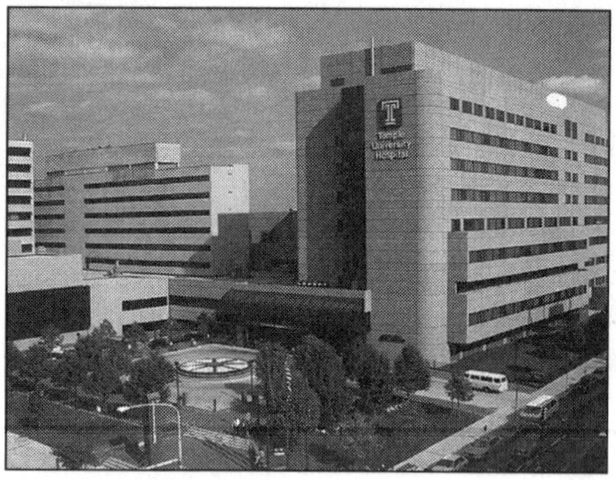

Temple University School of Medicine

Philadelphia, Pennsylvania

Dr. Leon S. Malmud, *Dean and Vice President*
Dr. Richard J. Kozera, *Executive Dean*
Dr. Audrey B. Uknis, *Assistant Dean for Admissions*

ADDRESS INQUIRIES TO:

Office of Admissions
Temple University
School of Medicine
3400 N. Broad Street
Philadelphia, Pennsylvania 19140
(215) 707-3656; 707-6932 (FAX)
Web Site: http://www.temple.edu/medschool/

GENERAL INFORMATION

The Temple University School of Medicine opened as a college of Temple University in 1901. The School of Medicine shares a campus with Temple Hospital, Temple University Children's Medical Center, other health-related schools of the university, and the Student/ Faculty Center. Clinical experience and instruction are given at the new Temple University Hospital, the new Temple University Children's Medical Center, Crozer-Chestnut Medical Center, Fox Chase Cancer Center, and 23 other affiliated hospitals, in both Philadelphia and other Pennsylvania cities. A new clinical campus has been established in Pittsburgh at Western Pennsylvania Hospital.

CURRICULUM

The curriculum is designed to prepare students for graduate medical education by providing them with a background of basic factual knowledge and concepts, a command of the language of biomedical science, a mastery of the skills necessary for clinical problem solving and therapy, and a habit of continued self-education.

In the first two years, although primary emphasis is on the basic sciences taught in large measure in a small-group format, attention is also given to the clinical application of this material. In addition, courses on clinical medicine and primary care concepts prepare the students to assume initial clinical responsibilities. The third year includes clerkships in family practice, internal medicine, obstetrics-gynecology, pediatrics, psychiatry, and surgery, which provide experience in clinical diagnosis, problem solving, therapeutic planning, and patient relationships. In the fourth year, there are required rotations in emergency medicine, neuroscience, and a subinternship and 20 weeks of individually planned electives that permit students to explore career choice, correct deficits, and expand clinical knowledge.

There is an honors/high pass/pass/conditional/fail grading system.

M.D.-Ph.D. and M.D.-M.P.H. programs are available.

REQUIREMENTS FOR ENTRANCE

The MCAT and a minimum of 90 semester hours in an accredited college or university are required for admission. Applicants need not major in science, and a strong background and preparation in the humanities with particular emphasis on expository writing are essential. Students who have not completed the baccalaureate degree but who have demonstrated exceptional academic capability and evidence of unusual maturity may apply. The undergraduate program must include:

	Sem. hrs.
Biology (with lab)	8
Inorganic chemistry (with lab)	8
Organic chemistry (with lab)	8
General physics (with lab)	8
Humanities	6

Applicants are asked to have recommendations from their undergraduate premedical committee or faculty in two of the following three subjects: biology, chemistry, and physics.

It is suggested that the MCAT be taken in the spring of the calendar year of application and that all courses required for medical school be completed by the time of application.

SELECTION FACTORS

A variety of objective and subjective factors are considered in making decisions. Among these are the academic record and the college attended, MCAT scores, recommendations from faculty, extracurricular activities, and work experience. Those candidates who are to be given very serious consideration are invited for personal interviews with a member of the Admissions Committee.

As a state-related school, Temple shows preference to residents of Pennsylvania; however, a significant percentage of matriculants may be residents of other states. Nonresidents with a particular interest in Temple and strong credentials are encouraged to apply.

Temple University School of Medicine does not discriminate on the basis of race, sex, creed, national origin, age, or handicap.

Selected characteristics of the 1999 entering class are as follows: *average science GPA,* 3.4; *average MCAT: sciences,* 10; *sex,* 37 percent women; *minorities,* 17 percent.

FINANCIAL AID

With the exception of a restricted number of scholarships, all financial aid is in the form of loans and is based solely on need. Need is established by the use of a national standard financial aid application through GAPSFAS, which details financial resources of students (or their families) and balances them against a standard budget plus special need factors. A modicum of relatively low-cost financial aid comes from Temple University-based moneys as part of the federal programs for the Health Professions Student Loan and the Perkins Loan. The initial source of assistance for most students will be the Stafford Student Loan Program; in fact, all eligible students are expected to secure the first $7,500 of aid from this source. Other sources of assistance may come from medical societies, fraternal organizations, church groups, and, in the case of minority students, from the National Medical Fellowships, Inc. In selected instances students have applied to the scholarship programs of the Armed Forces and the National Health Service Corps. Approximately 80 percent of the students receive financial aid.

INFORMATION FOR MINORITY STUDENTS

An active program, Recruitment, Admission, and Retention (RAR), meets the special needs of minority applicants. RAR provides exceptional resources for professional academic guidance and personal counseling. Participation in the Summer Educational Reinforcement Activity is encouraged for accepted minority students and others.

Private Institution

APPLICATION AND ACCEPTANCE POLICIES FOR 2001–2002 FIRST-YEAR CLASS

School participates in AMCAS. See Chapter 6.

Filing of AMCAS application
  Earliest date: June 1, 2000
  Latest date: Dec. 1, 2000
School application fee to all applicants: $55
Oldest MCAT scores considered: 1998
Does have Early Decision Program (EDP)
  EDP application period: June 1–Aug. 1, 2000
  EDP applicants notified by: Oct. 1, 2000
Acceptance notice to regular applicants
  Earliest date: Oct. 15, 2000
  Latest date: Until class is filled
Applicant's response to acceptance offer
  Maximum time: 2 weeks
Requests for deferred entrance considered: Yes
Deposit to hold place in class (applied to tuition):
  $100, due with response to acceptance offer
Deposit refundable prior to: May 15, 2001
Estimated number of new entrants: 200 (5 EDP)
Starting date: Aug. 2001

TUITION AND STUDENT FEES PER YEAR FOR 1999–2000 FIRST-YEAR CLASS

Tuition
  Resident: $23,708
  Nonresident: $28,900

Student fees: $407

INFORMATION ON 1998–99 FIRST-YEAR CLASS

Number of	*In-State*	*Out-of-State*	*Total*
Applicants	1,041	6,441	7,482
Applicants Interviewed	337	455	792
New Entrants*	131	75	206

*All took the MCAT and had baccalaureate degrees.

CHAPTER 11

Universidad Central del Caribe School of Medicine

Bayamón, Puerto Rico

Dr. Helen Rosa, *Acting Dean of Medicine*
Dr. Nereida Diaz, *Dean of Admissions and Student Affairs*
Vivian Cintron, *Financial Aid Officer*

ADDRESS INQUIRIES TO:

Office of Admissions
Universidad Central del Caribe
School of Medicine
P.O. Box 60-327
Bayamón, Puerto Rico 00960-6032
(787) 740-1611 Ext. 210; 269-7550 (FAX)
Web Site: http://www.uccaribe.edu

GENERAL INFORMATION

The Universidad Central del Caribe School of Medicine was founded in 1976 as a nonprofit private institution chartered under the laws of the Commonwealth of Puerto Rico. The new building for the basic sciences, library, animal house, and central administration was inaugurated in 1990 adjacent to Dr. Ramón Ruíz Arnau University Hospital, which serves as the principal teaching hospital. The school facilities are located in a 56-acre academic health center in the city of Bayamón.

CURRICULUM

The educational goal of the medical school is to develop an individual who is oriented toward the provision of primary health care. In line with this goal, the medical school experience emphasizes community health, family medicine, and primary medical care aspects of internal medicine, surgery, pediatrics, obstetrics and gynecology, and psychiatry.

The medical curriculum is organized in two years of preclinical and two years of clinical experiences. Clinical correlations are included in the basic science courses. Introduction to clinical medicine has as its foundation the biopsychosocial model. This is a problem-based course structured around prevalent problems encountered in primary care. The third-year learning experience evolves around the required clerkships in internal medicine, pediatrics, obstetrics-gynecology, general surgery, and family and community medicine. The latter takes place in the ambulatory setting. Also, during the third year, students enroll in the surgical subspecialties and psychiatry clerkships. Sixteen weeks of electives are provided in the fourth year, plus three months in required courses in Neurology, Emergency Medicine, and Primary Care.

Individual student evaluation in all requisite basic science and clinical science courses is based on letter grade and pass/fail systems. Student evaluation in all elective courses is based on an honors/pass/fail system.

REQUIREMENTS FOR ENTRANCE

The MCAT and a minimum of 90 credits of satisfactory work in an accredited undergraduate institution are required. A baccalaureate degree is highly recommended. All premedical course requirements must either be completed or be in progress prior to consideration for admission.

Required premedical courses and minimum required credits are:

	Sem. hrs.
General biology or zoology	8
General chemistry	8
Organic chemistry	8
General physics	8
College mathematics	6
English	12
Spanish	6
Behavioral/Social sciences	12

The applicant must demonstrate proficiency in both Spanish and English. Teaching in basic sciences and clinical sciences is conducted mainly in Spanish.

A strong background and preparation in the humanities and behavioral sciences is highly encouraged so that the applicant may obtain a well-rounded undergraduate education. This background should provide the applicant with a broad cultural foundation, and it will allow our institution to produce physicians with a humanistic approach to the practice of the profession. As long as students fulfill the basic requirements for admission, they may obtain a baccalaureate degree in any field of learning.

Applicants are strongly urged to take the MCAT in the spring prior to application and to have completed the required courses by the time of application since applications are not reviewed by the Admissions Committee until the MCAT scores and grades are available. Taking the fall MCAT or having required courses in process may delay consideration of an application, thus reducing the applicant's chances of acceptance.

SELECTION FACTORS

The selection of candidates for admission is made exclusively by the Admissions Committee. The admission process does not discriminate against any individual on the basis of sex, age, race, religion, economic status, political ideology, or national origin. Major factors considered in the selection of candidates for admission include undergraduate academic record, general GPA and science GPA, performance in all areas of the MCAT, results of a personal interview, and letters of recommendation. A personal interview is required prior to consideration for admission. All interviews are arranged by the Office of Admissions and are conducted at the medical school facilities in Bayamón. Rejected applicants are given the opportunity to reapply for admission.

For the 1999 entering class the *mean undergraduate general GPA* was 3.30, and 53 percent of the entering students were women.

FINANCIAL AID

The Office of the Dean for Student Affairs provides financial aid counseling to all prospective students. Incoming freshmen qualify for application to all pertinent federal and commonwealth scholarship and loan programs. Economic status of the applicant is not a consideration during the selection of candidates for admission.

Private Institution

APPLICATION AND ACCEPTANCE POLICIES FOR 2001–2002 FIRST-YEAR CLASS

School participates in AMCAS. See Chapter 6.

Filing of AMCAS application
  Earliest date: June 1, 2000
  Latest date: Dec. 15, 2000
School application fee to all applicants: $50
Oldest MCAT scores considered: 1999
Does not have Early Decision Program
Acceptance notice to regular applicants
  Earliest date: Dec. 15, 2000
  Latest date: Until class is filled
Applicant's response to acceptance offer
  Maximum time: 10 days
Requests for deferred entrance considered: No
  Deposit to hold place in class: $500, due with response to acceptance offer (of which, $400 is applicable to tuition); nonrefundable
Estimated number of new entrants: 60
Starting date: Aug. 2001

TUITION AND STUDENT FEES PER YEAR FOR 1999–2000 FIRST-YEAR CLASS

Tuition
  Resident: $17,000
  Nonresident: $24,000

Student fees: $2,695

INFORMATION ON 1999–2000 FIRST-YEAR CLASS

Number of	*In-State*	*Out-of-State*	*Total*
Applicants	352	578	930
Applicants Interviewed	144	27	171
New Entrants*	51	9	60

*All took the MCAT; 90% had baccalaureate degrees.

CHAPTER 11

Ponce School of Medicine

Ponce, Puerto Rico

Dr. Manuel Martinez-Maldonado, *President and Dean*
Dr. Carmen M. Mercado, *Assistant Dean for Admissions*
Rosalia Martinez, *Financial Aid Director*

ADDRESS INQUIRIES TO:

Admissions Office
Ponce School of Medicine
P.O. Box 7004
Ponce, Puerto Rico 00732
(787) 840-2511; 840-9756 (FAX)

GENERAL INFORMATION

The Ponce School of Medicine of the Ponce Medical School Foundation, Inc., formerly Catholic University of Puerto Rico School of Medicine, took over the operations on July 1, 1980, under the government of a board of trustees. The school graduated its first class in June 1981.

Clinical training is offered at the following facilities in Ponce: Damas Hospital, a private institution with 356 beds; La Playa Diagnostic Center, which serves as the main training area for community and family practice; Ponce District Hospital with 550 beds; Dr. Pila Hospital with 160 beds; and St. Luke's Hospital with 160 beds. Clinical training is also offered at the Concepción Hospital with 188 beds, located in San Germán, and at Yauco Regional Hospital with 140 beds.

CURRICULUM

The medical program's basic objective is to provide the Commonwealth of Puerto Rico, especially the southern region of the island, with ethically motivated, professionally competent primary care physicians. The curriculum provides students with an early experience in family and community health needs. During the first two years the basic medical sciences are thoroughly emphasized. Clinical experience takes precedence during the third and fourth years. The correlation between the basic and clinical sciences is achieved in a multidisciplinary program. Throughout the four-year program great emphasis is placed on the student's contact with patients and their families, as a complement to the student's academic-hospital experience.

Every academic semester contains, in addition to the regular curriculum, a series of supplementary seminars dealing with the ethical and social components of medical practice and with additional specific subjects that are incidental and relevant to the profession. A problem-based learning program has been introduced in clinical correlation sessions in the first year of medical studies and in the pathophysiology course, in which it is presented as a student-centered integrative exercise.

The program seeks to develop well-balanced, mature general practitioners, equally well qualified in the professional ethical aspects of medicine.

Students must pass the USMLE before being promoted to the third year.

Students work is graded according to an honors/pass/fail/incomplete.

REQUIREMENTS FOR ENTRANCE

The MCAT and a minimum of three years (90 semester hours) of accredited college work are required. Accredited courses should include the following minimum requirements:

	Sem. hrs.
Biology	8
Inorganic chemistry	8
Organic chemistry	8
Physics	8
College mathematics or trigonometry	6
Humanities*	12
English	12
Spanish	6

*Course work must be in sociology, psychology, political science, economics, or anthropology.

Academic requirements should be met not later than during the academic year immediately preceding the applicant's anticipated entrance to the school. Applicants are required to submit written evaluations from three faculty members of the institution where they have recently studied or one from their premedical advisory committee.

SELECTION FACTORS

Selection of applicants is made by the Admissions Committee on the basis of academic achievement, MCAT scores, evaluation letters, and personal interviews. The interviews are used to determine the motivation and character of the applicants. Only those who pass a preliminary screening, based on MCAT scores and college grades, are interviewed. Careful consideration is given to all applicants regardless of racial or ethnic background, religious affiliation, sex, or national origin. Residents of Puerto Rico are given preference, although a limited number of applicants who live in the United

States are accepted. Candidates who do not have a functional knowledge of both English and Spanish are not encouraged to apply, since instruction is given in both languages.

The 1999 entering class had the following profile: *average GPA,* 3.44 (100 percent above 3.0); *sex,* 43 percent female; *residence,* 77 percent from Puerto Rico, 24 percent from the continental United States; *undergraduate major,* 70 percent in biology and general science.

FINANCIAL AID

Students are admitted to the School of Medicine without regard to financial circumstances. After acceptance, prospective students are mailed the necessary forms to complete the financial aid process. The school participates in federal scholarship and loan programs.

Financial Aid Awards are based on need. Students must submit data either of the Renewal or FAFSA (Free Application for Federal Student Aid) to apply for aid from Federal programs.

About 92 percent of 1999 entrants received financial aid. Financial Aid applications are mailed in February, and awards are made in July. Students are informed about financial aid opportunities prior to acceptance at the School of Medicine.

Private Institution

APPLICATION AND ACCEPTANCE POLICIES FOR 2001–2002 FIRST-YEAR CLASS

School participates in AMCAS. See Chapter 6.

Filing of AMCAS application
- Earliest date: June 1, 2000
- Latest date: Dec. 15, 2000

School application fee to all applicants: $100
Oldest MCAT scores considered: 1998
Does have Early Decision Program (EDP)
- EDP is for residents of Puerto Rico only.
- EDP application period: June 1–Aug. 1, 2000
- EDP applicants notified by: Oct, 1, 2000

Acceptance notice to regular applicants
- Earliest date: Oct. 15, 2000
- Latest date: Until class is filled

Applicant's response to acceptance offer
- Maximum time: 20 working days

Requests for deferred entrance considered: No
Deposit to hold place in class (applied to tuition):
- $1,000, due with response to acceptance offer; nonrefundable

Estimated number of new entrants: 60 (3 EDP)
Starting date: July 2001

TUITION AND STUDENT FEES PER YEAR FOR 1999–2000 FIRST-YEAR CLASS

Tuition
- Resident: $17,312
- Nonresident: $25,810

Student fees: $2,025

INFORMATION ON 1999–2000 FIRST-YEAR CLASS

Number of	*In-State*	*Out-of-State*	*Total*
Applicants	378	616	994
Applicants Interviewed	167	34	201
New Entrants*	14	46	60

*All took the MCAT; 92% had baccalaureate degrees.

CHAPTER 11

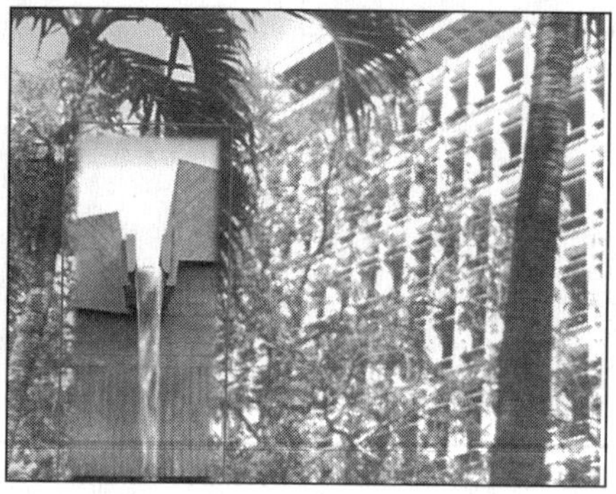

University of Puerto Rico School of Medicine

San Juan, Puerto Rico

Dr. Francisco Joglar, *Acting Dean*
Rita Aponte-Rodríguez, *Director of Admissions*
Zoraida Cruz, *Acting Director, Financial Aid Office*

ADDRESS INQUIRIES TO:

Central Admissions Office
School of Medicine
Medical Sciences Campus
University of Puerto Rico
P.O. Box 365067
San Juan, Puerto Rico 00936-5067
(787) 758-2525, Ext. 5213; 282-7117 (FAX)
Web Site: http://www.rcm.upr.clu.edu

MISSION STATEMENT

The mission of the University of Puerto Rico School of Medicine is to transmit, enrich, and increase knowledge in the medical sciences through teaching, research, and clinical service. The school is committed to achieve the ideals of personal and academic excellence through the interdisciplinary model for providing education and health services, especially at the primary level. An academic and institutional environment conducive to personal and professional development of both students and faculty will be provided by the school.

GENERAL INFORMATION

The University of Puerto Rico School of Medicine was established in 1949. The affiliated hospitals of the Puerto Rico Medical Center and the Hospital Consortium, which include the main health care facilities in other cities, serve the medical school for teaching purposes. On the Medical Sciences Campus, the School of Medicine works in close relation with the School of Dentistry, the College of Allied Health Professions, the Faculty of Biosocial Sciences and Graduate School of Public Health, the School of Nursing, and the School of Pharmacy, in an interdisciplinary team approach. Its location, adjacent to the University District Hospital, permits integration of basic and clinical departments and an improved utilization of all Medical Sciences Campus Resources.

CURRICULUM

The new curriculum has been designed to last four academic years. The first two years include the fundamentals of biological, behavioral, and clinical sciences and are mostly handled by the basic sciences departments. Part of the sophomore year is dedicated to pathophysiology, physical diagnosis, and basic clerkship, which are offered by a multidisciplinary faculty. Small-group sessions utilizing the problem-based learning approach are introduced at the beginning of the medical studies. Human behavior, environmental factors, and public health concepts are integrated into the curriculum. The third and fourth years are dedicated to required clinical experiences and elective courses. The use of diverse educational strategies, increased use of educational technology, and diversification of teaching exercises are emphasized. Through the Hispanic Center of Excellence, the curriculum has been focused toward community-oriented primary care exposure. Support services, counseling, tutorials, and other services are provided to students to assist in retention. Students are graded on a letter grade system during all four years.

REQUIREMENTS FOR ENTRANCE

Applicants are required to take the MCAT not later than August of the year before admission, and complete a minimum of 90 semester hours of accredited college work with no less than 2.50 general and science GPA, which must be completed no later than the academic year (not summer session) preceding admission. Since our curriculum is conducted in English and Spanish, demonstrated fluency in speaking, reading, and writing both languages is required. College work must include the following courses.

	Sem. hrs.
Biology	8
General chemistry (with lab)	8
Organic chemistry (with lab)	8
Physics (with lab)	8
English	12
Spanish	12
Behavioral and social sciences	12

(Course work must be in sociology, psychology, political sciences, economics, or anthropology.)

In addition to the above requirements, course work in biochemistry, anatomy, cell biology, liberal arts, and humanities are strongly recommended. Working knowledge in computers and its applications is required, given the integration of computer technology in the medical curriculum.

The School of Medicine accepts CLEP and advanced placement examinations toward the fulfillment of admission requirements if credits are offically granted and clearly indicated on the college transcript as having been accepted by that college.

Since the preclinical courses in the School of Medicine are largely scientific in nature, it is to the student's advantage to obtain a well-rounded undergraduate education.

SELECTION FACTORS

Since the University of Puerto Rico School of Medicine is a state-supported institution, strong first preference will be given to qualified applicants who are legal residents of Puerto Rico. Highly qualified non-Puerto Rico residents must demonstrate strong ties to Puerto Rico. To determine strong residential ties to Puerto Rico, the Admissions Committee will review the applicant's birthplace, legal residence at the time of application, high school attended, college attended, and parent's legal residence. Only those applicants who meet three out of the five categories demonstrate strong ties to Puerto Rico and will be forwarded secondary applications. Foreign national applicants with an established residence in Puerto Rico will be considered only if, at the time of application, they are either U.S. citizens or have been granted a permanent resident visa in the United States.

In selecting students the Admissions Committee considers the candidate's academic performance, MCAT scores, recommendations of instructors, attitudinal and other personality factors assessed in personal interviews, extracurricular activities, and any other pertinent information. Personal interviews are conducted only by invitation from the Admissions Committee to those students with high numerical ranks according to the admissions formula. Interviews are conducted only on the site of the medical school, or the affiliated hospitals at the Puerto Rico Medical Center. The admissions formula gives equal weight to academic indices and MCAT scores, with somewhat less weight given to ratings derived from evaluations by premedical committees and interviewers. Rejected applicants are given the opportunity to reapply for admission. Applicants, without exception, must submit all application material and supporting documents by December 1 of the year preceding the school year for which they request admission.

The School of Medicine has the policy of giving equal opportunity for education and training in the practice of the health professions without regard to race, creed, sex, national origin, age, or handicap

The school accepts transfer applications into the third-year class from residents of Puerto Rico who are presently enrolled and have satisfactorily completed the first two years of the medical curriculum at an LCME-accredited medical school. Promotion into the third year must be recommended by the original school. In addition to completing the same requirements for admissions into the first-year class, they must pass Step I of the USMLE. Deadline to submit application and supporting documents is May 1 of the same year of admission.

Accepted students for the 1998 class had the following credentials: *mean GPA,* 3.65 (range 2.98–4.00; 99 percent above 3.00); *mean science grade index,* 3.55 (range 2.85–4.00; 91 percent above 3.00); *mean and range MCAT scores, VR*-7 (4–11), *PS*-7 (5–12), *WS*-K/L (J–R), *BS*-8 (5–12); *sex,* 50 percent female; *residence,* 97 percent from Puerto Rico; *overall acceptance rate,* 970 applications were received, and 120 offers of acceptance were made to obtain a class of 115 freshmen.

FINANCIAL AID

Financial aid is available to students. Awards are made on the basis of confidential applications submitted by students. Financial need is the major criterion. Applicants who require scholarship assistance may make application in conjunction with the application for admission or before April 30. Financial need will not influence the selection process. Forms are available from the Financial Aid Office upon request. We do not offer financial assistance to foreign students.

Public Institution

APPLICATION AND ACCEPTANCE POLICIES FOR 2001–2002 FIRST-YEAR CLASS

School participates in AMCAS. See Chapter 6.

Filing of AMCAS application
- Earliest date: June 1, 2000
- Latest date: Dec. 1, 2000

School application fee to all applicants: $15
Oldest MCAT scores considered: 1997
Does not have Early Decision Program
Acceptance notice to regular applicants
- Earliest date: Dec. 2000
- Latest date: March 31, 2001

Applicant's response to acceptance offer
- Maximum time: 2 weeks

Requests for deferred entrance considered: Yes
Deposit to hold place in class (applied to tuition): $100, due with response to acceptance offer; nonrefundable
Estimated number of new entrants: 110
Starting date: Aug. 2001

TUITION AND STUDENT FEES PER YEAR FOR 1999–2000 FIRST-YEAR CLASS

Tuition
- Resident: $5,000
- Nonresident: $10,500; Pays according to a standardized fee scale (U.S. mainland and foreign residents)

Student fees: $901

INFORMATION ON 1999–2000 FIRST-YEAR CLASS

Number of	*In-State*	*Out-of-State*	*Total*
Applicants	361	532	893
Applicants Interviewed	146	0	146
New Entrants*	110	0	110

*All took the MCAT; 75% had baccalaureate degrees.

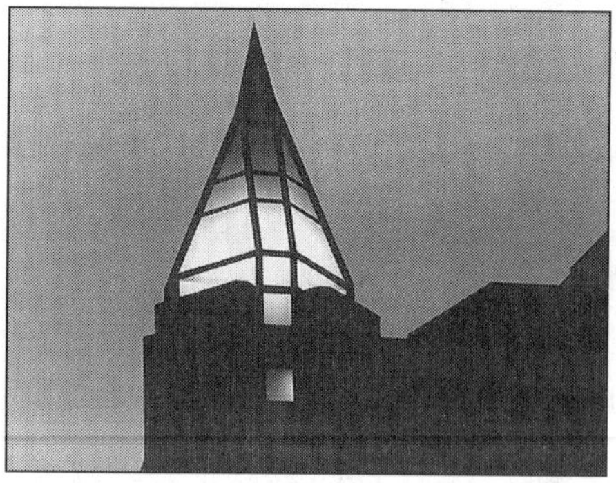

Brown University School of Medicine

Providence, Rhode Island

Dr. Donald J. Marsh, *Dean of Medicine and Biological Sciences*
Kathleen A. Baer, *Director of Admissions and Financial Aid*
Dr. Stephen R. Smith, *Associate Dean for Medical Education*

ADDRESS INQUIRIES TO:

Office of Admissions and Financial Aid
Brown University
School of Medicine
97 Waterman St., Box G-A212
Providence, Rhode Island 02912-9706
(401) 863-2149; 863-3801 (FAX)
E-mail: MedSchool_Admissions@brown.edu
Web Site: http://www.brown.edu

GENERAL INFORMATION

Important Note. *The Brown University program is an eight-year continuum of college and medical school (Program in Liberal Medical Education) that offers admission to high school seniors (see Chapter 10). However, limited spaces are available for admission into the first year of medical school. Please read carefully the information provided below regarding eligibility for admission before requesting an application.*

GENERAL INFORMATION

Brown University, founded in 1764, is the seventh oldest college in America and the third oldest in New England. In 1963 a Master of Medical Science Program, a six-year course of study emphasizing the basic sciences and encompassing the four years of premedical education and the first two years of medical school, was inaugurated. A program in medicine leading to the M.D. degree was accredited in 1975 as a four-year medical school. In 1981 the trustees of Dartmouth College and the Corporation of Brown University approved the Brown-Dartmouth Medical Program to which 15 medical students are admitted jointly. Students spend the first two years at Dartmouth Medical School and transfer to the Brown University School of Medicine for the last two years.

Entry into the first year of the Brown University School of Medicine is available only to individuals applying to the M.D.-Ph.D. program; to students enrolled in postbaccalaureate premedical study at Brown University, Bryn Mawr College, or Columbia University; to students enrolled in the Early Identification Program at Providence College, Tougaloo College, Rhode Island College, or the University of Rhode Island; and to undergraduate or graduate students at Brown University. Individuals who are ineligible to apply through these routes may apply to the Brown-Dartmouth Program and are encouraged to contact Dartmouth Medical School directly for further information. Students attending any school accredited by the Liaison Committee on Medical Education and Rhode Island residents attending foreign medical schools accredited by the W.H.O. may apply for advanced standing admission into the School of Medicine.

CURRICULUM

The School of Medicine is based on Brown's campus and in the university's affiliated hospitals (Bradley, Butler, Memorial, Miriam, Rhode Island (including Hasbro Children's Hospital), Women and Infants, and Veterans Administration hospitals).

The first year is devoted to courses in human morphology, mammalian physiology, human histology, social and behavioral sciences, medical microbiology, general pathology, molecular and regulatory biochemistry, human neurobiology, epidemiology, medical interviewing, and the brain and human behavior.

The second-year curriculum consists of pathophysiology, neurosciences, systemic pathology, organ-system pharmacology, neurologic pathophysiology, and introductory courses in psychiatry and clinical medicine, including physical diagnosis.

First- and second-year students also participate in the Affinity Group Program in which students are matched with physicians and other health care professionals in small mentoring groups around areas of common interest. Affinity Groups provide a format for early clinical experiences, community interactions, and the pursuit of creative opportunities.

Students in the third and fourth years are required to satisfactorily complete 48 weeks of clinical clerkships and 32 weeks of electives. The clinical clerkships include internal medicine (12 weeks), surgery (12 weeks), psychiatry (6 weeks), obstetrics and gynecology (6 weeks), pediatrics (6 weeks), family medicine (6 weeks), and community health, which is integrated into the clerkships in medicine and family medicine. Additional requirements include a four-week advanced clinical clerkship in medicine or pediatrics, an ambulatory longitudinal clerkship (one-half day per week for six months), and an eight-week selective clerkship.

The graduate programs offered to M.D.-Ph.D. candidates are artificial organs, biomaterials, and cellular technology; ecology and evolutionary biology; epidemiology; biostatistics and health services research, molecular biology, cell biology and biochemistry; molecular pharmacology and physiology; neuroscience; and pathobiology.

REQUIREMENTS FOR ENTRANCE

The MCAT is required only if the applicant is applying to the Brown-Dartmouth Program. Students admitted to the Brown University School of Medicine must attain competence in the sciences basic to medicine and sufficient to provide adequate preparation for medical school. Applicants are expected to demonstrate competence by successfully completing courses in the following areas of study:

	Semesters
Biology	2
Biochemistry	1
Calculus	1
Probability and statistics	1
General chemistry	2
Organic chemistry	1
Physics	2
Social and behavioral sciences	2

SELECTION FACTORS

Candidates are selected on the basis of academic achievement, faculty evaluations, evidence of maturity, motivation, leadership, integrity, and compassion. Candidates must also present a 3.0 minimum grade-point average (on a 4.0 scale). In addition, applicants must have completed requirements for the baccalaureate degree upon matriculation into the School of Medicine.

Applicants also must be capable of meeting the competency requirements expected of all graduates, with reasonable accommodation. These requirements are sent to applicants following their acceptance.

Applicants are assessed without regard to race, religion, national or ethnic origin, sexual preference, age, or physical handicap. Applications from minority groups and Rhode Island residents are especially encouraged.

FINANCIAL AID

The School of Medicine makes every effort to assist students in meeting the cost of their medical education through a combination of low-interest loans and scholarships. Approximately 68 percent of the students receive some type of financial assistance. Employment during the school year is discouraged. Financial aid may be awarded to foreign national students on an extremely limited basis. M.D.-Ph.D. students are eligible for a graduate fellowship (tuition and stipend) during the Ph.D. portion of their studies and a full tuition scholarship during the last two years of medical school following successful completion of Ph.D. work.

INFORMATION FOR MINORITY STUDENTS

Brown University particularly invites applications from individuals who are members of ethnic and racial groups traditionally underrepresented in American medicine. Established in 1981, the Office of Minority Affairs (OMA) has as its primary objective the recruitment, retention, and graduation of minority students. The OMA provides academic and personal counseling, workshops on test-taking approaches, information and guidance on special prizes and scholarship awards, and a program that links minority students with minority alumni/ae.

Private Institution

APPLICATION AND ACCEPTANCE POLICIES FOR 2001–2002 FIRST-YEAR CLASS

Filing of application
  Earliest date: July 15, 2000
  Latest date: March 1, 2001 (Nov. 15, 2000 for M.D.–Ph.D. applicants)
School application fee to all applicants: $65
Oldest MCAT scores considered: Not required
Does not have Early Decision Program
Acceptance notice to regular applicants
  Earliest date: Jan. 1, 2001
  Latest date: April 1, 2001
Applicant's response to acceptance offer
  Maximum time: 3 weeks
Requests for deferred entrance considered: Yes
Deposit to hold place in class: None
Estimated number of new entrants: 68
Starting date: Sept. 2001

TUITION AND STUDENT FEES PER YEAR FOR 1999–2000 FIRST-YEAR CLASS

Tuition: $27,704   Student fees: $1,323

INFORMATION ON 1999–2000 FIRST-YEAR CLASS

Number of	*In-State*	*Out-of-State*	*Total*
Applicants	56	1,970	2,026
Applicants Interviewed*	3	8	11
New Entrants†	9	56	65

*Interviews are required only for M.D.-Ph.D.

†All had baccalaureate degrees; 21% took the MCAT.

CHAPTER 11

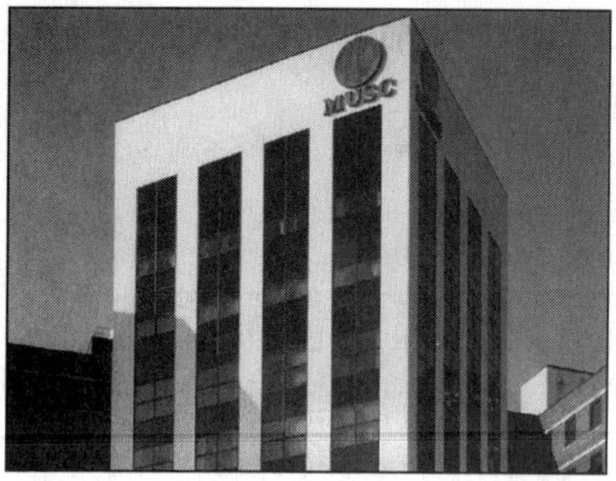

Medical University of South Carolina College of Medicine

Charleston, South Carolina

Dr. Layton McCurdy, *Dean*
Dr. Paul B. Underwood, *Assistant Dean for Admissions*
Wanda L. Taylor, *Director of Admissions*

ADDRESS INQUIRIES TO:

Office of Enrollment Services
Medical University of South Carolina
171 Ashley Avenue
Charleston, South Carolina 29425
(803) 792-3283; 792-4262 (FAX)
E-mail: taylorwl@musc.edu
Web Site: http://www2.musc.edu

MISSION STATEMENT

The College is committed to maintaining an educational environment for all students which prepares them for a career of excellence in the practice of medicine and service to their communities. It is concerned with ensuring optimal opportunities or all students, faculty, and administration, including all backgrounds and levels of diversity, to achieve full potential.

GENERAL INFORMATION

The College of Medicine of the Medical University of South Carolina (MUSC) was founded in Charleston in 1824 and is the South's oldest medical school. Its major clinical facilities comprise the MUSC Medical Center, which consists of the Medical University Hospital, the Children's Hospital, the Storm Eye Institute, the Psychiatric Institute, the Hollings Cancer Center, and the Gazes Cardiac Research Institute-Thurmond Biomedical Research Building. The adjacent Veterans Administration Hospital and Charleston Memorial Hospital, along with consortium and community hospitals in Greenville, Spartanburg, Columbia, and Florence, supply additional facilities for clinical teaching.

In addition to the classical basic science and clinical departments, there is a Department of Family Medicine, which conducts a model program in the clinical area.

CURRICULUM

The goal of the College of Medicine is to produce a caring and competent physician capable of choosing any postgraduate career. The curriculum during the first two years addresses four major objectives: provision of basic science concepts; acquisition of problem-solving strategies; development of skills which permit the performance of an adequate history and physical examination; and an introduction to the role of the physician in society. During these years emphasis is placed on small-group instruction. The curriculum was changed in fall 1999, to expand and improve opportunities for independent self-directed learning. Students are being exposed earlier to certain clinical skills and approaches.

The junior year consists of seven core clerkships. The clinical core consists of eight weeks each of internal medicine, obstetrics-gynecology, pediatrics, and surgery, as well as four weeks each of family medicine, psychiatry, and neurology. In addition, all students take a block of 40 hours of clinical nutrition. During these experiences, emphasis is placed on the development of clinical, interpersonal, and professional competence.

During the senior year, students take a minimum of seven 4-week rotations. The student is required to take a clinical externship (in general medicine, pediatrics, or surgery) and one month each of ambulatory surgery and internal medicine. The remaining four blocks are elective and, depending on previous academic performance, can be taken at approved sites throughout the state and country.

The two-year parallel curriculum or problem-based learning program is a method of teaching and learning that emphasizes reflective critical thinking and sound clinical reasoning. The content emphasis is on the basic sciences, as in the traditional curriculum; however, the methodology of learning is self-directed study with small-group interaction. Learning groups, composed of six students and two faculty members, are encouraged to use multiple learning resources—textbooks, journals, videotapes, computer databases, and other faculty members—to investigate learning issues. This program is open to all accepted applicants at the time of acceptance to the College of Medicine, and selection is made on a random basis. Currently, there are twenty-four students selected for the parallel curriculum each year.

The College of Graduate Studies and the College of Medicine offer a combined program leading to both the M.D. and Ph.D. degrees. The purpose of this combined program is to provide competence in medicine plus detailed knowledge and research training in one of the related sciences without sacrificing the customary requirements for either degree. A student interested in the combined program must apply simultaneously to the College of Medicine and the College of Graduate Studies.

REQUIREMENTS FOR ENTRANCE

The MCAT and a minimum of three years of college (90 semester hours) are required. Preference is given to applicants who have completed four years of college and earned a baccalaureate degree. Only those applicants with extremely unusual circumstances are admitted after 90 hours. There are no specific course requirements. Students are advised to construct courses of study that are intellectually interesting and challenging for them individually. Any education that engenders curiosity and enthusiasm for learning is desirable. Students who choose to major in a science should select a broad range of studies outside the sciences as well.

SELECTION FACTORS

Selection is based on a total evaluation of the student. Objectively derived data allow the College of Medicine to set a minimum level for academic performance, above which students can do the work of medical school without academic difficulty. These data are based on the cumulative GPA and total MCAT scores. Students who pass this academic level are invited for interviews. Acceptance into medical school from the selection pool is then based on evaluation of noncognitive traits and personal characteristics that are desirable in future physicians. These traits include emotional stability, integrity, reasoning skills, enthusiasm, brightness, and genuine concern for others. Nonresident applications are considered, but superior credentials are necessary for acceptance. Application through the Early Decision Program is encouraged for those applicants who have the academic credentials of the preceding entering medical class.

South Carolina residency is a primary admission consideration. Nonresident applicants are considered; however, due to limited facilities, few are selected and superior credentials are necessary for acceptance. Foreign students without a South Carolina permanent residence visa are unable to be considered.

FINANCIAL AID

Scholarship funds, including some state scholarships, are available to entering freshmen. The James B. Edwards Scholars Program provides full tuition, fees, and living expenses for the entire medical education of a few select entering freshmen. Loan programs are also available.

INFORMATION FOR MINORITY STUDENTS

Minority students are strongly encouraged to apply, and there is an active recruitment program in place. The Postbaccalaureate Reapplication Education Program (PREP) is an integrative, individually tailored course of undergraduate study prescribed for underprepared but promising South Carolina students who seek admission to MUSC. The full-time, 12-month curriculum may include undergraduate courses in the areas of biology, physics, chemistry, and mathematics, a learning strategies course, human gross anatomy, and a course in critical thinking/reasoning skills. Minority applicants who apply to the College of Medicine, but do not meet the minimum academic requirements for interview, automatically will be considered for the PREP. Three students are usually chosen for PREP each year.

The Office of Diversity provides counseling and support services; academic assistance is provided to students through tutorial programs, test-taking skills, training, and the like.

TRANSFER

Because of limited space, the College of Medicine does not accept transfer students from U.S. or foreign medical schools.

Public Institution

APPLICATION AND ACCEPTANCE POLICIES FOR 2001–2002 FIRST-YEAR CLASS

School participates in AMCAS. See Chapter 6.

Filing of AMCAS application
Earliest date: June 1, 2000
Latest date: Dec. 1, 2000
School application fee to all applicants: $55
Oldest MCAT scores considered: 1995
Does have Early Decision Program (EDP)
For South Carolina residents only.
EDP application period: June 1–Aug. 2000
EDP applicants notified by: Oct. 1, 2000
Acceptance notice to regular applicants
Earliest date: Oct. 15, 2000
Latest date: March 15, 2001 or until class is filled
Applicant's response to acceptance offer
Maximum time: 2 weeks
Requests for deferred entrance considered: Yes
Deposit to hold place in class: $160, due with response to acceptance offer
Deposit refundable prior to: May 15, 2001
Estimated number of new entrants: 135 (17 EDP)
Starting date: Aug. 22, 2001

TUITION AND STUDENT FEES PER YEAR FOR 1999–2000 FIRST-YEAR CLASS

Tuition	Student fees:
Resident: $3,104	Resident: $6,444
Nonresident: $9,974	Nonresident: $16,426

INFORMATION ON 1999–2000 FIRST-YEAR CLASS

Number of	*In-State*	*Out-of-State*	*Total*
Applicants	498	1,555	2,053
Applicants Interviewed	315	33	348
New Entrants*	136	3	139†

*All had baccalaureate degrees; 99% took the MCAT (students entering through the Early Assurance Program are not required to take the MCAT).

† Includes 4 M.D.-Ph.D. students.

CHAPTER 11

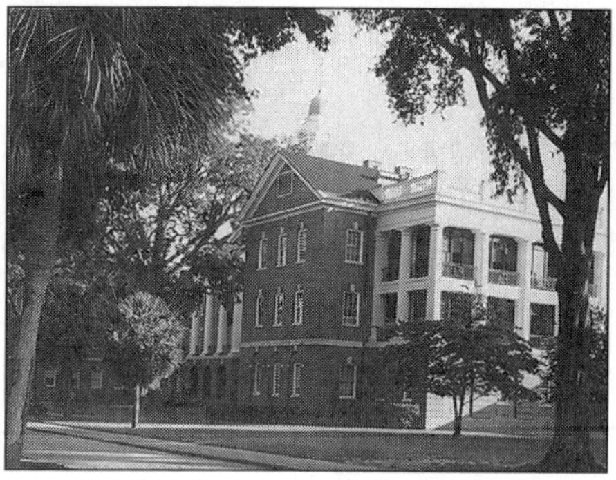

University of South Carolina School of Medicine

Columbia, South Carolina

Dr. Larry R. Faulkner, *Vice President for Medical Affairs and Dean*
Dr. Robert F. Sabalis, *Associate Dean for Medical Education and Academic Affairs*
Peggy Lynch, *Assistant Director of Student Services/Financial Aid*

ADDRESS INQUIRIES TO:

Associate Dean for Medical Education and Academic Affairs
University of South Carolina
School of Medicine
Columbia, South Carolina 29208
(803) 733-3325; 733-3328 (FAX)
Web Site: http://www.med.sc.edu

MISSION STATEMENT

The mission of the University of South Carolina School of Medicine is to improve the health of the people of the state of South Carolina through the development and implementation of programs for medical education, research, and the delivery of health care. Programs will be developed in collaboration with affiliated institutions, and allocation of resources will be based upon the physician manpower and health care needs of South Carolina, the effectiveness and efficiency of specific programs, and the accreditation requirements of all appropriate organizations. Medical education and graduate education at all levels are conducted in a highly personal atmosphere that emphasizes a balance among scientific disciplines, humanistic concerns, and societal needs.

GENERAL INFORMATION

The University of South Carolina School of Medicine was established in 1974 by the South Carolina General Assembly in conjunction with the Veterans Administration. The charter class matriculated in 1977 and graduated in 1981. Initially housed on the main campus of the University of South Carolina, the School of Medicine moved its administrative and faculty offices, teaching and research laboratories, and first- and second-year educational facilities in 1983 to completely renovated historic buildings on a 93-acre campus adjacent to the Dorn Veterans Hospital. The 90,000-volume medical library is accessible to medical students on a 24-hour-a-day basis.

Clinical instruction takes place in a variety of area hospitals that provide an ample number of teaching beds and extensive outpatient facilities. These include the 649-bed Palmetto Richland Memorial Hospital, the major regional medical center; the 270-bed William S. Hall Psychiatric Institute, the teaching and research division of the South Carolina Department of Mental Health; the 447-bed Dorn Veterans Affairs Medical Center; and the 60-bed Moncrief Army Hospital, a short-term general hospital located at Fort Jackson, the regional army training center. In addition, core clinical training can be pursued at the Greenville Memorial Hospital, while elective opportunities are available throughout South Carolina at community hospitals affiliated with the Area Health Education Consortium (AHEC), at other medical centers in the United States, and abroad.

CURRICULUM

The School of Medicine offers a program of study designed to provide education and training in the art and science of medicine and to prepare students for a wide variety of medical career choices. Each of the first two years of the regular four-year medical program consists of two academic semesters composed of both basic science and clinically relevant course work in which students are exposed to patients in various inpatient, outpatient, community, and rural settings. The correlation between basic and clinical science information in the first two years is emphasized by means of an interdisciplinary, four-semester Introduction to Clinical Practice course continuum.

The third year consists of required clinical clerkships in medicine, surgery, pediatrics, obstetrics-gynecology, family medicine, and psychiatry. The fourth year is devoted to advanced clinical work, including 20 weeks each of required and elective rotations, during which students have the opportunity to strengthen their clinical skills and pursue individual academic interests and career goals in preparation for the lifelong study of medicine.

A six- to seven-year combined M.D.-Ph.D. program in biomedical sciences is available to students interested in careers in academic medicine and medical research. A five-year combined M.D.-M.P.H. program is also available.

REQUIREMENTS FOR ENTRANCE

The MCAT and the equivalent of three years of undergraduate work are required. Strong preference is given to those applicants who will have earned their baccalaureate degrees prior to matriculation. Specific minimum course work requirements are:

	Sem. hrs.
General biology or zoology (with lab)	8
Inorganic chemistry (with lab)	8
Organic chemistry (with lab)	8

General physics (with lab) 8
College mathematics 6
A minimum of college algebra is required; calculus is recommended.
English composition and literature. 6

The science and mathematics requirements must be acceptable for continued study by departmental majors.

With the exception of these specific courses, applicants are encouraged to pursue their personal educational interests without regard to any specific field of study. Quality of course work rather than the field in which it is taken is the most important consideration.

Applicants are required to take the MCAT by the fall of the year of application. Applicants enrolled in advanced degree programs must complete their degrees prior to matriculation.

SELECTION FACTORS

The selection process involves the comparative evaluation and review of all available application data, including MCAT scores, undergraduate academic performance, comments contained in letters of evaluation, and the results of personal interviews with members of the Admissions Committee. The opportunity for admission is greatest for legal residents of South Carolina. Competitive nonresidents must have superior credentials. The ultimate selection of a student is based upon a total and comparative appraisal of the applicant's suitability for the successful practice of medicine.

The AMCAS application is used for preliminary screening. After this initial review, the Admissions Committee may request the applicant to submit additional material for the final application, such as letters of evaluation, a personal essay, and a photograph, as well as extend an invitation for personal interviews at the medical campus in Columbia. Each applicant is evaluated on the basis of individual qualifications without regard to age, race, creed, national origin, sex, or handicap.

The School of Medicine can accept an application for transfer from any student who is currently enrolled, and in good standing, in a medical school accredited by the Liaison Committee on Medical Education and who meets the prerequisite requirements.

FINANCIAL AID

The School of Medicine participates in all federally funded loan and scholarship programs. Additionally, there is a School of Medicine-sponsored low-interest loan program available to students with proven need. Over 86 percent of enrolled students receive financial assistance in the form of scholarships, loans, and/or grants. The Office of Student Services makes every effort to provide information and assistance to help students meet their financial obligations. Ultimate responsibility for arranging the financing of his/her medical education must rest with the student. Students seeking part-time employment during medical school should have the prior approval of the director of student services.

INFORMATION FOR MINORITY STUDENTS

The School of Medicine actively encourages applications from members of groups underrepresented in the medical profession. Minority faculty members are represented on the Admissions Committee. For additional information, contact the assistant dean for minority affairs at (803) 733-3319.

Public Institution

APPLICATION AND ACCEPTANCE POLICIES FOR 2001–2002 FIRST-YEAR CLASS

School participates in AMCAS. See Chapter 6.

Filing of AMCAS application
Earliest date: June 1, 2000
Latest date: Dec. 1, 2000
School application fee after screening: $45
Oldest MCAT scores considered: 1998
Does have Early Decision Program (EDP)
EDP application period: June 1–Aug. 1, 2000
EDP applicants notified by: Oct. 1, 2000
Acceptance notice to regular applicants
Earliest date: Oct. 15, 2000
Latest date: Until class is filled
Applicant's response to acceptance offer
Maximum time: 2 weeks
Requests for deferred entrance considered: Yes
Deposit to hold place in class (applied to tuition):
$100, due with response to acceptance offer
Deposit refundable prior to: May 15, 2001
Estimated number of new entrants: 75 (10 EDP)
Starting date: Aug. 2001

TUITION AND STUDENT FEES PER YEAR FOR 1999–2000 FIRST-YEAR CLASS

Tuition
Resident: $8,572
Nonresident: $24,836

Student fees: $45

INFORMATION ON 1999–2000 FIRST-YEAR CLASS

Number of	*In-State*	*Out-of-State*	*Total*
Applicants	435	869	1,304
Applicants Interviewed	267	53	320
New Entrants*	69	5	74

*All took the MCAT and had baccalaureate degrees.

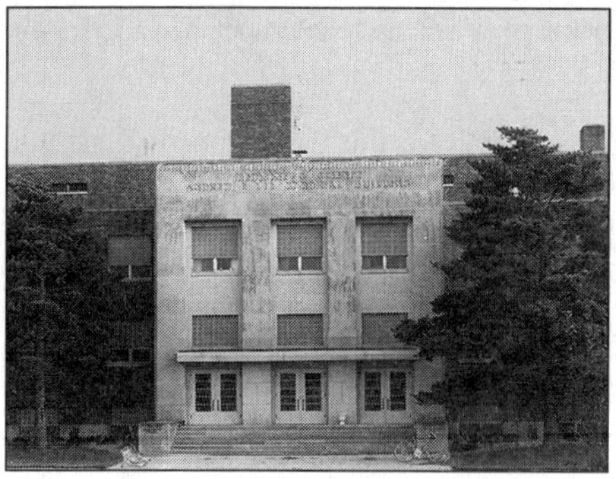

University of South Dakota School of Medicine

Vermillion, South Dakota

Dr. Robert C. Talley, *Dean*
Dr. Paul C. Bunger, *Dean, Medical Student Affairs*
Carol Hemmingson, *Financial Aid Assistant*

ADDRESS INQUIRIES TO:

Medical School Admissions
University of South Dakota
School of Medicine
414 East Clark Street
Vermillion, South Dakota 57069
(605) 677-6886; 677-5109 (FAX)
E-mail: usdsmsa@usd.edu
Web Site: http://www.usd.edu/med/md

MISSION STATEMENT

The mission of the University of South Dakota School of Medicine is to provide the opportunity for South Dakota residents to receive a quality, broad-based medical education with an emphasis on family practice. The curriculum is to be established to encourage graduates to serve people living in medically underserved areas of South Dakota and to require excellence in the basic sciences and in all clinical disciplines. The School of Medicine is to provide to its students and to the people of South Dakota excellence in education, research, and service. To these ends, the school provides educational pathways leading to the Doctor of Medicine and the Doctor of Philosophy degrees. Quality health care for the people of South Dakota is addressed by undergraduate, graduate, and continuing education programs, as well as by basic and applied medical research. The School of Medicine serves as a technical resource in the development of health care policy in the state and provides extension and research initiatives to improve the health care of the citizens of South Dakota.

GENERAL INFORMATION

The School of Medicine was established in 1907 as a two-year school for the basic medical sciences and has been in continuous operation since that time. The school was physically expanded in 1960 and again in 1969 and houses modern teaching facilities and research laboratories.

In 1974, a degree-granting program began with the first third-year class beginning in 1975 at two clinical training sites, one in Yankton and one in Sioux Falls. Both sites are within 60 minutes of Vermillion. A West River clinical training site in Rapid City has been added. The primary objective of the medical school is the training of family practice physicians for South Dakota.

In 1994, the School of Medicine opened the USDSM Health Science Center on the Sioux Falls campus. The Health Science Center houses the School of Medicine's clinical departments and administrative offices, provides teaching space for medical students and other health professions students, and houses the South Dakota Health Research Foundation's Cardiovascular Research Institute. This Institute provides quality laboratory research experience for faculty and students. In 1998, the Karl and Mary Jo Wegner Health Science Information Center was opened as a regional biomedical information library.

CURRICULUM

A thorough knowledge of the basic medical sciences is emphasized during the first two years. An understanding of these basic concepts provides fundamental knowledge of the human body and hence a rational approach to the diagnosis and treatment of disease. Students are also introduced to patients in the affiliated hospitals. At the end of year two, each student spends four weeks with a physician in a primary care setting in a South Dakota community. For the Sioux Falls and West River sites, the third year is hospital based and consists of six major clerkships: Family Medicine, Internal Medicine, Pediatrics, Obstetrics/Gynecology, Psychiatry, and Surgery. Each site also has significant ambulatory clinic experience throughout the year. For the Yankton site, the third year is a clinic based program with students rotating through all six of the clerkships throughout the year and following patients during hospitalizations. During year four, students have required clerkships in Rural Family Medicine, Emergency Medicine, and Surgical subspecialties as well as having elective clerkships available both within and outside South Dakota. Primary care medicine is emphasized throughout all four years.

Student progress is recorded each semester using the conventional letter grading system (A, B, C, D, F). Students must pass both Step 1 and Step 2 of the USMLE.

REQUIREMENTS FOR ENTRANCE

The MCAT and at least three years of college are required. The baccalaureate degree is very desirable. Each applicant must have completed at least 64 semester hours from an accredited college to be considered for admission and have completed at least 90 semester hours to matriculate. At matriculation, a baccalaureate degree from an accredited undergraduate institution is preferred. The following courses are required, although specific courses may be waived under certain conditions:

	Years
General biology or zoology (with lab)	1
General chemistry (with lab)	1
Organic chemistry (with lab) or second-semester biochemistry	1
General physics (with lab)	1
College mathematics	1

Analytical geometry and calculus are preferred.

All science courses should involve extensive lab work. Chemistry courses should include qualitative analysis and the study of aliphatic and aromatic compounds.

Additional courses in genetics, cell biology, statistics, behavioral sciences, and computer science are recommended.

All required courses should be the same courses taken by majors in each area. Applicants are encouraged to arrange their premedical studies around an undergraduate major. Students are encouraged to obtain a broad background in the natural and social sciences and in the humanities, and they should develop good oral and written communication skills. In the case of courses waived by examination or by advanced placement, it is expected that students will enroll in advanced courses that would be more stimulating and challenging. The School of Medicine does not consider CLEP or AP courses to be sufficient to fulfill the premedicine requirements.

The MCAT is required and must be taken no later than the fall of the year of application. No application is reviewed until the AMCAS application, letters of recommendation, and supplementary application have been received.

SELECTION FACTORS

Applicants are chosen on the basis of intellect, character, and motivation. Information about the applicant considered by the Committee on Admissions includes: academic achievement as indicated by the student's scholastic records; retentiveness and ability to perform under pressure as reflected by MCAT scores; curiosity, learning habits, and fitness for a career in medicine as viewed by the applicant's former instructors; and assessments of personal factors of the applicant as determined by interviews conducted by the Admissions Committee. Applicants are invited to participate in required personal interviews with members of the Admissions Committee. All interviews are conducted at the office or clinic of the interviewer.

Accepted applicants for the 1999 entering class had the following credentials: *science GPA,* 3.61; *nonscience GPA,* 3.72; *total/overall GPA,* 3.65; *gender,* 42 percent women; *undergraduate major,* 90 percent in science and 10 percent in nonscience. *MCAT scores* (mean): *VR*-9.1; *PS*-8.7; *BS*-9.1.

The school does not discriminate on the basis of race, gender, creed, national origin, age, or disability. Priority for secondary applications is shown to legal residents of South Dakota, nonresidents with strong ties to South Dakota, and Native Americans, affiliated with federally recognized tribes in the region. The School of Medicine does not participate in an Early Assurance Program. An Alumni Student Scholars Program (ASSP) offers a limited number of provisional acceptances to high school seniors who meet strict criteria.

The School of Medicine will consider applications for transfer only into Year 2 or Year 3 and only from students who are currently in good standing at an LCME-accredited medical school. Transfer opportunities are very limited, and priority is given to South Dakota residents.

FINANCIAL AID

Economic status plays no role in the admissions process. Low-interest loans are available to students on the basis of demonstrated financial need. Applications from first-year medical students for this financial aid are considered only after fall classes begin. Students are discouraged from seeking outside employment during academic periods. Approximately 93 percent of the student body receive financial aid.

Public Institution

APPLICATION AND ACCEPTANCE POLICIES FOR 2001–2002 FIRST-YEAR CLASS

School participates in AMCAS. See Chapter 6.

Filing of AMCAS application
Earliest date: June 1, 2000
Latest date: Nov. 15, 2000
School application fee after screening: $15
Oldest MCAT scores considered: 1997
Does not have Early Decision Program
Acceptance notice to regular applicants
Earliest date: Dec. 15, 2000
Latest date: Until class is filled
Applicant's response to acceptance offer
Maximum time: 2 weeks
Requests for deferred entrance considered: Yes
Deposit to hold place in class (applied to tuition): $100, due with response to acceptance offer
Deposit refundable prior to: June 1, 2001
Estimated number of new entrants: 50
Starting date: Aug. 2001

TUITION AND STUDENT FEES PER YEAR FOR 1999–2000 FIRST-YEAR CLASS

Tuition
Resident: $10,125
Nonresident: $24,254

Student fees: $2,415

INFORMATION ON 1999–2000 FIRST-YEAR CLASS

Number of	*In-State*	*Out-of-State*	*Total*
Applicants	124	519	643
Applicants Interviewed	124	25	149
New Entrants*	44	6	50†

* 94% took the MCAT and had baccalaureate degrees.
†3 students admitted through ASSP did not take MCAT.

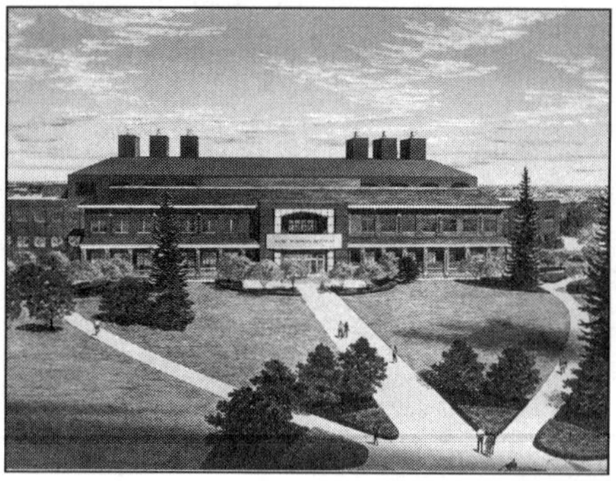

East Tennessee State University James H. Quillen College of Medicine

Johnson City, Tennessee

Dr. Ronald D. Franks, *Dean of Medicine and Vice President for Health Affairs*
Edwin D.Taylor, *Assistant Dean for Admissions and Records*
Ruth Angle, *Assistant Director for Financial Aid*

ADDRESS INQUIRIES TO:

Assistant Dean for Admissions and Records
East Tennessee State University
James H. Quillen College of Medicine
P.O. Box 70580
Johnson City, Tennessee 37614-0580
(423) 439-4753; 439-8206 (FAX)
E-mail: sacom@etsu.edu
Web Site: http://qcom.etsu.edu

MISSION STATEMENT

To educate students to become responsible, enlightened, and productive citizens; conduct scholarship that improves the human condition; serve business, education, government, health care systems, and community; and enhance the cultural environment of the region.

To provide primary care physicians and medical care for the people in the surrounding region.

GENERAL INFORMATION

The ETSU College of Medicine opened its doors to its first class of 24 students in 1978. Emphasizing primary care medicine, the medical school has continued to develop, improve, and expand each year.

The school is located in Tennessee's fourth largest metropolitan area (population 1.2 million) and on the campus of the state's fourth largest university (enrollment 12,000 plus). It is supported by modern and convenient medical centers and clinics throughout the Tri-Cities, as well as hospitals and clinics located in small, rural communities like Rogersville and Mountain City. To enhance training in primary care medicine, ETSU successfully competed for and received a sizable grant from the W.K. Kellogg Foundation under their Community Partnership Program. This provided the opportunity to plan and execute an innovative interdisciplinary curriculum for training primary care physicians—the Rural Primary Care Track.

The school enrolls one class of 60 new students in August of each year. Residency training programs are available in family medicine, internal medicine, surgery, psychiatry, pediatrics, pathology, and Ob-Gyn. Accelerated residency training programs in family medicine and internal medicine are also available.

CURRICULUM

The Quillen College of Medicine offers a semitraditional four-year medical program with the basic sciences being taught the first two years and intensive clinical application occurring throughout the last two years. Our curriculum is under constant review and modified as needed to keep pace with the rapid and constant changes in medicine. The Rural Primary Care Track was designed to promote exposure to and training in rural locations and leads to an unrestricted M.D. degree. Over 60 percent of Quillen College of Medicine graduates have initially chosen residency training in primary care.

The curriculum includes a wide range of well-presented educational experiences, varied patient populations and hospitals, a small class size, and a highly diversified, caring faculty. Patient contact comes early in the curriculum and continues throughout. Flexibility is attained by allowing students to decelerate a portion of the curriculum for elective courses including research and advanced clinical studies.

Student input is a key component in curricular change, along with the rapidly changing body of knowledge and the needs of the profession. The goals of the curriculum are to prepare students to be well grounded in the sciences and art of medicine, capable practitioners of their profession, and self-directed, lifelong learners.

Computers are an essential part of the learning process. Due to their importance, a basic working knowledge of computers will prove very beneficial to the student while at the Quillen College of Medicine. The campus provides the largest open-access computer lab in the Tennessee Board of Regents System.

REQUIREMENTS FOR ENTRANCE

The MCAT and a minimum of 90 semester hours of credit, applicable toward a B.A. or B.S. degree at a regionally accredited institution, make up the minimum requirement, although most selected students complete the entire four years. Specific required courses are:

	Sem. hrs.
Biology (with lab)	8
General or inorganic chemistry (with lab)	8
Organic chemistry (with lab)	8
Physics (with lab)	8
Communications skills courses	9

Applicants are urged to follow their personal interests in developing their premedical courses of study with the exception of the courses noted above. Preference is not given to any undergraduate major, but a broadly based education that prepares the student to be a self-directed, lifelong learner is suggested. CLEP credit in any of the required premedical courses is acceptable, provided that one or more advanced courses in the same area are successfully completed later.

The acquisition of important skills is further suggested, such as the ability to read with speed, comprehension, and retention; the ability to understand concepts and draw logical conclusions; the ability to adapt; the ability to communicate effectively; and the ability to apply knowledge effectively.

Most courses and clerkships are graded on the standard A, B, C system with P/F grades used where appropriate.

Flexibility in the curriculum is allowed for those with research interest or those seeking the masters or Ph.D. in biomedical science or other programs.

SELECTION FACTORS

Admission to the College of Medicine is based upon a competitive selection process involving those applicants who meet the minimum requirements for admissions consideration. The responsibility of the Admissions Committee is to select those students who give the promise of being not merely satisfactory medical students but also capable, responsible physicians of high ethical standards. The Admissions Committee screens applicants on the basis of academic achievement, MCAT scores, letters of recommendation, pertinent extracurricular research and work experiences, and evidence of nonscholastic accomplishments.

After a general screening, the Admissions Committee may request supplementary information and a personal interview with the applicant. Interviews are held only on the campus and are at the applicant's expense.

Admission preferences are for residents of the state of Tennessee who are U.S. citizens, veterans of U.S. military service, and students with baccalaureate degrees prior to enrollment. Marginally qualified nonresidents should not apply.

Some characteristics of the students accepted for the 1999 entering class were: *mean GPA,* 3.5; *mean MCAT score,* (*VR*–9.6, *PS*–8.9, *BI*–9.3); *sex,* 53 percent women; *minorities,* 18 percent.

FINANCIAL AID

The need for student financial assistance is not a consideration in the selection process. Scholarships, grants, and loans are available for students who demonstrate need as defined by a federal needs analysis and who meet the specific criteria set forth by the various agencies.

Further information may be obtained by writing directly to the medical school director for financial aid. Practice-related scholarships may be available through the Financial Aid Office.

INFORMATION FOR MINORITY STUDENTS

The College of Medicine actively seeks applicants of both sexes and members of minority groups. A limited number of state grants are available for black matriculants who are state residents. Support services are available to matriculants to assist in the timely completion of the medical curriculum. ETSU does not discriminate on the basis of race, sex, creed, national origin, age, or disability. The university is an equal opportunity/affirmative action employer.

Public Institution

APPLICATION AND ACCEPTANCE POLICIES FOR 2001–2002 FIRST-YEAR CLASS

School participates in AMCAS. See Chapter 6.

Filing of AMCAS application
- Earliest date: June 1, 2000
- Latest date: Dec. 1, 2000

School application fee after screening: $25
Oldest MCAT scores considered: 1998
Does have Early Decision Program (EDP)
- EDP application period: June 1–Aug. 1, 2000
- EDP applicants notified by: Oct. 1, 2000

Acceptance notice to regular applicants
- Earliest date: Oct. 15, 2000
- Latest date: Until class is filled

Applicant's response to acceptance offer
- Maximum time: 14 days

Requests for deferred entrance considered: Yes
Deposit to hold place in class (applied to tuition): $100, due with response to acceptance offer
Deposit refundable prior to: May 15, 2001
Estimated number of new entrants: 60 (6 EDP)
Starting date: Aug. 2001

TUITION AND STUDENT FEES PER YEAR FOR 1999–2000 FIRST-YEAR CLASS

Tuition
- Resident: $10,342
- Nonresident: $21,080

Student fees (include microscope rental): $782

INFORMATION ON 1999–2000 FIRST-YEAR CLASS

Number of	*In-State*	*Out-of-State*	*Total*
Applicants	569	895	1,464
Applicants Interviewed	192	72	264
New Entrants*	52	8	60

*All took the MCAT; 97% had baccalaureate degrees.

CHAPTER 11

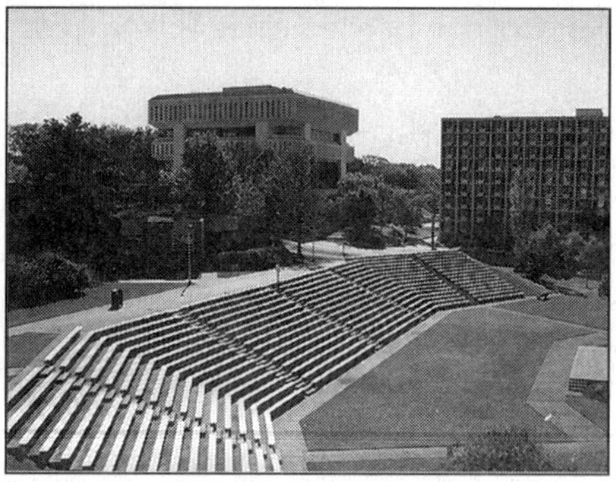

Meharry Medical College School of Medicine

Nashville, Tennessee

Dr. A. Cherrie Epps, *Dean*
Allen D. Mosley, *Director, Admissions and Records*
Vickie L. Johnson, *Director, Student Financial Aid*

ADDRESS INQUIRIES TO:

Director, Admissions and Records
Meharry Medical College
1005 D. B. Todd Boulevard
Nashville, Tennessee 37208
(615) 327-6223; 327-6228 (FAX)
Web Site: http://www.mmc.edu

GENERAL INFORMATION

In October 1876, Meharry Medical College was founded and established as the Meharry Medical Department of Central Tennessee College by the Freedmen's Aid Society of the Methodist Episcopal Church. Meharry's inception was part of the society's continuing effort to educate freed slaves and to provide health care services for the poor and underserved. Today, the School of Medicine continues to provide excellent educational opportunities to promising African Americans and other ethnic minority students.

Clinical teaching facilities include the Metropolitan Nashville General Hospital, York Veterans Administration Medical Center, Blanchfield Community Hospital, and the Elam Community Mental Health Center. In addition, clinical instruction is carried out at the Murfreesboro Veterans Administration hospital and a number of affiliated hospitals and clinics.

The provision of primary care, particularly in medically underserved areas, is a special emphasis, as is biomedical research into areas of concern to underserved populations.

CURRICULUM

There are two programs leading to the M.D. degree, a traditional four-year program, and a five-year program. Both programs are divided into the preclinical and clinical years.

The preclinical years begin with gross anatomy, microanatomy, neuroscience, biochemistry, introduction to clinical medicine I, and physiology during the freshman year; they conclude with behavioral sciences, microbiology, pharmacology, pathology, introduction to clinical medicine II (includes pathophysiology, clinical correlations, and physical diagnosis), and medical genetics during the sophomore year.

The five-year curricular program differs from the four-year program in that the freshman year is split into two segments, which span a two-year period. The first segment (Freshman I) consists of a summer prematriculation program known as the Mini Academic Program for Success (MAPS), which prepares students for the rigors of medical school and provides an introduction to freshman course work. This is followed in the fall and spring semesters by gross anatomy, microanatomy, neuroscience, and introduction to clinical medicine. The Freshman II segment consists of biochemistry, introduction to clinical medicine, and physiology. The sophomore year is the same as that of the four-year program.

The clinical years consist of three 4-week blocks of family medicine, preventative medicine, and psychiatry; three 8-week blocks of obstetrics and gynecology, pediatrics, and surgery; and one 12-week block of internal medicine during the junior year that spans 48 weeks. The 32-week senior year consists of five 4-week blocks of surgery, psychiatry, internal medicine, Area Health Education Center exposure (ambulatory rotation, served in an urban or rural underserved area), and radiology; and three 4-week blocks of guided electives.

Internal and external examinations are used in the assessment of student performance in addition to standardized patients. Passage of USMLE Steps 1 and 2 is required for graduation. A letter grading system (A, B, C, F) is used in all segments of the curriculum to report student achievement.

REQUIREMENTS FOR ENTRANCE

The MCAT is required. The baccalaureate degree is desirable; however, three years of college work is acceptable. Premedical work must include:

	Sem./Qtr. hrs
General biology or zoology (with lab)	8/12
General chemistry (with lab)	8/12
Organic chemistry (with lab)	8/12
General physics (with lab)	8/12
English (composition and literature)	6/9

All premedical education must be taken at an approved college in the United States, including the courses listed as requirements for admission.

Applicants are urged to take the MCAT in the spring of the year of application to permit earlier consideration of their applications.

SELECTION FACTORS

Applicants are selected on a competitive basis with regard to cognitive and noncognitive skills that denote probable success in medical school. Performance in the basic science prerequisite subjects (general biology, inorganic chemistry, organic chemistry, and physics) and MCAT scores form the basis for screening for the interview process in which the noncognitive aspects of the applicant are assessed. Meharry accepts students from all parts of the country, with preferential consideration given to equally qualified applicants from states that contract to subsidize the education of their citizens at Meharry. While special empathy is held for minority and disadvantaged applicants of all origins, Meharry Medical College seeks to attract a wide demographic, cultural, and educational population to reflect the caliber of social interchange in which the eventual practice of medicine will occur.

Early Decision Program applicants must have their complete application on file by August 1 for consideration.

Meharry Medical College does not discriminate on the basis of race, sex, creed, national origin, age, or handicap.

FINANCIAL AID

Financial aid awards are based on analyses of student needs and academic achievement. The limited financial aid program includes scholarships, grants-in-aid, loans, and fellowships.

Because of fluctuation in federal and private support for financial aid programs, the types and amounts of awards are revised and adjusted on a continuing basis. Therefore, it is necessary for applicants to plan their financial program as carefully as their academic program.

INFORMATION FOR MINORITY STUDENTS

For over 120 years, Meharry has produced a large percentage of the minority health professionals in the United States and abroad. Of the 1999 entering class, 64 percent were women and 78 percent were minority students.

Private Institution

APPLICATION AND ACCEPTANCE POLICIES FOR 2001–2002 FIRST-YEAR CLASS

School participates in AMCAS. See Chapter 6.

Filing of AMCAS application
- Earliest date: June 1, 2000
- Latest date: Dec. 15, 2000

School application fee after screening: $45
Oldest MCAT scores considered: 1998
Does have Early Decision Program (EDP)
- EDP application period: June 1–Aug. 1, 2000
- EDP applicants notified by: Oct. 1, 2000

Acceptance notice to regular applicants
- Earliest date: Oct. 15, 2000
- Latest date: Until class is filled

Applicant's response to acceptance offer
- Maximum time: 3 weeks

Requests for deferred entrance considered: Yes
Deposit to hold place in class (applied to tuition): $300, due with response to acceptance offer; nonrefundable
Estimated number of new entrants: 80 (0 EDP)
Starting date: June 2001

TUITION AND STUDENT FEES PER YEAR FOR 1999–2000 FIRST-YEAR CLASS

Tuition: $21,824 Student fees: $3,998

INFORMATION ON 1999–2000 FIRST-YEAR CLASS

Number of	*In-State*	*Out-of-State*	*Total*
Applicants	221	4,117	4,338
Applicants Interviewed	58	574	632
New Entrants*	18	62	80

*All took the MCAT; 98% had baccalaureate degrees.

CHAPTER 11

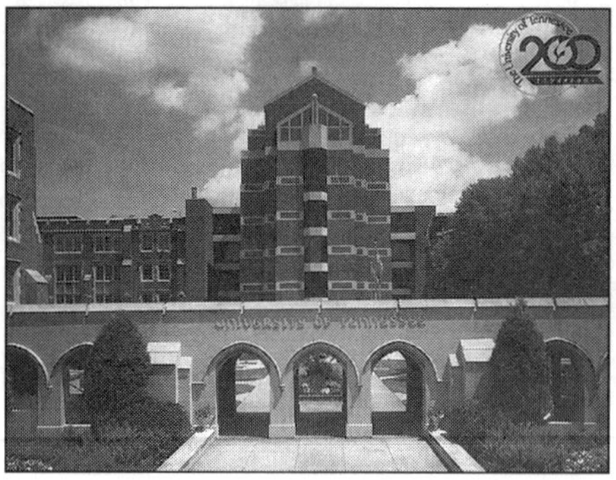

University of Tennessee, Memphis College of Medicine

Memphis, Tennessee

Dr. Henry G. Herrod, *Dean*
Dr. Hershel P. Wall, *Associate Dean for Admissions and Student Affairs*
E. Nelson Strother, Jr., *Assistant Dean for Admissions and Student Affairs*

ADDRESS INQUIRIES TO:

University of Tennessee, Memphis
College of Medicine
790 Madison Avenue
Memphis, Tennessee 38163-2166
(901) 448-5559; 448-1740 (FAX)
Web Site: http://www.utmem.edu/medicine

GENERAL INFORMATION

Founded in 1851, the College of Medicine, the colleges of dentistry, pharmacy, nursing, allied health, and the College of Graduate Health Sciences make up the University of Tennessee, Memphis. Within the 41-acre campus, there are over 6,000 patient beds and 15 hospitals and clinics affiliated with the University of Tennessee College of Medicine, including the University of Tennessee William F. Bowld Hospital, St. Jude Children's Hospital, LeBonheur Children's Hospital, Veterans Administration Hospital, Baptist Memorial Hospital, Regional Medical Center, LePasses Rehabilitation Center, and Campbell Clinic.

CURRICULUM

The course of study at the University of Tennessee College of Medicine is designed to develop knowledge, skills, and attitudes appropriate to all doctors of medicine. It is sufficiently broad to allow the graduates to enter any graduate training programs designed for primary care specialties, medical and surgical specialties, or research and academic pursuits.

The medical curriculum is a 45-month program consisting of two major components: (1) biomedical science and (2) clinical clerkships and electives. The biomedical science portion of the curriculum includes, during the first year, gross anatomy, histology, biochemistry, fundamentals of cellular and molecular biology, medical genetics, physiology, and neuroanatomy. The second year includes microbiology, pharmacology, neurosciences, pathology, and pathophysiology. Students are introduced to clinical medicine beginning their first semester through the Longitudinal Community Program (LCP), which is presented in each year. The LCP exposes students to the real-life practice of medicine by placing them in a community physician's office and emphasizing professionalism. Students may elect to take three years for the biomedical science portion of the curriculum (optional expanded academic program). Application may be made at matriculation or in the first academic year.

The clerkship and the elective portion of the curriculum consist of 20 months of required and elective experiences. In general, students proceed from the biomedical sciences portion of the curriculum to the junior year of clerkship rotations. Selected clerkships and electives may be taken in Chattanooga, Knoxville, Jackson, Memphis, and Nashville. Junior-year clerkships include rotations in medicine, surgery, pediatrics, obstetrics-gynecology, psychiatry, and family medicine. The senior year consists of one-month required clerkships in neurology, ambulatory medicine, surgical subspecialties, junior internship (medicine), junior internship (any third-year clerkship discipline), and three months of electives.

All students enrolled in the College of Medicine are required to pass both Step 1 and Step 2 of the USMLE as candidates.

REQUIREMENTS FOR ENTRANCE

A minimum of 90 semester hours and the MCAT are required. However, with rare exception, the completion of an undergraduate degree will be necessary in order to meet educational expectations. The Committee on Admissions is particularly impressed by students whose education has provided a broad range of intellectual experience, including opportunities for analytical thinking and independent study. Furthermore, prospective candidates are strongly encouraged to major in their area of greatest interest; there is no requirement that a student major in the sciences. Regardless of choice of major, applicants are encouraged to pursue a course of study that achieves balance between both science and nonscience course work. The required courses are:

	Sem. hrs.
Biology (with lab)	8
Inorganic chemistry (with lab)	8
Organic chemistry (with lab)	8
General physics (with lab)	8
English composition and literature	6
Electives	52

SELECTION FACTORS

The criteria the Committee on Admissions uses in the selection process are the academic record, MCAT scores, preprofessional evaluations, and personal interviews. The required personal interviews by members of the Committee on Admissions provide the candidates with an opportunity to review their curriculum and extracurricular activities. More importantly, the interviewers gain insights into the character of the applicants as well as how they have formulated individual plans for the study and practice of medicine.

Applicants must be citizens or permanent residents of the United States at the time of application. Applications are considered from a nine-state region consisting of Tennessee and its contiguous states (Mississippi, Arkansas, Missouri, Kentucky, Virginia, North Carolina, Georgia, and Alabama). In addition, children of University of Tennessee alumni may be considered regardless of their state of residence. Since priority is given to qualified Tennesseans, out-of-state applicants must possess superior qualifications to be considered by the Committee on Admissions. Currently, only 10 percent of the entering class may be non-resident students. Upon initial review of the AMCAS application, a supplemental application will be forwarded to applicants considered competitive for further review by the Committee on Admissions.

Transfer or advanced standing applications will be considered for the **third** year only. Applicants must be residents of Tennessee at the time of admission to the medical school in which the student has been enrolled, must be enrolled in an LCME-accredited institution, and must pass the United States Medical Licensing Examination, Step 1. In addition, the applicant must provide evidence of circumstances necessitating a transfer. **Deadline for application is April 1**.

Some characteristics of the 1999 entering class were the following: *mean GPA*, 3.55; *mean MCAT scores, VR*-9, *PS*-9, *WS*-0, *BS*-10; *women*, 37 percent; *minorities*, 12 percent.

FINANCIAL AID

Various loan funds and scholarships are available for students who have demonstrated financial need. The College Scholarship Service is utilized in the determination of need. Information packets concerning all available financial assistance are mailed to accepted students. The various academic scholarships are competitive and include a full tuition stipend awarded for each of the four years in school. Loans and scholarships are used in combination whenever possible. Part-time employment during the first two years is discouraged. The Underserved Areas Program offers, through private sponsorship, grants to students who agree to practice in a designated underserved area in the state after residency. Residencies must be completed in family medicine, general internal medicine, general pediatrics, medicine/pediatrics or obstetrics-gynecology. The conditional grant covers tuition, and fees, and also provides additional funding for living expenses. The grant carries a year-for-year service obligation.

INFORMATION FOR MINORITY STUDENTS

The University of Tennessee College of Medicine seeks applications from members of minority groups. The Committee on Admissions evaluates nonacademic as well as academic factors in the selection process, with consideration being given to the unique backgrounds and problems of minority and disadvantaged applicants. Academic support and retention programs are provided for students from minority and/or disadvantaged backgrounds. Scholarship support is available to minority students who are Tennessee residents and residents of contiguous states.

Public Institution

APPLICATION AND ACCEPTANCE POLICIES FOR 2001–2002 FIRST-YEAR CLASS

School participates in AMCAS. See Chapter 6.

Filing of AMCAS application
Earliest date: June 1, 2000
Latest date: Nov. 15, 2000
School application fee after screening: $50
Oldest MCAT scores considered: 1996
Does not have Early Decision Program
Acceptance notice to regular applicants
Earliest date: Oct. 15, 2000
Latest date: April 1, 2001
Applicant's response to acceptance offer
Maximum time: 2 weeks
Requests for deferred entrance considered: Yes
Deposit to hold place in class (applied to tuition):
$100, due with response to acceptance offer
Deposit refundable prior to: May 15, 2001
Estimated number of new entrants: 165
Starting date: Aug. 2001

TUITION AND STUDENT FEES PER YEAR FOR 1999–2000 FIRST-YEAR CLASS

Tuition
Resident: $10,398
Nonresident: $21,834
Student fees: $213

INFORMATION ON 1999–2000 FIRST-YEAR CLASS

Number of	*In-State*	*Out-of-State*	*Total*
Applicants	628	1,009	1,637
Applicants Interviewed	338	63	401
New Entrants*	150	15	165

*All took the MCAT; 98% had baccalaureate degrees.

CHAPTER 11

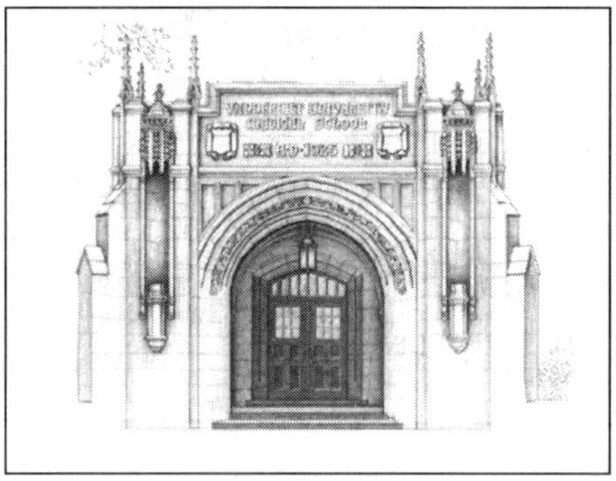

Vanderbilt University School of Medicine

Nashville, Tennessee

Dr. John E. Chapman, *Dean*
Dr. John N. Lukens, *Chairman, Committee for Admissions*
Vicky L. Cagle, *Director of Financial Aid*

ADDRESS INQUIRIES TO:

Office of Admissions
209 Light Hall
Vanderbilt University
School of Medicine
Nashville, Tennessee 37232-0685
(615) 322-2145; 343-8397 (FAX)
E-mail: medsch.admis@mcmail.vanderbilt.edu
Web Site: http://www.mc.vanderbilt.edu/medschool/

MISSION STATEMENT

Vanderbilt University School of Medicine's mission is to educate physicians at all levels of their professional experience: medical school; postgraduate education, including basic science and clinical training; and continuing education for the practicing physician. The faculty seeks to provide students with the attitudes and background, based on sound biomedical science, to continue their education lifelong. At Vanderbilt, every medical student has access to examples of the highest standards of biomedical investigation and clinical practice. The desired end is a graduate who has been challenged and stimulated in as many areas of medicine as are feasible within the limits of a four-year course of study.

GENERAL INFORMATION

Vanderbilt University School of Medicine is a private medical school located on the campus of Vanderbilt University. The Vanderbilt University Medical Center and affiliated hospitals provide a total of over 5,000 beds for diversified, comprehensive clinical experience. These hospitals share common goals of education, research, patient care, and community service. Participation in fundamental and clinical research is encouraged.

CURRICULUM

Medical education at Vanderbilt is oriented toward promoting the intellectual development of students and equipping them with the disciplined approach, knowledge, and skills required of both a physician and scientist. The curriculum provides the student with a fundamental knowledge of basic medical principles, but flexibility is stressed. Changes in curriculum content and teaching methods continually evolve from Vanderbilt's focus upon new ways to assist students in their preparation for a lifetime of learning. While sufficient structure is maintained for adequate guidance, the curriculum offers a productive blend of required and elective courses throughout all four years of the program.

Vanderbilt encourages students to develop their full intellectual talents and places great emphasis upon acquiring a sympathetic understanding of the behavior of the human being in health and sickness. The school's education is comprehensive, encompassing the entire span of medicine. In addition to providing a thorough basic education, the curriculum is designed to emphasize the relationship of emotional, social, and environmental factors to medical disorders.

To provide well-balanced exposure to both clinical and research experiences, Vanderbilt allows students wide latitude in their learning process and encourages self-motivation. Research experience is part of the required curriculum for first-year students and is also available during the elective and summer periods. The Vanderbilt Medical Scientist Training Program in the Biomedical Sciences allows the student to engage in research and study in a basic discipline while pursuing studies toward the M.D. degree. For interested select students, this combined M.D.-Ph.D. program broadens the scope of training so that graduates may choose to assume positions of responsibility and leadership as investigators and medical educators.

The School of Medicine is organized to ensure opportunity for excellence by providing unusual opportunities for close association with the faculty.

REQUIREMENTS FOR ENTRANCE

The MCAT is required. A bachelor's degree is recommended, and most successful candidates have earned the bachelor's degree by the time they enroll in the medical school. Required courses are:

	Sem. hrs.
Biology and/or zoology (with 2 hrs. of lab)	8
Not more than half may be in botany.	
Inorganic chemistry (with 2 hrs. of lab)	8
Organic chemistry (with 2 hrs. of lab)	8
Must cover aliphatic and aromatic compounds.	
Physics (with 2 hrs. of lab)	8
English and composition	6

No preference is given to any one college major. Besides meeting the specific requirements, students should devote their time to strengthening their educational foundation of fundamental knowledge and broadening their cultural background.

SELECTION FACTORS

Applications are invited without regard to race, sex, creed, national origin, or state of residence. Applicants must possess sufficient intellectual ability, emotional stability, and sensory and motor functions to meet the academic requirements of the school of medicine, without fundamental alteration in the nature of this program. Applications are reviewed in two stages. The initial review is made from material provided through AMCAS. Competitive strength of credentials reflecting preparation for medical studies, motivation, personal qualities, and educational background, as these relate to career promise in medicine, is evaluated by the Admissions Committee and determines the recipients of secondary applications. Applicants receiving favorable initial review are invited to file a secondary application, which requires a $50 application fee, except in demonstrated circumstances of serious financial hardship. Those who are sent a secondary application also are invited for an interview. Applicants are encouraged to have their interviews at Vanderbilt, and more than 90 percent do so. For those unable to visit Vanderbilt, arrangements are made for regional interviews.

The 104 members of the 1999 first-year class graduated from 52 different colleges and universities. They hail from 29 states. Nine are enrolled in the Medical Scientist Training Program. The *mean GPA* for the class is 3.73 and the *mean composite MCAT score* is 11.2.

Vanderbilt undergraduates, with at least a 3.5, are eligible to apply for early acceptance during the spring of the sophomore year. Those accepted are encouraged to broaden their curricular experiences. The number of early acceptance candidates in the school's current classes ranges from 4 to 12.

Opportunities for transfer are rarely available because of the low attrition rate and are limited to the third year. Those students who have completed the second year in good standing at LCME-accredited U.S. or Canadian medical schools are eligible to apply.

FINANCIAL AID

Limited scholarships, fellowships, loans, and other financial aid are available. Most scholarships, awards, and all loans are given on the basis of demonstrated financial need. The G. Canby Robinson Scholars Program uses a combination of academic excellence and financial need as the basis for selection of scholars. Foreign students are eligible for support from this program.

Students selected for medical study at Vanderbilt should give careful attention to financial planning and are expected to utilize their own financial resources to the fullest extent possible. Financial aid will be heavily related to available federal programs.

The telephone number for the financial aid office is (615) 343-6310.

INFORMATION FOR MINORITY STUDENTS

Vanderbilt invites applicants from a broad spectrum of student backgrounds to submit an application for admission. Applications are sought from members of groups presently not adequately represented in medicine who feel a commitment to helping resolve the special problems of health care delivery to minority and underprivileged groups.

Private Institution

APPLICATION AND ACCEPTANCE POLICIES FOR 2001–2002 FIRST-YEAR CLASS

School participates in AMCAS. See Chapter 6.

Filing of AMCAS application
- Earliest date: June 1, 2000
- Latest date: Oct. 15, 2000

School application fee after screening: $50
Oldest MCAT scores considered: 1997
Does have Early Decision Program (EDP)
- EDP application period: June 1–Aug. 1, 2000
- EDP applicants notified by: Oct. 1, 2000

Acceptance notice to regular applicants
- Earliest date: Oct. 15, 2000
- Latest date: Until class is filled

Applicant's response to acceptance offer
- Maximum time: 2 weeks

Requests for deferred entrance considered: Yes
Deposit to hold place in class: None
Estimated number of new entrants: 104 (5 EDP)
Starting date: Aug. 2001

TUITION AND STUDENT FEES PER YEAR FOR 1999–2000 FIRST-YEAR CLASS

Tuition: $25,250 Student fees: $1,360

INFORMATION ON 1999–2000 FIRST-YEAR CLASS

Number of	*In-State*	*Out-of-State*	*Total*
Applicants	273	4,151	4,424
Applicants Interviewed	47	774	821
New Entrants*	10	93	103

*All had baccalaureate degrees; 96% took the MCAT.

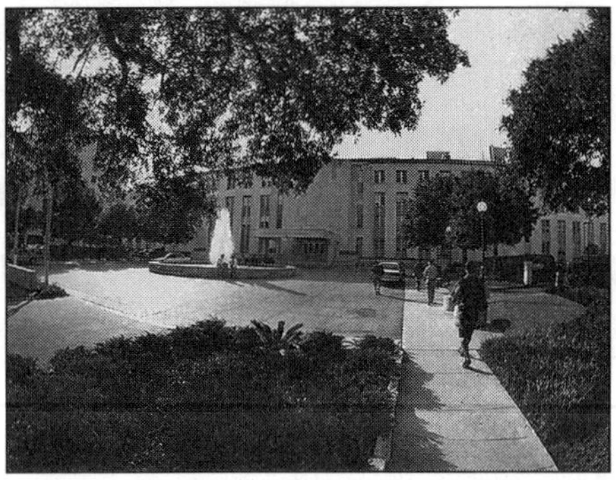

Baylor College of Medicine

Houston, Texas

Dr. Ralph D. Feigin, *President*
Dr. Major Bradshaw, *Dean of Education*
Dr. L. Leighton Hill, *Senior Associate Dean, Admissions*

ADDRESS INQUIRIES TO:

Office of Admissions
Baylor College of Medicine
One Baylor Plaza
Houston, Texas 77030
(713) 798-4842
E-mail: melodym@bcm.tmc.edu
Web Site: http://www.bcm.tmc.edu/bcm-admissions.html

MISSION STATEMENT

The mission of Baylor College of Medicine is to promote health for all people through education, research, and public service.

The college pursues this mission by sustaining excellence in educating medical and graduate students, primary care and specialty physicians, biomedical scientists and allied health professionals; by advancing basic and clinical biomedical research; by fostering public awareness of health and the prevention of disease; and by promoting patient care of the highest standard.

GENERAL INFORMATION

Baylor College of Medicine is a private, nonsectarian institution governed by an independent Board of Trustees of community leaders. Baylor College of Medicine is the academic center around which the 356-acre Texas Medical Center was developed. The Baylor faculty currently is composed of 1,570 full-time members and another 1,672 on a part-time and voluntary basis. Facilities include teaching and research buildings and seven affiliated teaching hospitals (including private, county, and Veterans Administration hospitals), which together have approximately 5,000 beds. The Texas Medical Center is located in a university, residential, and park area in the southwest section of Houston.

CURRICULUM

The goal of the educational program at Baylor College of Medicine is to provide the highest-quality educational experience in the art and science of medicine, fostering a drive for excellence among all students. The curriculum is structured to prepare graduates to pursue careers as primary care physicians, specialists, research scientists, academic physicians, or physicians involved in public health policy. After major reform in 1995, the Baylor curriculum integrates basic and clinical sciences throughout the four-year program. This integration includes direct patient-care experiences early in the first year and a focus on core basic science topics prior to graduation. This integration also includes special courses featuring problem-based learning and clinical skills training that encourage application of content learned in lectures and labs.

The Baylor curriculum is unique in that the basic sciences are taught in slightly less than 1½ years, giving students more time to take advantage of a wealth of clinical experiences. During the preclinical curriculum, study and vacation periods are scheduled prior to exams approximately every 8-10 weeks. During the clinical curriculum, students have flexibility in organizing their schedules to complete 56 weeks of required clinical clerkships, 4 weeks of selectives, and 20 weeks of elective experiences. Approximately 200 discrete electives are available at Baylor and throughout the Texas Medical Center. Interested students are given opportunity to do research or to apply for a combined M.D.-Ph.D. program.

The Baylor/Rice program in Health Sciences Management consists of two dual-degree programs of M.D.-M.B.A. and Ph.D.-M.B.A., as well as an M.B.A. with a health care focus. The programs are sponsored jointly by the Jones School of Management at Rice University and by Baylor College of Medicine.

REQUIREMENTS FOR ENTRANCE

The MCAT is required. Applicants are strongly advised to take the MCAT in the spring of the year of application and to have their science course requirements completed at the time of application.

The baccalaureate degree is highly desirable. In recent years very few students matriculated without a baccalaureate degree. Applicants must have satisfactorily completed a minimum of 90 undergraduate semester hours (or an equivalent number of quarter hours) at a fully accredited college or university in the United States prior to enrollment. Courses must include:

	Years
General biology (with lab)	1
General chemistry (with lab)	1
Organic chemistry (with lab)	1
English	1

SELECTION FACTORS

All applicants offered places in the class are interviewed on the Baylor College of Medicine campus. The Admissions

Committee selects for interview applicants whose files are complete and who are considered to be competitive for admission. All information available is utilized in the selection process. In evaluating the applicant's academic record, attention is paid to course selections, academic challenge imposed by the student's curriculum, and the extent to which extracurricular activities and employment may have broadened a student's experiences or limited the applicant's opportunity for high academic achievement.

Intellectual ability and academic achievement alone are not sufficient to support the development of the ideal physician. To work effectively in a profession dependent upon interpersonal relationships, physicians should possess those traits of personality and character which permit them to communicate effectively with warmth and compassion.

There are 168 students in each first-year class; approximately 70–75 percent are residents of Texas.

Requests for deferred entrance (delayed matriculation) from accepted students will be considered but are not encouraged. Such requests must be in writing and will be reviewed on an individual basis.

Students matriculating in 1999 had the following credentials: *mean GPA,* 3.8; *average MCAT score* was 33, *sex,* 48 percent women; *undergraduate major,* 77 percent in sciences, with the remainder from a variety of fields.

Baylor College of Medicine does not discriminate on the basis of race, sex, creed, national origin, age, or disability.

FINANCIAL AID

Financial need is not a factor in the selection of students. Aid funds are provided by private donors, the Board of Trustees, and various state and federal loan, scholarship, and work-study programs. Employment for spouses and part-time employment for students is also available. Financial aid information and application materials are sent to all accepted applicants and a financial aid officer is available for consultation with students and parents.

INFORMATION FOR MINORITY STUDENTS

Baylor College of Medicine encourages applications from members of groups not adequately represented in medicine.

Students from minority groups comprise a substantial portion of the student body, and the Admissions Committee has members from these groups as well.

Private Institution

APPLICATION AND ACCEPTANCE POLICIES FOR 2000–2001 FIRST-YEAR CLASS

Filing of application
- Earliest date: June 1, 2000
- Latest date: Nov. 1, 2000

School application fee to all applicants: $35
Oldest MCAT scores considered: 1997
Does have Early Decision Program (EDP)
- EDP application period: June 1–Aug. 1, 2000
- EDP applicants notified by: Oct. 1, 2000

Acceptance notice to regular applicants
- Earliest date: Oct. 15, 2000
- Latest date: Until class is filled

Requests for deferred entrance considered: Yes
Deposit to hold place in class (applied to tuition):
$300, due May 15, 2001; nonrefundable
Estimated number of new entrants: 168 (5 EDP)
Starting date: Aug. 2001

TUITION AND STUDENT FEES PER YEAR FOR 1999–2000 FIRST-YEAR CLASS

Tuition
- Resident: $6,550
- Nonresident: $19,650

Student fees: $963

INFORMATION ON 1999–2000 FIRST-YEAR CLASS

Number of	*In-State*	*Out-of-State*	*Total*
Applicants	1,290	1,067	2,357
Applicants Interviewed	413	200	613
New Entrants	129	38	167

*All had baccalaureate degrees; 96% took the MCAT.

CHAPTER 11

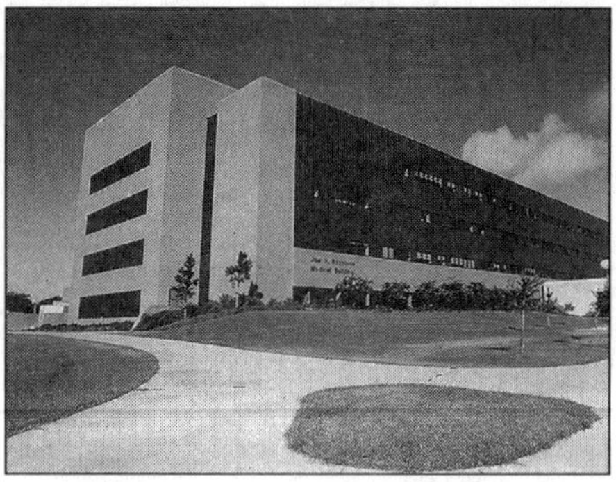

Texas A&M University System Health Science Center College of Medicine

College Station, Texas

Dr. Roderick E. McCallum, *Interim Dean of Medicine*
Dr. Kathleen F. Williams, *Associate Dean for Student Affairs and Admissions*
Filomeno G. Maldonado, *Assistant Dean for Admissions*

ADDRESS INQUIRIES TO:

Office of Student Affairs and Admissions
Texas A&M University System Health Science Center
College of Medicine
159 Joe Reynolds Medical Bldg.
College Station, Texas 77843-1114
(409) 845-7743; 845-5533 (FAX)
E-mail: med-stu-aff@tamu.edu
Web Site: http://tamushsc.tamu.edu

MISSION STATEMENT

The Texas A&M University System Health Science Center and College of Medicine are explicit about their commitment to excellence in improving the health and public health needs of Texans, particularly rural and underserved populations, through integrated education, research, and the use of community-focused health education and public service programs. This mission is the foundation on which the Admissions Committee makes important individual admissions decisions and strives to admit students whose goals and attitudes are consistent with this philosophy and mission of the Texas A&M University System Health Science Center and College of Medicine.

GENERAL INFORMATION

Established in 1973, Texas A&M University College of Medicine is part of the Texas A&M University System Health Science Center, a public institution. The College of Medicine's administrative offices and basic science campus are located in College Station on the campus of Texas A&M University. Texas A&M University, whose research budget is among the top five in the nation, is a comprehensive land, sea, and space grant university with a total enrollment of 36,082 undergraduate students and 6,861 graduate and professional students. The clinical campus consists of the Central Texas Medical Centers, a consortium of Veterans Administration hospitals and outpatient clinics, that serves veterans in a 35-county-wide primary care service area of central Texas, the Olin E. Teague Veterans' Center in Temple, Texas; the Scott and White Clinic and Hospital in Temple, Texas; Darnall Army Community Hospital at nearby Fort Hood in Killeen, Texas; and Driscoll Children's Hospital in Corpus Christi, Texas. These comprehensive facilities provide 1,976 teaching beds and aggregate annual outpatient visits in excess of 2 million.

The College of Medicine is chartered to grant the degrees of doctor of medicine, master of science, and doctor of philosophy.

CURRICULUM

The primary goal of the curriculum is to produce undifferentiated physicians of the highest caliber. A second principal mission is the systematic utilization of the vast intellectual and technological resources available within other disciplines of the parent university in collaborative research and instructional programs.

The College of Medicine offers a four-year program leading to the M.D. degree. The first two years are taught on the Texas A&M University campus in College Station and include, besides the traditional basic science disciplines, instruction in behavioral science, humanities in medicine, community medicine, and leadership in medicine. Although the faculty is organized along disciplinary lines, courses are scheduled to assure a high degree of integration of subject matter across disciplines. Correlation of the basic sciences with clinical medicine is achieved from the start, with clinical correlation experiences in all courses and regularly scheduled sessions for clinical instruction and practice in both years 1 and 2.

The third- and fourth-year clinical programs, conducted predominantly on the Temple campus at the Scott and White Clinic and Hospital and the Olin E. Teague Veterans' Center, consist of traditional clerkships and a mixed rotation of ambulatory care experiences. In addition, each student spends a minimum of six weeks in an approved family medicine clerkship in a nonurban location.

Electives are available in both basic and clinical sciences. A standardized letter grading system (A, B, C, F) is utilized.

Selected students may participate in the combined M.D.-Ph.D. program.

REQUIREMENTS FOR ENTRANCE

The MCAT and 90 semester hours of appropriate undergraduate study from an accredited U.S. institution are required. Required courses are:

	Credit Hrs./Years
General biology (with lab)	8/1
Additional advanced biological science	3/½
Inorganic chemistry (with lab)	8/1

Organic chemistry (with lab) 8/1
General physics (with lab) 8/1
Calculus 3/½
English 6/1

Applicants are urged to take the MCAT in the spring of the year of application. Early application is encouraged.

SELECTION FACTORS

Academic ability, as evidenced by grades in college courses and performance on the MCAT, is an important selection criterion. Equally important are personal traits such as interpersonal and communication skills, maturity, motivation, and compassion. In addition, it is critical for members of the Admissions Committee to understand the circumstances of applicants and give careful consideration to other factors such as dedication to service, circumstances indicative of some hardship, need to work, support from faculty and mentors, evidence of interest in primary care, rural or an underserved area, and knowledge of cultural factors as they may impact health care. It is also important for applicants to have some knowledge and experience of the profession of medicine. However, it must be understood that not all of the applicants under review will be either interviewed or offered admission. Competitive applicants are invited for personal interviews, which are conducted between the College Station and Temple campuses over two days—Thursday and Friday. Each applicant is scheduled for two 30-minute individual interviews with some combination of faculty Admissions Committee members, Medical Student Admissions Committee members, and faculty guest interviewers. Admission to the College of Medicine is open to qualified individuals regardless of race, color, religion, gender, age, national origin, or disability.

Some characteristics of the 1999 entering class were: *mean GPA*, 3.64; *mean MCAT*, 9.7; *gender*, 56 percent women; *minorities*, 7.7 percent; *residents*, 96 percent; *undergraduate major*, 89 percent in sciences; and the remainder were nonscience degrees varying from accounting to international relations.

FINANCIAL AID

Scholarship and loan funds are available to students with financial need from local, state, and national sources. In addition, three full-tuition scholarships, which pay for resident tuition over four years, may be awarded to the year's top-ranked applicants and outstanding students with financial need. Financial needs of the applicant are not a consideration in the admission process, and after acceptance, every effort is made to assist students in meeting their financial requirements. Approximately 90 percent of the students currently in the program are receiving some form of financial aid. For further information, contact the director of student financial aid.

INFORMATION FOR DISADVANTAGED AND MINORITY STUDENTS

The College of Medicine is committed to identifying and recruiting qualified students from minority and disadvantaged backgrounds. As part of its commitment to this effort, the College of Medicine administers several programs for disadvantaged students. The Bridge to Medicine summer program is open to students from minority and disadvantaged backgrounds who have completed the requirements for medical school. It offers college students an intensive academic program to reinforce their knowledge of the basic sciences and prepare them for the MCAT. In addition, the Office of Special Programs facilitates the adjustment and the retention of disadvantaged and minority students attending the College of Medicine.

Public Institution

APPLICATION AND ACCEPTANCE POLICIES FOR 2001–2002 FIRST-YEAR CLASS

Application must be made through the Texas Medical and Dental Schools Application Service, Suite 620, 702 Colorado, Austin, Texas 78701.

Filing of Application:
Earliest date: May 1, 2000
Latest date: Oct. 15, 2000
School application fee to all applicants: $45
Oldest MCAT scores considered: 1996
Does not have Early Decision Program
Acceptance notice to regular applicants
Earliest date: Jan. 15, 2001
Latest date: Until class is filled
Applicant's response to acceptance offer
Maximum time: 2 weeks
Requests for deferred entrance considered: Yes
Deposit to hold place in class: None
Estimated number of new entrants: 64
Starting date: Aug. 2001

TUITION AND STUDENT FEES PER YEAR FOR 1999–2000 FIRST-YEAR CLASS

Tuition
Resident: $6,550
Nonresident: $19,650

Student fees: $1,216

INFORMATION ON 1999–2000 FIRST-YEAR CLASS

Number of	*In-State*	*Out-of-State*	*Total*
Applicants	1,131	311	1,442
Applicants Interviewed	525	28	553
New Entrants*	75	3	78

*All took the MCAT; 96% had baccalaureate degrees.

CHAPTER 11

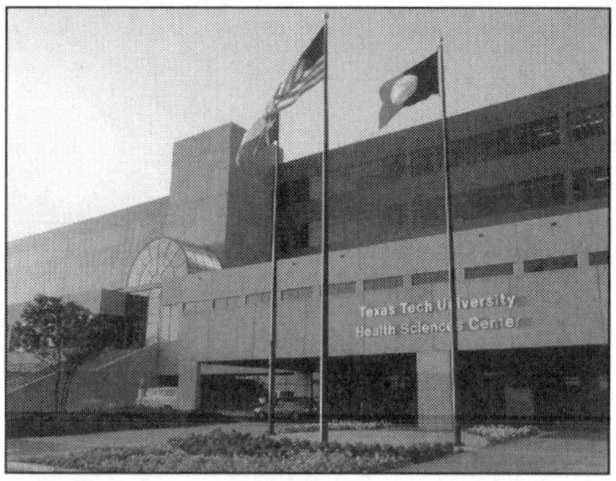

Texas Tech University Health Sciences Center School of Medicine

Lubbock, Texas

Dr. Joel Kupersmith, *Dean and Vice President for Clinical Affairs*
Dr. Bernell K. Dalley, *Assistant Dean, Admissions and Student Affairs*
E. Marcus Wilson, *Director, Financial Aid*

ADDRESS INQUIRIES TO:

Texas Tech University Health Sciences Center
School of Medicine
Office of Admissions, Room 2B116
3601 4th Street, Lubbock, Texas 79430
(806) 743-2297; 743-2725 (FAX)
Web Site: http://www.ttuhsc.edu

MISSION STATEMENT

Texas Tech University Health Sciences Center School of Medicine provides the highest standard of excellence in higher education, while pursuing continuous quality improvement. The medical school is committed to medical education and health care delivery for its 135,000 square mile serving area of West Texas via regional academic health centers in Lubbock, Amarillo, El Paso, and Odessa; to prepare graduates of the institution for real world medicine. At the same time and as part of improvement of health care, its efforts include support of meaningful academic research for the betterment of future health care.

GENERAL INFORMATION

Texas Tech University School of Medicine, established in 1969, is part of the Texas Tech University Health Sciences Center. The School of Medicine is adjacent to Texas Tech University, which has an enrollment of 24,000 students. All medical students spend the first two years at the Lubbock campus; junior and senior students receive their clinical training in Lubbock, Amarillo, or El Paso. At each academic health center the primary teaching hospital is located in close proximity to the medical school facility. Affiliations with the primary teaching hospital and other community hospitals provide over 2,900 beds for clinical teaching. The medical school has 485 full-time faculty members and more than 1,000 volunteer clinical faculty members.

CURRICULUM

The four-year curriculum provides a broad introduction to medical knowledge while developing the student's analytical, problem-solving skills. The first two years are divided into four terms, with an emphasis on basic sciences. Introduction to clinical material begins in the first year with preceptorial experiences, including shadowing of community physicians and training in patient history and interviewing. These experiences may be augmented by doing summer preceptorships following the first year of medical school. It continues in the second year with the introduction to patient assessment course, which integrates pathophysiology and physical diagnosis. The clinical curriculum includes clerkships in family medicine, internal medicine, neurology, obstetrics-gynecology, pediatrics, psychiatry, and surgery. It also includes experience with family medicine in the community setting. The electives program consists of five electives chosen by the students in consultation with their advisors.

Research opportunities are available in the summer following the first year. In addition, there is a Research Honors Program in which the student devotes a full year to research between the second and third years. An integrated M.D.-Ph.D. program providing stipends and tuition scholarships to especially qualified candidates is also available.

Students are graded on a numerical system and must maintain a numerical average of 75 for promotion and graduation.

A dually accredited joint M.B.A.–M.D. program is offered in which qualified students may earn both degrees within a four-year period beginning the summer before entry to medical school. Students will complete a 51-hour M.B.A. in Health Organization Management in addition to the M.D.

REQUIREMENTS FOR ENTRANCE

At least three years of study (90 semester hours) with recorded grades in a U.S.- or Canadian-accredited college or university are required. All prerequisite courses must be taken in a U.S. or Canadian school. The completion of four years of college and a B.S. or B.A. degree is highly desirable before entrance into medical school.

Specific course requirements have been kept at a minimum to permit maximum flexibility in the selection of well-rounded students. Graded prerequisite courses require a grade of "C" or better.

	Sem. hrs.
Biology or zoology	12
Biology lab (minimum)	2
Inorganic chemistry (with lab)	8
Organic chemistry (with lab)	8
Physics (with lab)	8
Calculus	3
English	6

The MCAT is also a requirement for admission. It is recommended that students take the MCAT in the spring of the year in which application will be made.

SELECTION FACTORS

Applications are invited from qualified residents of the state of Texas and service area counties of New Mexico and Oklahoma. Only U.S. citizens or applicants with permanent resident visas are considered. Application forms and procedural information may be obtained from the Texas Medical and Dental Schools Application Service (http://dpweb1.dp.utexas.edu/mdac/homepage.htm). A secondary application to Texas Tech University Health Sciences Center School of Medicine is also required and is linked to the main application *or* via www.ttuhsc.edu/medicine.

The Admissions Committee carefully reviews the applications of all individuals meeting the entrance requirements. Although evidence of high intellectual ability and a record of strong academic achievement are essential for success in the study of medicine, the committee also looks for such qualities as compassion, motivation, the ability to communicate with people, maturity, and personal integrity. There is no discrimination on the basis of race, sex, creed, national origin, age, or disability.

Personal interviews are offered to those candidates deemed competitive for admission. Interviews are conducted only at the Lubbock campus.

Students in the 1999 entering class had the following credentials: *mean GPA,* 3.58; 36 percent *women;* 14 percent *Hispanic/Mexican American;* 33 percent *Asian;* 80 percent *science majors;* 99 percent Texas *residents,* and includes one African-American and two non-Texas residents.

FINANCIAL AID

Financial aid is available for students who demonstrate need. Applications for financial assistance are processed after an applicant has been accepted. Detailed information on the available programs can be obtained from the Office of Student Financial Aid. Over 91 percent of the student body receive some type of financial assistance. Employment, other than during the summer, is discouraged.

INFORMATION FOR DISADVANTAGED STUDENTS

The School of Medicine takes disadvantaged status into account in evaluation of an applicant's overall status. Qualified students from educationally and/or socioeconomically disadvantaged backgrounds are encouraged to apply.

SPECIAL PROGRAMS

Agreements have been developed with Texas Tech University Health Sciences Center School of Medicine, Texas Tech University, West Texas A&M University, and Austin College to provide early acceptance of qualified students into TTUHSC School of Medicine. In order to qualify for an interview in the third semester of college, applicants must meet entrance requirements, including an established performance on the SAT/ACT, and maintenance of a high grade point average (GPA), including a specified number of prerequisite courses. All coursework must be taken at the college/university through which the applicant is applying. The applicant will then be invited to the Lubbock campus for an interview. If the Admissions Committee recommends acceptance of the applicant, and provided the applicant maintains the required GPA for the remainder of their undergraduate education, candidates are guaranteed admission to Texas Tech School of Medicine in the fall following graduating with a Bachelor's degree. The Medical College Admissions Test (MCAT) is waived for these applicants.

Public Institution

APPLICATION AND ACCEPTANCE POLICIES FOR 2001–2002 FIRST-YEAR CLASS

Filing of application
- Earliest date: May 1, 2000
- Latest date: Oct. 15, 2000

Main application fee to all applicants: $55 plus $10 for each additional school. (Nonresidents–$100 plus $10 for each additional school.)

Secondary application fee to TTUHSC School of Medicine–$40 (required)

Oldest MCAT scores considered: 1996

Does have Early Decision Program (EDP)
- For Texas residents only
- EDP application period: May 1–August 12, 2000
- EDP applicants notified by: Oct. 1, 2000

Acceptance notice to regular applicants
- Earliest date: Jan. 15, 2001
- Latest date: Until class is filled

Applicant's response to acceptance offer
- Maximum time: 2 weeks

Requests for deferred entrance considered: Yes

Deposit to hold place in class:
- $100, due April 1, 2001 (nonrefundable)

Estimated number of new entrants: 120 (6 EDP)

Starting date: Aug. 2001

TUITION AND STUDENT FEES PER YEAR FOR 1999–2000 FIRST-YEAR CLASS

Tuition
- Resident: $7,251*
- Nonresident: $20,351*

Student fees: $757

INFORMATION ON 1999–2000 FIRST-YEAR CLASS

Number of	*In-State*	*Out-of-State*	*Total*
Applicants	1,453	31	1,484
Applicants Interviewed	642	6	648
New Entrants†	121	2	123

*Includes $701 general use fee.

†All took the MCAT and had baccalaureate degrees.

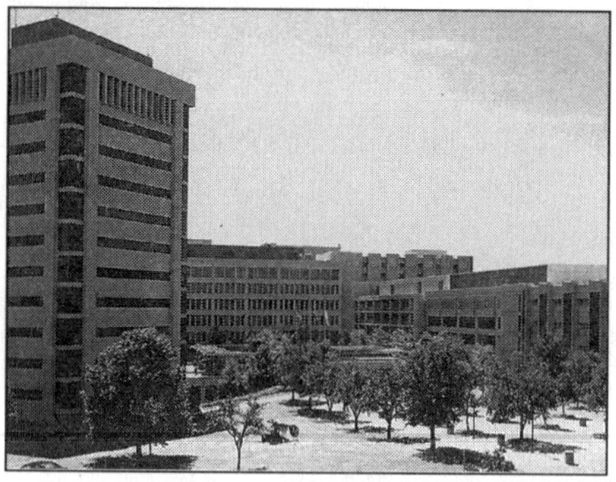

University of Texas Southwestern Medical Center at Dallas Southwestern Medical School

Dallas, Texas

Dr. Robert J. Alpern, *Dean, UT Southwestern Medical School*
Dr. James Wagner, *Associate Dean for Student Affairs*
Dr. J. Scott Wright, *Director of Admissions*

ADDRESS INQUIRIES TO:

University of Texas
Southwestern Medical Center at Dallas
5323 Harry Hines Boulevard
Dallas, Texas 75390-9162
(214) 648-5617; 648-3289 (FAX)
Web Site: http://www.swmed.edu/medapp
E-mail: admissions@mednet.swmed.edu

MISSION STATEMENT

The central purpose of Southwestern Medical School is to produce physicians who will be inspired to maintain lifelong medical scholarship and who will apply the knowledge gained in a responsible and humanistic manner to the care of patients. An important focus of the educational effort of UT Southwestern is training primary care physicians and preparing doctors who will practice in underserved areas of Texas. Additionally, the medical school seeks to fully prepare students who seek careers in academic medicine and research.

GENERAL INFORMATION

Southwestern Medical School, founded in 1943, is a part of the University of Texas Southwestern Medical Center at Dallas, a multifaceted academic institution nationally recognized for its excellence in educating physicians, biomedical scientists, and health care professionals. Located just north of downtown Dallas, the 100-acre campus includes modern classrooms and laboratories and an extensive medical library, as well as a recreation center, tennis and basketball courts, jogging paths, and a six-acre wooded bird sanctuary. Clinical training takes place at university sites and affiliated institutions including Parkland Memorial Hospital, the James Aston Ambulatory Care Center, Zale Lipshy University Hospital, Children's Medical Center, Dallas Veterans Affairs Medical Center, Southwestern Institute of Forensic Sciences, Baylor University Medical Center, Presbyterian Hospital of Dallas, Methodist Hospitals of Dallas, St. Paul Medical Center, Texas Scottish Rite Hospital for Children, and John Peter Smith Hospital in Fort Worth.

CURRICULUM

Southwestern Medical School offers a four-year curriculum based on departmental as well as interdisciplinary teaching. The purpose of the first two years is to provide a strong background in the basic sciences as well as an introduction to clinical medicine.

The first-year curriculum is designed to begin the study of the normal human body and its processes at the molecular and cellular levels. Biochemistry, anatomy, and genetics are presented concurrently for the first portion of the year, building together the concepts of macromolecular and cellular interactions within tissues. The spring term is composed of courses in physiology and neurosciences, cell biology, and human behavior. At the completion of the first year, a vertical course in human reproduction and endocrinology provides an overall synthesis, based on the previous course work. A year-long, problem-based introduction to clinical medicine course introduces first-year students to taking histories from standardized patients along with content in ethics, human behavior, and prevention.

The second year begins a study of disease processes and provides insight into how man may interfere with those processes therapeutically. The material is presented in a block fashion similar to that of the freshman year. The year begins with microbiology and immunology and concludes with pharmacology. Extending throughout most of the year are pathology and introduction to clinical medicine, which serve to correlate the basic sciences with clinical medicine. Contact with patients begins early in the second year with history taking and physical examination as well as visits to outpatient clinics. The basic concepts of psychiatry are presented over the first two years in a series of conferences and lectures.

The third and fourth years provide intense clinical experiences involving the student in direct inpatient and outpatient care. The junior year is composed of 12 weeks of internal medicine, 6 weeks each of psychiatry and obstetrics/gynecology, 8 weeks each of surgery and pediatrics, and 4 weeks of family practice. The fourth year provides a series of one-month clinical rotations; required months in neurology, subinternship in internal medicine on a ward or an intensive care unit, an ambulatory care rotation, and a women's health care rotation; two selectives from the departments of obstetrics/gynecology, surgery, pediatrics, or family practice; and at least two months of electives.

Every year the curriculum becomes more computer based. Learning material in multimedia format is presently provided by direct network connection as well as CD-ROM. Therefore, UT Southwestern requires each student to own a personal computer for use during the first two years of medical school.

Purchase and support of student computers are facilitated by the medical school. Additionally, several computer labs dedicated exclusively to student use are available on campus.

REQUIREMENTS FOR ENTRANCE

The MCAT (taken within the last five years) and at least three years (90 semester hours) of accredited college work are required. Preference is given to applicants who have or will have earned a bachelor's degree. Minimum course requirements are:

	Years
Biology	2
One year must include lab.	
Inorganic chemistry (with lab)	1
Organic chemistry (with lab)	1
Physics (with lab)	1
Calculus	½
English	1

Sound preparation in basic science is essential, but a broad background in the humanities and an understanding of people and their problems are equally necessary. Applicants are urged to take the MCAT in the spring of the year of application and to complete required course work before applying if possible.

SELECTION FACTORS

The Admissions Committee considers all of the following in evaluating each applicant's acceptability: scores from the MCAT; academic performance in college as reflected in the GPA; the rigor of the undergraduate curriculum; recommendations from the college premedical committee or college faculty; extracurricular activities; socioeconomic background; time spent in outside employment; personal integrity and compassion for others; the ability to communicate; other personal qualities and individual factors such as leadership, social/family support, self-appraisal, maturity/coping skills, and determination; as well as motivation for a career in medicine. In addition, applicants are evaluated with regard to the mission of Southwestern Medical School. State law requires that at least 90 percent of the class be residents of Texas. Therefore, the minimum credentials for nonresidents are more stringent than those for Texas residents.

Early application is strongly advised. A personal on-campus interview is required and is initiated by invitation from the Admissions Committee. Interviews are held on Saturdays from early September until mid-December.

FINANCIAL AID

UT Southwestern works directly with students to obtain funding for their medical education. Most of the financial aid available is obtained through federal and state loan programs. However, a limited number of scholarships from private sources are available. No student has ever discontinued school for financial reasons.

INFORMATION FOR MINORITY STUDENTS

The Admissions Committee at Southwestern Medical School recognizes the need for increased numbers of physicians from racial minorities and encourages applications from Texas residents who are members of these groups.

Public Institution

APPLICATION AND ACCEPTANCE POLICIES FOR 2001–2002 FIRST-YEAR CLASS

Application must be made through the
University of Texas System Medical and Dental Application Center, Suite 620, 702 Colorado, Austin, Texas 78701

Filing of application
Earliest date: May 1, 2000
Latest date: Oct. 15, 2000

School application fee to all applicants: $55

Oldest MCAT scores considered: 1996

Does not have Early Decision Program

Acceptance notice to regular applicants
Earliest date: Jan. 15, 2001
Latest date: Varies

Applicant's response to acceptance offer
Maximum time: 2 weeks

Requests for deferred entrance considered: Yes

Deposit to hold place in class: None

Estimated number of new entrants: 200

Starting date: Aug. 2001

TUITION AND STUDENT FEES PER YEAR FOR 1999–2000 FIRST-YEAR CLASS

Tuition
Resident: $6,550
Nonresident*: $19,650

Student fees: $796

INFORMATION ON 1999–2000 FIRST-YEAR CLASS

Number of	*In-State*	*Out-of-State*	*Total*
Applicants	2,118	473	2,591
Applicants Interviewed	592	92	684
New Entrants†	183	20	203

*Nonresidents are eligible to pay resident tuition on receipt of a competitive academic scholarship worth at least $1,000 per year.

†All took the MCAT; 98% had baccalaureate degrees.

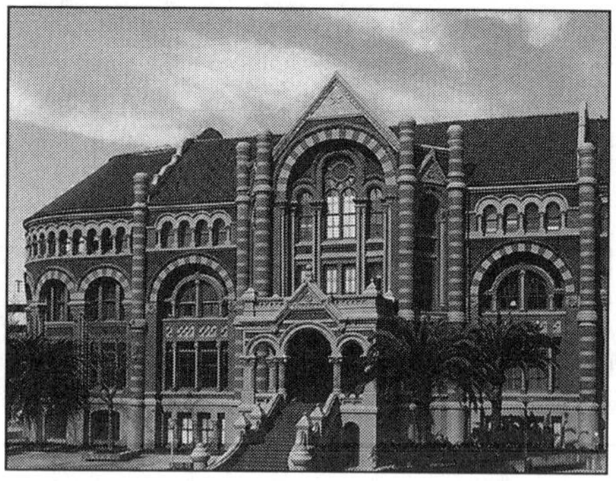

University of Texas Medical School at Galveston

Galveston, Texas

Dr. Stanley Lemon, *Dean Pro-tem*
Dr. Billy R. Ballard, *Associate Dean for Admissions and Student Affairs*
Betty Hazelbaker, *Director, Student Financial Aid*

ADDRESS INQUIRIES TO:

Office of Admissions
G-210, Ashbel Smith Building
University of Texas Medical Branch at Galveston
School of Medicine
Galveston, Texas 77555-1317
(409) 772-3517; 772-5753 (FAX)
E-mail: pwylie@utmb.edu
Web Site: http://www.utmb.edu

GENERAL INFORMATION

The University of Texas Medical Branch (UTMB) at Galveston was established in 1891 and graduated its first class in 1892. It is a state-owned medical center with the Medical Branch hospitals under direct supervision of the UTMB administration. The Medical Branch has 8 hospitals with 923 open beds, 75 hospital clinics, and 93 outpatient clinics. The Shriners Burn Institute, the Marine Biomedical Institute, and the Institute for the Medical Humanities also serve as teaching and research facilities.

CURRICULUM

The University of Texas Medical School at Galveston has two distinct curricula—the Integrated Medical Curriculum (IMC) and the Interactive Learning Track (ILT). Both curricula are integrated, centrally governed by the Curriculum Committee, and heavily committed to active learning. The ILT is limited to 24 students, and the remaining 176 students enter the IMC. After acceptance into medical school, students may submit an application to the ILT. Selections are made on a random basis.

The goals and objectives of the IMC are to produce knowledgeable and skillful physicians who possess professional attitudes and are committed to lifelong learning. The 1998 entering class is the first cohort to progress through the IMC. The first two years of the IMC utilize a fully integrated basic science core followed by a multidisciplinary approach organized by organ systems (such as cardiovascular/pulmonary, renal/electrolytes) rather than by individual disciplines (e.g., biochemistry, physiology, or pharmacology). The IMC emphasizes self-directed active learning stimulated by actual clinical cases. Varieties of educational methods are utilized including small-group, problem-based learning, formal lecture, laboratory, demonstrations, and computer-assisted education. Early community-based clinical experiences are a feature of this curriculum. The social, cultural, and ethical issues of the medical profession and the introduction of the student to clinical medicine are addressed longitudinally across the curriculum in the Practice of Medicine course, in years one and two. The final weeks of the second year are devoted to the great syndromes, which are integrated case studies of complex multi-organ problems.

The ILT is an alternative medical curriculum that relies almost exclusively on group tutorial-based learning. The ILT utilizes problem-based learning as the primary method of education, and emphasizes integration and retention of basic science knowledge through early application to clinical problems, problem-solving skills, group interaction, self-directed learning, and personal and professional development.

During the third year all students have required rotations in family medicine, internal medicine, obstetrics-gynecology, pediatrics, psychiatry, surgery, and a multidisciplinary ambulatory clerkship, which includes family medicine, internal medicine, and pediatrics. In the fourth year, the required clerkships are neurology, senior surgery, emergency medicine and advanced cardiac life support, radiology, dermatology, and an acting internship selective. The remaining 20 weeks are electives and depending on previous academic performance may be taken at approved U.S. or international sites. The grading systems for the required core courses are honors, high pass, pass, and fail, and pass/fail for elective courses.

REQUIREMENTS FOR ENTRANCE

The MCAT and a minimum of 90 semester hours of college work including specific courses are required. The baccalaureate degree is highly desirable. Course work is acceptable only if completed at U.S. colleges and universities with accreditation from one of the regional accrediting agencies.

Applicants are encouraged to take the MCAT in the spring of the year of application. Results from the MCAT taken in the spring of the year of anticipated matriculation will not be received in time to be considered. Applicants are encouraged to complete the required courses and/or take the MCAT by the time they submit an application.

The required courses are:

	Years
Biology	2

One year must include lab.

Inorganic chemistry (with lab)	1
Organic chemistry (with lab)	1
General physics (with lab)	1
Calculus	½
English	1

Science courses should be equivalent to course work required for college science majors. A broad background in the humanities is encouraged.

SELECTION FACTORS

All information available is utilized in the selection process. The most significant factors are intellect, achievement, character, interpersonal skills, and motivation. In evaluating candidates, consideration is given to the total academic record, the results of aptitude and achievement tests, college preprofessional committee evaluations, and the personal interview. Only those applicants whose personal qualifications, academic records, aptitude and achievement test scores, and preprofessional evaluations are considered sufficiently competitive and are invited for personal interviews. Only U.S. citizens or applicants with permanent visas are considered. Preference is given to legal residents of Texas. Up to 10 percent of the class may be filled with residents of other states.

Accepted applicants for the 1999 entering class had the following credentials: *average GPA,* 3.57; MCAT 27: *residence,* 98 percent from Texas.

FINANCIAL AID

Long-term, low-interest loans and short-term loans of varying interest rates are available to students with financial need. A number of scholarships funded by private donors are available. Most of these are based on need; some are based on academic achievement. A number of scholarships are available to disadvantaged students. Considerable individual attention is provided to students to help them with their fiscal planning, with debt management, and with exploring the various funding options. Applications for financial assistance are provided to students who have been accepted for admission and have indicated that they will attend the University of Texas Medical School at Galveston. There are no fixed deadlines. Inquiries must be directed to the Office of Student Fiscal Planning and Management.

INFORMATION FOR ECONOMICALLY AND DISADVANTAGED STUDENTS

The University of Texas Medical Branch at Galveston is committed to increasing the number of disadvantaged students in medicine. Each applicant is reviewed by experienced members of the Committee on Admissions with particular emphasis on the applicant's potential. Both cognitive and noncognitive qualifications are considered. There are no quotas, and all applicants are considered on the basis of individual achievement and promise. Following admission, a broad range of support services are available to assist students in completing the medical curriculum. Specific information about the services provided to applicants can be obtained by contacting the Office of Student Affairs. The University of Texas Medical Branch does not discriminate on the basis of race, sex, creed, national origin, age, or handicap.

Public Institution

APPLICATION AND ACCEPTANCE POLICIES FOR 2001–2002 FIRST-YEAR CLASS

Application must be made through the University of Texas System Medical and Dental Application Center, Suite 620, 702 Colorado, Austin, Texas 78701
Filing of application
- Earliest date: April 15, 2000
- Latest date: Oct. 15, 2000

School application fee: None
Application Center fees
- Resident: $45 for application to one school plus $5 for each additional school applied to in the University of Texas system
- Nonresident: $80 for application to one school plus $10 for each additional school applied to in the University of Texas system

Oldest MCAT scores considered: April 1, 1997
Does not have Early Decision Program
Acceptance notice to regular applicants
- Earliest date: Jan. 15, 2001
- Latest date: Until class is filled

Applicant's response to acceptance offer
- Maximum time: 2 weeks

Requests for deferred entrance considered: Yes
Deposit to hold place in class: None
Estimated number of new entrants: 200
Starting date: Aug. 2001

TUITION AND STUDENT FEES PER YEAR FOR 1999–2000 FIRST-YEAR CLASS

Tuition
- Resident: $6,550
- Nonresident: $19,650

Student fees: $530

INFORMATION ON 1999–2000 FIRST-YEAR CLASS

Number of	*In-State*	*Out-of-State*	*Total*
Applicants	2,287	378	2,665
Applicants Interviewed	1,223	66	1,289
New Entrants*	195	5	200

*All took the MCAT; 98% had baccalaureate degrees.

CHAPTER 11

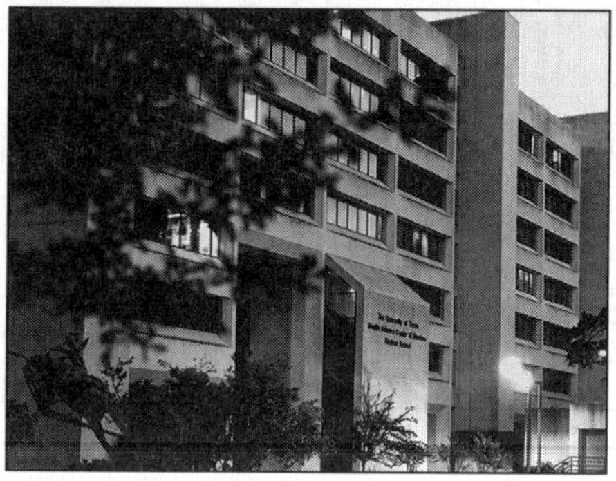

University of Texas—Houston Medical School

Houston, Texas

Dr. L. Maximilian Buja, *Dean*
Dr. Albert E. Gunn, *Associate Dean for Admissions*
Carolyn B. Sherman, *Coordinator of Admissions*

ADDRESS INQUIRIES TO:

Office of Admissions-Room G-024
University of Texas—
Houston Medical School
P.O. Box 20708
Houston, Texas 77225
(713) 500-5116; 500-0604 (FAX)
Web Site: http://www.med.uth.tmc.edu

MISSION STATEMENT

The mission of the University of Texas—Houston Medical School is to provide the highest quality of education and training of future physicians for the state of Texas, in harmony with the state's diverse population, and to conduct the highest caliber of research in the biomedical and health sciences.

We aim to provide an educational environment stressing primary care and quality care, and to prepare our students to serve all patients in need whatever their means; to make contributions to the understanding, prevention, and treatment of disease and injury; and to pursue a lifetime of study so that they will remain the best possible practitioners of medicine. The fulfillment of the academic mission requires the provision of exemplary clinical services, primacy in prevention, leadership in research and research training, and continuing education of graduates and other health care providers.

GENERAL INFORMATION

The University of Texas—Houston Medical School was authorized in May 1969 by the Texas Legislature. The Medical School is part of the University of Texas System.

The Medical School is located in the Texas Medical Center in Houston in order to take advantage of the many other medical institutions in the area. The major teaching hospital is Hermann Hospital, a 650-bed general medical and surgical hospital. Other major teaching hospitals include the University of Texas, M.D. Anderson Cancer Center, St. Joseph Hospital, San Jose Clinic, Southwest Memorial Hospital, and the Lyndon Baines Johnson Hospital, a facility of the Harris County Hospital District.

CURRICULUM

In September 1977 a four-year educational program began. The first two academic years are divided into four semesters. Three months of vacation time are provided for first-year students between the first and second academic years. The initial four semesters are devoted to preparing the student for the specific clerkship experiences that constitute the clinical years. During the first two academic years the student becomes familiar with the basic and applied biomedical sciences. As the student progresses from a study of the morphology of the human body and the fundamentals of molecular and cellular biology to that of the normal and abnormal structure and function of the various organ systems, the techniques of interviewing, history taking, and performance of physical and mental status examinations are introduced. Appropriate material from the behavioral sciences is presented concomitantly, as are opportunities to become familiar with the realities and problems of human medicine and family practice.

After completion of this educational sequence, the student progresses through a series of clinical clerkships in the major clinical disciplines for the next 12 months. In the remaining year, there are four months of required clerkships, four periods of electives, and one period reserved for additional instruction in medical jurisprudence, clinical epidemiology, medical ethics, and technical skills. In consultation with faculty, each student devises an educational sequence that relates specifically to ultimate career goals and postgraduate educational plans.

Problem-based learning is extensively employed in achieving the school's educational objectives.

REQUIREMENTS FOR ENTRANCE

Students must take the MCAT and complete at least 90 undergraduate credit hours at a U.S. or Canadian university. A baccalaureate degree is highly desirable and recommended. The specific premedical credits listed below are required.

	Sem. hrs.
Biology	14
One year must include lab.	
Inorganic chemistry (with lab)	8
Organic chemistry (with lab)	8
Physics (with lab)	8
Calculus	3
English	6

While the applicant should demonstrate aptitude for and achievement in the basic sciences, it is essential that an in-depth experience in some area of the humanities be obtained. Liberal arts majors are encouraged.

Applicants should take the MCAT in the spring of the year of application.

SELECTION FACTORS

Applicants are selected on the basis of motivation and potential for service, especially in the state of Texas. Academic ability is evaluated to ensure those who are accepted can complete medical studies. Emphasis is given to students who have a broad education and who display intellectual interest. A command of the language with ability to write and speak well is essential. The applicant's academic record is evaluated with special attention to the subjects taken and the demonstration of a broadly based comprehensive educational experience. The overall philosophy is that knowledge is an end in itself; while vocational-type curricula are not ruled out, liberal arts are preferred. Universities with core curricula generally provide the type of diversity sought in subject distribution. Significant attention is given to humanitarian endeavors, achievement in a nonacademic field of activity, and specific interest by the applicant in the University of Texas—Houston Medical School. Applicants are invited for personal interviews based on the admissions criteria. In the interview, which is an important element in the selection process, applicants are expected to cogently discuss their motivation and the experiences that led them to a medical career. It is also anticipated they will discuss their intellectual interests and generally demonstrate their suitability to enter a learned profession. Admission decisions are made in light of the school's mission, with preference given to Texas residents and those who will practice in shortage areas and specialties in the state. The University of Texas—Houston Medical School does not discriminate on the basis of race, sex, creed, national origin, age, or handicap.

Accepted students for the 1999 entering class had the following credentials: *mean GPA*, 3.60; *residence*, 99 percent from Texas; *mean MCAT*, 28.3, WS–P. For additional information concerning admissions criteria for the University of Texas—Houston Medical School, go to http://www.med.uth.tmc.edu/.

FINANCIAL AID

Scholarship and loan funds are available to students with financial need from local, state, federal, and national sources. Financial independence is not a criterion for admission as indicated by the fact that 60 percent of the students enrolled at present have received financial aid.

Public Institution

APPLICATION AND ACCEPTANCE POLICIES FOR 2001–2002 FIRST-YEAR CLASS

Application must be made through the
 Texas Medical and Dental Schools Application
 Center, Suite 6400,
 702 Colorado, Austin, Texas 78701
Filing of application
 Earliest date: June 15, 2000
 Latest date: Oct. 1, 2000
School application fee: None
Application Center fees
 Resident: $55 for application to one school plus $5 for each additional school applied to of those participating
 Nonresident: $90 for application to one school plus $10 for each additional school applied to of those participating
Oldest MCAT scores considered: 1995
Does not have Early Decision Program
Acceptance notice to regular applicants
 Earliest date: Jan. 15, 2001
 Latest date: Until class is filled
Applicant's response to acceptance offer
 Maximum time: 2 weeks
Requests for deferred entrance considered: No
Deposit to hold place in class: None
Estimated number of new entrants: 200
Starting date: Aug. 2001

TUITION AND STUDENT FEES PER YEAR FOR 1999–2000 FIRST-YEAR CLASS

Tuition
 Resident: $7,300
 Nonresident: $20,400

Student fees: $778

INFORMATION ON 1999–2000 FIRST-YEAR CLASS

Number of	*In-State*	*Out-of-State*	*Total*
Applicants	2,293	207	2,500
Applicants Interviewed	1,249	11	1,260
New Entrants*	200	2	202

*All took the MCAT; 99% had baccalaureate degrees.

CHAPTER 11

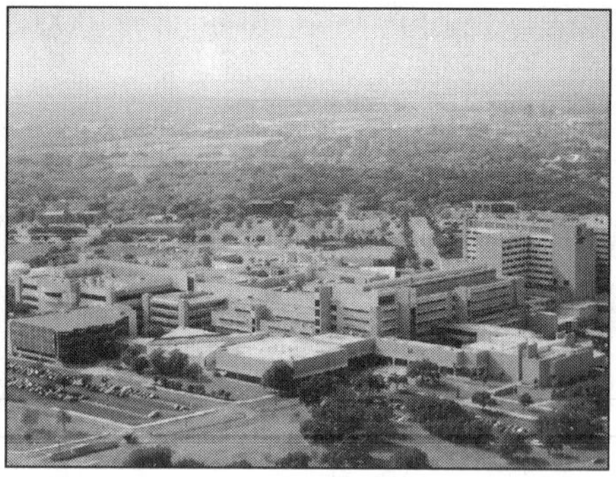

University of Texas Medical School at San Antonio

San Antonio, Texas

Dr. Stephen A. Wartman, *Dean*
Dr. David J. Jones, *Associate Dean for Admissions*

ADDRESS INQUIRIES TO:

Medical School Admissions
Registrar's Office
University of Texas Health Science Center at San Antonio
7703 Floyd Curl Drive
San Antonio, Texas 78229-7702
(210) 567-2665; 567-2685 (FAX)
E-mail: msprospect@uthscsa.edu
Web Site: http://www.uthscsa.edu

MISSION STATEMENT

The mission of the UTHSCSA Medical School is to serve the needs of the citizens of Texas by: providing medical education and training to medical students and physicians at all career levels with special commitment to the preparation of physicians for careers in the practice of primary health care; conducting biomedical and other health-related research; delivering exemplary quality health care; and providing a responsive resource in health-related affairs for the nation and the state, with particular emphasis on south Texas.

GENERAL INFORMATION

The University of Texas Medical School at San Antonio was created by the Texas Legislature in 1959 as a four-year school of medicine and graduated its first class in 1970. In late 1972 the Medical School and its fellow institutions, the Dental School, and the Graduate School of Biomedical Sciences were designated the University of Texas Health Science Center at San Antonio. Clinical instruction is carried out at the University Hospital, University Health Center, Audie Murphy Veterans Hospital, and affiliated hospitals, which include Wilford Hall USAF Hospital, Brooke Army Hospital, the Aerospace Medical Division of USAF, Baptist Memorial Hospital System, and Santa Rosa Medical Center.

CURRICULUM

A four-year curriculum is offered. The first month is devoted to an introduction to patient care, and throughout the first two years one-half day per week is devoted to clinical integration activities. In the first year, the traditional basic science courses are taught. The second year is anchored by the pathology course, and it incorporates pharmacology, medicine, pediatrics, obstetrics and gynecology, and surgery coordinated by organ systems. Behavioral sciences and an introduction to psychiatry are also included. The third academic year is spent entirely in the clinical setting in eight consecutive assignments of six weeks each in family practice, medicine, the medical specialties, surgery, the surgical specialties, obstetrics and gynecology, psychiatry, and pediatrics. The senior year includes a didactic period of two months, with the rest of the academic year consisting of elective courses. Some time is also available to the students for interviews for postgraduate training or for vacation. A letter grading system is used.

REQUIREMENTS FOR ENTRANCE

The MCAT and the equivalent of three academic years (90 semester hours) are required for admission. Courses specifically required (with a grade of C or better) are:

	Sem. Hrs.
Biology	14
One year must include lab.	
Inorganic chemistry (with lab)	8
Organic chemistry (with lab)	8
General physics (with lab)	8
Calculus	3
English	6

Science courses should be equivalent to course work as required for college science majors. Candidates are desired who have a broad humanities background.

SELECTION FACTORS

Ranking of applicants is done with consideration for GPA; separate MCAT component scores; evaluation by premedical advisors; the candidate's potential relative to society's health care needs; and judgment by the Committee on Admissions of the candidate's nonacademic achievements and personal qualifications such as responsibility, integrity, maturity, and motivation. No person shall be excluded from participation in, denied the benefits of, or subject to discrimination under any program or activity sponsored or conducted by the University of Texas System on the basis of age, race, national origin, religion, or sex. Although legal residents of Texas are preferred, up to 10 percent of entrants may be nonresidents if their credentials are especially outstanding.

Accepted students for the 1999 entering class had the following credentials: *mean GPA,* 3.45 (range 2.9–4.0); *mean*

MCAT 28 (range 20–35); *sex*, 52 percent women; *residence*, 4 percent nonresidents; *overall acceptance rate*, 250 acceptances were offered to obtain a class of 200 first-year students.

Application forms and any procedural information should be obtained from the Texas Medical and Dental Schools Application Service in the adjacent box.

Questions related to completeness of an application or other information should be directed to the Office of Student Services, Medical Admissions at the Health Science Center.

FINANCIAL AID

Financial assistance for students in need is available in the form of loans and a limited number of scholarships. Student employment, though not encouraged, is permissible provided a satisfactory level of achievement is maintained. Part-time student employment opportunities are available at the Health Science Center as well as in the hospitals located in close proximity. Financial considerations do not influence admission decisions, although the school recognizes that many families are unable to bear the full cost of medical education. Accepted applicants can obtain complete information regarding financial assistance from the financial aid administrator in the Office of Student Services (http://www.uthscsa.edu/students.html).

Public Institution

APPLICATION AND ACCEPTANCE POLICIES FOR 2001–2002 FIRST-YEAR CLASS

Application must be made through the
Texas Medical and Dental Schools Application Service, Suite 6400, 702 Colorado, Austin, Texas 78701
via: http://dpweb1.dp.utexas.edu/mdac
Filing of application
Earliest date: May 1, 2000
Latest date: Oct. 15, 2000
School application fee: None
Application Center fees
Resident: $55 for application to one school plus $5 for each additional school
Nonresident: $90 for application to one school plus $10 for each additional school
Oldest MCAT scores considered: 1997
Does not have Early Decision Program
Acceptance notice to regular applicants
Earliest date: Jan. 15, 2001
Latest date: Until class is filled
Applicant's response to acceptance offer
Maximum time: 2 weeks
Requests for deferred entrance considered: Yes
Deposit to hold place in class: None
Estimated number of new entrants: 200
Starting date: July 2001

TUITION AND STUDENT FEES PER YEAR FOR 1999–2000 FIRST-YEAR CLASS

Tuition
Resident: $6,550
Nonresident: $19,650

Student fees: $670

INFORMATION ON 1999–2000 FIRST-YEAR CLASS

Number of	*In-State*	*Out-of-State*	*Total*
Applicants	2,248	399	2,647
Applicants Interviewed	948	199	1,147
New Entrants*	196	8	204

*All took the MCAT; 98% had baccalaureate degrees.

CHAPTER 11

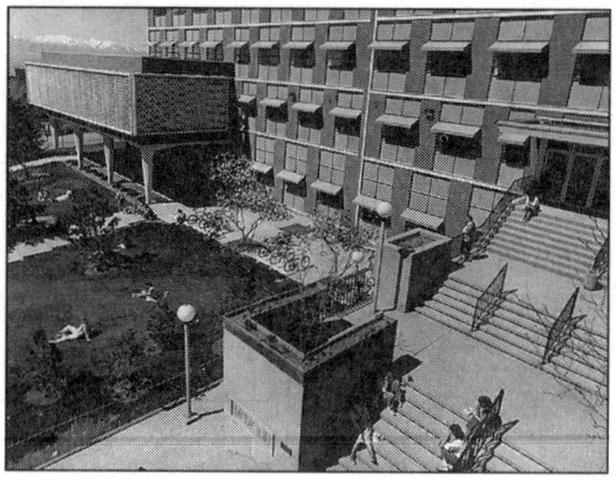

University of Utah School of Medicine

Salt Lake City, Utah

Dr. Lorris Betz, *Sr. Vice President for Health Sciences and Dean, School of Medicine*
Dr. Samuel Shomaker, *Sr. Assoc. Dean, Academic Affairs*
Dr. Victoria E. Judd, *Associate Dean, Admissions and Community Outreach*

ADDRESS INQUIRIES TO:

Kathy Z. Doulis
Director, Admissions
University of Utah
50 North Medical Drive Room 1C029
Salt Lake City, Utah 84132
(801) 581-7498; FAX (801) 585-3300
E-mail: deans.admissions@hsc.utah.edu
Web Site: http://med.utah.edu/som

GENERAL INFORMATION

The School of Medicine was founded as a two-year school in 1904 and expanded to a four-year program in 1942. It is one of the 17 colleges of the University of Utah. The medical school is a component of the University of Utah Health Sciences Center, which also includes colleges of pharmacy, nursing, and health; a health sciences library; Howard Hughes Medical Institute; Eccles Program in Human Molecular Biology and Genetics; Utah Genome Center; Utah Cancer Center; Huntsman Cancer Institute; several other centers for special studies; the Moran Eye Center; and the University of Utah Hospitals and Clinics.

CURRICULUM

The University of Utah School of Medicine implemented a new curriculum during the 1997–1998 academic year, which emphasizes active learning approaches, critical thinking skills, and information management techniques. Our curriculum builds upon the strengths of the traditional one and, in addition, explores areas of study opened up by the explosion of biomedical knowledge and the transformation of America's health-care delivery system. The goal of the curriculum is to produce highly skilled physicians who are technically proficient, caring, and compassionate, and flexible enough to adapt to the changing demands they will face in the 21st-century medical environment.

In the first two years of medical school, students will receive a solid foundation in the sciences basic to medicine, including gross anatomy, embryology, histology, psychiatry, biochemistry, pharmacology, immunology, microbiology, genetics, physiology, pathology, and organ system pathophysiology. Courses cover such topics as health-care financing and delivery, community and public health, research methodology and medical literature analysis, biostatistics, and epidemiology. The critical skills of communicating with, examining, and diagnosing patients are also covered in depth.

The third year of the curriculum centers on clinical clerkships in internal medicine, surgery, obstetrics and gynecology, pediatrics, family practice, psychiatry, and neurology.

During the fourth year a preceptorship in primary care medicine gives students a broader perspective on the health-care issues facing medically underserved rural and urban areas; students generally live in the underserved area during the six-week preceptorship. Ample elective time is available for students to pursue areas of particular interest. Finally, a required sub-internship will serve as a transition to residency. Students with the help of faculty advisors will apply to various postgraduate residency-training programs through the National Resident Matching Program.

REQUIREMENTS FOR ENTRANCE

The MCAT is required and must be taken within three years of application. The Admissions Committee is eager to admit students with a broad perspective of life. The school believes that the true physician not only is skilled in medicine and the allied sciences but also is a person of culture and broad intelligence.

In addition to a bachelor's degree the applicant must have subject matter competence in the following courses:

Chemistry: Two years; the general chemistry series including quantitative and qualitative analysis (AP credit accepted if at a level 4 or 5), and the organic series (AP credit not accepted), both with a laboratory.
Physics: One year with a laboratory (AP credit not accepted).
English: One year of English writing/speech courses. The courses taken must fulfill the institution writing/composition classification (AP credit not accepted).
Biology: Two college courses in biology. One course must be in cellular biology or biochemistry (No substitutions, AP credit not accepted).
Social Science: A college course in social science (AP credit not accepted).
Humanities: A college course in humanities (AP credit not accepted).

With the exception of advanced placement credit for general chemistry at a level of 4 or 5, CLEP, advanced placement, and home study credit will not be accepted for completion of required course work. All premedical courses must be completed at an accredited college or university in the United States or Canada.

Completion of four years of college work and a bachelor's degree are required before entering the School of Medicine.

Only those students who have completed most of their undergraduate training in a U.S. or Canadian school will be considered.

SELECTION FACTORS

Students are considered on the basis of scholarship; extracurricular activities including volunteer work, research, and community work; letters of recommendation; and assessment of personality, character, maturity, motivation, and exposure to medicine. The School of Medicine is state-assisted, and a majority of its admissions are Utah residents. The medical school has special arrangements with the state of Idaho to provide six positions for certified residents of this state. Competition for the few remaining nonresident positions is very keen. Nonresident applicants, excluding Idaho, and those who qualify to apply with the diversity initiative, are required to apply through the Early Decision Program. Nonresidents with background or ties to Utah, or who are applying to the M.D.-Ph.D. program, may petition to have their application considered during the regular process.

The School of Medicine does not discriminate on the basis of age, color, gender, sexual orientation, race, national origin, religion, veteran status, or disability. The selection process conducted by the committee is the same for all applicants. The University of Utah provides reasonable accommodations to the known disabilities of applicants.

Applications should be filed no later than October 15 through AMCAS. The Admissions Committee will notify eligible candidates concerning interview appointments. Final selections are made by majority vote of the committee.

No more than three consecutive applications will be accepted from any one candidate. Transfer positions are not available unless the transfering student's spouse is on the medical school faculty or in a postgraduate residency training program.

FINANCIAL AID

In addition to the Federal subsidized and unsubsidized Stafford Loans and the Federal Perkins Loan, a limited number of institutional loans and scholarships are awarded each year. All awards are based on the student's need as determined by the university's Financial Aid Office. However, remember that financial aid is supplementary to the contribution that can be made by the student and/or family. The student and family are expected to provide the maximum assistance possible.

THE OFFICE OF DIVERSITY AND COMMUNITY OUTREACH

Under the direction of the associate dean of diversity and community outreach, this office assists the School of Medicine in fulfilling its commitment to recruiting, admitting, and graduating a diverse student body. The office works closely with students from diverse backgrounds, including students from rural Utah communities; students who are educationally, socially, or financially disadvantaged; and students from those minority groups specifically recognized by the Association of American Medical Colleges: African Americans, American Indians, mainland Puerto Ricans, Mexican Americans, and native Hawaiians. The office provides academic advising and assistance to these students in their preparation for and application to medical school, and presents a series of precollege and premedical educational outreach programs throughout the state. The office also seeks to assure retention of matriculated students through counseling, academic guidance, and support services.

Public Institution

APPLICATION AND ACCEPTANCE POLICIES FOR 2001–2002 FIRST-YEAR CLASS

School participates in AMCAS. See Chapter 6.

Filing of AMCAS application
  Earliest date: June 1, 2000
  Latest date: Oct. 15, 2000
School application fee to all applicants: $60
Oldest MCAT scores considered: 1997
Does have Early Decision Program (EDP)
  Nonresidents must apply through EDP
  EDP application period: June 1–Aug. 1, 2000
  EDP applicants notified by: Oct. 1, 2000
Acceptance notice to regular applicants
  Earliest date: Nov. 1, 2000
  Latest date: Until class is filled
Applicant's response to acceptance offer
  Maximum time: 2 weeks
Requests for deferred entrance considered: No
Deposit to hold place in class (applied to tuition):
  $100, due with response to acceptance offer
Deposit refundable prior to: May 15, 2001
Estimated number of new entrants: 100 (5 EDP)
Starting date: Aug. 2001

TUITION AND STUDENT FEES PER YEAR FOR 1999–2000 FIRST-YEAR CLASS

Tuition
  Resident: $9,629
  Nonresident: $18,229

Student fees: $545

INFORMATION ON 1999–2000 FIRST-YEAR CLASS

Number of	*In-State*	*Out-of-State*	*Total*
Applicants	414	896	1,310
Applicants Interviewed	275	166	441
New Entrants*	75	27	102

*All took the MCAT and had baccalaureate degrees.

CHAPTER 11

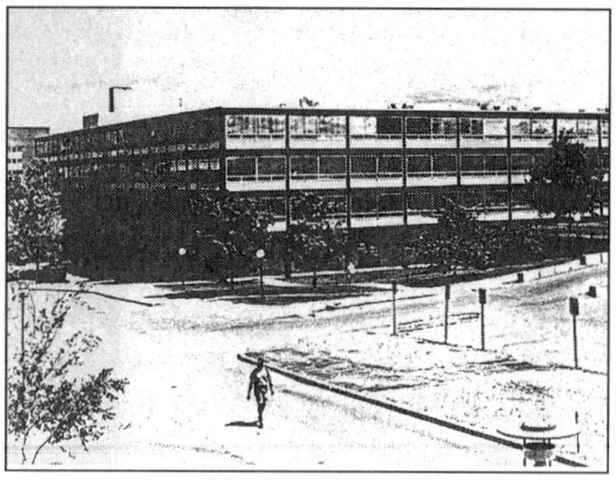

University of Vermont College of Medicine

Burlington, Vermont

Dr. John Frymoyer, *Dean*
Dr. Cathleen J. Gleeson, *Director of Admissions*
Sean McGivney, *Financial Aid Officer*

ADDRESS INQUIRIES TO:

Admissions Office
C-225 Given Building
University of Vermont
College of Medicine
Burlington, Vermont 05405
(802) 656-2154
Web Site: http://www.med.uvm.edu

GENERAL INFORMATION

The University of Vermont College of Medicine is located on the eastern shore of Lake Champlain in the city of Burlington, Vermont, a community of about 38,000 people. Established in 1822, it is the seventh oldest medical school in the United States. The College of Medicine recognizes the need for primary care physicians, clinical specialists, and research scientists. Our curriculum provides a general professional education in both basic and clinical sciences, followed by a period structured to meet each student's individual goals.

Our principal teaching hospital is Fletcher Allen Health Care's Medical Center Hospital of Vermont Campus, a 500-bed hospital adjacent to the College of Medicine. The hospital provides community care for Burlington and the surrounding communities and tertiary referral care for patients from the entire state of Vermont and from the northern Adirondack region of New York State.

CURRICULUM

The College of Medicine is committed to preparing students to become excellent practicing physicians, teachers, and scientific investigators.

The curriculum is divided into three phases. The first phase consists of one and one-half years of instruction in the basic sciences. A clinical course called Doctoring Skills, which prepares the student for the study of medicine by the study of patients, is presented throughout this portion of the curriculum. The second phase, 12 months in length, is devoted to the clinical sciences of medicine. These two segments are designed to provide students with a broad, general professional education. The final phase of the curriculum, the Senior Selective Program, extends through the one and one-half years prior to graduation. This program enables students to select a course of study and experience best suited to their career objectives. Twelve months of this final period are available for electives at Fletcher Allen Health Care, elsewhere in the United States, or abroad.

We use an honors/pass/fail method of grading, coupled with individual narrative evaluations of performance in clinical rotations.

During the Basic Science Core, a parallel program called the Vermont Generalist Curriculum helps students translate classroom learning into clinical practice—especially primary care practice.

The Vermont Generalist Curriculum consists of three courses. The Physician and Society course explores the human issues of being a physician as well as the ethical, social, cultural, and psychological factors affecting health and illness. The Doctoring Skills course provides training in physical examination, interviewing patients, and technical skills such as drawing blood and starting intravenous lines. Beginning in the second semester, a year-long course called Doctoring in Vermont places each student in the office of a generalist physician from family practice, internal medicine, or pediatrics for four hours every other week. Doctoring in Vermont also involves a community project in which students learn about community agencies and see firsthand how agencies influence health care in the community.

The University of Vermont is developing an integrated, competency-based, patient-centered curriculum. Students are involved in all aspects, including new project development. The fall curriculum will be in place in 2002.

REQUIREMENTS FOR ENTRANCE

The MCAT is required and must be taken by August of the application year. Applicants must have completed at least three years of undergraduate study in an accredited college or university in the United States or Canada; the baccalaureate degree is highly desirable. Applicants are urged to take the MCAT in the spring of the year of application and to have their basic premedical requirements completed at the time of application. The undergraduate program must include the following course work:

	Years/Credit Hours
Biology (with lab)	1/8
General chemistry (with lab)	1/8
Organic chemistry (with lab)	1/8
General physics (with lab)	1/8

Secondary school advanced placement courses will be recognized only if credit for them appears on the college transcript.

SELECTION FACTORS

The Committee on Admissions seeks a heterogeneous student body. We look for evidence of the promise of excellence accompanied by genuine concern for the welfare of others. Effective interpersonal skills are considered especially important. Significant experience in health care or other direct human services, either as an employee or as a volunteer, is expected of all applicants. The University of Vermont does not discriminate on the basis of race, color, sex, sexual orientation, religion, age, handicap, national origin, or Vietnam veteran status. All applicants receive a secondary application.

Selection of an applicant for admission is based upon the past pattern of academic performance plus an assessment of the applicant's fitness for the study and practice of medicine in terms of aptitude, interests, experience, motivation, attitudes, and maturity. Letters of recommendation and a personal interview form an important part of the application process. The interview is required and is by invitation. We do not offer off-campus interviews.

Preference for admission is given to well-qualified residents of Vermont and states that have contractual arrangements with the university (currently Maine). However, significant numbers of openings remain for qualified residents of other states. Members of minority groups are encouraged to apply for admission.

Transfer Students—The unique structure of the curriculum, and the minimal student attrition, generally precludes accepting transfer students. However, after January 1, students wishing to explore the possibility of transferring may request an application that outlines requirements for transfer. Students who transfer generally complete two years of school elsewhere and then enroll at the beginning or middle of the second year at the University of Vermont. Decisions may be delayed until August.

The 1999 entering class had the following characteristics: *mean GPA,* 3.4; *mean MCAT,* 9.0; *sex,* 54 percent female; 46 percent male; *residence,* 31 from Vermont, 10 from Maine, 54 from other states; *undergraduate major,* 72 percent in the natural or biological sciences; *overall acceptance rate:* 5,805 applications received, 516 applicants interviewed, 177 acceptances offered to obtain a class of 95 students.

Because of the November 1 deadline, early application is recommended. Extensions are not granted.

FINANCIAL AID

Financial aid funds are limited and are primarily in the form of loans. Funds are distributed according to relative need. Entering students are considered for awards on the same basis as those already enrolled. An applicant's financial status has no bearing on admission determination.

Public Institution

APPLICATION AND ACCEPTANCE POLICIES FOR 2001–2002 FIRST-YEAR CLASS

School participates in AMCAS. See Chapter 6.

Filing of AMCAS application
  Earliest date: June 1, 2000
  Latest date: Nov. 1, 2000
School application fee to all applicants: $80
Oldest MCAT scores considered: 1997
Does have Early Decision Program (EDP)
  EDP application period: June 1–Aug. 1, 2000
  EDP applicants notified by: Oct. 1, 2000
Acceptance notice to regular applicants
  Earliest date: Dec. 10, 2000
  Latest date: Until class is filled
Applicant's response to acceptance offer
  Maximum time: 2 weeks
Requests for deferred entrance considered: Yes
Deposit to hold place in class (applied to tuition):
  $100, due with response to acceptance offer
Deposit refundable prior to: May 15, 2001
Estimated number of new entrants: 93 (15 EDP)
Starting date: Aug. 2001

TUITION AND STUDENT FEES PER YEAR FOR 1999–2000 FIRST-YEAR CLASS

Tuition
  Resident: $19,060
  Nonresident: $33,360

Student fees: $717

INFORMATION ON 1999–2000 FIRST-YEAR CLASS

Number of	*In-State*	*Out-of-State*	*Total*
Applicants	86	5,719	5,805
Applicants Interviewed	49	467	516
New Entrants*	31	64	95

*All took the MCAT and had baccalaureate degrees.

CHAPTER 11

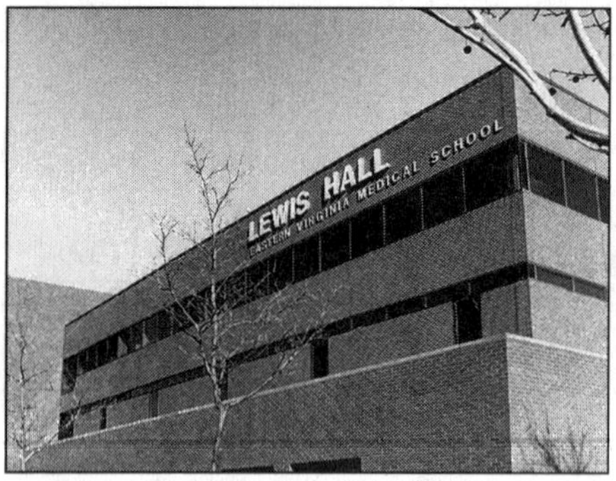

Eastern Virginia Medical School of the Medical College of Hampton Roads

Norfolk, Virginia

Dr. James E. Etheridge, Jr., *Interim Dean/Provost*
Dr. Donald W. Lewis, *Associate Dean for Admissions*
Susan L. Castora, *Director of Admissions*

ADDRESS INQUIRIES TO:

Office of Admissions
Eastern Virginia Medical School
721 Fairfax Avenue
Norfolk, Virginia 23507-2000
(757) 446-5812; 446-5896 (FAX)
Web Site: http://www.evms.edu

MISSION STATEMENT

The Eastern Virginia Medical School is a private community-based academic institution dedicated to medical and health education, biomedical research, and the enhancement of health care in the Commonwealth of Virginia.

GENERAL INFORMATION

The Eastern Virginia Medical School (EVMS) was established in 1973 in response to the desire of the Hampton Roads community to enhance the quality and diversity of health care throughout the region. Because of its history, the mission of EVMS is deeply rooted in the education and training of primary care physicians. This mission has been recently revitalized through a series of innovative programs established through the Center for Generalist Medicine. The additional benefit achieved by the creation of an academic health center has been the promotion and expansion of medical research and the development of several centers of excellence such as the Jones Institute for Reproductive Medicine, the Center for Pediatric Research, the Strelitz Diabetes Institute, and the Glennan Center for Geriatric Medicine.

Through its affiliation with over 33 health care facilities, including Sentara Norfolk General Hospital, the Children's Hospital of the Kings Daughters, the U.S. Naval Medical Center in Portsmouth, and the Veteran's Administration Hospital in Hampton, EVMS provides health care for more than one quarter of Virginia's population as well as neighboring regions of North Carolina. EVMS provides a community-based educational program arming students with the requisite scientific, academic, and humanistic skills most relevant to practicing medicine into the twenty-first century. Two hundred and ninety full-time faculty and over a thousand community faculty provide students with exposure to a broad range of clinical experiences and to the diversity of medical care delivery systems.

CURRICULUM

The curriculum has been designed to educate students in both the science of human biology and art of the practice of medicine. Throughout the first two years, students are introduced to clinical medicine through two vehicles: the nationally recognized Theresa A. Thomas Professional Skills Teaching and Assessment Center laboratory utilizing standardized patients and a one-on-one longitudinal mentorship with a generalist physician in community practice. Careful coordination between basic sciences and generalist disciplines permits an integrated curriculum, so that students can appreciate the clinical correlation to their scientific studies. Weekly small-group sessions, facilitated by basic scientists and clinical scholars, introduce students to clinical problem solving. Areas covered relate to clinical skills development, including medical interviewing, doctor-patient relationships, and medical ethics. In sum, through this early introduction to clinical medicine, students learn the medical art of history taking and physician examination along with the application of basic science knowledge to patient care.

A substantial part of clinical clerkships focus on ambulatory care in community-based sites in balance with basic inpatient care experiences. In addition to the required clerkships in family medicine, internal medicine, pediatrics, obstetrics and gynecology, psychiatry, and surgery are rotations in substance abuse, geriatrics, and surgical subspecialties. For those interested in generalist medicine, electives are offered in special populations, rural health care, and an elective honors track in generalist medicine. For those interested in research or subspecialty care, at least six months are available in elective opportunities. The Jones Institute for Women's Health, the Diabetes Center, and the Center for Pediatric Research are but a few of the excellent resources to enhance skills in research.

Evaluation of clinical skills is a central component of the education process through the use of standardized patients. Overall, students are graded as honors, high pass, pass, or fail.

EVMS offers combined programs (B.S.-M.D.) with several colleges and universities within the state allowing outstanding high school and undergraduate students the opportunity to explore varied educational and life experiences as they prepare for a career in medicine.

REQUIREMENTS FOR ENTRANCE

The MCAT and a minimum of 100 college semester hours at an accredited American or Canadian college or university are required. Course work must include the following subjects:

	Years
Biology (with lab)	1

General chemistry (with lab) 1
Organic chemistry (with lab) 1
Physics (with lab) 1

Applicants are expected to have grades of C or better in all required courses. Credits earned through advanced placement programs or CLEP are acceptable. Applicants may enhance their chances of acceptance by taking graduate course work in a natural science. In recent years, students matriculating at EVMS have had a *mean GPA* of 3.41 and have averaged 10 in each subject area of the MCAT.

SELECTION FACTORS

EVMS does not discriminate on the basis of sex, race, creed, age, national origin, marital status, or handicap. After obtaining a completed AMCAS application, a supplementary application packet is sent to those applicants receiving a favorable initial screening, based on both objective and subjective factors, including grades, MCAT scores, medical exposure, and life experience.

For each applicant, the Admissions Committee considers the entire academic record, including science and overall GPA, MCAT scores, exposure to the medical field, maturity, character, and motivation. The application fee will be waived if a fee waiver is granted by AMCAS. Foreign nationals without permanent visas cannot be considered.

Preference is given to legal residents of Virginia. In addition, recognizing the goals set by the Virginia legislature, EVMS is seeking persons with personal and background traits, that indicate a high potential for becoming a family physician, general pediatrician, general internist, or general obstetrician.

Applicants who have completed one or more years in a medical school accredited by the Association of American Medical Colleges can be considered for transfer into the second or third year of our curriculum only to fill vacancies that may arise with the withdrawal of previously enrolled students. All transfers must meet the requirements stated for general admission.

FINANCIAL AID

The ability of a student to provide for the costs of education is not a factor in the admissions selection process. Over 90 percent of the student body receives financial assistance. Scholarships are limited, and loans constitute the majority of aid received. Students may fully meet the costs of medical school at EVMS, providing they meet all federal criteria, meet citizenship requirements, are creditworthy, and maintain satisfactory academic progress. For those interested in a primary care obligation, there are numerous federal and state scholarships available. Virginia residents also benefit from the state-funded Tuition Assistance Grant Program (TAGP), which provides annual grants of approximately $2,700.

Applicants for financial assistance must file the cost-free FAFSA and other additional required forms. For additional details and assistance in financial planning, please contact the Office of Financial Aid at (757) 446-5813.

INFORMATION FOR MINORITY STUDENTS

Minority students are strongly encouraged to apply. Every effort is made to evaluate these applicants giving due consideration to variances in educational and socioeconomic backgrounds. Academic scholarships are available each year for black students. EVMS has college-endorsed student organizations and faculty liaison committees that actively address minority concerns. Information is available from the minority affairs counselor and the assistant dean for minority affairs.

Private Institution

APPLICATION AND ACCEPTANCE POLICIES FOR 2001–2002 FIRST-YEAR CLASS

School participates in AMCAS. See Chapter 6.

Filing of AMCAS application
  Earliest date: June 1, 2000
  Latest date: Nov. 15, 2000
School application fee after screening: $85
Oldest MCAT scores considered: 1998
Does have Early Decision Program (EDP)
  EDP application period: June 1–Aug. 1, 2000
  EDP applicants notified by: Oct. 1, 2000
Acceptance notice to regular applicants
  Earliest date: Oct. 15, 2000
  Latest date: Until class is filled
Applicant's response to acceptance offer
  Maximum time: 2 weeks
Requests for deferred entrance considered: Yes
Deposit to hold place in class (applied to tuition):
  $200, due with response to acceptance offer
Deposit refundable prior to: May 15, 2001
Estimated number of new entrants: 100 (8 EDP)
Starting date: Aug. 2001

TUITION AND STUDENT FEES PER YEAR FOR 1999–2000 FIRST-YEAR CLASS

Tuition
  Resident: $15,000
  Nonresident: $27,500
Student fees: $2,390

INFORMATION ON 1999–2000 FIRST-YEAR CLASS

Number of	*In-State*	*Out-of-State*	*Total*
Applicants	819	3,116	3,935
Applicants Interviewed	310	212	522
New Entrants*	77	25	102

*All had baccalaureate degrees; 92% took the MCAT.

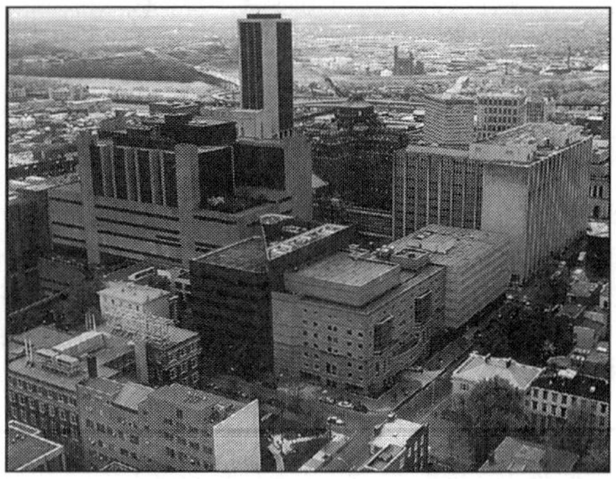

Virginia Commonwealth University School of Medicine

Richmond, Virginia

Dr. Hermes A. Kontos, *Dean*
Dr. Cynthia M. Heldberg, *Associate Dean for Admissions*
Sean Bates, *Assistant Director for Financial Aid*

ADDRESS INQUIRIES TO:

Virginia Commonwealth University
School of Medicine
P.O. Box 980565
Richmond, Virginia 23298-0565
(804) 828-9629; 828-1246 (FAX)
Web Site: http://www.medschool.vcu.edu

GENERAL INFORMATION

The School of Medicine, which has been in continuous operation since 1838, is the founding institution of the Medical College of Virginia, Campus of Virginia Commonwealth University. The health science campus includes not only the school of medicine but also the only school of dentistry in the state plus schools of nursing, pharmacy, and allied health professions. The vitality of the Medical College of Virginia's campus research programs is reflected in the caliber of its faculty, the success of its patient care programs, and the level of research funding generated. Since the mid-1970s, federally funded research has shown a straight-line growth rate, due in part to the MCV Clinical Research Center, a program funded by the federal government since 1961. With 1,000 hospital beds at the main campus, the largest emergency room, and the largest neonatal intensive care unit in the state, plus 800 beds at one of the newest VA hospitals in the South, the Medical College of Virginia campus is one of the largest university-owned medical centers in the United States and affords its students an unparalleled clinical experience. The campus is located near the financial and governmental areas of downtown Richmond, the capital of Virginia and one of the South's most historic and cosmopolitan cities.

CURRICULUM

The first year is spent studying normal structure and function in a traditional discipline format. The second year emphasizes pathogenesis of disease and its manifestations and is taught in an organ system manner. Pathogenesis, pathology, pharmacology, and the major manifestations and principles of management are discussed in each of the major body systems.

There is a longitudinal experience in clinical medicine for first- and second-year students. Students spend two afternoons per month in a small group learning the fundamentals of clinical medicine. This is supplemented by a clinical experience in the office of a primary care physician two afternoons per month. This unique clinical experience is integrated with the basic science curriculum in a way that enhances and enriches the student's learning. There is a computer lab with over 40 workstations and a full array of commercial and in-house, faculty-developed educational software.

In the third year, the clinical rotations are at the University and Veterans Administration Hospitals, with ambulatory care rotations at nonuniversity primary care sites. Computer educational workstations, distributed throughout the hospitals and clinics, give students access to the university library databases, expert decision support systems, and educational software programs.

During the fourth year, the student may choose from a wide variety of electives both at the university and throughout the United States. Additionally there are elective programs serving the first and second years.

REQUIREMENTS FOR ENTRANCE

The MCAT is required. A demonstrated competence in basic science is essential, although a science major is not required. Each matriculant must have at least 90 semester hours or equivalent in an accredited college. Courses must include:

	Semesters
Biology (with lab)	2
General chemistry (with lab)	2
Organic chemistry (with lab)	2
General physics (with lab)	2
College mathematics	2
English	2

Applicants are urged to take the MCAT in the spring of the year of application and no later than the fall of that year. Early Decision Program applicants must have MCAT scores available when applying. The school has a guaranteed admissions program with Virginia Commonwealth University's undergraduate honors program. High school seniors who have 1270 or better on their SATs and a GPA of 3.5 may apply. They must complete the usual premed requirements, all honors program requirements, and maintain a 3.5 GPA throughout their undergraduate years.

SELECTION FACTORS

Applicants are selected on the basis of their potential as prospective physicians as well as students of medicine. Attributes of character, personality factors, academic skills, and exposure to medicine are considered along with academic performance, GPA, MCAT scores, letters of recommendation, and personal interviews at the School of Medicine.

The school gives preference to bona fide residents of the Commonwealth of Virginia and does not discriminate on the basis of age, race, sex, creed, national origin, or handicap. Foreign nationals must be permanent residents at the time of application.

The 1999 entering class of 172 students had the following credentials: *undergraduate major,* 25 percent in arts or humanities, 65 percent in sciences; *degrees,* 10 percent with graduate degrees, including one doctorate degree; *residence,* 70 percent Virginia residents; *minorities,* 4.65 percent black; *sex,* 43 percent women; *overall undergraduate GPA,* 3.48; *MCAT average score,* 9.9.

The uniform acceptance date is October 15 with additional selections in December, January, and February. Applicants who have been rejected in previous years should demonstrate significant improvement in their academic credentials before reapplying.

FINANCIAL AID

Assistance to students in meeting the cost of their medical education is available in the form of loans and scholarships, and financial counseling offered by the Financial Aid Office of the School of Medicine. The Free Application for Federal Student Aid (FAFSA) is used in awarding need-based aid (see Part 1). Parent information should be included on this form to be considered for the Department of Health and Human Services programs.

The School of Medicine's Financial Aid Office administers all major federal aid programs and coordinates with the School of Medicine in the administration of state, private, and institutional scholarships and loans. The Financial Aid Office responds to requests for information within 24 hours. Application forms and aid fact sheets are available in mid-January of each year. Applications for aid may be made prior to notification of acceptance by the School of Medicine. The Federal Identification number for VCU is 003735. This must appear on the FAFSA. Applicants are encouraged to seek all resources available to them and apply as early as feasible to maximize the possibility of obtaining funding. Ninety-one percent of the medical students receive some aid, and 42 percent receive School of Medicine scholarships of varying amounts. Financial assistance is not available to students who are not U.S. citizens or permanent residents.

Information may be obtained from the following address: Financial Aid Office, VCU School of Medicine, P.O. Box 980565, Richmond, Virginia 23298; the location is 11th and Broad Streets in Richmond.

Public Institution

APPLICATION AND ACCEPTANCE POLICIES FOR 2001–2002 FIRST-YEAR CLASS

School participates in AMCAS. See Chapter 6.

Filing of AMCAS application
  Earliest date: June 1, 2000
  Latest date: Nov. 15, 2000
School application fee after screening: $75
Oldest MCAT scores considered: 1997
Does have Early Decision Program (EDP)
  EDP application period: June 1–Aug. 1, 2000
  EDP applicants notified by: Oct. 1, 2000
Acceptance notice to regular applicants
  Earliest date: Oct. 15, 2000
  Latest date: Until class is filled
Applicant's response to acceptance offer
  Maximum time: 2 weeks
Requests for deferred entrance considered: Yes
Deposit to hold place in class (applied to tuition):
  $100, due with response to acceptance offer
Deposit refundable prior to: May 15, 2001
Estimated number of new entrants: 172 (20 EDP)
Starting date: Aug. 2001

TUITION AND STUDENT FEES PER YEAR FOR 1999–2000 FIRST-YEAR CLASS

Tuition
  Resident: $10,428
  Nonresident: $26,734

Student fees: $1,198

INFORMATION ON 1999–2000 FIRST-YEAR CLASS

Number of	*In-State*	*Out-of-State*	*Total*
Applicants	882	3,245	4,127
Applicants Interviewed	355	216	571
New Entrants*	121	51	172

*All had baccalaureate degrees; 94% took the MCAT.

CHAPTER 11

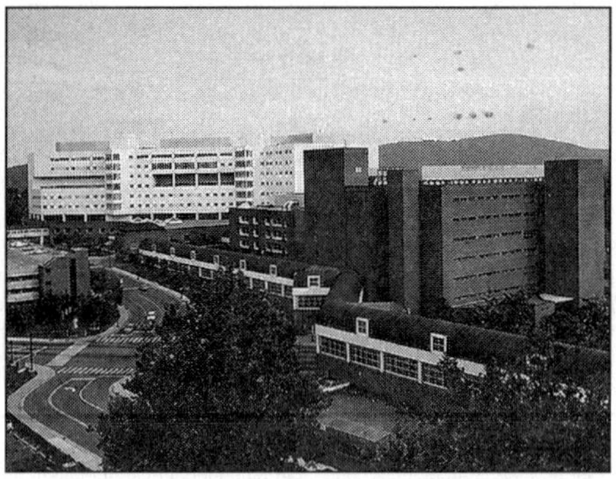

University of Virginia School of Medicine

Charlottesville, Virginia

Dr. Robert M. Carey, *Dean*
Dr. B. C. Sturgill, *Associate Dean for Admissions*
Beth A. Bailey, *Director of Admissions*

ADDRESS INQUIRIES TO:

Medical School Admissions Office, Box 235
University of Virginia
School of Medicine
Charlottesville, Virginia 22908
(804) 924-5571; 982-2586 (FAX)
Web Site: http://www.med.virginia.edu/home.html

MISSION STATEMENT

The mission of the University of Virginia School of Medicine is:

- To educate students in the health sciences in order to fulfill the need for practitioners and scientists;
- To provide cost-effective, high-quality patient care at primary, secondary, and tertiary levels as needed by the citizens of the region and nation;
- To produce new knowledge required to advance health by conducting research in the basic, clinical, and social sciences; and,
- To provide public service as needed by citizens or by public jurisdictions.

GENERAL INFORMATION

Authorized by Thomas Jefferson, the University of Virginia School of Medicine was opened for instruction in 1825, making it one of the oldest medical schools in the South.

Both the School of Medicine and the University of Virginia Hospital are located on the grounds of the University of Virginia in Charlottesville. The University of Virginia Medical Center cares for 27,000 inpatients and 400,000 outpatients annually. The University Hospital staffs 552 beds, 61 infant bassinets, and 7 separate intensive care units.

CURRICULUM

Courses in the first year focus on the basic and clinical sciences that are requisite to understanding physical and psychological aspects of human health. The second-year curriculum focuses on disease and is coordinated with the problem-oriented Introduction to Clinical Medicine course.

The remainder of the curriculum consists of 12 months of required clinical clerkships and 8 months of elective opportunities. During the clerkships, the learning experience focuses on the social, ethical, and biomedical factors required for excellence in patient care. Teaching occurs primarily at the bedside; small tutorial seminars, lectures, and group discussions are also conducted. In addition to the clinical clerkships at the University of Virginia Hospital, all students can expect to have part of their clerkship experience at an affiliated hospital under the direction of full-time faculty members.

Students selected for the Generalist Scholars Program receive enhanced training in disease prevention, health promotion, subtance abuse, family therapy, clinical epidemiology, and office procedural skills. The elective program of the fourth year offers students the opportunity to pursue widely their own interests and abilities and to sample diverse training experiences in medical centers from Alaska to South America. Students may choose from a variety of electives, including clinical experiences, graduate courses, and research activities.

Many opportunities exist for students who are interested in medical research. Prominent among these opportunities are the Summer Research Program and the M.D.-Ph.D. program. This accelerated program leads to both M.D. and Ph.D. degrees and utilizes the facilities of both the School of Medicine and the Graduate School of Arts and Sciences. It is designed specifically to prepare a limited number of highly qualified men and women for careers in both research and clinical medicine. Medical students may also elect to extend their education to include a year of basic science or clinical research.

REQUIREMENTS FOR ENTRANCE

The MCAT is required and must be taken no later than the fall of the year of application and no earlier than spring of 1998. The minimum undergraduate college requirement for admission is 90 semester hours of graded course work in a U.S. or Canadian school; however, it is unusual to accept students who will not have received the baccalaureate degree by the time of enrollment. Without exception the following courses are required:

	Years
Biology (with lab)	1
General chemistry (with lab)	1
Organic chemistry (with lab)	1
General physics (with lab)	1

Other than these courses, the college curriculum for the premedical student should be planned in accord with individual interests and aptitudes to gain as broad an educational background as possible.

Advanced placement credit is acceptable if such credit is indicated on the undergraduate college transcripts as having been accepted by the college toward fulfillment of requirements for the bachelor's degree. Students are expected to pursue advanced courses if advanced placement credit was awarded for any of the required science courses (including laboratory work).

SELECTION FACTORS

Preference is given to residents of Virginia. Applications from well-qualified nonresidents are welcomed, but early application is advised. Foreign nationals should have baccalaureate degrees from American or Canadian colleges or universities; reapplicants should show significant improvement in their applications. The Committee on Admissions does not discriminate on the basis of race, gender, sexual preference, creed, national origin, age, or disability.

Numerical criteria, work and volunteer experience, interpersonal and communication skills, letters of recommendations, and the interview influence committee decisions. The Admissions Committee does not grant regional interviews or interviews by applicant request.

Outstanding applicants are encouraged to apply for admission to the combined M.D.-Ph.D. program. This program offers training for those individuals who plan a career that combines medical research with clinical activities.

The class entering in 1999 had a *mean GPA* of 3.67 and a *mean MCAT score* of 10.73.

FINANCIAL AID

In addition to Ford Federal Direct Loans comparable to Stafford Loans, the University of Virginia School of Medicine provides school-funded scholarships and loans to students who demonstrate need via the Free Application for Federal Student Aid. Parental financial information is required for all applicants who wish to receive aid from school funds. Approximately 85 percent of the student body receive financial aid. Student employment is not encouraged. Financial aid applications should be requested by January 1 or immediately after acceptance. For more information, contact Ms. Catharine Anas, financial aid director.

INFORMATION FOR MINORITY STUDENTS

This institution is committed to increasing the representation of minority physicians in medicine. To this end, we welcome applications from competitive out-of-state and in-state minority students. Structures in place to facilitate preparation and success of students include: (1) content-based MCAT program; (2) pre-matriculation academic advancement summer program for those accepted into the School of Medicine; (3) extensive tutorial and other academic support programs upon admission; and (4) need-based financial assistance. Early completion of application for admission is strongly recommended. The Admissions Committee includes minority members, and a team of committed faculty and administrators provides support at all levels for minority students.

Public Institution

APPLICATION AND ACCEPTANCE POLICIES FOR 2001–2002 FIRST-YEAR CLASS

School participates in AMCAS. See Chapter 6.

Filing of AMCAS application
  Earliest date: June 1, 2000
  Latest date: Nov. 1, 2000
School application fee to all applicants: $60
Oldest MCAT scores considered: 1998
Does not have Early Decision Program
Acceptance notice to regular applicants
  Earliest date: Oct. 15, 2000
  Latest date: Until class is filled
Applicant's response to acceptance offer
  Maximum time: 3 weeks
Requests for deferred entrance considered: Yes
Deposit to hold place in class: None
Estimated number of new entrants: 139
Starting date: Aug. 2001

TUITION AND STUDENT FEES PER YEAR FOR 1999–2000 FIRST-YEAR CLASS

Tuition
  Resident: $11,968
  Nonresident: $23,949

Student fees: $1,186

INFORMATION ON 1999–2000 FIRST-YEAR CLASS

Number of	*In-State*	*Out-of-State*	*Total*
Applicants	796	3,355	4,151
Applicants Interviewed	211	285	496
New Entrants*	93	46	139

*All took the MCAT and had baccalaureate degrees.

CHAPTER 11

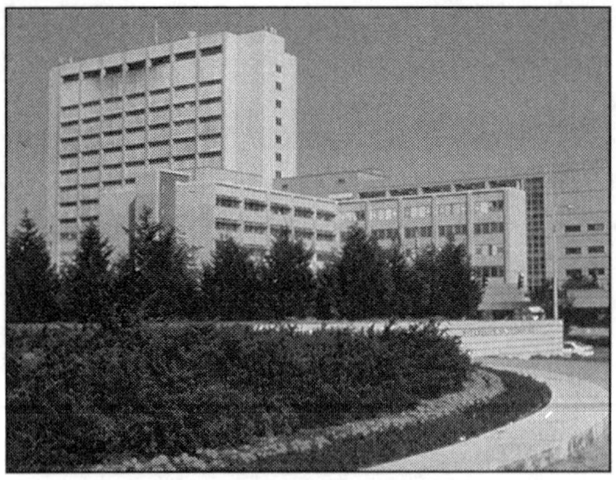

University of Washington School of Medicine

Seattle, Washington

Dr. Paul G. Ramsey, *Dean*
Dr. Werner E. Samson, *Assistant Dean for Admissions*
Patricia T. Fero, *Admissions Officer*

ADDRESS INQUIRIES TO:

Admissions Office
Health Sciences Center A-300, Box 356340
University of Washington
Seattle, Washington 98195-6340
(206) 543-7212
E-mail: askuwsom@u.washington.edu
Web Site: http://www.washington.edu/medical/som/

GENERAL INFORMATION

The University of Washington School of Medicine was established in 1945. For complete information about policies, procedures, and programs, candidates are referred to the current University of Washington General Catalog available from the University Bookstore at (206) 634-3400 or on-line at http://www.washington.edu/students/crscat/index.html.

CURRICULUM

The first two years of the curriculum are identified as the basic organ system curriculum. It consists of three phases or groups of courses: pre-organ system courses; organ systems taught by basic and clinical disciplines; and introduction to clinical medicine and health care. The academic demands of the basic curriculum are scaled so that most students will be able to take elective courses.

The clinical curriculum is pursued predominantly in the third and fourth years. It includes three elements: prescribed clerkships to be completed by all students in family medicine, obstetrics-gynecology, pediatrics, psychiatry, and surgery; a clinical selective series requiring a minimum number of credits in two clinical areas (rehabilitation medicine/chronic care and emergency care/trauma); and clinical clerkships elected by the student. The Independent Study in Medical Science requirement enables students to gain an understanding of the philosophy and methods of science as they relate to their chosen field of medicine.

One aspect of the curriculum is the WWAMI program of decentralized medical education (see Chapter 5). All students enrolled at the University of Washington School of Medicine may receive as part of this program a portion of training at sites away from the University of Washington campus. Offers of acceptance, therefore, are conditional upon agreement to participate in the WWAMI program.

REQUIREMENTS FOR ENTRANCE

The MCAT taken in the spring of 1998 or thereafter is required. This exam must be taken no later than the autumn of the year before possible matriculation. Under exceptional circumstances, the GRE may be considered during the admissions process; however, if accepted, the applicant will be required to take the MCAT prior to matriculation. The following course requirements must be completed before matriculation:

	Sem. hrs.
Biology	8
Chemistry	12

(May be satisfied by taking any combination of inorganic, organic, biochemistry, or molecular biology courses.)

The understanding of certain basic biochemistry/molecular biology concepts is a matriculation requirement. Applicants are urged to contact the office of Admissions for an outline of the concepts (generally covered in a first semester biochemistry course) the matriculant is expected to master.

Physics	4
Other science	8

(May be satisfied by taking other courses in any of the above categories.)

Proficiency in English, basic mathematics, and information technologies is also essential. Entering students are required to have a personal computer.

Under exceptional circumstances, certain course requirements may be waived for individuals with unusual achievements and academic promise.

A minimum of three years of college is required; however, all entrants in recent years have fulfilled requirements for a bachelor's degree. No major is preferred, but a broad educational background is encouraged.

Applicants who are seriously considered will be requested to submit supplemental information, one part of which will be a premedical committee evaluation or three individual letters submitted from instructors who have taught the candidate in a collegiate course (a mixture of evaluations from the sciences and humanities is recommended). In addition, signed documentation indicating the student's ability to meet our essential requirements (with or without reasonable accommodations) for graduation, as well as authorization for a criminal background check (necessitated by Washington state law) is required.

All supplemental materials must be submitted by January 15, 2000. Early submission of application and supplemental materials is encouraged.

Candidates who wish to be considered for the M.D.-Ph.D. program must submit the Medical Scientist Training Program (MSTP) application. This application is sent to all eligible candidates along with the acknowledgment of receipt of the medical school application. All candidates considered eligible for this program after initial review of the MSTP application will be requested to send further supplementary materials.

SELECTION FACTORS

Candidates for admission are considered comparatively on the basis of academic performance, motivation, maturity, personal integrity, and demonstrated humanitarian qualities. Research experience, disadvantaged background, and interest in serving the underserved are other important considerations. A knowledge of the needs of individuals and society and an awareness of health care delivery systems are essential. Extenuating circumstances in an applicant's background are evaluated as they relate to these selection factors.

Students entering in the fall of 1999 had a *mean GPA* of 3.59. *Mean scores on the MCAT* were as follows: *VR*-9.9, *PS*-10.1, *BS*-10.4, *WS*-P.

Residents of the states of Washington, Wyoming, Alaska, Montana, or Idaho are eligible to apply. Individuals with a demonstrated interest in research may apply for the M.D.-Ph.D. program (MSTP) regardless of residency. Applicants from outside this five-state region who come from disadvantaged backgrounds or who have demonstrated a commitment to serving underserved populations will be considered. Foreign applicants, in addition to the above requirements, must also have a permanent resident visa.

After the completed applications are screened, applicants considered to be competitive will be invited to Seattle for an interview.

FINANCIAL AID

Financial status has no bearing on chances for admission. All applicants for aid must submit data for an analysis of need through the FAFSA (see Part 1). The application receipt deadline of February 28 must be met, regardless of admission date, in order to receive highest priority for aid; applicants should mail this form mid-February or earlier. Approximately 83 percent of the student body receives some form of aid, most of which is in the form of loans. Financial aid applications are available in January. Contact the School of Medicine's Financial Aid Office at (206) 685-2520.

Public Institution

APPLICATION AND ACCEPTANCE POLICIES FOR 2001–2002 FIRST-YEAR CLASS

School participates in AMCAS. See Chapter 6.

Filing of AMCAS application
  Earliest date: June 1, 2000
  Latest date: Nov. 1, 2000
School application fee to all applicants: $35
Oldest MCAT scores considered: 1998
Does not have Early Decision Program
Acceptance notice to regular applicants
  Earliest date: Nov. 1, 2000
  Latest date: Until class is filled
Applicant's response to acceptance offer
  Maximum time: 2 weeks
Requests for deferred entrance considered: Yes
Deposit to hold place in class (applied to tuition):
  $100, due with response to acceptance offer; nonrefundable
Estimated number of new entrants: 176
Starting date: Sept. 2001

TUITION AND STUDENT FEES PER YEAR FOR 1999–2000 FIRST-YEAR CLASS

Tuition:
  Resident: $8,823
  Nonresident: $22,869

Student fees: $387

INFORMATION ON 1999–2000 FIRST-YEAR CLASS

Number of	*In-State**	*Out-of-State*	*Total*
Applicants	946	2,085	3,031
Applicants Interviewed	658	104	762
New Entrants	154†	21	175

*In-state figures include Washington, Wyoming, Alaska, Montana, and Idaho residents.

†All took the MCAT and had baccalaureate degrees.

CHAPTER 11

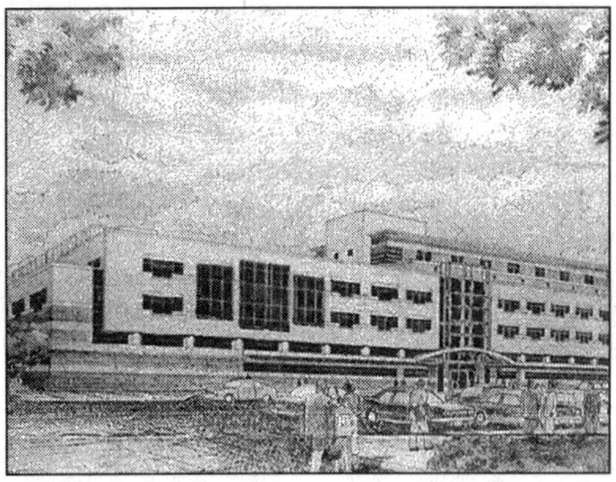

Marshall University School of Medicine

Huntington, West Virginia

Dr. Charles H. McKown, Jr., *Vice President and Dean*
Cynthia A. Warren, *Director of Admissions and Student Affairs*
Dr. Jack L. Toney, *Director of Student Financial Assistance*

ADDRESS INQUIRIES TO:

Admissions Office
Marshall University
School of Medicine
1600 Medical Center Drive, Suite 3400
Huntington, West Virginia 25701-3655
(304) 691-1738; (800) 544-8514; (304) 691-1744 (FAX)
Web Site: www.musom.marshall.edu

MISSION STATEMENT

The Marshall University School of Medicine has a special mission to respond to the health care needs of West Virginians. We emphasize training in the primary care specialties and encourage graduates to practice in the state's underserved rural areas. Marshall now ranks second in the nation in the percentage of graduates who choose to enter a primary care specialty.

GENERAL INFORMATION

The Marshall University School of Medicine was developed under the Veterans Administration Medical Assistance and Health Training Act passed by Congress in 1972. The School of Medicine was granted full accreditation and graduated its first class in 1981.

The School of Medicine is a community-based program. The school's many affiliations provide the opportunity to experience medical practice in varied settings: a new $32 million ambulatory care center, the Veterans Affairs Medical Center, successful rural clinics, highly specialized tertiary-care services in community hospitals, offices of private physicians, and others.

CURRICULUM

In the first year, the basic sciences courses of anatomy, physiology, neurosciences, medical cell and molecular biology, and biochemistry are supplemented by medical ethics and a clinical interdepartmental course entitled Introduction to Patient Care, which covers early physical diagnosis and behavioral medicine. The second year includes pharmacology, pathology, microbiology, genetics, psychopathology, community medicine, physical diagnosis, immunology, medical ethics, and introduction to clinical medicine. During the third and fourth years, students are rotated through clerkships at participating community hospitals and other locations in the clinical fields of medicine, surgery, pediatrics, psychiatry, family practice, and obstetrics-gynecology. Several rural health care programs are available for students who demonstrate special interest in primary care medicine. Twenty-seven weeks are devoted to electives in the senior year. A standard letter grading system (A, B, C, D, F) is utilized.

REQUIREMENTS FOR ENTRANCE

The MCAT is required. The baccalaureate degree is preferred. However, exceptionally well qualified students with three years of college education or the equivalent may be considered for admission. Minimum course requirements are:

	Sem. hrs.
General biology or zoology (with lab)	8
Inorganic chemistry (with lab)	8
Organic chemistry (with lab)	8
Physics (with lab)	8
English composition and rhetoric	6
Behavioral or social sciences	6

With the exception of these specific courses, applicants are encouraged to pursue their personal educational interests. Quality of course work rather than the field in which it is taken is the more important consideration.

It is urged that applicants take the MCAT in the spring of the year of application but no later than the fall of that year.

SELECTION FACTORS

There is no discrimination because of race, sex, religion, age, handicap, sexual orientation, or national origin. Qualified members of minority groups are encouraged to apply.

Applicants are evaluated on the basis of their academic records, MCAT scores, recommendations from instructors, and personal qualifications as judged through interviews. Interviews are arranged only by invitation of the Admissions Committee.

Academic achievement alone is not a sufficient foundation for success in the profession of medicine. Applicants must exhibit excellence in character, motivation, and ideals. Behavioral qualities deemed essential for a career in medicine include, but are not limited to, good judgment, integrity, responsibility, and sensitivity.

As a state-assisted institution, the School of Medicine gives preference in selection of students to West Virginia residents.

A limited number of positions will be available to well-qualified nonresidents from states contiguous to West Virginia or to nonresidents who have strong ties to West Virginia. Other nonresidents are not considered. Only applicants who are U.S. citizens or who have permanent resident visas are eligible for admission.

The August 1999 entering class had the following profile: *resident,* 98 percent West Virginia residents; *mean overall GPA,* 3.5; *gender,* 50 percent women; *undergraduate major,* 85 percent in biological sciences, chemistry, or preprofessional curriculum; *degrees,* 37 bachelor's degrees, 3 master's degrees, 1 doctoral degree, and 7 students without baccalaureate degrees; *undergraduate schools,* 31 students attended West Virginia schools.

The School of Medicine considers for transfer admissions those applicants who are currently in good standing at an allopathic medical school. Positions are limited by attrition and are rarely available. The residency policy for regular admissions also applies to transfer admissions. Only U.S. citizens are considered.

FINANCIAL AID

The financial needs of the applicant are not a consideration in the admissions process. There are a variety of resources for financial assistance available to medical students. Currently 90 percent of the students are receiving financial assistance. Further information and applications for financial aid may be obtained from Marshall at the following address: Office of Financial Assistance, Marshall University, Huntington, West Virginia 25755.

Because of the rigorous nature of the medical program, students are advised not to attempt outside employment during the academic year.

The supplemental application fee will be waived for individuals who have been granted an AMCAS fee waiver.

Public Institution

APPLICATION AND ACCEPTANCE POLICIES FOR 2001–2002 FIRST-YEAR CLASS

School participates in AMCAS. See Chapter 6.

Filing of AMCAS application
- Earliest date: June 1, 2000
- Latest date: Nov. 15, 2000

School application fee to all applicants:
- Residents: $40
- Nonresidents: $80

Oldest MCAT scores considered: 1998

Does not have Early Decision Program (EDP)

Acceptance notice to regular applicants
- Earliest date: Oct. 15, 2000
- Latest date: Until class is filled

Applicant's response to acceptance offer
- Maximum time: 2 weeks

Requests for deferred entrance considered: Yes

Deposit to hold place in class: None

Estimated number of new entrants: 48

Starting date: Aug. 2001

TUITION AND STUDENT FEES PER YEAR FOR 1999–2000 FIRST-YEAR CLASS

Tuition
- Resident: $9,030
- Nonresident: $23,010

Student fees: $446

INFORMATION ON 1999–2000 FIRST-YEAR CLASS

Number of	*In-State*	*Out-of-State*	*Total*
Applicants	293	648	941
Applicants Interviewed	221	10	231
New Entrants*	47	1	48

*All took the MCAT; 85% had baccalaureate degrees.

CHAPTER 11

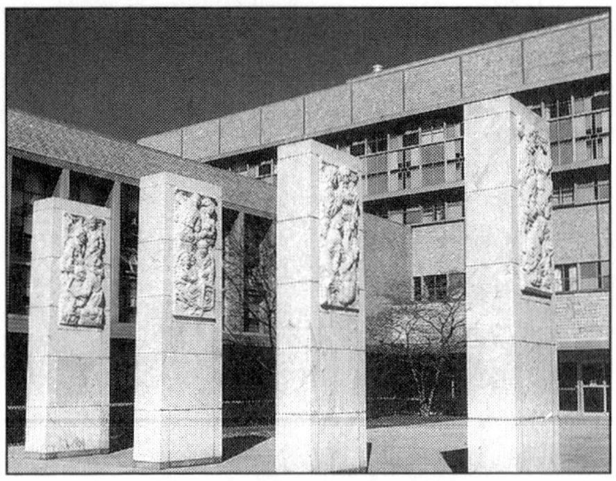

West Virginia University School of Medicine

Morgantown, West Virginia

Dr. Robert D'Alessandri, *Dean*
Dr. Anne C. Cutlip, *Associate Dean for Student Services and Professional Development*
Candace Hostutler, *Financial Aid Officer*

ADDRESS INQUIRIES TO:

Office of Admissions and Records
West Virginia University
Health Sciences Center
P.O. Box 9815
Morgantown, West Virginia 26506
(304) 293-3521; 293-7968 (FAX)
Web Site: http://www.hsc.wvu.edu/som/

MISSION STATEMENT

The mission of the West Virginia University School of Medicine is to improve the health of West Virginians through the education of health professionals, through basic/clinical scientific research and research in rural health care delivery, through the provision of continuing professional education, and through participation in the provision of direct and supportive health care.

GENERAL INFORMATION

West Virginia University, a public institution, has offered the first two years of the medical curriculum continuously since 1902. Four decades ago the Health Sciences Center was established, including the School of Medicine and the schools of dentistry, nursing, and pharmacy. A modern physical plant provides facilities for the schools, including three hospitals—the 400-bed Ruby Memorial Hospital, the 80-bed Chestnut Ridge Psychiatric Hospital, and the 80-bed Health South Mountainview Regional Rehabilitation Hospital—and a cancer center. Clinical instruction is also provided in the Charleston Division of the Health Sciences Center.

Some university housing is available for both married and unmarried students.

CURRICULUM

The educational program of the School of Medicine is designed to provide students with a foundation upon which they can base further preparation for any branch of medicine, specifically primary care, other specialty practice, teaching, research, or a combination of these career objectives.

In the first and second years the plan of study is directed toward the principles and methodology of the basic medical sciences. However, the basic courses are designed so that the student begins to synthesize concepts of patient care. The first-year basic science courses are integrated through common test methods and through problem-based learning clinical applications. Clinical experiences are introduced the first semester of the first year. Summer externships are available in all primary care fields. Additional early exposure to patient-oriented instruction is through the introduction to clinical medicine, community medicine, and other behavioral medicine courses during the second basic science year.

A traditional third-year curriculum gives the student a foundation in history taking, examination, patient relations, laboratory aids, diagnosis, treatment, and use of medical literature in the major clinical disciplines.

The fourth year is composed of requirements (60 percent) and electives (40 percent). Requirements include critical care medicine; primary care ambulatory medicine; surgical subspecialties; and a medicine, family practice, or pediatrics subinternship.

Students with exceptional interest in research will be considered for the Medical Scientist M.D.-Ph.D. program. The Ph.D. is offered in eight disciplines. An M.D.-M.P.H. program is also offered.

An honors/satisfactory/unsatisfactory grading system is used in the School of Medicine.

REQUIREMENTS FOR ENTRANCE

The MCAT and a minimum of three years of college (minimum of 90 semester hours or equivalent) are required. All required courses must be passed with a grade of C or better. College work must include:

	Sem. hrs.
Biology (with lab)	8
Inorganic chemistry (with lab)	8
Organic chemistry (with lab)	8
General physics (with lab)	8
English	6
Behavioral or social sciences	6

The best-prepared applicants will have completed a course in biochemistry and in cell/molecular biology. Fundamental competence in communication skills is emphasized as a great need. Additional course work should be designed to provide breadth leading toward a bachelor's degree in a major field of the applicant's own choosing, not necessarily in the natural sciences or in a premedical curriculum. Computer literacy is required.

Applicants are strongly encouraged to (and Early Decision applicants must) take the MCAT no later than April of the year before they hope to enter medical school. Applicants may apply as early as June 1 and normally should apply no later than mid-August. Interviews are held on site only beginning in September. No applicant is admitted without an interview. Acceptances will be issued periodically throughout the interview period.

Transfer applications are accepted from medical students who are in good academic and professional standing. Students from other doctoral-level programs (dental, podiatric, graduate, etc.) are ineligible for advanced standing. With the exception of West Virginia residents, advanced standing applicants must transfer from LCME-accredited medical schools.

SELECTION FACTORS

As a state-supported school, the School of Medicine gives preference in selection of students to West Virginia residents, but places may be available each year to well-qualified nonresidents, especially those who have strong ties to the state of West Virginia. Choice of students is based upon scholarship, MCAT scores, and personal qualifications as judged by interviews and recommendations from qualified persons. Although most students present a bachelor's degree at matriculation, a small number of carefully selected individuals are admitted at the end of three years (90 semester hours) of college work.

The School of Medicine does not discriminate on the basis of race, sex, creed, national origin, age, or handicap. Qualified members of minority groups are encouraged to apply. The Health Careers Opportunity Program is available for minority or disadvantaged students.

A select number of students will be required to spend their clinical years at the Charleston Division of the West Virginia University School of Medicine.

The 1999 entering class had the following profile: *residence,* 95 percent West Virginia residents; *mean overall GPA,* 3.68; *mean MCAT scores, VR*-9.0, *PS*-8.9, *WS*-P, *BS*-9.1; *sex,* 42 percent women; *undergraduate major,* 83 percent in biological sciences, chemistry, or preprofessional curriculum; *degrees,* 81 bachelor's degrees, 6 graduate degrees; *undergraduate schools,* 60 students attended West Virginia schools.

FINANCIAL AID

Approximately 90 percent of the school's medical students receive financial aid. A limited number of scholarship awards are available to well-qualified students based on financial need. In addition, multiple loan funds are also available. Students' spouses with reasonable training and experience ordinarily have no difficulty in finding work near the medical school, the university, or Morgantown. Medical students themselves cannot seek outside employment while enrolled. There is no provision for financial assistance to foreign students (who are not eligible to apply unless they have strong ties to the state of West Virginia).

Public Institution

APPLICATION AND ACCEPTANCE POLICIES FOR 2001–2002 FIRST-YEAR CLASS

School participates in AMCAS. See Chapter 6.

Filing of AMCAS application
  Earliest date: June 1, 2000
  Latest date: Nov. 15, 2000
School application fee to all applicants: $45
Oldest MCAT scores considered: 1999
Does have Early Decision Program (EDP)
  For West Virginia residents only
  EDP application period: June 1–Aug. 1, 2000
  EDP applicants notified by: Oct. 1, 2000
Acceptance notice to regular applicants
  Earliest date: Oct. 15, 2000
  Latest date: Until class is filled
Applicant's response to acceptance offer
  Maximum time: 2 weeks
Requests for deferred entrance considered: Yes
Deposit to hold place in class (applied to tuition):
  $100, due with response to acceptance offer
Deposit refundable prior to: June 1, 2001
Estimated number of new entrants: 88 (10 EDP)
Starting date: Aug. 2001

TUITION AND STUDENT FEES PER YEAR FOR 1999–2000 FIRST-YEAR CLASS

Tuition
  Resident: $8,618
  Nonresident: $22,556
Student fees: $2,486

INFORMATION ON 1999–2000 FIRST-YEAR CLASS

Number of	*In-State*	*Out-of-State*	*Total*
Applicants	291	707	998
Applicants Interviewed	215	40	255
New Entrants*	83	5	88

*All took the MCAT; 97% had baccalaureate degrees.

CHAPTER 11

Medical College of Wisconsin

Milwaukee, Wisconsin

Dr. Michael J. Dunn, *Dean and Executive Vice President*
Sharon A. Carpenter, *Director of Admissions*
Linda L. Pascal, *Director of Student Financial Services*

ADDRESS INQUIRIES TO:

Office of Admissions
Medical College of Wisconsin
8701 Watertown Plank Road
Milwaukee, Wisconsin 53226
(414) 456-8246
Web Site: http://www.mcw.edu/acad/admission

GENERAL INFORMATION

With roots going back to the last century, the Medical College of Wisconsin became an independent, freestanding school of medicine in 1967. Located on the campus of the Milwaukee Regional Medical Center, it is a private medical school with a public mission of education, research, patient care, and community service. Strong relationships and special educational programs are maintained with other educational institutions throughout Wisconsin. Major affiliated teaching hospitals include the Froedtert Memorial Lutheran Hospital, Clement J. Zablocki Veterans Affairs Medical Center, and the Children's Hospital of Wisconsin. Additional affiliations with both private and community hospitals bring the number of teaching beds available for clinical education to over 7,000.

CURRICULUM

The curriculum is designed to provide a solid foundation for a career in any discipline of medicine. In the first two years, students acquire a thorough knowledge of the basic medical sciences. Courses in anatomy, neuroscience, biochemistry, physiology, biostatistics, and psychiatry comprise the first year. The second-year courses include microbiology, pathology, pharmacology, and psychiatry. The clinical continuum provides first- and second-year students with integrated early generalist experiences, the fundamental skills and attitudes of professional development, and knowledge in the following disciplines: human behavior, bioethics and care of the terminally ill, information management, physical diagnosis, and health care systems.

The third year consists of a brief introduction to clinical skills course, followed by two-month clerkships in medicine, surgery, obstetrics-gynecology, pediatrics, and a combination of psychiatry and anesthesiology. In addition, students have a one-month clerkship in family medicine, with continuing longitudinal experience in the same clinic setting. Students may also select a four-week, non-graded elective experience.

During the fourth year, students complete three one-month rotations in surgery: a medical selective; a subinternship (internal medicine, pediatrics, or family medicine); and six one-month electives.

Students with a particular interest in research can pursue a variety of options, including the Honors in Research program or joint M.S.-M.D. or M.D.-Ph.D. degree programs. Two students are selected annually for the Medical Scientist Training Program, which culminates with the awarding of both the M.D. and Ph.D. degrees at the end of a seven-year period of study. A five-year extended curriculum is available to students who wish to carry out their studies in the M.D. program over a longer period of time.

REQUIREMENTS FOR ENTRANCE

The MCAT is required and must be taken no more than three years prior to matriculation. A minimum of three years of undergraduate work (90 semester hours) at an accredited college or university in the United States or Canada is required; however, almost all students entering the Medical College of Wisconsin have completed a baccalaureate degree. Because the school accepts students from a variety of major fields of study, students are encouraged to determine their fields of major study according to their personal interest. Each prospective medical student must take the following courses for graded credit at an accredited college or university in the United States or Canada:

	Graded Credit
Biology (with lab)	8
General chemistry (with lab)	8
Organic chemistry (with lab)	8
Physics	8
English	6
Should stress composition	
Mathematics	
Completion of a course in algebra in high school or college.	

Officially granted Advanced Placement (AP) credit will only be accepted to fulfill 3 graded credits of English.

Applicants to the Medical College of Wisconsin who attend undergraduate colleges/universities, who do not give graded credit for coursework, will not be considered for admission.

Students must be capable of expressing themselves effectively, both orally and in writing.

SELECTION FACTORS

The college seeks students who are well suited to a competent and ethical practice of medicine. Successful applicants will have a mature sense of values, sound motivation, demonstrated academic achievement, willingness and ability to assume responsibility, and be of high moral and ethical character.

The selection of students is based on a careful analysis of each candidate's suitability for the profession of medicine. Undergraduate achievement and MCAT scores are carefully evaluated, but academic excellence alone does not assure acceptance. Subjective factors, including the candidate's statement in the AMCAS application, academic recommendations, and personal interviews are also important.

Interviews are an integral part of the admissions process, and all applicants being seriously considered are interviewed before being offered an acceptance. Interviews are scheduled only at the request of the Admissions Committee, following a review of the application and are done only at the College.

The Medical College of Wisconsin accepts about half of its entering class from Wisconsin, with the remainder coming from other states. Women represented 38 percent of the 1999 entering class. The Medical College of Wisconsin does not discriminate on the basis of race, gender, creed, disability, age, national origin, or sexual orientation.

FINANCIAL AID

Most financial assistance available through the college, including federal and institutional scholarships and loans, is awarded solely on the basis of need. The Financial Aid Office develops a financial aid package for each student, based upon individual needs. The office helps direct students to additional sources of support. Applicants are strongly encouraged to initiate their financial aid application as soon as they have been interviewed. *A stipulation of acceptance for all applicants includes documentation of a current credit report, and compliance with the Medical College's credit guidelines.* Because of restrictions placed on loan and scholarship funds, foreign citizens are not eligible for financial aid. All foreign applicants must file proof of financial support before they are eligible for acceptance.

INFORMATION FOR MINORITY STUDENTS

The Medical College of Wisconsin actively seeks applications from talented minority students, particularly those who are Wisconsin residents. In addition to academic achievement, MCAT scores, letters of recommendation, and personal interviews, the Admissions Committee carefully considers the student's motivation and cultural and educational background. Through the Office of Minority Student Affairs, a variety of programs exist to assist minority students, demonstrating the college's strong commitment to the recruitment, retention, and graduation of minority students. Further information concerning programs for minority students may be obtained from the associate dean for minority student affairs.

Private Institution

APPLICATION AND ACCEPTANCE POLICIES FOR 2001–2002 FIRST-YEAR CLASS

School participates in AMCAS. See Chapter 6.

Filing of AMCAS application
  Earliest date: June 1, 2000
  Latest date: Nov. 1, 2000
School application fee to all applicants: $60
Oldest MCAT scores considered: 1998
Does have Early Decision Program (EDP)
  EDP application period: June 1–Aug. 1, 2000
  EDP applicants notified by: Oct. 1, 2000
Acceptance notice to regular applicants
  Earliest date: Oct. 15, 2000
  Latest date: Until class is filled
Applicant's response to acceptance offer
  Maximum time: 3 weeks
Requests for deferred entrance considered: Yes
Deposit to hold place in class (applied to tuition):
  $100, due with response to acceptance offer
Deposit refundable prior to: May 15, 2001
Estimated number of new entrants: 204 (30 EDP)
Starting date: Aug. 2001

TUITION AND STUDENT FEES PER YEAR FOR 1999–2000 FIRST-YEAR CLASS

Tuition
  Resident: $17,314
  Nonresident: $27,405

Student fees: $95

INFORMATION ON 1999–2000 FIRST-YEAR CLASS

Number of	*In-State*	*Out-of-State*	*Total*
Applicants	540	4,795	5,335
Applicants Interviewed	228	391	619
New Entrants*	97	107	204

*All took the MCAT; 99% had baccalaureate degrees.

CHAPTER 11

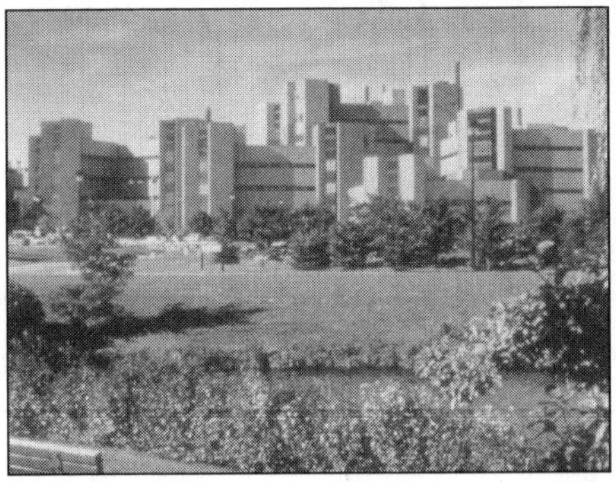

University of Wisconsin Medical School

Madison, Wisconsin

Dr. Philip M. Farrell, *Dean*
Janice Waisman, *Director of Admissions*
John Selbo, *Student Financial Aid*

ADDRESS INQUIRIES TO:

Admissions Committee
Medical Sciences Center, Room 1140
University of Wisconsin Medical School
1300 University Avenue
Madison, Wisconsin 53706
(608) 263-4925; 262-2327 (FAX)
Web Site: http://www.biostat.wisc.edu

MISSION STATEMENT

The University of Wisconsin Medical School is committed to meeting the health needs of Wisconsin and beyond through excellence in education, research, patient care, and service. The UW Medical School seeks to be one of the preeminent medical schools by excelling in the creation, integration, and transfer of knowledge through a combination of basic, translational, and clinical research; a greater emphasis on active learning; and consistently outstanding patient care.

GENERAL INFORMATION

The University of Wisconsin Medical School initiated a two-year program in 1907 and expanded to a full four-year program in 1924. The present University of Wisconsin Center for Health Sciences—which includes the Medical School, University Hospital and Clinics—is located on the university campus in Madison. The medical school basic science departments, first- and second-year teaching facilities, and administrative offices are located in the Medical Sciences Center. The Clinical Science Center houses the clinical departments, University Hospital and Clinics, School of Nursing, and Wisconsin Clinical Cancer Center. In addition to the University Hospital and Clinics, other clinical sites in Madison and throughout the state are utilized in the educational program.

CURRICULUM

The educational and research programs have been developed to educate students to become qualified to undertake any career in medicine. Our curriculum introduces students to the generalist practice of medicine by exposing students to community-based settings in the first and second years. The curriculum emphasizes: active learning; case-based problem-solving; interdisciplinary teaching by the basic science and clinical faculty throughout the first and second years; a four-year curriculum that prepares students for either a primary care or specialty career; diverse clinical clerkship experiences around the state, including inner-city and rural sites; and an eight-week one-on-one preceptorship with an experienced clinician in Year 4. The senior year provides elective opportunities for study at other institutions and abroad.

Opportunities for research are available to medical students in individually arranged programs leading to the M.S. and Ph.D. degrees or by nondegree arrangements. Competitive support is offered to resident and nonresident students entering as M.D.-Ph.D. candidates. Letter grades are used to evaluate students' academic performance throughout the four-year curriculum.

REQUIREMENTS FOR ENTRANCE

The MCAT is required. Applicants are strongly encouraged to take the MCAT in the spring before application. Consideration of applicants who indicate they are taking the fall MCAT will be delayed, without detriment, until receipt of those scores.

Applicants must have a minimum of three years (90 semester hours) of college work by the time of matriculation. However, applicants are encouraged to obtain a baccalaureate degree before matriculation. Courses in English, biochemistry, quantitative analysis, and calculus and electives in the humanities and social sciences are recommended. College work must include:

	Semesters
General zoology or biology (with lab)	1
Advanced zoology or biology (with lab)	1
Inorganic chemistry (with lab)	2
Organic chemistry (with lab)	2
General physics (with lab)	2
Mathematics	2
Minimum requirement of college algebra and trigonometry.	

SELECTION FACTORS

Breadth of academic and nonacademic interests and experiences, ability to communicate with others, motivation for medicine, personal characteristics, and intellectual ability are some of the factors considered by the Admissions Committee. The Admissions Committee seeks students with diverse backgrounds and interests, which is of value in training professionals for good health care delivery. A preprofessional committee evaluation or three academic letters of recommendation plus one nonacademic letter of recommendation are required and must be submitted no later than December 1. Following the initial screening process, applicants will be invited for personal interviews to complete the application process.

The University of Wisconsin Medical School does not discriminate on the basis of race, sex, creed, national origin, age, or handicap. Women, minorities and/or disadvantaged students, and students from rural areas are encouraged to apply since these groups are presently underrepresented in both the applicant pool and the medical profession. Preference is given to residents of Wisconsin. Nonresident applicants are competing for relatively few places. Secondary applications are sent only to eligible applicants, following a screening of the AMCAS application, who are academically qualified. Applications are accepted from foreign nationals who have a permanent resident visa in the United States. The 1998 entering class had an *average GPA* of 3.73; *average MCAT* scores were VR–9.8, PS–10.1, WS–P, BS–10.3.

FINANCIAL AID

All financial aid allocated by the University of Wisconsin Medical School is awarded on the basis of proven need. Need is calculated as the necessary expenses incurred while attending medical school minus the resources provided to the student by outside agencies, personal resources, and available parental resources. Priority for financial aid, especially grant awards, will be given to students with the greatest need. The major proportion of total financial aid is available in the form of loans. Approximately 90 percent of the students receive financial assistance.

INFORMATION FOR MINORITY STUDENTS

The University of Wisconsin Medical School is committed to increasing the number of physicians from minority groups and those showing evidence of socioeconomically and educationally disadvantaged backgrounds. Applications are encouraged from resident and nonresident Black Americans, mainland Puerto Ricans, Mexican Americans, American Indians, Alaskan Natives, and Native Hawaiians. Applications are also encouraged from persons with socioeconomic disadvantages.

Public Institution

APPLICATION AND ACCEPTANCE POLICIES FOR 2001–2002 FIRST-YEAR CLASS

School participates in AMCAS. See Chapter 6.

Filing of AMCAS application
- Earliest date: June 1, 2000
- Latest date: Oct. 15, 2000

School application fee after screening: $45
Oldest MCAT scores considered: 1997
Does have Early Decision Program (EDP)
- For Wisconsin residents only
- EDP application period: June 1–Aug. 1, 2000
- EDP applicants notified by: Oct. 1, 2000

Acceptance notice to regular applicants
- Earliest date: Oct. 15, 2000
- Latest date: Varies

Applicant's response to acceptance offer
- Maximum time: 2 weeks

Requests for deferred entrance considered: Yes
(for Wisconsin residents only)
Deposit to hold place in class: None
Estimated number of new entrants: 143 (EDP varies)
Starting date: Aug. 2001

TUITION AND STUDENT FEES PER YEAR FOR 1999–2000 FIRST-YEAR CLASS

Tuition:
- Resident: $16,558
- Nonresident: $25,268

Student Fees: $448

INFORMATION ON 1999–2000 FIRST-YEAR CLASS

Number of	*In-State*	*Out-of-State*	*Total*
Applicants	589	1,592	2,181
Applicants Interviewed	220	40	260
New Entrants*	130	14	144

*99% had baccalaureate degrees; 76% took the MCAT.

CHAPTER 11

Information About Canadian Medical Schools
Accredited by the LCME and by the CACMS

12

The 16 medical schools in Canada are affiliate institutional members of the Association of American Medical Colleges (AAMC) and participate in the Association's activities. The Canadian medical schools are accredited jointly by the Liaison Committee on Medical Education (LCME) and the Committee on Accreditation of Canadian Medical Schools (CACMS) of the Association of Canadian Medical Colleges. All are M.D. degree-granting schools with high-quality educational programs.

Admission policies and procedures of the Canadian schools are in many respects similar to policies and procedures followed in U.S. schools. Thus, many of the suggestions in chapters 1 through 7 are applicable also to students applying to these schools. Differences exist, however, in the relative importance given by the schools to various factors considered relevant in the selection process. Reference should be made to the individual school entries for details on these differences.

Fourteen Canadian medical schools have four-year programs. McMaster and Calgary have three-year programs. In 1992, the University of Montreal changed from a five-year to a new four-year curriculum. With the introduction of the four-year curriculum some students are now admitted into a one-year preparatory program prior to commencing the four-year M.D. curriculum. Laval University allows students, after admission, to opt to extend the four-year program over five years. Thus there is some variation in the duration of medical curricula in different Canadian faculties of medicine.

SELECTION CRITERIA

Pre-university education differs in Canada from the straight elementary-secondary 12-year system in the United States. There are also significant differences from province to province within Canada. As reflected in the individual entries, these differences affect the number of years of college/university instruction required of applicants to medical schools located in the different provinces. Individual schools also impose their own requirements independent of the differences that arise out of the educational system itself. Table 12-A shows that physics, inorganic and organic chemistry, biology, humanities, and English are the most common subjects required in undergraduate education by the Canadian schools. Medical schools are drifting away from rigid course prerequisites.

Language of Instruction

Three Canadian medical schools require fluency in French as all instruction is given in French. These schools are Laval, Montreal, and Sherbrooke—all located in the province of Quebec. Instruction in the other 13 schools is given in English. Students at the University of Ottawa have the option to write their examinations in French and instruction in French is gradually being introduced into the curriculum. It is planned that, by the year 2000, all instruction will be available in both languages.

Residence Requirements

Most medical schools give preference to citizens and landed immigrants residing in the province in which the medical school is located, because universities are a provincial responsibility in Canada. Individual schools within a province may prefer to select students from specific regions within the province. Prospective applicants should be aware of these preferences to maximize their chances of success.

A number of foreign students are accepted into Canadian medical schools each year. In this context, "foreign" refers to persons who are neither citizens of Canada nor landed immigrants in Canada at the time of application.

Some medical schools have a specific quota of places for applicants from the United States. In particular, students from the United States who are contemplating enrollment in Canada should study the admission requirements of Memorial University in St. John's, Newfoundland; and McGill University in Montreal, Quebec. Other faculties of medicine in Canada either have or are currently considering the introduction of U.S. or other foreign student-specific quotas.

Foreign students, including U.S. students, pay substantially higher tuition fees.

Applicants from outside Canada should check with the particular school in which they are interested to ascertain whether that school considers applications from non-Canadian citizens or nonimmigrants.

Academic Record/Suitability

Although it is probably fair to state that an excellent academic record is a very important factor in gaining admission to a Canadian medical school, a great deal of effort goes into devising means of assessing suitability for a medical career based on factors other than academic ability. Personal suitability is assessed in a variety of ways by the schools, and so appli-

TABLE 12-A

Subjects Required by Three or More Canadian Medical Schools 2001–2002 Entering Class

Required Subject	No. of Schools (*n = 8*)
Physics	4
Inorganic Chemistry	6
Organic Chemistry	6
Biology	6
English	4

NOTE: Figures based on data provided fall 1999. Eight of the 16 medical schools (Calgary, Dalhousie, McMaster, Queen's, Toronto, Western Ontario, Laval, and Saskatchewan) did not indicate specific course requirements and are not included in the tabulations.

cants able to demonstrate the qualities considered important in the practice of medicine may occasionally gain access to medical school even if their academic record is not outstanding. Also, applicants with outstanding records who fail to demonstrate the personal qualities considered important may not gain a place in medical school.

Most successful applicants to Canadian medical schools are interviewed prior to acceptance. The discussion of the interview in Chapter 7 also applies in the context of admission to Canadian schools.

MCAT

Eleven Canadian medical schools require applicants to take the Medical College Admission Test (MCAT). These schools are Alberta, British Columbia, Calgary, Dalhousie, Manitoba, McGill, Memorial, Queen's, Saskatchewan, Toronto, and Western Ontario.

Other Considerations

Applicants and entrants to Canadian schools today are often older than their counterparts of the past.

Most medical schools no longer have admissions policies related to age, although older applicants are not quite as successful in gaining admission as younger ones. Prospective candidates who are concerned about this should check the statistics of the schools to which they wish to apply.

Canadian faculties of medicine do not use race, religion, or sex as criteria in selection. The admission and enrollment of native Indian and Inuit students are encouraged in several Canadian medical schools. The number of female applicants has risen dramatically in recent years, and correspondingly larger proportions of the entering classes have been made up of women. Women comprised 52 percent of the 1998–99 applicant pool. Overall, 22.2 percent of the applicants received at least one offer of admission. The success rate of women was higher than that of men. The first year class at Canadian medical schools was 51.3 percent female in 1998–99.

EXPENSES/FINANCIAL AID

Tuition and student fees for Canadian and non-Canadian students in the 1999–2000 entering class are given in Table 12-B and in the individual school entries. Expenses will vary from school to school and from individual to individual. It should be noted that tuition in several Canadian schools is slightly lower for successive years than for the first year. Tuition and fees at all Canadian universities are expected to increase substantially in the next few years.

Some information about financial aid is given in the individual school entries. Eligible Canadian students may apply for a Canada Student Loan, or they may apply to the Department of Education of their own province for a provincial student loan.

ONTARIO MEDICAL SCHOOL APPLICATION SERVICE (OMSAS)

The Ontario Medical School Application Service (OMSAS) is a nonprofit, centralized application service for applicants to the five medical schools in the province of Ontario. OMSAS provides only the application processing service; each medical school is completely autonomous in reaching its own admission decisions. *All applications to the Ontario medical schools must be made through OMSAS.*

OMSAS application materials are available July 1. Completed application materials must be received by OMSAS no later than October 15. Official transcripts must be received by OMSAS no later than November 15. However, applicants are advised to submit their application materials in advance of the deadline. An instruction booklet, containing information about application procedures and admission requirements, and the OMSAS application on diskette, may be obtained from:

OMSAS
Ontario Universities' Application Centre
P.O. Box 1328
650 Woodlawn Road West
Guelph, Ontario N1H 7P4
Canada
Telephone: (519) 823-1940, Ext. 553
E-mail: omsas@ouac.on.ca

TABLE 12-B

Tuition and Student Fees for 1999–2000 First-Year Students at Canadian Medical Schools (In Canadian Dollars)

Categories of Students	Range	Median	Average
Canadian	2,528–10,918	5,906	6,340*
Non-Canadian, Regular*	9,525–32,893	16,403	18,981*
Non-Canadian, Contract*	25,225–35,722	28,280	28,785

NOTE: Figures based on data provided fall 1999.

*Average Canadian was derived from all 16 Canadian schools. Average non-Canadian (regular) was derived from 9 Canadian schools reporting (7 schools do not accept non-Canadians into regular quota positions). Average non-Canadian (contract) was derived from 8 schools that accept foreign students into above-quota positions on a cost-recovery, contract basis.

Source: Association of Canadian Medical Colleges

SOURCES OF FURTHER INFORMATION

Further information about admission requirements, curricula of Canadian medical schools, and medical education in Canada is in the catalogs available from each school and in *Admission Requirements to Canadian Faculties of Medicine and Their Selection Policies* (edited in 1998 for admission in 1999–2000 or 2000–01). Prices for this publication are $25 in Canada, $25 (U.S.) for requests from the United States, and $30 (U.S.) for requests from overseas and may be ordered from:

Association of Canadian Medical Colleges
774 Echo Drive
Ottawa, Ontario K1S 5P2
Canada
Telephone: (613) 730-0687
Fax: (613) 730-1196
Web Site: www.acmc.ca

ABBREVIATIONS

Listed below are the abbreviations used in the school entries in this chapter.

GPA—Grade-point average
MCAT—Medical College Admission Test
VR—Verbal Reasoning
PS—Physical Sciences
WS—Writing Sample
BS—Biological Sciences
OMSAS—Ontario Medical School Application Service

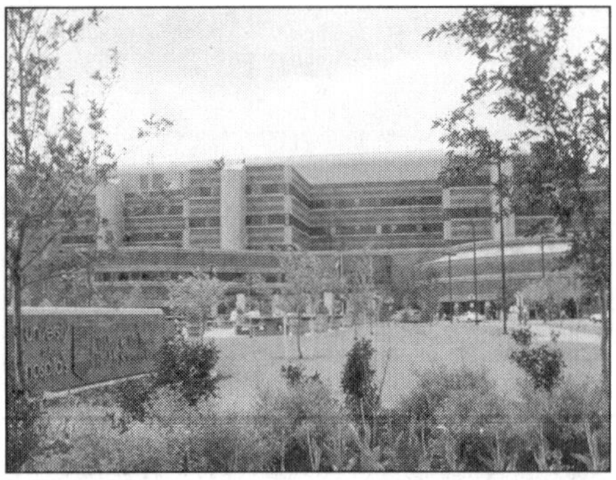

University of Alberta Faculty of Medicine and Dentistry

Edmonton, Alberta

Dr. D. L. J. Tyrrell, *Dean*
Dr. C. G. Baker, *Assistant Dean, Admissions*
M. Healey, *Admissions Officer*

ADDRESS INQUIRIES TO:

Admissions Officer, Admissions
2-45 Medical Sciences Building
University of Alberta
Faculty of Medicine and Dentistry
Edmonton, Alberta
Canada, T6G 2H7
(780) 492-9524; 492-9531 (FAX)
E-mail: admissions@med.ualberta.ca
Web site: http://www.med.ualberta.ca

GENERAL INFORMATION

The Faculty of Medicine at the University of Alberta was founded in 1913.

The Medical Sciences Building, the Clinical Sciences Building, the Walter C. Mackenzie Health Sciences Centre, and the University of Alberta Hospitals are located on the university campus. Clinical instruction is also given at the Royal Alexandra Hospital, Edmonton General Hospital, Misericordia Hospital, Alberta Hospital, Glenrose Hospital, Cross Cancer Institute, Grey Nuns Hospital, and Charles Camsell Hospital.

Student counseling services and student health services are available to all University of Alberta students.

CURRICULUM

The Faculty of Medicine conducts a fully accredited, four-year program leading to the degree of doctor of medicine. Each of the first two years consists of 33 weeks of instruction, from early September until mid-May. The final two years are conducted as a continuum, during which each student has a four-week holiday period.

The first two years of the curriculum are an integrated systems-based program covering the basic and clinical sciences. It is primarily case based and uses a mixture of lectures and small-group sessions with some problem-based learning. The last two years are composed of a student internship of at least 56 weeks, during which the student is assigned to hospitals affiliated with the faculty for clinical study and experience, a selective program in medicine and surgery, and an elective program that allows students to develop their own curriculum and spend a minimum of 12 weeks in one or more subject areas of their choice.

Throughout the program, emphasis is on self-education; much instruction is on a small-group basis.

A graduate training program leading to eligibility for specialist qualifications by the Royal College of Physicians and Surgeons of Canada is offered in most clinical specialties. Programs leading to the degree of master of science or doctor of philosophy in any of the basic medical sciences and in most of the clinical medical sciences are conducted under the direction of the Faculty of Graduate Studies and Research of the university.

Opportunity for research in the basic medical sciences is available to those students interested in spending a year or more in this type of work and obtaining a bachelor of science in medicine degree.

REQUIREMENTS FOR ENTRANCE

The MCAT is compulsory. All students considering medicine must register in a degree program and maintain good standing in that program. Irrespective of the degree program, the student must take courses in the following subjects:

Biological sciences: General biology
Biochemistry
Chemistry: Inorganic and organic chemistry
General physics
Statistics
English

These courses must be full-year courses (equivalent to six-credit courses at the University of Alberta) or two single-term courses (equivalent to three-credit courses at the University of Alberta) with the exception of statistics and biochemistry, in which a single three-credit course is acceptable.

Students are encouraged to obtain a baccalaureate degree prior to admission but may apply after two or three years in a degree program. To be considered for early selection, a student must have all the prerequisites as well as exceptional academic (minimum GPA of 8.4 on a 9.0 scale) and personal qualifications. Mature applicants may be given special consideration.

SELECTION FACTORS

Selection is based upon quality of scholastic achievement, personal suitability, and performance on the MCAT. Alberta residents are preferred, although each year out-of-province applicants are considered for 15 percent of first-year places.

An interview, résumé, essay, and letter(s) of reference are required. All information on each candidate is considered by the Admissions Committee, and the quota is filled by the best candidates available.

ABORIGINAL APPLICANTS

The Faculty of Medicine and Dentistry may provide up to two positions over the regular quota of 102 for the M.D. program to Aboriginal applicants. For clarification, it is noted that students who are Aboriginal ancestry within the meaning of the Constitution Act of 1982, Section 35. (2) will be considered in this category.

Candidates will be subject to normal minimum admission requirements and approval by the Faculty of Medicine and Dentistry Admissions Committee. If there are no qualified Aboriginal students in any given year, these positions will not be allocated to other applicants.

Aboriginal student applicants and prospective premedical students are encouraged to contact the Coordinator, Native Health Care Careers, Faculty of Medicine and Dentistry, for individual counseling and career planning.

M.D.–PH.D. PROGRAM

Highly qualified students motivated toward a career in medical research may wish to consider the M.D.-Ph.D. program.

FINANCIAL AID

Loans are available under the Canada Student Loan Plan or the Province of Alberta Loan Plan to Canadian citizens or permanent residents who have been in Canada and in Alberta for 12 months prior to the beginning of the academic term.

Public Institution

APPLICATION AND ACCEPTANCE POLICIES FOR 2001–2002 FIRST-YEAR CLASS

Fees and expenses are in Canadian dollars.

Filing of application
  Earliest date: July 1, 2000
  Latest date: Nov. 1, 2000
School application fee to all applicants: $60
Oldest MCAT scores considered: 1997
Does not have Early Decision Program
  Acceptance notice to regular applicants
  Earliest date: May 1, 2001
  Latest date: July 1, 2001
Applicant's response to acceptance offer
  Maximum time: 10 days
Requests for deferred entrance considered: Yes
Deposit to hold place in class (applied to tuition):
  $175, due with response to acceptance offer; nonrefundable
Estimated number of new entrants: 102
Starting date: Aug. 2001

TUITION AND STUDENT FEES PER YEAR FOR 1999–2000 FIRST-YEAR CLASS

Tuition*
  Canadian: $7,289
  Non-Canadian: N/A

INFORMATION ON 1999–2000 FIRST-YEAR CLASS

Number of	*In-Province*	*Out-of-Province*	*Total*
Applicants	580	515	1,095
Applicants Interviewed	—	—	415
New Entrants†	90	14	104

*Includes student fees; no longer broken down into tuition and fees.

†All took the MCAT; 80% had baccalaureate degrees.

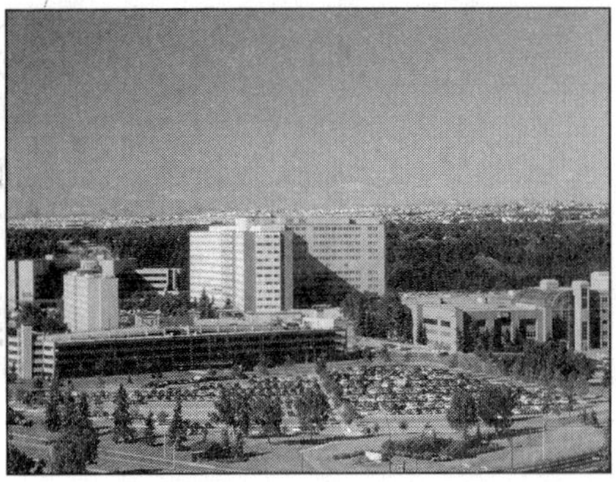

University of Calgary Faculty of Medicine

Calgary, Alberta

Dr. Grant Gall, *Dean of Medicine*
Adele Meyers, *Admissions Officer*
Joan Van Housen, *Director, Awards and Financial Aid*

ADDRESS INQUIRIES TO:

Office of Admissions
University of Calgary
Faculty of Medicine
3330 Hospital Drive, N.W.
Calgary, Alberta
Canada T2N 4N1
(403) 220-4262
E-mail: staylor@ucalgary.ca
Web Site: http://www.med.ucalgary.ca/admissions

MISSION STATEMENT

What kind of medical school do we wish to be?

- A medical school responsive to community and societal needs—not only of the present but of the future.
- A medical school determined to shape the future of society, i.e., a medical school that leads with vision, developing new ideas, resources, technology, health care, and scientific professionals that will ensure that the preferred or desired future will become a reality.
- A medical school rooted in basic research and discovery, the creation of new knowledge, and the transfer of that knowledge and discovery to benefit society.
- A medical school committed to excellence and pursuit of excellence, to high quality and standards, to continuous evaluation of status quo, to assurance of quality, to effective and efficient outcomes, and to continuous improvement in all endeavours.
- A medical school committed to innovation and creativity in education, research, clinical service, administration and management, and development of human resources and technology.
- A medical school with a sense of values, principles, and priorities.

GENERAL INFORMATION

The Faculty of Medicine at the University of Calgary accepted its first students in September 1970. In 1972 the Faculty of Medicine moved into its permanent facilities in the Calgary Health Sciences Centre. The centre has been designed to complement the objectives of the faculty's integrated teaching program.

CURRICULUM

The curriculum is based on clinical presentations the way patients present to physicians. One hundred twenty clinical presentations have been defined ranging from simple to complex and are grouped by body system and human development. The first course offered is principles for medicine, which serves to introduce the different modes of solving clinical problems and the basic concepts essential to an understanding of human structure, function, and growth as well as provision of comprehensive medical care to the individual, the family, and society. Introductory clinical skills of communication and physical examination also commence in the first weeks of the curriculum. Following principles of medicine is the first of the interdisciplinary body systems courses. Approximately two-thirds of the student's time is allocated to these regularly scheduled courses. The remaining period is available for elective study and the independent study or tutorial program. Each academic year lasts about 11 months. The problem-solving approach, combined with the curriculum design, is intended to facilitate the integration between the conventional basic and clinical sciences. As well, students have the opportunity to reinforce in a clinical setting what they have learned in the body systems as they progress through each of the systems. The curriculum also focuses on the relevance of the family and the community in health and disease.

The school employs a pass/fail grading system. Interested students may apply for the combined M.D.-M.Sc. or M.D.-Ph.D. program. At the end of the three years, students will be granted the M.D. degree. The school's philosophy is to produce generalist physicians who can proceed to further training in specialty, family medicine, or research.

REQUIREMENTS FOR ENTRANCE

All students are required to take the new MCAT by the fall of the year before anticipated enrollment. Most students have a B.A. or B.Sc. degree before entering the Faculty of Medicine, although a few extremely well qualified students have been admitted after two years in an arts or science program. There is some advantage to majoring in a science area, but the student who has excelled in behavioral science or any other undergraduate area may be accepted.

The following undergraduate courses are recommended: general biology, cell biology, mammalian physiology, organic and inorganic chemistry, biochemistry, English, physics, calculus, and one course of psychology, sociology, or anthropology.

SELECTION FACTORS

The Admissions Committee selects applicants without discrimination to gender, race, religion, or age and attempts to apply six criteria: undergraduate academic achievement, employment history, extracurricular activities, an essay, letters of recommendation, and the MCAT. Final applicants will be required to attend an interview at the University of Calgary at their own expense. Final applicants will also be required to write an on-site essay on a topic assigned by the Admissions Committee. Preference is given to Alberta residents. The Faculty of Medicine has a policy on admission of candidates who are neither Canadian citizens nor landed Immigrants. This policy is available on the school's Web Site at <http://www.ucalgary.ca/md/>. Rejected applicants are given the opportunity to reapply for admission. Applicants who have been asked to withdraw or who have been suspended or expelled from any medical school will not normally be considered.

ADMISSION OF STUDENTS BY TRANSFER

The University of Calgary Faculty of Medicine will consider application by students for transfer only from other LCME-accredited medical schools and only under special circumstances. Approval of transfer will be based on evaluation of the candidate and his/her past performance and on the availability of positions. Because the first and second years of the three-year M.D. program at the University of Calgary are regarded as a continuum of course work, transfers will only be considered in the final or clerkship year.

FINANCIAL AID

The majority of students obtain financial aid through student loans. Because the students attend school 11 months each year, summer employment is unlikely, and, therefore, financial support must be sufficient to meet their requirements over the subsequent three years. The student awards officer will provide information about student loans, bursaries, and awards. The financial status of the applicant does not affect acceptance into the program.

Students receive a total stipend of $3,420 for the third (final) year.

Public Institution

APPLICATION AND ACCEPTANCE POLICIES FOR 2001–2002 FIRST-YEAR CLASS

Fees and expenses are in Canadian dollars.

Filing of application
  Earliest date: July 15, 2000
  Latest date: Nov. 15, 2000
School application fee to all applicants: $65
Oldest MCAT scores considered: 1991
Does not have Early Decision Program
Acceptance notice to regular applicants
  Earliest date: May 15, 2001
  Latest date: Varies
Applicant's response to acceptance offer
  Maximum time: 15 days
Requests for deferred entrance considered: No
Deposit to hold place in class (applied to tuition):
  $100, due with response to acceptance offer
Deposit refundable prior to: June 15, 2001
Estimated number of new entrants: 69*
Starting date: Aug. 2001

TUITION AND STUDENT FEES PER YEAR FOR 1999–2000 FIRST-YEAR CLASS

Tuition
  Canadian: $5,836
  Non-Canadian: $30,000

Student fees: $333.50

INFORMATION ON 1999–2000 FIRST-YEAR CLASS

Number of	*In-Province*	*Out-of-Province*	*Total*
Applicants	516	798	1,314
Applicants Interviewed	91	130	221
New Entrants†	31	38‡	69

*Negotiations are underway to raise this but exactly how much and when is unknown at this time.

†All took the MCAT; 81% had baccalaureate degrees.

‡38 Canadian; 10 International

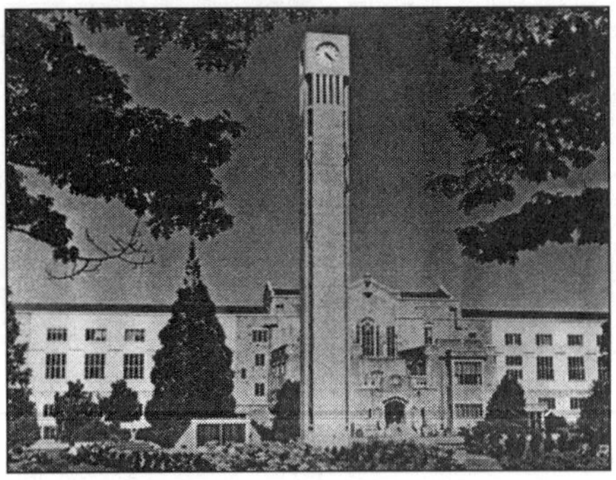

University of British Columbia Faculty of Medicine

Vancouver, British Columbia

Dr. J.A. Cairns, *Dean*
Dr. Joanna Bates, *Associate Dean, Admissions*
Carol Gibson, *Director, Awards and Financial Aid*

ADDRESS INQUIRIES TO:

Office of the Dean, Faculty of Medicine
Admissions Office
University of British Columbia
317-2194 Health Sciences Mall
Vancouver, British Columbia
Canada V6T 1Z3
(604) 822-4482; 822-6061 (FAX)
Web Site: http://www.med.ubc.ca

MISSION STATEMENT

Our mission is to advance the knowledge, understanding, and health of our society through education, scholarship, and health care with excellence as the most important criterion.

GENERAL INFORMATION

The Faculty of Medicine of the University of British Columbia received its first students in 1950 and graduated its first class in 1954. It is an integral part of a large provincial university comprising a variety of faculties and schools with a total enrollment of over 30,000 students.

Teaching in the preclinical subject areas is based in the basic medical science departments. Clinical teaching is currently carried out at the Vancouver Hospital and Health Sciences Center, St. Paul's and Children's Hospitals, BC Women's Hospital and Health Centre, and a number of other institutions.

The health sciences complex on the university campus comprises a large Instructional Resources Center providing lecture theaters, small group seminar rooms, audiovisual facilities, and student lounge and snack bar areas; a 60-bed psychiatric hospital with additional day care facilities; a 300-bed extended care unit; and a 240-bed acute care Hospital. New off-campus hospital facilities at Children's Hospital and an adjoining obstetrical and gynecological unit at BC Women's Hospital and Health Centre were opened in 1982.

CURRICULUM

In the fall of 1997, a case-based curriculum was introduced. The four years of instruction are broadly divided into three phases: an initial 18-month period with emphasis on the basic medical sciences, a 12-month clinical clerkship, and the final 9 months are directed to advanced clinical clerkships, as well as a return to the basic medical sciences. Teaching in the first year is carried out largely on campus, but during the second year it is transferred in part to the teaching hospitals; in the third and fourth years it is largely hospital based.

Earlier introduction of students to patients in a clinical setting, the integration and coordination of learning experiences in the basic medical sciences and clinical practice, provision of increased elective and self-study time, and the development of more effective measures for evaluation of students and of the educational program are among the major objectives of the Faculty of Medicine.

REQUIREMENTS FOR ENTRANCE

The MCAT, a minimum of three years (90 semester hours) of accredited college course work, and a minimum of a B average or second class standing (70 percent) are required. The faculty recommends that students take courses in behavioral sciences, biometrics and statistics, and physics. A baccalaureate degree is not a prerequisite.

The minimum subject requirements are:

	Years
General biology	1
General biochemistry	1
General chemistry	1
Organic chemistry	1
English literature and composition	1

SELECTION FACTORS

Selection is not contingent upon an applicant's sex, age, race, religion, or national origin. Those accepted are generally within the age range of 20 to 30 years. Preference is given to well-qualified British Columbia residents; small numbers of candidates with superior qualifications from other Canadian provinces may be admitted. No applicant is considered who has been required to withdraw from another medical school.

Admission is based on intellectual achievement and potential, as demonstrated by overall academic records and MCAT scores, and on qualities of personality, character, and motivation, evaluated by interviews, preprofessional committee reports, letters of reference, and an autobiographical statement submitted with the application. Applicants will be advised if personal interviews are required.

FINANCIAL AID

Scholarships are awarded to students showing proficiency and promise in their medical school studies. Generally they are available to only those students who have been in attendance in a university in British Columbia for at least one year. These scholarships are provided through the generosity of various medical and other organizations in British Columbia. Bursaries and loans may be applied for in any academic year.

It is recommended that students devote themselves entirely to the full-time demands of the medical course. Students' spouses may find employment through the university's personnel office.

Public Institution

APPLICATION AND ACCEPTANCE POLICIES FOR 2001–2002 FIRST-YEAR CLASS

Fees and expenses are in Canadian dollars.

Filing of application
Earliest date: Aug. 15, 2000
Latest date: Dec. 1, 2000
School application fee: $105 British Columbia applicants; $155 out-of-province applicants; additional $30 to evaluate out-of-province transcripts
Oldest MCAT scores considered: 1995
Does not have Early Decision Program
Acceptance notice to regular applicants
Earliest date: May 1, 2001
Latest date: Until class is filled
Applicant's response to acceptance offer
Maximum time: 10 days
Requests for deferred entrance considered: Yes
Deposit to hold place in class (applied to tuition): $300, due with response to acceptance offer; nonrefundable
Estimated number of new entrants: 120
Starting date: Aug. 2001

TUITION AND STUDENT FEES PER YEAR FOR 1999–2000 FIRST-YEAR CLASS

Tuition: $4,000 Student fees: $256

INFORMATION ON 1999–2000 FIRST-YEAR CLASS

Number of	*In-Province*	*Out-of-Province*	*Total*
Applicants	469	141	610
Applicants Interviewed	—	—	229
New Entrants*	120	0	120

*All took the MCAT; 84% had baccalaureate degrees.

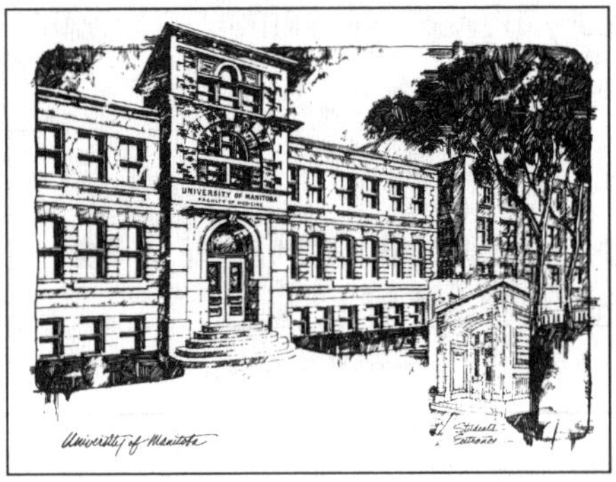

University of Manitoba Faculty of Medicine

Winnipeg, Manitoba

Dr. B. Hennen, *Dean*
Dr. L. J. Elliott, *Associate Dean, Admissions*
C. K. Paragg, *Registrar*

ADDRESS INQUIRIES TO:

Chair, Admissions Committee
University of Manitoba
Faculty of Medicine
753 McDermot Avenue
Winnipeg, Manitoba
Canada R3E 0W3
(204) 789-3569; 789-3929 (FAX)
E-mail: registrar_med@umanitoba.ca
Web Site: http://www.umanitoba.ca/faculties/medicine

GENERAL INFORMATION

The Manitoba Medical College was established in 1883 and from its beginning was affiliated with the University of Manitoba. The first class of six graduated in 1886. In 1918 the Manitoba Medical College became the Faculty of Medicine of the University of Manitoba. In 1924 it received approval as a Class A medical school. The medical buildings are adjacent to the Health Sciences Centre in Winnipeg, which is some distance from the main university campus.

Teaching hospitals affiliated with the Faculty of Medicine are the Health Sciences Centre (Children's, Adults', Women's, and Respiratory and Rehabilitation hospitals—1,064 beds); St. Boniface General Hospital (900 beds); Deer Lodge Veterans Hospital (500 beds); Grace Hospital (306 beds); Seven Oaks Hospital (336 beds); Victoria Hospital (254 beds); and Misericordia Hospital (409 beds).

CURRICULUM

Medicine is a four-year course at the University of Manitoba. In the first and second years there are, on the average, 30 hours of formal instruction per week for 39 weeks. The first- and second-year curriculum covers the basic and clinical sciences, clinical and communication skills, and professional attitudes and behavior pertinent to the practice of medicine. It is composed of six instructional blocks that address the core concepts of health and medicine, human growth and development, and four organ systems-based blocks. The third and fourth years are devoted to preclerkship (9 weeks); clerkship (eight clerkships of 7 weeks duration each); electives (13 weeks); and basic science review. A pass/fail system of evaluating student performance has been adopted, and, consequently, no rank in class or grades is given.

REQUIREMENTS FOR ENTRANCE

The MCAT and a bachelor's degree are mandatory. The academic requirements for admission are clear senior matriculation (comparable with sophomore matriculation in U.S. colleges) and the completion of three premedical years of 32 weeks each (15 full courses) in the Faculty of Arts and Science of the University of Manitoba or its equivalent.

The following subjects must be included in the course of study:

	Credit hrs.
Biochemistry	6
English	6

In other respects, the content of the course work must satisfy either the university's B.A. or B.Sc. degree requirements, with a minimum of 18 hours in the social sciences/humanities and 18 hours in the natural/physical sciences. Applicants must write the MCAT no later than August of the year preceding entry.

SELECTION FACTORS

Selection by the Committee on Admissions is made primarily on the basis of a composite score, calculated as follows: (i) adjusted grade-point score: maximum, 10 percent; (ii) MCAT score: maximum, 50 percent; and (iii) personal assessment score: maximum, 40 percent. The personal assessment score is based on an autobiographical essay of approximately 800 words, the MCAT writing sample, a standardized questionnaire sent to references named by the applicant, and the results of an interview with a panel of three interviewers. Ninety percent of the 70 places available in the entering class normally are filled in this way. However, about 10 percent of successful applicants with acceptable but noncompetitive undergraduate performance may be selected on the basis of special premedical experience (educational or occupational) of relevance to the study and practice of medicine. Preference is given to undergraduates and graduates of the universities in Manitoba who are Canadian citizens or permanent residents of Canada. At the discretion of the committee, a limited number of places may be made available to undergraduates of other universities. The school does not discriminate on the basis of race, sex, creed, or national origin. Special efforts are made to recruit and retain applicants from the aboriginal populations.

Applicants for the 1999 entering class with a minimum GPA of 3.6 were interviewed, and 39 percent of those interviewed were enrolled.

Advanced standing consideration is given to candidates in Medicine I and II attending schools formally accredited by the joint LCME/CACMS accreditation committee to bring a class up to its first-year enrollment limit.

FINANCIAL AID

Under the Canadian Students Loan Act, Canadians can obtain interest-free loans during their undergraduate course in medicine. Bursaries from the university and from the provincial government are available to deserving students. Students may also obtain assistance from the W. K. Kellogg Student Loan Program and from the Gordon Bell/College of Physicians and Surgeons (Manitoba) Loan Fund. A few scholarships of smaller amounts are also available.

OTHER PROGRAMS

Most graduates of the University of Manitoba Faculty of Medicine gain licensure by completing the two-part Medical Council of Canada Qualifying Examination (MCCQE), plus earning certification by either the Royal College of Physicians and Surgeons of Canada or the College of Family Physicians of Canada.

Specialty training is approved by the Royal College of Physicians and Surgeons of Canada and is conducted in the Affiliated Teaching Hospitals of the University of Manitoba. The University of Manitoba currently holds Royal College approval for 45 specialty training programs.

The Family Medicine Program is a two-year integrated training program leading to certification by the College of Family Physicians of Canada. The program is conducted in the affiliated teaching hospitals as well as in rural settings.

Continuing Medical Education is provided for practicing physicians. The Faculty of Medicine also provides opportunities for graduate studies in all the basic science departments as well as in selected clinical departments. Vibrant research activities are conducted by dedicated basic science and clinical staff.

A formal Bachelor of Science in the Medicine Research Program is offered to selected medical students in the summers following first- and second-year medicine. Summer opportunities are also available for rural medicine placements as well as placements with the Northern Medical Unit. The faculty offers M.Sc. and Ph.D. programs in all of its major departments.

Public Institution

APPLICATION AND ACCEPTANCE POLICIES FOR 2001–2002 FIRST-YEAR CLASS

Fees and expenses are in Canadian dollars.

Filing of application
  Earliest date: July 15, 2000
  Latest date: Nov. 15, 2000
School application fee to all applicants: $60
Oldest MCAT scores considered: 1997
Does not have Early Decision Program
Acceptance notice to regular applicants
  Earliest date: June 7, 2001
  Latest date: Until class is filled
Applicant's response to acceptance offer
  Maximum time: 10 days
Requests for deferred entrance considered: No
Deposit to hold place in class (applied to tuition):
  $100, due with response to acceptance offer
Deposit refundable prior to: Aug. 1, 2001
Estimated number of new entrants: 70
Starting date: Aug. 2001

TUITION AND STUDENT FEES PER YEAR FOR 1999–2000 FIRST-YEAR CLASS

Tuition: $7,791 Student fees: $41

INFORMATION ON 1999–2000 FIRST-YEAR CLASS

Number of	*In-Province*	*Out-of-Province*	*Total*
Applicants	187	324	511
Applicants Interviewed	170	24	194
New Entrants*	68	8	76

*All took the MCAT and had baccalaureate degrees.

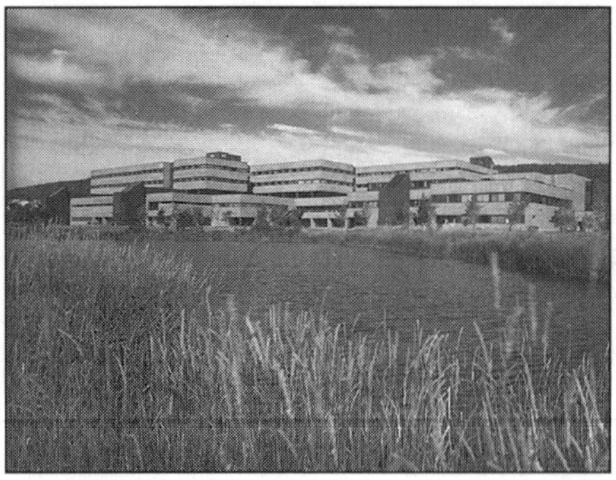

Memorial University of Newfoundland Faculty of Medicine

St. John's, Newfoundland

Dr. M.I. Bowmer, *Dean of Medicine*
Dr. W.L. Parsons, *Assistant Dean for Admissions*
Janet McHugh, *Admissions Officer*

ADDRESS INQUIRIES TO:

Janet McHugh, Admissions Officer
Memorial University of Newfoundland
Faculty of Medicine
St. John's, Newfoundland
Canada A1B 3V6
(709) 737-6615; 737-5186 (FAX)
E-mail: munmed@morgan.ucs.mun.ca
Web Site: http://www.med.mun.ca/admissions

MISSION STATEMENT

A primary objective of the medical school is to teach medical students to be physicians; and to provide such learning experiences as will inspire all medical graduates of the school to be prepared to practice medicine at the highest standards, serving all individuals and societies in the pursuit of health.

GENERAL INFORMATION

Memorial is the only university in the province of Newfoundland. The university was established as Memorial College in 1925 and incorporated as a university in 1949. In 1959 campus buildings were erected on a 1,000-acre site. There are some 12,000 undergraduates and a faculty of about 1,000 (including visiting professors) working on the campus, which is situated on the periphery of St. John's. The medical school is one of the four most recently established in Canada. It is housed in the Health Sciences Centre with General Hospital (531 beds) and a biomedical library. The medical school is fully accredited by the Committee on Accreditation of Canadian Medical Schools (CACMS) of the Association of Canadian Medical Colleges and the Canadian Medical Association, the Liaison Committee on Medical Education (LCME) of the Association of American Medical Colleges, and the American Medical Association. These accreditations mean that the medical school is equivalent in every respect to other medical schools in Canada and the United States.

Approved teaching programs for interns and residents are under the direction of the medical school. These programs are based at associate hospitals in St. John's and other provincial centers with a total bed complement of 3,116 covering inpatient and outpatient services in virtually all branches of medicine. Research work is being conducted both in the hospitals and in the Health Sciences Centre.

Residences for single and married students are provided on the campus, and the university maintains a list of approved off-campus accommodations. A health service is open to all students.

CURRICULUM

The curriculum, the physical structure, and the administrative organization of the school were planned to allow for maximum cooperation among the various basic science and clinical disciplines. The M.D. degree is granted upon completion of the fourth year, at which time Medical Council of Canada Examinations may be taken. The third and fourth years are clinical clerkship years, similar to the traditional internship.

During the first year of the medical program, students take introductory courses in cell structure and functions, biochemistry, physiology, molecular genetics, pharmacology, microbiology, anatomy, behavioral science, ethics, interviewing skills, and community medicine. These opportunities are provided in a wide range of medical settings—family practice, general hospital, rural hospital, and public health programs.

In the second half of the first year and the second year, teaching has a systems approach; material from anatomy, physiology, pathology, and clinical medicine is presented in an integrated manner. The third year is a structured clinical clerkship that includes eight weeks of electives, and the fourth year is made up of electives and selectives. Rotations for Rural Medicine take place in the first, third, and fourth years.

A pass/fail system is used for grading.

Although no formal medical/graduate (i.e., M.D.-Ph.D.) program exists, arrangements may be made for medical students to pursue, either concurrently or sequentially, both clinical and research training programs.

REQUIREMENTS FOR ENTRANCE

A bachelor's degree is required. In exceptional circumstances, an application may be considered from someone who does not hold a bachelor's degree; such an applicant will have completed at least 20 one-semester courses and be a student who has work-related or other experience acceptable to the admissions committee. The course of study must include two courses in English. All applicants must take the new MCAT (revised in 1991) prior to the application deadline.

Because of the limited number of places available and the intense competition for entry, applicants are advised to pursue a degree program of their choice and prepare for the MCAT. Although science courses are not required, a basic knowledge of the physical and life sciences may be helpful in writing the MCAT and in the medical program.

SELECTION FACTORS

The school admits students on the basis of residency priority as follows: bona fide residents of Newfoundland and Labrador, the rest of Canada, and non-Canadian applicants. In every case a high academic standard is required. Memorial University does not discriminate on the basis of race, marital status, sex, creed, national origin, or disability. Age by itself is not used as a basis for selection or rejection. However, both age and length of time away from full-time academic studies may be taken into consideration.

Normally, the medical school does not accept transfer students from other medical schools. In rare circumstances, a transfer may be considered if there is space available.

FINANCIAL AID

Financial assistance is available to medical students through government student loan programs. Information can be obtained by contacting the Student Affairs Office at: Student Affairs Office, Faculty of Medicine, Memorial University of Newfoundland, St. John's, NF, A1B 3VC; telephone (709) 737-6690; or E-mail mdray@morgan.ucs.mun.ca.

INFORMATION FOR MINORITIES, DISADVANTAGED, AND/OR NONTRADITIONAL APPLICANTS

Although there is no formal affirmative action process at this medical school, the Admissions Committee does take into consideration the background of all applicants in making its decisions.

Public Institution

APPLICATION AND ACCEPTANCE POLICIES FOR 2001–2002 FIRST-YEAR CLASS

Fees and expenses are in Canadian dollars.

Filing of application
  Earliest date: July 3, 2000
  Latest date: Nov. 15, 2000
School application fee to all applicants: $75
Oldest MCAT scores considered: 1991
Does not have Early Decision Program
Acceptance notice to regular applicants
  Earliest date: March 1, 2001
  Latest date: Until class is filled
Applicant's response to acceptance offer
  Maximum time: 14 days
Requests for deferred entrance considered: Yes
Deposit to hold place in class (applied to tuition):
  $200, due with response to acceptance offer; nonrefundable
Estimated number of new entrants: 60
Starting date: Sept. 2001

TUITION AND STUDENT FEES PER YEAR FOR 1999–2000 FIRST-YEAR CLASS

Tuition	Student fees:
Resident: $6,250	Resident: $227
Nonresident: $30,000	Nonresident: $553

INFORMATION ON 1999–2000 FIRST-YEAR CLASS

Number of	*In-Province*	*Out-of-Province*	*Total*
Applicants	187	460	647
Applicants Interviewed	147	45	192
New Entrants*	46	13	59

*All took the MCAT and had baccalaureate degrees.

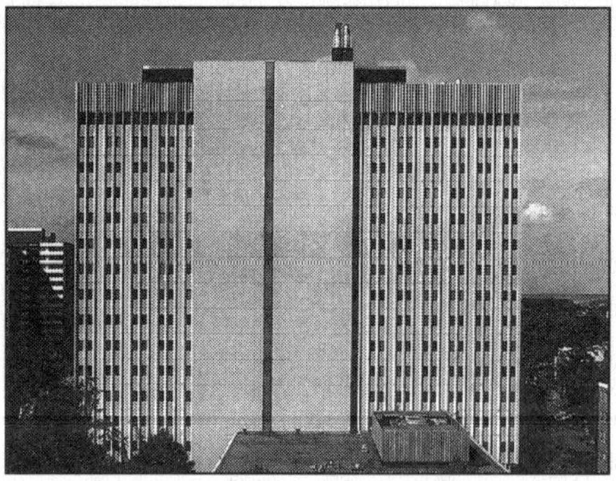

Dalhousie University Faculty of Medicine

Halifax, Nova Scotia

Dr. Noni MacDonald, *Dean*
Dr. Margaret Casey, *Director of Admissions*

ADDRESS INQUIRIES TO:

Brenda L. Detienne, Admissions Coordinator
Room C-132, Lower Level, Clinical Research Centre
Dalhousie University
Halifax, Nova Scotia
Canada B3H 4H7
(902) 494-1083; 494-8884 (FAX)
E-mail: brenda.detienne@tupdean2.med.dal.ca
Web Site: http://www.mcms.dal.ca/

GENERAL INFORMATION

Dalhousie University, a privately endowed institution founded in 1838, established the Faculty of Medicine in 1868. The main responsibility of the Faculty of Medicine is to the three Maritime Provinces of Canada (Nova Scotia, New Brunswick, and Prince Edward Island), which have a population of some 1.7 million.

The teaching hospitals located in the immediate vicinity of the medical school have a total of 2,300 beds covering inpatient and outpatient services in all branches of medicine.

University housing and a comprehensive Student Health Service are available.

CURRICULUM

The aim of the four-year course of study in medicine is to provide a basic education that would permit a graduate to enter any branch of postgraduate training.

The academic year for Medicine One and Medicine Two begins in early September and extends to the end of May. Medicine Three begins in late August/early September and ends in March. Medicine Four begins in March and extends until May of the following year. The M.D. degree is granted upon successful completion of the fourth year.

During the first two years of the curriculum, students will learn predominantly in small groups, working with a tutor. The curriculum is organized around clinical problems to provide an integrated context for students to learn both basic and clinical science, and to begin the development of clinical reasoning skills. The third and fourth years are predominantly clinical, with the years being broken into a series of rotations within the various clinical disciplines. Starting in the first year, Dalhousie students have extensive patient contact hours, as the school places great emphasis on the development of clinical skills. In addition to small-group teaching, which emphasizes independent learning, teaching methods include lectures, laboratories, and bedside teaching.

In addition to the basic M.D. program, Dalhousie offers a bachelor of science in medicine program and an M.D.-Ph.D. program.

Dalhousie University through its Faculty of Medicine offers university-arranged and university-supervised clinical training, which meets national accreditation standards, for postgraduate medical trainees.

In all provinces with the exception of Quebec, the basis for licensure for the majority of trainees in a postgraduate training program affiliated with a CACMS/LCME medical school is successful completion of the two-part Medical Council of Canada Qualifying Examination (MCCQE), plus certification by either the College of Family Physicians of Canada or the Royal College of Physicians and Surgeons of Canada. There is great competition for entry into all programs.

The family medicine program at Dalhousie is a two-year integrated training experience following the M.D. leading to certification by the College of Family Physicians of Canada.

Specialty training is approved by the Royal College of Physicians and Surgeons of Canada and is conducted in affiliated teaching hospitals in both Halifax and Saint John. Dalhousie University currently holds Royal College approval for 41 specialty training programs.

The Faculty of Medicine maintains an active program of continuing medical education for practicing physicians in the Maritime Provinces. Research and graduate education are in all the basic science departments and in most of the clinical departments.

REQUIREMENTS FOR ENTRANCE

A university degree and the writing of the MCAT are absolute requirements. Students applying in the fall of 2000 for admission in September 2001 must have written either the April 1996 or subsequent MCAT. The April writing of the MCAT will not be considered for entry in September of the same year. There are no absolute prerequisite courses required. The major objective is that premedical education encompasses broad study in the physical, life, and social sciences and the humanities. The minimum requirement for entry, however, is a baccalaureate degree.

All applicants must meet the following minimum academic requirements:

Maritime Applicants: A minimum academic average of B+ (77 percent or higher) or a GPA of 3.30 based on a full course load of 5 full courses in the last two undergraduate years, or three out of four good years plus MCAT scores of 10 and above, with a minimum score of 24.

Non-Maritime Applicants: A minimum academic average of A– (80 percent or higher) or a GPA of 3.70 based on a full course load of 5 full courses in the last two undergraduate years, or three out of four good years plus MCAT scores of 10 and above, with a minimum score of 30.

Background in the physical and life sciences will help a student deal with the considerable load of scientific information involved in undergraduate medical study. Courses in the social sciences and humanities will be helpful in understanding human behavior in health and illness. The ability to communicate effectively, both orally and in writing, is essential. The committee believes that attracting students with a rich variety of educational backgrounds is in the interest of all students. Such preparation supports the training of outstanding physicians.

The medical undergraduate student has to deal with a great deal more information per unit of time than is usually the case in university undergraduate programs in arts and science. Therefore, the Admissions Committee will consider not only the academic grades of applicants but the type and degree of difficulty of university courses completed.

Applications from very well qualified students from other provinces and countries will be considered for up to 10 percent of the entering places in each class. Unless such nonresident applicants have reasonable prospects of being accepted at their local medical school, they should not expect to be accepted at Dalhousie and would be well advised not to apply.

SELECTION FACTORS

Sources of information and factors considered by the Admissions Committee include academic requirements, ability as judged on university records and on the MCAT, confidential assessments received from referees of the applicant's choice and from any others the committee may wish to consult, interviews (selected applicants only), and place of residence. Detailed comments and explanations on these selection factors may be obtained in the Faculty of Medicine Calendar.

Dalhousie does not discriminate on the basis of race, sex, creed, national origin, age, or handicap.

FINANCIAL AID

A few entrance scholarships and entrance bursaries are awarded to students in the first year who are residents of the Maritime Provinces. The Dalhousie Medical Alumni Association Entrance Scholarship, the Dr. E. James Gordon Scholarship, and the Halifax Medical Society Entrance Scholarship are available to anyone regardless of residency. A number of bursaries and prizes are available in each year. The university maintains a loan fund, which is interest-free until graduation. Applicants are advised not to plan to earn money in time-consuming work, which may jeopardize their academic standing.

INFORMATION FOR MINORITY STUDENTS

Students from minority groups will be considered on their individual merits.

Dalhousie University is an affirmative action and equal-opportunity educational institution.

Private Institution

APPLICATION AND ACCEPTANCE POLICIES FOR 2001–2002 FIRST-YEAR CLASS

Fees and expenses are in Canadian dollars.

Filing of application
  Earliest date: Oct. 1, 2000
  Latest date: Nov. 15, 2000
School application fee to all applicants: $60
Oldest MCAT scores considered: 1996
Does not have Early Decision Program
Acceptance notice to regular applicants
  Earliest date: Feb. 1, 2001
  Latest date: June 30, 2001
Applicant's response to acceptance offer
  Maximum time: 4 weeks
Requests for deferred entrance considered: Yes
Deposit to hold place in class (applied to tuition): $200, due with response to acceptance offer; nonrefundable
Estimated number of new entrants: 82
Starting date: Aug. 2001

TUITION AND STUDENT FEES PER YEAR FOR 1999–2000 FIRST-YEAR CLASS

Tuition
  Canadian: $6,670
  Non-Canadian: $9,760
Student fees: $352

INFORMATION ON 1999–2000 FIRST-YEAR CLASS

Number of	*Maritime*	*Non-Maritime*	*Total*
Applicants	269	300	569
Applicants Interviewed	215	45	260
New Entrants*	76	10	86

*All took the MCAT and had baccalaureate degrees.

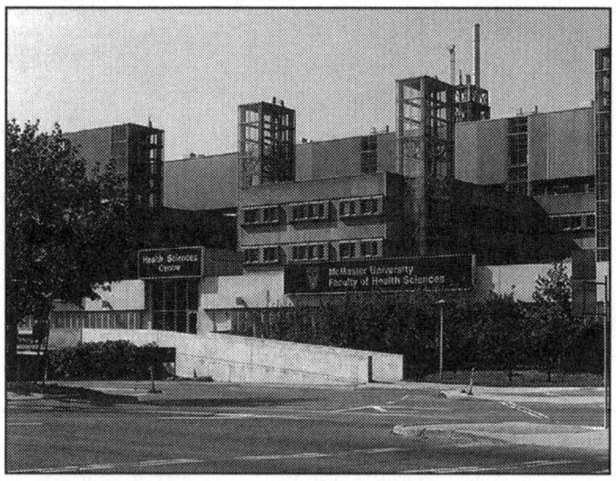

McMaster University Undergraduate Medical Programme School of Medicine

Hamilton, Ontario

Dr. Russell T. Joffe, *Dean (Health Sciences)*
Dr. Claude Nahmias, *Chair, M.D. Admissions*
Debbie Martin, *M.D. Programme Administrator*

ADDRESS INQUIRIES TO:

Admissions and Records
HSC 1B7-Health Sciences Centre
McMaster University
1200 Main Street West
Hamilton, Ontario
Canada L8N 3Z5
(905) 525-9140, Ext. 22235; 527-2707 (FAX)
E-mail: mdadmit@fhs.mcmaster.ca
Web Site: http://www.fhs.mcmaster.ca/mdprog

GENERAL INFORMATION

The Faculty of Health Sciences at McMaster University offers programs in health sciences education, including undergraduate and postgraduate medical education, and in health sciences research. The clinical programs use the teaching hospital and extensive ambulatory facilities of the McMaster Division of the Hamilton Health Sciences Corporation, but also involve clinical teaching units at the major Hamilton hospitals and community health care centers. The Undergraduate Medical Programme was initiated in 1969, and the first class of students graduated in May 1972.

CURRICULUM

The three-year program (130 weeks of instruction) in medicine at McMaster uses an approach to learning that will apply throughout the physician's career. The components have been organized in a relevant and logical manner with early exposure to patients. Flexibility is ensured to allow for the variety of student backgrounds and career goals.

The graduates of McMaster's Undergraduate Medical Programme will have developed the knowledge, ability, and attitudes necessary to qualify for further education in any medical career. The general goals for students in the program include the following: the development of competency in problem-based learning and in problem solving, the development of the personal characteristics and attitudes compatible with effective health care, the development of clinical and communication skills, and the development of the skills to be a lifelong, self-directed learner.

To achieve the objectives of the Undergraduate Medical Programme, students are introduced to patients and their problems within the first unit. They are presented with a series of health care problems and questions requiring the understanding of principles and data collection. Much of the students' learning occurs within the setting of the small-group tutorial. Faculty members serve as tutors/facilitators or as sources of expert knowledge.

The Undergraduate Medical Programme is arranged as a four-unit preclerkship sequence followed by a clerkship; there are additional elective opportunities, both in block periods (totaling 26 weeks) and horizontal electives taken concurrently with ongoing units. Unit 1 is a 12-week introduction to concepts and information from three knowledge perspectives: population, behavior, and biology. In addition, a major theme of the entire curriculum, the life cycle, is developed as a perspective and anchors the three subunits of Unit 1: Early Development, Maturation, and Aging. Units 2, 3, and 4 are 14-week units organized on the basis of organ systems, where biomedical and health care problems are analyzed in depth. The clerkship emphasizes the clinical application of concepts learned in the earlier units and consists of experience in inpatient and ambulatory settings. These include internal medicine, family medicine, surgery, psychiatry, obstetrics-gynecology, and pediatrics. Unit 6, which follows the clerkship, is an interactive unit in which students will tackle issues derived from societal expectations of a practicing physician.

REQUIREMENTS FOR ENTRANCE

Completion of a minimum of three years at an accredited university with at least an overall second class (B) average is required. There are no course prerequisites. The MCAT is not required.

Applicants who are not Canadian citizens or landed immigrants in Canada will be invited to interview only when they are considered to be clearly more suitable on all criteria than Canadian candidates.

Both academic achievement and personal qualities are considered. Academic achievement is assessed on the basis of course grades. Personal qualities and attributes are assessed on the basis of a submission written by the applicant, an autobiographical sketch, three references, a personal interview, and the performance in a simulated tutorial. The Faculty does not accept applications for transfer into the programme.

SELECTION FACTORS

Students and members of the community and faculty are involved in the assessment of applicants. The aim is to select students who not only have the necessary academic standards but also display characteristics that are deemed to be important for the study and practice of medicine. These include characteristics that suggest sensitivity to the needs of the community; sensitivity to the emotional, psychological, and physical aspects of patients; the ability to detect and solve problems; the ability to learn independently; the ability to function as a member of a small group; and the ability to plan one's career in a way that reflects the needs of the community.

Applicants rating highest in academic achievement and in personal qualities will be invited for an interview. Some weighting according to bona fide residence may be applied according to the following priorities: Ontario, other Canadian provinces, and other countries. From these applicants, 100 students will be selected to fill the entering class.

The M.D. programme has a policy on admission of candidates who are neither Canadian citizens nor land immigrants. This policy is available on the school's Web site at www.fhs.mcmaster.ca/mdprog.

FINANCIAL AID

Medical students at McMaster, in addition to facing the general scarcity of financial assistance, are unable to rely on summer employment as a source of funds. In this situation, it is incumbent on students admitted to the Undergraduate Medical Programme to clarify immediately their fiscal situations and to secure or identify sufficient support to meet their financial obligations over the subsequent three years.

There are some government programs (available only to Canadians) and private agencies that offer financial assistance to medical students. The M.D. Programme and the central University Financial Aid Program offer quite a large bursary program to supplement financial resources of students in financial need. As well, the M.D. Programme administers a small loans program for students in need.

Public Institution

APPLICATION AND ACCEPTANCE POLICIES FOR 2001–2002 FIRST-YEAR CLASS

Fees and expenses are in Canadian dollars.
School participates in OMSAS. See Chapter 12.

Application must be made through Ontario Medical School Application Service (OMSAS), Ontario Universities' Application Centre, P.O. Box 1328, Guelph, Ontario Canada N1H 7P4

Filing of OMSAS application
- Earliest date: July 1, 2000
- Latest date: Oct. 15, 2000 (4:30 p.m. E.S.T.)

OMSAS fee: $175 for one school applied to in Ontario; $75 for each additional school

Oldest MCAT scores considered: None

Does not have Early Decision Program

Acceptance notice to regular applicants
- Earliest date: Last Business Day in May
- Latest date: Until class is filled

Applicant's response to acceptance offer
- Maximum time: 2 weeks

Requests for deferred entrance considered: Yes

Deposit to hold place in class: None

Estimated number of new entrants: 100

Starting date: Sept. 2001

TUITION AND STUDENT FEES PER YEAR FOR 1999–2000 FIRST-YEAR CLASS

Tuition:
- Resident: $13,092
- Non-resident: $38,970

INFORMATION ON 1999–2000 FIRST-YEAR CLASS

Number of	*In-Province*	*Out-of-Province*	*Total*
Applicants	1,880	627	2,507
Applicants Interviewed	352	32	400
New Entrants*	94	6	100

*92% had baccalaureate degrees.

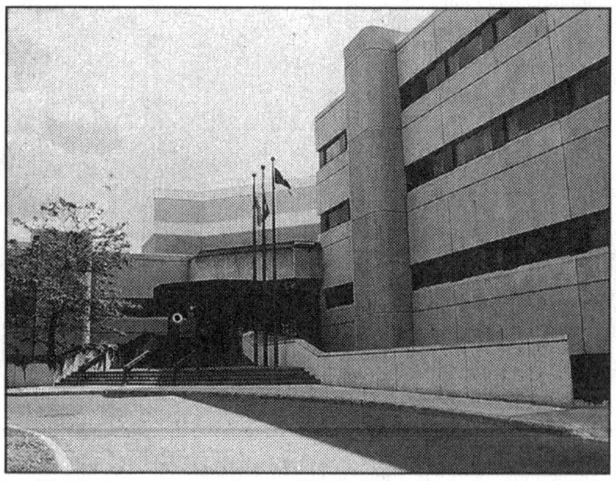

University of Ottawa Faculty of Medicine

Ottawa, Ontario

Dr. Peter Walker, *Dean*
Pierre Soucy, *Assistant Dean, Admissions*
Nicole Racine, *Admissions Officer*

ADDRESS INQUIRIES TO:

Admissions
University of Ottawa
Faculty of Medicine
451 Smyth Road
Ottawa, Ontario
Canada K1H 8M5
(613) 562-5409; 562-5420 (FAX)
E-mail: admissmd@uottawa.ca
Web Site: www.uottawa.ca/academic/med

GENERAL INFORMATION

The University of Ottawa received its charter from the province of Ontario in 1866. It was founded by the Missionary Oblates of Mary Immaculate, who were its administrators until 1965, when important structural reforms were introduced through an act of the legislative assembly of the province of Ontario. The management of the university is now under the Board of Governors consisting of members from various sectors of the community. The management, discipline, and control of the university are free from the restrictions and control of any outside body, whether lay or religious. The Faculty of Medicine was established in 1945. In 1978 the health sciences were regrouped into the Faculty of Health Sciences comprising the School of Medicine, the School of Nursing, and the School of Human Kinetics. In 1989, however, the Faculty of Medicine regained its status as a separate academic unit.

CURRICULUM

During their undergraduate training, students acquire the knowledge, skills, and attitudes necessary to recognize, understand, and apply effective, efficient strategies for the prevention and treatment of common and important health problems. The program integrates the basic and clinical sciences throughout the four years of study. Emphasis is placed on self-learning principles, and facts are assimilated in a multidisciplinary fashion, within the context of clinical problems. Lectures and seminars are used to discuss basic concepts, explore new developments, and provide overviews of the biomedical sciences fundamental to the practice of medicine. Training occurs in ambulatory, primary, secondary, and tertiary settings, with students functioning as members of the medical team in collaboration with other health professionals. The program emphasizes health promotion and disease prevention and is responsive to individual needs and abilities and to the changes occurring in society and the health care system.

The program fosters the qualities of trust and compassion, communication skills, ethical professional conduct, and patient advocacy.

The program is scheduled over four calendar years and is divided into two stages. The first stage includes 70 weeks of study of essential biomedical principles and consists of 13 multidisciplinary blocks. The students learn communication and clinical skills in an integrated fashion with the study of body systems. The second stage, of two years duration, is devoted to clinical clerkships; an extended period of 16 weeks is available for elective study.

REQUIREMENTS FOR ENTRANCE

Applicants are not required to write the MCAT to be eligible to apply.

Students in the following categories are eligible to apply for admission to the first year of the four-year program in the Faculty of Medicine.

(1) Students who have completed successfully in a university three years (full-time studies) of a bachelor's degree program. Required course work must include:

	Years
Biochemistry* (without laboratory)	1
General chemistry* (with laboratory)	1
Organic chemistry* (with laboratory)	1
General biology or zoology (with laboratory)	1
Humanities	1

**Two of the three chemistries are required.*

(2) Students of other universities who have completed studies equivalent to those listed above. (Equivalence is determined by the University of Ottawa Faculty of Medicine.)

SELECTION FACTORS

Academic excellence and interview rating are the main selection criterion used by the Admissions Committee. Academics are measured by an assessment of marks and by a comparison of the applicant's academic record in relationship with those of the other applicants.

Consideration for admission will be given primarily to those eligible candidates who have maintained an overall academic average during the university years of at least B + (or the equivalent GPA). Due to the limited class size, it is to be noted that meeting the above minimum standard does not guarantee admission. No preference is given to academic achievement in one program over another as long as the prerequisites for eligibility have been met. Furthermore, in selecting the students, the Admissions Committee reserves the right to assess, in the applicant's program, the level of difficulty of the courses and/or their pertinence for future medical studies at the University of Ottawa and the performance achieved by the candidate in these courses. No quota is predetermined before the selection is made; each file meeting the requirements is studied individually.

No candidate will be admitted without an interview, and the rating of the interview and of other nonacademic data will be taken into account in the admission process.

It is highly desirable that the candidate who has a broad exposure to biology and physical sciences also have a broad exposure to the arts, humanities, and social sciences.

In view of the limited number of places available, a candidate whose GPA is below 3.4 (scale of 4.0) has considerably less chance of being admitted, depending on the year's competition.

Sex, race, age, religion, and socioeconomic status play no part in the selection process. Only applications from Canadian citizens or permanent residents or applications from children of alumni of the University of Ottawa can be considered.

The courses are given in English. Problem-based tutorials and introduction to clinical skills are also offered in French. Knowledge of both official languages of the university will be an asset (but not a prerequisite).

Applicants who are in the third year of a program at the time they apply must, before June 1, submit an official transcript.

FINANCIAL AID

Students may apply to the Student Financial Aid Office of the university and to their respective provincial governments for loan assistance. The Ontario Medical Association Bursaries and Loan Fund, the Kellogg Foundation Loan Fund, and a special bursaries fund are administered by the Awards Committee of the Faculty of Medicine. The Association of Professors of the University also provides a limited number of bursaries. Most of these awards are made on the basis of demonstrable financial need and good academic standing.

Public Institution

APPLICATION AND ACCEPTANCE POLICIES FOR 2001–2002 FIRST-YEAR CLASS

Fees and expenses are in Canadian dollars.
School participates in OMSAS. See Chapter 12.

Application must be made through Ontario Medical School Application Service (OMSAS), Ontario Universities' Application Centre, P.O. Box 1328, Guelph, Ontario Canada N1H 7P4
Filing of OMSAS application
  Earliest date: July 1, 2000
  Latest date: Oct. 15, 2000
OMSAS fee: $175; $75 for each school
School application fee: $75
Oldest MCAT scores considered: None required
Does not have Early Decision Program
Acceptance notice to regular applicants
  Earliest date: End of May 2001
  Latest date: Until class is filled
Applicant's response to acceptance offer
  Maximum time: 2 weeks
Requests for deferred entrance considered: Yes
Deposit to hold place in class (applied to tuition)
  $100; nonrefundable
Estimated number of new entrants: 84
Starting date: Sept. 2001

TUITION AND STUDENT FEES PER YEAR FOR 1999–2000 FIRST-YEAR CLASS

Tuition: $7,000 Student fees: $372.75

INFORMATION ON 1999–2000 FIRST-YEAR CLASS

Number of	*In-Province*	*Out-of-Province*	*Total*
Applicants	1,711	680	2,391
Applicants Interviewed	*	*	587
New Entrants†	73	11	84

*Data not available.

66.6% had baccalaureate degrees.

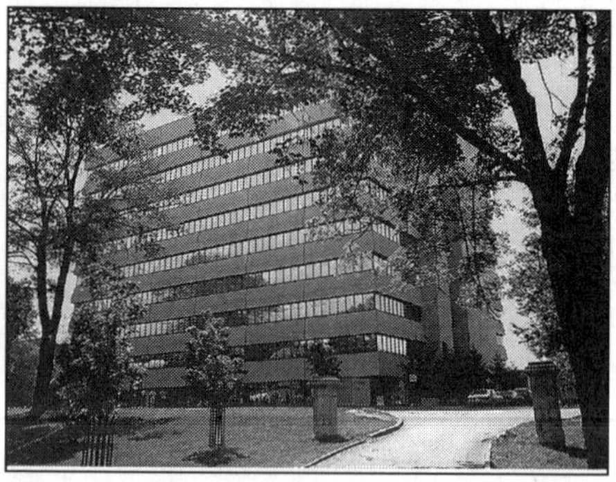

Queen's University Faculty of Health Sciences School of Medicine

Kingston, Ontario

Dr. R.V. Birtwhistle, *Associate Dean, Undergraduate Medical Education*
Thelma C. Rikley, *Manager, Undergraduate Medical Education*

ADDRESS INQUIRIES TO:

Admissions Office
Queen's University
Faculty of Health Sciences
School of Medicine
Kingston, Ontario
Canada K7L 3N6
(613) 533-2542; 533-6884 (FAX)
Web Site: http://meds.queensu.ca/medicine/calendar/toc.html

MISSION STATEMENT

Our mission is to educate health professionals and students in the biomedical sciences by conducting research, by generating a spirit of enquiry, and by serving the health needs of the people of southeastern Ontario, drawing on Queen's learning environment to enable our graduates to become the leading clinicians of Canada's rural, northern, and urban communities and the researchers and educators of the nation's future.

GENERAL INFORMATION

Queen's University School of Medicine, established in 1854, is an integral part of a university of more than 10,000 full-time students. The campus is situated within the city of Kingston, which is located on Lake Ontario at the origin of the St. Lawrence River and has a population of 135,000.

The provision of health care services in Kingston is presently being restructured and will change over the next two years. The Kingston General Hospital will provide most in-patient care for the region. There will be a site for ambulatory care, which, at the present, is centered at the Hotel Dieu Hospital. Chronic care, geriatrics, palliative care, and rehabilitation services are currently provided at St. Mary's of the Lake Hospital.

CURRICULUM

The curriculum is integrated throughout with faculty from different departments contributing to each course. The program is a four-year curriculum with three sequential phases:

Phase I—Introduction to the Sciences Relevant to Medicine	16 weeks
Phase II—System-oriented Clinically based Learning	63 weeks
Phase III—Clinical Clerkship	68 weeks

The Medicine in Society Phase extends throughout the four years and includes information literacy, medical ethics, law in medicine, psychosocial aspects of medicine, and history of medicine as well as topics in family medicine, rehabilitation medicine, growth and development, geriatrics, and community health and epidemiology. These subjects have been chosen to relate to, and enhance, the material that the students will learn in the respective Phases I-III.

Students are introduced in their first year to communication and physical examination. Clinical Skills runs throughout the curriculum to provide the students with opportunities to learn and practice interviewing, history taking, physical examination, clinical reasoning, medical record keeping, and approaches to diagnosis and management. There is an eight-week Critical Enquiry Elective at the end of the second year. This time provides an opportunity for students to investigate a medical question in depth and may involve data collection and analysis. Self-directed learning is emphasized in the curriculum, and learning formats include whole class lectures, tutorials, seminars, symposia, and problem-based learning. Assessment is done using criterion-referenced examinations, small-group evaluation, and objective-structured clinical examinations (OSCE) for clinical skills. Evaluation is honors/pass/fail.

REQUIREMENTS FOR ENTRANCE

The minimum academic requirement for admission is three years of study in any university program (a minimum of 15 full courses).

Candidates are required to successfully complete the equivalent of a full-year (2 semesters) university-level course in each of the following:

	Years
Biological sciences	1
Physical sciences	1
Humanities or social sciences	1

As a requirement for admission, the student must have completed Hepatitis B immunization, and documentation of Hepatitis B serological status must be provided to the School's Undergraduate Office. A student seeking admission will be required to provide documentation of serological status for Hepatitis B, and to undergo further testing as required, after being offered a place. The offer of a place will only be confirmed after this documentation is presented, but the presence of *Hepatitis B Antigen postivity* will not influence the student's acceptance for admission.

All applicants are required to write the MCAT prior to the deadline date for submission of applications to OMSAS.

To be eligible for admission, candidates must be Canadian citizens, Canadian permanent residents (landed immigrants) by February 1 following submission of the OMSAS application, or the children of Queen's University alumni who are residents outside Canada. Verification must be sent to the Admissions Office at the time of application.

SELECTION FACTORS

Seventy-five students are admitted annually into the first medical year and are selected on the basis of a strong academic record and assessment of personal characteristics considered to be most appropriate for the study of medicine at Queen's University and for the subsequent practice of medicine. The following steps are used to identify the group to be invited for interview and for assessment of personal qualities: the cumulative converted GPA based on all years of undergraduate study, and the results of the MCAT. Applications of those below the cutoff will be reviewed by members of the Admissions Committee, who will utilize specific guidelines to identify any unusual circumstances.

Candidates who do not make the academic cut based on their undergraduate grade-point average but who have completed graduate work are considered in this group. The cutoff is based on the median grade-point average of all candidates for the given year.

Given that it is practicable to interview approximately 400 candidates for 75 positions, the Admissions Committee attempts to include as many highly qualified candidates as it can while taking into consideration as many anomalous situations as possible in attempting to give maximum benefit to the applicant population without discriminating against any sector. Unfortunately, it is not possible to interview all of the many highly qualified candidates that apply to our program.

The personal assessment score for those candidates who meet the criteria for steps 1 and 2 is determined from the assessment of the confidential letters of reference, the personal information form, the autobiographic sketch (50 percent), and the personal interview (50 percent), from which candidates will be ranked for offers and placement on the waiting list.

The Admissions Committee does not give preference to applicants who have studied in any particular university program. Applicants are encouraged to consider all of the undergraduate programs available to them and to embark on the course of studies in which they have the greatest interest and that would prepare them for an alternate career should they not gain a place in medicine.

No preference is shown to applicants at any particular level of training.

Place of residence and location of the university where studies have been undertaken are not criteria in selection. Age, gender, race, and religion are not factors considered in the selection process.

Because of the unique structure of the medical curriculum, candidates are not normally considered for admission with advanced standing or transfer.

Students entering in 1999 presented the following *MCAT profile (mean score and range): BS*-11.14 (9-14), *PS*-11.6 (9-14), *VR*-10.77 (10-13), *WS-Q(N-T)*.

INFORMATION FOR MINORITY STUDENTS

There is an alternate admissions process available to Aboriginal candidates.

Public Institution

APPLICATION AND ACCEPTANCE POLICIES FOR 2001–2002 FIRST-YEAR CLASS

Fees and expenses are in Canadian dollars.
School participates in OMSAS. See Chapter 12.

Application must be made through Ontario Medical School Application Service (OMSAS),
Ontario Universities' Application Centre,
P.O. Box 1328, Guelph, Ontario
Canada N1H 7P4

Filing of OMSAS application
Earliest date: July 1, 2000
Latest date: Oct. 15, 2000

OMSAS fee: $175 plus an institutional levy of $75 for each medical school selection

Oldest MCAT scores considered: 1991

Does not have Early Decision Program

Acceptance notice to regular applicants
Earliest date: May 31, 2001
Latest date: Until class is filled

Applicant's response to acceptance offer
Maximum time: 2 weeks

Requests for deferred entrance considered: Yes

Deposit to hold place in class: None

Estimated number of new entrants: 75

Starting date: August 2001

TUITION AND STUDENT FEES PER YEAR FOR 1999–2000 FIRST-YEAR CLASS

Tuition
Canadian: $9,200
Non-Canadian: $16,800

Student fees: $548

INFORMATION ON 1999–2000 FIRST-YEAR CLASS

Number of	*In-Province*	*Out-of-Province*	*Total*
Applicants	1,002	446	1,448
Applicants Interviewed	N/A	N/A	406
New Entrants*	56	22	78

*All took the MCAT; 81% had baccalaureate degrees.

CHAPTER 12

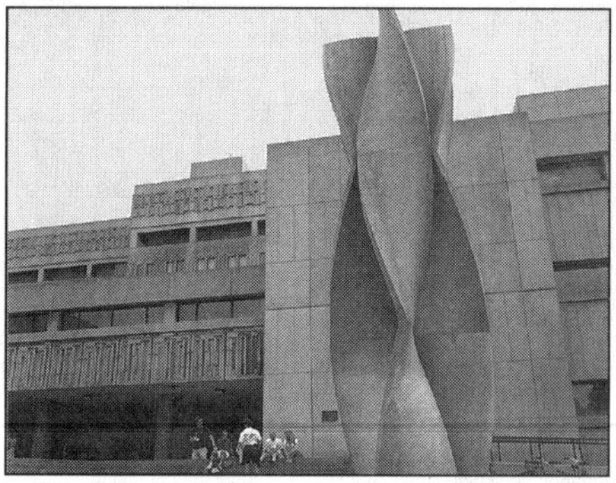

University of Toronto Faculty of Medicine

Toronto, Ontario

Dr. C. David Naylor, *Dean*
Dr. M. Rossi, *Associate Dean, Student Affairs*
Judy Irvine, *Coordinator, Admissions, Awards and Registrarial Affairs*

ADDRESS INQUIRIES TO:

University of Toronto
Faculty of Medicine
Toronto, Ontario
Canada M5S 1A8
(416) 978-2717; 971-2163 (FAX)
Web Site:
http://utll.library.utoronto.ca/www/medicine/ume.htm

GENERAL INFORMATION

The medical school was founded in 1843 as part of King's College, which later became the University of Toronto. The school is a faculty of the university and, as such, receives support from the government of Ontario.

CURRICULUM

The four-year curriculum is focused on student-centered learning. The preclerkship phase (approximately 82 weeks) consists of six multidisciplinary courses, each of which is built upon a series of patient-based cases. Selected lectures, seminars, and laboratory exercises will complement small-group, problem-based learning sessions. Themes for the courses will include the following: the determinants of health; structure and function; the brain, behavior, and communication; metabolism and nutrition; pathobiology of disease; and the foundations of medical practice. Students are required to fulfill specific learning objectives for each course and will be assessed both within and at the completion of each course. In addition, longitudinal clinical and community experiences—beginning in Year 1—are intended to provide students with the opportunity to acquire knowledge and skills through direct interaction with patients.

Following the preclerkship, students spend approximately 78 weeks as clinical clerks. This phase of medical education enables the student to participate in the study and care of patients as a member of a clinical team, which includes residents and the attending staff physician or surgeon. As clerks, medical students rotate for defined periods through hospital services, including medicine, surgery, obstetrics, paediatrics, family medicine, and psychiatry. Each rotation includes community experiences as well as elements of problem-based learning and basic science.

As part of the clerkship, students spend a total of 18 weeks in elective rotations to allow them to explore areas of medicine of particular interest. Clerks may choose to participate in the most technically sophisticated medical units or medical research, work with family physicians in a rural setting, or spend part of their elective working in another country.

During the clerkship, students apply to the Canadian Resident Matching Service to select the program with which they wish to do their postgraduate training. Applications must be submitted in the fall, and students are notified in March as to the program to which they have been matched.

A joint M.D.-Ph.D. program is offered in the Faculty of Medicine and the School of Graduate Studies for individuals wishing to make a commitment to research in addition to the practice of clinical medicine. Students accepted into the combined program may pursue the dual degrees via either a sequential or an integrated route. Interested individuals must apply to the M.D. program at the Faculty of Medicine in the normal manner and request an application from the coordinator of the M.D.-Ph.D. program. Entry into the M.D.-Ph.D. program is dependent upon acceptance into the M.D. program.

REQUIREMENTS FOR ENTRANCE

All applicants are required to write the revised (1991) MCAT prior to the deadline date for submission of applications to OMSAS. A minimum of three years in a degree program at a Canadian university or, for applicants enrolled at a non-Canadian university, an honours bachelor's degree is required.

The faculty does not accept applications for transfer into the program.

Enrollment in the first-year class is currently 177 students.

All applicants are required to have satisfactorily completed the following courses: two full-course equivalents in life sciences plus one full-course equivalent in social sciences or humanities or languages.

It is recommended, although not required, that applicants complete a university-level course in biometrics or statistics.

SELECTION FACTORS

Applicants are judged initially upon their academic and nonacademic records. In addition, attention is paid to the results of the MCAT, statements of referees, and an autobiographical essay. Applicants are also required to appear for an interview in Toronto. Definite preference is given to Canadian residents. A maximum of seven places will be offered to applicants with student visas. Sex, race, and religion are not considered in determining those applicants to whom places are offered.

Successful candidates must be deemed by the Admissions Committee to be acceptable in all aspects of the admissions process. This may include cumulative grade-point average, MCAT scores, published papers, supervisor's letters, nonacademic factors, English proficiency, performance on interview, and any other criteria put forward by the faculty.

FINANCIAL AID

Financial aid is available under the Province of Ontario Student Assistance Program and the Canada Student Loan Program. Applicants are referred to the publications of the Department of University Affairs for details of the regulations governing these awards. Applicants are advised not to plan to earn money in time-consuming work that may jeopardize their standing during the academic year.

Public Institution

APPLICATION AND ACCEPTANCE POLICIES FOR 2001–2002 FIRST-YEAR CLASS

Fees and expenses are in Canadian dollars.
School participates in OMSAS. See Chapter 12.

Application must be made through Ontario Medical
School Application Service (OMSAS),
Ontario Universities' Application Centre,
P.O. Box 1328, Guelph, Ontario
Canada N1H 7P4

Filing of OMSAS application
Earliest date: July 1, 2000
Latest date: Oct. 15, 2000

OMSAS fee: $75

School application fee to all applicants: $75

Oldest MCAT scores considered: within 5 years of application deadlines

Does not have Early Decision Program

Acceptance notice to regular applicants
Earliest date: May 31, 2001
Latest date: Until class is filled

Applicant's response to acceptance offer
Maximum time: 14 days

Requests for deferred entrance considered: Yes

Deposit to hold place in class: None

Estimated number of new entrants: 177

Starting date: Sept. 2001

TUITION AND STUDENT FEES PER YEAR FOR 1999–2000 FIRST-YEAR CLASS

Tuition	Student fees:
Canadian: $11,000	Canadian: $918.73
Non-Canadian: $23,750	Non-Canadian: $1,497.72

INFORMATION ON 1999–2000 FIRST-YEAR CLASS

Number of	*In-Province*	*Out-of-Province*	*Total*
Applicants	1,170	472	1,642
Applicants Interviewed	*	*	365
New Entrants†	150	27	177

*Data not available.
†All took the MCAT; 84% had baccalaureate degrees.

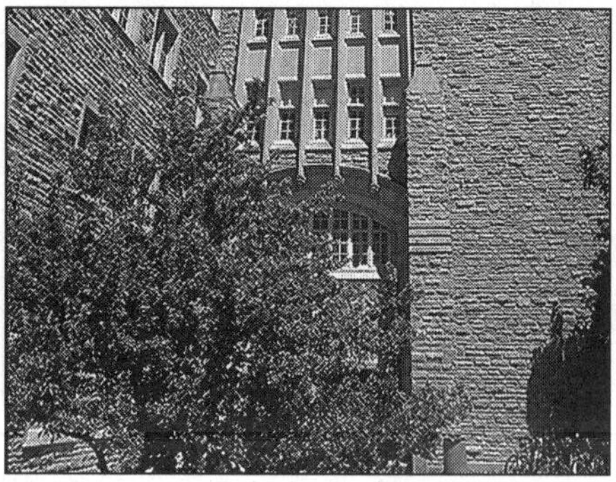

University of Western Ontario Faculty of Medicine & Dentistry Health Sciences Addition

London, Ontario

Dr. Carol P. Herbert, *Dean*
Dr. J.A. Silcox, *Associate Dean, Admissions/Student & Equity Affairs*
Darla McNeil, *Administrative Officer, Medicine Admissions Office*

ADDRESS INQUIRIES TO:

Admissions/Student & Equity Affairs
Faculty of Medicine & Dentistry
Medical Sciences Bldg.
The University of Western Ontario
London, Ontario
Canada N6A 5C1
(519) 661-3744; 661-3797 (FAX)
E-mail: Admissions@med.uwo.ca
Web Site: http://www.med.uwo.ca

GENERAL INFORMATION

The Faculty of Medicine of the University of Western Ontario had its origin in 1882 and came under the direct control of the university in 1912. The University of Western Ontario (U.W.O.) is a private university but in receipt of government grants in common with other universities of Ontario having faculties of medicine.

Students are free to choose any approved residency program. The teaching hospitals, incorporating the clinical science departments, are approved for the graduate training leading to certification in the Royal College of Physicians and Surgeons of Canada.

CURRICULUM

The undergraduate medical curriculum is a four-year program that is patient centred in its content, and student centred in its delivery. It is designed to provide each student with an opportunity to acquire the knowledge, skills, and attitudes required to advance to postgraduate training leading to clinical practice, research, or other medical careers. The educational format is a blend of lectures, laboratory experience, small group problem-based learning sessions, and supervised clinical experiences.

Years One and Two: The first two years of the curriculum provide the student with a solid grounding in the basic and clinical sciences. These two years are each divided into a series of blocks: "Introduction to Medicine," "The Thorax," "The Abdomen," "Head and Neck," "Back and Limbs," and "Systems." Within each block, various subject areas are presented, which integrate the basic and clinical sciences.

The weekly timetable is structured around a presenting case, which is introduced at the beginning of each week. The case provides the stimulus for instruction, and is designed to highlight a number of objectives of the M.D. program. Throughout the week, the student is exposed to a variety of teaching methods including small group tutorials, problem-based learning, lectures and large group discussions, self-instructional materials, and laboratories.

Students participate in early patient contact that emphasizes a patient-centred approach to medicine, beginning in year one. Part of being a good physician is understanding the community in which patients live, and the first two years of the program provide a variety of opportunities for student involvement in the community.

Years Three and Four: The third and fourth years of medicine include a 52-week integrated clerkship, clinical electives, and advanced basic science electives.

During the third-year clerkship, the student becomes an active member of clinical care teams in the following medical disciplines: family medicine, medicine, obstetrics and gynecology, pediatrics, psychiatry, and surgery. Under the supervision of faculty and more senior house staff, clerks are given graded responsibility in the diagnosis, investigation, and management of patients in hospital, clinic, and outpatient settings.

Beginning in year four, clinical electives are arranged entirely by the student in any area of medicine, at Western or in other centres. After completion of the clinical electives, students return to Western in February for the transition period, which includes: Advanced Basic Sciences (e.g., surgical anatomy, medical physiology), Advanced Communication Skills, General Review, Health Care Systems, etc. This permits students to further integrate the basic and clinical aspects of medicine in light of their clinical experience.

REQUIREMENTS FOR ENTRANCE

All applicants must submit results of the revised MCAT (April 1991 or later). The MCAT must be written prior to the application deadline of Oct. 15.

Individuals in the third year of study, or those who have successfully completed three full years of study (15 full or equivalent courses) in any degree program at a recognized university, are eligible to apply. A minimum of five full or equivalent courses must be included in the final undergraduate year and in one other undergraduate year. In addition, three full or equivalent senior-level courses must be included in each of two years (one being the final undergraduate year).

Individuals who have earned a degree from a recognized university may elect to continue in full-time undergraduate studies for the purpose of improving academic standing for application to medical school for a one-year period only. The special year must contain five full or equivalent honors courses. These courses must be equivalent to honors-level courses (200 or higher at Western).

Graduate students will be expected to have completed all requirements (including submission of the thesis, if one is required) for their graduate degree prior to registration in the M.D. Program.

Prior to being permitted to register in the M.D. Program, all applicants granted admission will be required to have successfully completed one full or equivalent laboratory course in biology and organic chemistry plus one other full or equivalent science course from a science discipline unrelated to biology and chemistry. In addition, three full or equivalent nonscience courses are required; two of these courses must be from different disciplines, one of which must be at the first-year level (one of these courses must be literature (English) or history, if the applicant does not have OAC1 English or equivalent from secondary school); and one other full or equivalent nonscience course must be at the senior level from one of the nonscience disciplines chosen above.

SELECTION FACTORS

Enrollment is limited. Admission to the Doctor of Medicine Program is competitive, and the possession of the minimum requirements does not assure acceptance. Admission consideration is based on academic achievement, MCAT scores, and a personal interview score. Only those applicants deemed competitive will be selected for an interview.

A limited number (not more than) ten international (student visa) admissions are available each year into the Doctor of Medicine Program. Interested individuals should contact the Admissions/Student & Faculty Affairs Office directly for application information.

FINANCIAL AID

Financial aid information may be obtained by contacting the Financial Aid Office, Somerville House, the University of Western Ontario, at (519) 661-3775.

Public Institution

APPLICATION AND ACCEPTANCE POLICIES FOR 2001–2002 FIRST-YEAR CLASS

Fees and expenses are in Canadian dollars.
School participates in OMSAS. See Chapter 12.

Application must be made through Ontario Medical School Application Service (OMSAS), Ontario Universities' Application Centre, P.O. Box 1328, Guelph, Ontario Canada N1H 7P4
Filing of OMSAS application
Earliest date: June 1, 2000
Latest date: Oct. 16, 2000
OMSAS fee: $175, plus $75 for each school (subject to change)
Oldest MCAT scores considered: 1991
Does not have Early Decision Program
Acceptance notice to regular applicants
Earliest date: May 31, 2001
Latest date: Until class is filled
Applicant's response to acceptance offer
Maximum time: 2 weeks
Requests for deferred entrance considered: No
Deposit to hold place in class: None
Number of new entrants: 96
Starting date: Sept. 2001

TUITION AND STUDENT FEES PER YEAR FOR 1999–2000 FIRST-YEAR CLASS

Tuition: $10,000* Student fees: $754*

INFORMATION ON 1999–2000 FIRST-YEAR CLASS

Number of	*In-Province*	*Out-of-Province*	*Total*
Applicants	†	†	1,725
Applicants Interviewed	†	†	420
New Entrants‡	†	†	96

*Subject to change
†Data not available.
‡All took the MCAT.

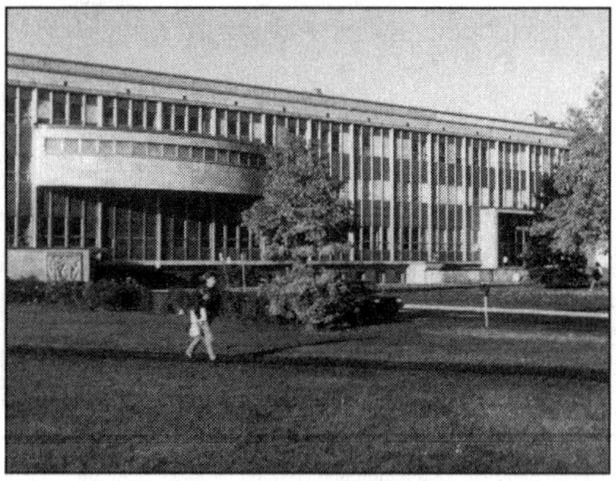

Université Laval Faculty of Medicine

Ste-Foy, Quebec

Dr. Marc Desmeules, *Dean*
Luc Côté, *Chairman, Admission Committee*
Dr. Guy Belanger, *Admission Officer*

ADDRESS INQUIRIES TO:

Secretary, Admissions Committee
Université Laval
Faculty of Medicine
Ste-Foy, Quebec
Canada G1K 7P4
(418) 656-2131, ext. 2492; 656-2733 (FAX)
E-mail: admission@fmed.ulaval.ca
Web Site: http://www.fmed.ulaval.ca

GENERAL INFORMATION

Université Laval was established in 1852 by a Royal Charter granted by Queen Victoria. It was named after Monsignor de Laval, first bishop of Quebec.

Research opportunities are provided in all the basic sciences and in many fields of clinical investigations. The clinical teaching is provided through a network of one academic health center, one affiliated hospital, and one institute. Residence accommodations are provided for many students. There is a University Health Service for students as well as vocational guidance and counseling services.

CURRICULUM

The curriculum aims to prepare students to undertake any career in medicine. During the first two years, the program provides early introduction to clinical problems and interdepartmental teaching by both basic science and clinical faculty. This part of the curriculum is designed to be flexible and can be spread over three calendar years. The basic clinical clerkships are given in the third and fourth years and provide a basic exposure to each major clinical discipline, including family medicine. The curriculum is monitored by both faculty and students.

REQUIREMENTS FOR ENTRANCE

Since all instruction is in French, fluency in the French language is an essential prerequisite.

Under the present Quebec educational system, the minimum requirements are two years of college (Health Sciences Program) and the diploma of collegial studies of the Ministry of Education (D.E.C.).

For other applicants, the degree in science is required.

Specific course requirements are:

	Sem. hrs.
General biology (with lab)	8
General or inorganic chemistry (with lab)	8
Organic chemistry	8
General physics (with lab)	2
Mathematics through calculus	2
Must include analytical geometry, college algebra, and trigonometry.	
French	
Humanities	
Behavioral and social sciences	

The MCAT is not required, although the scores are considered when available.

SELECTION FACTORS

Preference is given to applicants from the province of Quebec. Admission requirements for application from Quebec College (CEGEP) and universities include a standardized C.V. and a three-hour group session called Assessment by Simulation (APS). This test evaluates different personal characteristics of the candidates. A few outstanding French-speaking candidates are admitted from other Canadian provinces and the United States. These candidates are selected on the basis of different parameters: scholastic achievement, interview, and curriculum vitae. Sex, race, religion, age, and socioeconomic status are not considered in the selection process.

FINANCIAL AID

Financial aid is available to Quebec residents through the Bursaries Division of the Provincial Ministry of Education. Summer scholarships of $2,000 are also available to students who wish to devote their vacation period to research. There is no financial assistance for foreign applicants.

Public Institution

APPLICATION AND ACCEPTANCE POLICIES FOR 2001–2002 FIRST-YEAR CLASS

Fees and expenses are in Canadian dollars.

Filing of application
- Earliest date: Jan. 1, 2001
- Latest date: March 1, 2001 (for Quebec residents) Feb. 1, 2001 (for others)

School application fee to all applicants: $65
Oldest MCAT scores considered: 1997
Does not have Early Decision Program
Acceptance notice to regular applicants
- Earliest date: May 15, 2001
- Latest date: Until class is filled

Applicant's response to acceptance offer
- Maximum time: 10 days

Requests for deferred entrance considered: No
Deposit to hold place in class: None
Estimated number of new entrants: 130
Starting date: Sept. 2001

TUITION AND STUDENT FEES PER YEAR FOR 1999–2000 FIRST-YEAR CLASS

Tuition
- Resident: $1,964
- Nonresident: $7,927

Student fees: $200

INFORMATION ON 1999–2000 FIRST-YEAR CLASS

Number of	*In-Province*	*Out-of-Province*	*Total*
Applicants	1,385	85	1,470
Applicants Interviewed	350	5	355
New Entrants*	132	2	134

*35% had baccalaureate degrees.

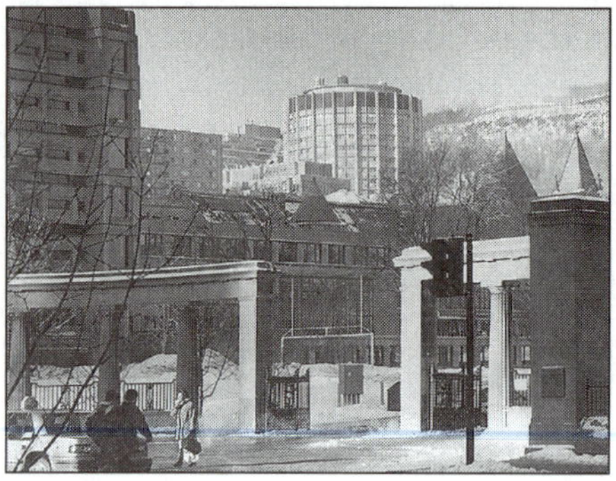

McGill University
Faculty of Medicine

Montreal, Quebec

Dr. Abraham Fuks, *Dean*
Dr. Philip R. Beck, *Associate Dean, Admissions*
Judy Stymest, *Director of Student Aid*

ADDRESS INQUIRIES TO:

Admissions Office
McGill University
Faculty of Medicine
3655 Drummond Street
Montreal, Quebec
Canada H3G 1Y6
(514) 398-3517; 398-4631 (FAX)
Web Site: http://www.med.mcgill.ca/admissions/

GENERAL INFORMATION

The Faculty of Medicine was established in 1829. It selects students from a variety of cultural and academic backgrounds and provides them with a medical education that places emphasis upon both basic medical sciences and clinical medicine. There are five university teaching hospitals, three specialty teaching hospitals, and 14 special research centers and units. The Quebec (Canadian) health care system has only one category of patient. All patients are available for the teaching of medical students. This gives McGill graduates the clinical skills for which they are renowned throughout the world. Research opportunities, available at the undergraduate and graduate levels, are provided in all of the basic medical sciences and in many fields of clinical medicine. The university offers residential facilities and provides student services, including a health service.

The language of instruction is English.

The faculty of medicine is accredited by the Liaison Committee on Medical Education of the AAMC and the AMA. Studying at McGill is identical to studying medicine in a U.S. medical school. U.S. students studying at McGill write the USMLE exams in the same way and at the same time as U.S. students studying in U.S. medical schools. These students return automatically to the United States for residency.

U.S. program directors recognize the high caliber of McGill graduates, and McGill students are very competitive in U.S. residency applications.

CURRICULUM

McGill University introduced a new curriculum for undergraduate medical education in August 1994. It recognizes the importance of a solid database and a multidisciplinary approach to medical education with interdigitation (integration) of clinical and basic science. It permits a variety of teaching and evaluation methods, emphasizing small-group teaching. Approximately 50 percent of the sessions are lectures. The other 50 percent include small-group teaching, computer-based instruction, and laboratories.

The curriculum is composed of four components entitled Basis of Medicine (BOM), Introduction to Clinical Medicine (ICM), Practice of Medicine (POM), and Back to Basics (BTB). The BOM component, occupying the first 18 months, introduces the fundamental pillars of medicine, such as anatomy and physiology. The students have extensive opportunities for "hands on" laboratory sessions and have patient contact sessions.

The clinical component is two phased. The initial portion, ICM, has a six-month duration. The student learns the techniques of physical examination and develops clinical reasoning strategies. Included are bedside teaching in the university hospitals, visits to community centers, exposure to family physicians in private offices, and the use of standardized patients for the teaching of specific skills.

The third component, POM, starts in the middle of the third year and provides exposure to the core disciplines of medicine: Internal Medicine, Pediatrics, Surgery, Obstetrics and Gynecology, Psychiatry, and Family Medicine. This component provides extensive clinical contact, under supervision by faculty members. The new curriculum has been structured so as to ensure that all core clerkship rotations are completed in time for the residency application process.

The ICM and POM components of the curriculum offer several opportunities for elective rotations, each at a four-week duration.

The last component is Back to Basics. It occupies the remainder of the fourth year. It is designed to reinforce the importance of the basic sciences in clinical practice.

The evaluation system at this faculty is multifaceted and includes small-group assessments, written examination, oral clinical examinations, assessment of written case reports, and others. The grading system is pass/fail.

McGill recently introduced an M.D.-M.B.A. program in response to the increasing need for doctors to acquire management skills that are unique to health care.

Similarly, a seven-year combined M.D.-Ph.D. program is offered for students interested in a research career in academic medicine.

REQUIREMENTS FOR ENTRANCE

Applicants to the four-year program must have received, or be in the final year of a course of study leading to, a bachelor's degree. Specific requirements include the MCAT and university-level courses in each of the following:

	Credit hrs.
General biology (with lab)	6
General chemistry (with lab)	6
Organic chemistry (with lab)	6
Physics (with lab)	6

Prerequisite courses completed more than eight years ago must be repeated. Exceptions may be made for applicants with advanced degrees in the material concerned.

University-level courses in biochemistry or cell biology and molecular biology are strongly recommended.

A Med-P program is restricted to residents of the province of Quebec who are attending the provincial colleges of general and professional education.

No places for transfer are available.

SELECTION FACTORS

Selection of students by the admissions committee is based upon academic achievement and an assessment of personal characteristics and accomplishments. Academic achievement is determined from the academic record in undergraduate studies and the result of the Medical College Admission Test. While completed graduate degrees are taken into consideration, applicants should know that the undergraduate CGPA is the major consideration in measuring academic performance. Applicants to the four-year program must have undergraduate CGPAs of 3.5 or better and a total of 30 or more in the MCAT scores.

The initial assessment of personal qualities and achievements is made from a study of the autobiographical letter and the letters of reference. Those applicants who are considered the most competitive will be invited for interviews. The files of candidates who are not invited for interviews are not considered further.

Following the interview the components of the application process—GPAs and MCAT scores for applicants to the four-year program, CEGEP averages for applicants to the Med-P program, the autobiographical letter, and interview performance—scores are aggregated. Places in the entering class are offered to those whose aggregated scores are most competitive.

The decisions are final and are not subject to appeal.

Students accepted into the 1998 entering class had the following academic profile: *mean GPA,* 3.77; *mean MCAT scores (new test) VR*-9.26, *PS*-10.83, *BS*-11.17.

FINANCIAL AID

Students who are U.S. citizens or U.S. permanent residents are normally eligible for funding from Subsidized Stafford Loans, Unsubsidized Stafford Loans, and TERI/PEP Loans.

The university offers modest levels of financial assistance to students with demonstrated need. Only students who have availed themselves of government funding will be considered for these awards. Pell Grants are not tenable at McGill University.

Information is available from: Student Aid Office, McGill University, 3637 Peel Street, Montreal, Quebec H3A 1X1; or call (514) 398-6013 or 6014.

Public Institution

APPLICATION AND ACCEPTANCE POLICIES FOR 2001–2002 FIRST-YEAR CLASS

Fees and expenses are in Canadian dollars.

Application for admission should be made through online admissions at **http://www.med.mcgill.ca/admissions/**. (Medical students are expected to have facility with computers and Internet access.)

Filing of application
- Earliest date: Sept. 1, 2000
- Latest date: Nov. 15, 2000 (out-of-province applicants applying to the regular four-year program and the M.D.-Ph.D. program); Nov. 15, 2000 (applicants to the M.D.-M.B.A. program); Jan. 15, 2001 (Quebec resident applicants to the four-year program); March 1, 2001 (Quebec resident applicants to the Med-P program)

School application fee to all applicants: $60 for electronic application; $100 for paper application

Oldest MCAT scores considered: 1997

Does not have Early Decision Program

Acceptance notice to regular applicants
- Earliest date: March 31, 2001
- Latest date: Varies

Applicant's response to acceptance offer
- Maximum time: 2 weeks

Requests for deferred entrance considered: Yes

Deposit to hold place in class (applied to tuition): $500, due with response to acceptance offer

Deposit refundable prior to: May 15, 2001

Estimated number of new entrants: 120

Starting date: Aug. 2001

TUITION AND STUDENT FEES PER YEAR FOR 1999–2000 FIRST-YEAR CLASS

First-year Tuition
- Resident: $3,559.04
- Non-Quebec Canadian: $7,335.04
- U.S. & International: $19,559.04

Student fees: $799.05

INFORMATION ON 1999–2000 FIRST-YEAR CLASS

Number of	*In-Province*	*Out-of-Province*	*Total*
Applicants	479	365	844
Applicants Interviewed	174	104	278
New Entrants*	90	30†	120

*All new entrants into four-year programs took the MCAT and had baccalaureate degrees.

†Seven additional students–2 U.S. students, 2 non-Quebec Canadian students, and 3 Quebec students–have been accepted into the first year of the M.D.-M.B.A. program. The first year of this program is spent in the Faculty of Management.

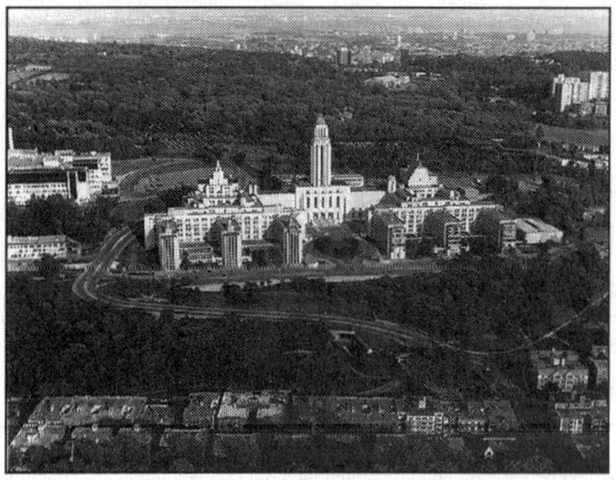

Université de Montréal School of Medicine

Montreal, Quebec

Dr. Patrick Vinay, *Dean of Faculty of Medicine*
Dr. Michel Gagnon, *President of Admission Committee*
Dr. Louise F. Charron, *Vice Dean*

ADDRESS INQUIRIES TO:

Committee on Admission
Université de Montréal
School of Medicine
P.O. Box 6128, Station Centre-Ville
Montreal, Quebec
Canada H3C 3J7
(514) 343-6265; 343-6629 (FAX)
E-mail: admmed@ere.umontreal.ca
Web Site: http://www-lercycle.med.umontreal.ca

GENERAL INFORMATION

The Faculty of Medicine of the University of Montreal can be traced back to a school first established in Montreal in 1843 and incorporated in 1845 under the name of Ecole de Médecine et de Chirurgie de Montréal. In 1891 the school merged with the Faculty of Medicine of the Montreal Branch of Laval University, which had been founded in 1877. In 1920, by an act of the Quebec legislature, the Montreal branch of Laval University was granted its independence, and the school of medicine became known by its present name.

All instruction is in French, and clinical instruction is carried out at 14 affiliated teaching hospitals and research centers.

CURRICULUM

In September 1993 a new four-year curriculum came into effect. The first year is devoted to basic biological and behavioral sciences. Clinical exposure begins with Year 1. It consists of two years (70 weeks) of problem-based learning during which students are exposed to biomedical and psychosocial sciences basic to medicine. Courses are interdisciplinary and system based. Introduction to clinical skills takes place in a continuous fashion throughout those two preclinical years. Ninety hours of electives are mandatory during the first two years. The third and fourth years consist of an 80-week clerkship.

In the new curriculum, formal lecturing is reduced to a minimum and replaced by active methods, especially problem-based learning and small-group discussion.

A premedical year is restricted to students having just graduated from the provincial colleges of general and professional education. Students who have completed one to three years at the university level in humanities are also eligible for the premedical year. Opportunities exist to pursue a combined M.D.-M.Sc. and M.D.-Ph.D. curriculum.

Residency training in the teaching hospitals is under the responsibility of the Faculty of Medicine. Various courses and symposia are organized by the continuing medical education division.

REQUIREMENTS FOR ENTRANCE

A thorough knowledge of the French language is a prerequisite. Under the present Quebec educational system, the minimum requirement is two years of college (Health Sciences Program) and the diploma of collegial studies of the Department of Education (D.E.C.).

The college curriculum should provide a wide cultural background. Course work must include: philosophy, behavioral and social sciences, French, English, mathematics (analytical geometry, calculus, college algebra, and trigonometry), and sciences (biology, inorganic and organic chemistry, and physics).

SELECTION FACTORS

Candidates accepted must be either Canadian citizens or landed immigrants, but due consideration will be given to French-speaking applicants from other provinces of Canada and from the United States. Selection of candidates is competitive and based on a global score derived from scholastic records and an interview. Interviews, conducted on the site of the medical school, are granted to about one-quarter of the applicants selected from their scholastic records. This interview can be eliminatory. For candidates holding a Ph.D. degree, performance in research may constitute an important selection factor. No consideration is given to race, sex, creed, or age.

FINANCIAL AID

Financial aid is available to students through the Bursaries Division of the Department of Education, the Kellogg Foundation Loan Fund, the Scholarships and Loan Committee of the university, and the Jean Frappier Fund. Summer scholarships are also available.

Public Institution

APPLICATION AND ACCEPTANCE POLICIES FOR 2000–2001 FIRST-YEAR CLASS

Fees and expenses are in Canadian dollars.

Filing of application
  Latest date: March 1, 2000
School application fee to all applicants: $30
Does not have Early Decision Program
Acceptance notice to regular applicants
  Earliest date: May 15, 2001
  Latest date: Until class is filled
Applicant's response to acceptance offer
  Maximum time: 14 days
Requests for deferred entrance considered: No
Deposit to hold place in class: None
Estimated number of new entrants: 165
Starting date: Aug. 2001

TUITION AND STUDENT FEES PER YEAR FOR 1998–99 FIRST-YEAR CLASS

Tuition
  Resident: $2,391
  Nonresident: $12,133

Student fees: $30

INFORMATION ON 1998–99 FIRST-YEAR CLASS

Number of	*In-Province*	*Out-of-Province*	*Total*
Applicants	1,656	260	1,916
Applicants Interviewed	425	11	436
New Entrants	158	4	162

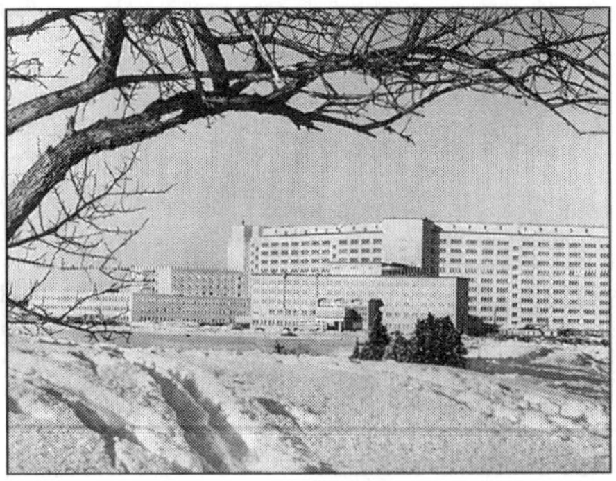

University of Sherbrooke Faculty of Medicine

Sherbrooke, Quebec

Dr. Michel Baron, *Dean*
Dr. Carolle Bernier, *Chair, Admissions Committee*

ADDRESS INQUIRIES TO:

Admission Office
University of Sherbrooke
Faculty of Medicine
Sherbrooke, Quebec
Canada J1H 5N4
(819) 564-5208; 564-5378 (FAX)
E-mail: admmed@courrier.usherb.ca
Web Site: http://www.usherb.ca

GENERAL INFORMATION

Officially founded in February 1961, the Faculty of Medicine at the University of Sherbrooke is a French-speaking institution. It admitted its first students in September 1966.

As required by modern medical teaching, the Faculty of Medicine is integrated into a developing Health Sciences Center to serve all members of the health team. This center includes a modern 700-bed teaching hospital. A Department of Nursing offers several programs of study at university level. The Faculty of Medicine offers residential facilities on campus. Twelve hospitals, many health centers, and CLSC are affiliated with the Faculty of Medicine.

CURRICULUM

Since 1987, a new four-year curriculum has begun. The form of teaching is now a problem-based learning program. Formal lecturing has been reduced to a minimum. Audiovisual facilities, seminars, small-group discussions, panels, field work, and case studies are used extensively. Most learning sessions integrate many disciplines representing various departments.

The M.D. degree is granted after successful completion of a four-year course. Students work in the hospital network from the beginning of their first year. The clerkship is a 16-month clinical training starting with the winter trimester of the third year.

Postgraduate programs are available in most departments leading to the M.Sc. or Ph.D. degree, and a diploma can be obtained in community health. Residency training is offered in all major specialties.

A joint M.D.-M.Sc. program is offered to students who are enrolled in an M.D. program with outstanding academic records. The medical student must have completed two years of the four-year M.D. program. The main objective of the joint program is to form doctors who will have achieved a scientific approach of medicine and who will also be able to pursue scientific activities among a team.

REQUIREMENTS FOR ENTRANCE

The minimum requirement for admission is two years of college under the present Quebec educational system—Collège d'enseignement général et professionnel (C.E.G.E.P.). B.A. or B.Sc. degrees are fully acceptable. The minimum science curriculum is as follows:

Candidates with a B.A. or B.Sc. degree:

	Semesters
General biology (with lab)	2
General chemistry (with lab)	2
Organic chemistry (with lab)	2
General physics (with lab)	3
Mathematics through calculus	3

Must include analytical geometry, college algebra, and trigonometry.

C.E.G.E.P. candidates:

College diploma (D.E.C.) with major in sciences.

The college curriculum should also provide a wide cultural background in the humanities (including philosophy and literature) and in the social and behavioral sciences (including history, psychology, and sociology). Since all instruction is in French, fluency and reading ability in the French language are essential prerequisites.

The MCAT is not required.

SELECTION FACTORS

Admission to the Faculty of Medicine is based primarily on ability and premedical achievement, as demonstrated by scholastic records. A learning skills test is included in selection for admission in 2000.

Eighty-six places are reserved for applicants from the province of Quebec. Fifteen additional places are reserved for applicants from New Brunswick for admission in 2000. There is also one place available for an applicant from Prince Edward Island, plus one from Nova Scotia. Two places are available for qualified foreign applicants with a student visa. Applicants must be fluent in both written and spoken French.

FINANCIAL AID

Financial aid is available to resident students through the Bursaries Division of the Provincial Ministry of Education, the Scholarships and Loans Committee of the university, and a few private foundations.

Public Institution

APPLICATION AND ACCEPTANCE POLICIES FOR 2001–2002 FIRST-YEAR CLASS

Fees and expenses are in Canadian dollars.

Filing of application
  Earliest date: Nov. 2000
  Latest date: March 1, 2001
School application fee to all applicants: $30
Oldest MCAT scores considered: Not required
Does not have Early Decision Program
Acceptance notice to regular applicants
  Earliest date: May 2001
  Latest date: Aug. 2001
Applicant's response to acceptance offer
  Maximum time: 15 days
Requests for deferred entrance considered: No
Deposit to hold place in class (applied to tuition):
  $200, due with response to acceptance offer; nonrefundable; Due Aug. 1, 2001
Estimated number of new entrants: 104
Starting date: Aug. 2001

TUITION AND STUDENT FEES PER YEAR FOR 1999–2000 FIRST-YEAR CLASS

Tuition and student fees:
  Canadian: $3,019.38
  Non-Canadian: $15,019.38

INFORMATION ON 1999–2000 FIRST-YEAR CLASS

Number of	*In-Province*	*Out-of-Province*	*Total*
Applicants	1,202	199	1,401
New Entrants*	86	16	104

*6% had baccalaureate degrees.
Non-Canadian, 2

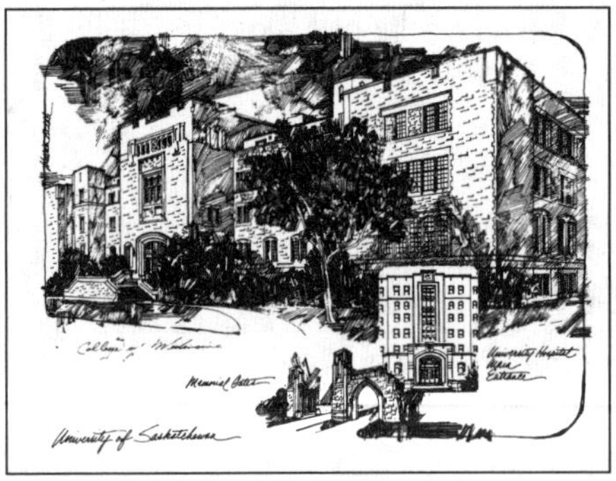

University of Saskatchewan College of Medicine

Saskatoon, Saskatchewan

Dr. D. R. Popkin, *Dean of Medicine*
M.D. Evered, *Director of Admissions and Student Affairs*
Joyce Pitzel, *Admissions Officer*

ADDRESS INQUIRIES TO:

Secretary, Admissions
University of Saskatchewan
College of Medicine
B103 Health Sciences Building, 107 Wiggins Road
Saskatoon, Saskatchewan
Canada S7N 5E5
(306) 966-8554; 966-6164 (FAX)
Web Site: http://www.usask.ca/medicine

GENERAL INFORMATION

The University of Saskatchewan began teaching medical students in a two-year medical sciences program in 1926. The present college was introduced in 1953 with a four-year curriculum leading to the M.D. degree. In 1968 the curriculum changed to five years with a one-year premedical university requirement. The curriculum reverted to a four-year program in 1988 with a minimum two-year premedical requirement.

Clinical teaching is based at the Royal University Hospital, St. Paul's and Saskatoon City Hospitals in Saskatoon, and the Plains Health Centre and General Hospital in Regina.

The maximum size of each entering class is 55 students.

CURRICULUM

The College of Medicine provides a curriculum leading to the general professional education of the physician: graduates may select careers in family medicine, specialty practice, public health, research, or teaching. During the course of the undergraduate M.D. curriculum, students may obtain a B.Sc. (Med.) degree in the basic medical sciences.

A "revised" curriculum was launched in the fall of 1997, Class of 2001. The classes of 1998–2000 will continue in the current curriculum, Phases 3-5.

Phase A: Revised Curriculum (33 weeks) provides students with an overview of the basic science disciplines appropriate to the study of medicine, as well as an introduction to professional skills (including primary clinical skills) within the context of developing the patient–doctor relationship. This phase includes a two-week clinical experience done in one of the Saskatchewan Health Districts. Phase B: Revised Curriculum (14 weeks) enables students to acquire specific knowledge in those subjects bridging the basic and clinical sciences and to enhance basic clinical skills. Phase 4 (47 weeks), enables learning of the principles and methods in core clinical knowledge. Phase 5 (52 weeks) of clinical clerkship provides an opportunity to apply the knowledge, skills, and attitudes students have acquired to the management of patients. Provision is made for clinical electives.

Learning in the basic and clinical sciences has been organized by body systems with a problem-solving emphasis. Significant time blocks have been reserved in Phases A–4 for independent study.

REQUIREMENTS FOR ENTRANCE

Two full years of university study are required after graduation from secondary school. The following courses or their equivalent are required:

	Credit hrs.
Biochemistry	6
General biology (with lab)	6
General chemistry (with lab)	3
General physics (with lab)	6
Organic chemistry (with lab)	3
English (lit. and comp.)	6
Social sciences or humanities (full course)	6

Standard First Aid Certificate.

The MCAT is required, and scores must be available at time of application.

The applicant must be a Canadian citizen or landed immigrant of at least three years at the time of application.

SELECTION FACTORS

The Admissions Committee considers academic ability and personal qualities assessed through scholastic records, letters of recommendation, and results of a personal interview by a team of four persons. All eligible candidates are interviewed during a weekend in March. At the time of selection, academic ability and personal qualities are weighted approximately 3 to 1. For the 1999 entering class, the average GPA was 87.2 percent, and the average interview score was 19 of a possible 24 points.

FINANCIAL AID

Various loan funds and scholarships are available. A limited number of bursaries enable students to engage in research between the end of one academic year and the beginning of another.

INFORMATION FOR MINORITY STUDENTS

There is an Aboriginal Access Program for Saskatchewan residents.

Public Institution

APPLICATION AND ACCEPTANCE POLICIES FOR 2001–2002 FIRST-YEAR CLASS

Fees and expenses are in Canadian dollars.

Filing of application
- Earliest date: Aug. 1, 2000
- Latest dates
  - In-province: Jan. 15, 2001
  - Out-of-province: Dec. 1, 2001

School application fee:
- Saskatchewan residents: $40
- Non-Saskatchewan residents: $75 plus transcript fee*

Oldest MCAT scores considered: 1995

Does not have Early Decision Program

Acceptance notice to regular applicants
- Earliest date: June 25, 2001
- Latest date: Varies

Applicant's response to acceptance offer
- Maximum time: 2 weeks

Requests for deferred entrance considered: Yes

Deposit to hold place in class (applied to tuition): $100, due with response to acceptance offer; nonrefundable

Estimated number of new entrants: 55

Starting date: Aug. 2001

TUITION AND STUDENT FEES PER YEAR FOR 1999–2000 FIRST-YEAR CLASS

Tuition: $6,400 Student fees: $110

INFORMATION ON 1999–2000 FIRST-YEAR CLASS

Number of	*In-Province*	*Out-of-Province*	*Total*
Applicants	70	173	243
Applicants Interviewed	55	32	87
New Entrants†	43	8	51

*Transcript fees are $25 for Canadian universities and $50 for non-Canadian universities.

†66.6% had baccalaureate degrees.

Publications of Interest

MCAT Student Manual

1995, 126 pages
$20, MCAT

The 1995 MCAT Student Manual provides detailed information about the format and content of the Medical College Admission Test. The manual contains science content listings and describes the science problem-solving, critical thinking, and communications/writing skills tested by the examination. Preparation and test-taking strategies are described. The manual includes sample items with response explanations, plus a full-length practice test (Practice Test I) with scoring key. The practice test alone is available in bulk packages of 10 for $50.00, MPT to undergraduate health professions advisors.

MCAT Practice Test II, (Book Set)

$20, MPT2 for the three-booklet set

This set includes:

- MCAT Practice Test II, 1991, 100 pages
- MCAT Practice Items: Verbal Reasoning and Writing Sample, 1991, 81 pages; and
- MCAT Practice Items: Physical Science and Biological Sciences, 1991, 112 pages

MCAT Practice Test II is an operational test form from the 1991 administration of the MCAT. This is a full-length MCAT examination with an answer key and scoring guide. The Practice Items booklets contain 263 Verbal Reasoning questions, four sample essay prompts, 199 Physical Sciences questions, and 223 Biological Sciences questions with answer keys for the multiple-choice questions. College or university health professions advisors may purchase Practice Test II alone in bulk packages of 10 for $50.

MCAT Practice Test III and Solutions Booklet

Practice Test III, 1995, 135 pages
Practice Test III Solutions Booklet, 1999, 70 pages
$35, MPT3

MCAT Practice Test III is full-length practice exam with an answer key and raw-to-scaled score conversion tables for each multiple-choice test section. It is a released version of a test form that was administered operationally. Supplementary work sheets are included to allow the user to analyze performance strengths and weaknesses on the test. An appendix at the end of the practice test booklet contains supplementary information on how the Writing Sample essays are scored, with critiques of sample essays. A separate, newly-developed Solutions Booklet for Practice Test III is included in this booklet-set. The Solutions Booklet provides detailed explanations and rationales for the correct answers for each question in Practice Test III. (This practice test is not available in bulk.)

Preparing for the MCAT (Video)

approx. 25 mins., VHS
$12, MVID

Designed for use with the MCAT Student Manual, this tape provides information about the knowledge and skills tested by the MCAT and discusses preparation strategies for each of the four test sections. (Other formats are available at a slightly higher price by special order.)

Scoring the MCAT Writing Sample: Examples of Writing Sample Responses and Explanations of Their Scores

1995, 28 pages
$10, SMWN * Free to Members

This publication is intended for use by examinees as they prepare to take the Writing Sample section of the MCAT and by health professions advisors, medical school admissions committee members, and other test score users when interpreting Writing Sample scores. The publication describes the process by which essays are scored and provides examples of actual essays written by examinees during operational administrations. Critiques discuss essays' strengths and weaknesses, explain the reasons for their scores, and offer suggestions for improvement. The material in this publication is also included in MCAT Practice Test III. AAMC Members may call 202-828-0690 for a free copy.

MCAT Practice Test IV and Solutions Booklet

1998, 115 pages Practice Test IV,
68 pages for Solutions Book
$35, MPT4

MCAT Practice Test IV is an additional full-length practice exam with a scoring key and raw-to-scaled score conversion table. The test is a released operational test form that was administered subsequent to the operational test forms released in Practice Test II and Practice Test III. Supplementary worksheets are included to allow the user to analyze performance strengths and weaknesses on the test. A separate Solutions Booklet, which provides a detailed explanation for the correct answers to the questions in the practice test, is included in the packet. Authorized undergraduate health professions advisors may purchase Practice Test IV alone in bulk packages of 10 for $75 for use in group practice sessions with their advisees.

ASSOCIATION OF AMERICAN MEDICAL COLLEGES

Order Form

Send Order To:
Association of American Medical Colleges
Department 66
Washington, DC 20055

(202) 828-0416 • Fax (202) 828-1123

Qty	Item Code	Title	Unit Price	Total

Subtotal	
Shipping/ Handling	
Total Amount Enclosed	

Total Number of Books Ordered:

	U.S.	CANADA*	MEXICO EASTERN EUROPE	WESTERN EUROPE	PACIFIC RIM	MIDDLE EAST
1 Book	$6.00	$20.00	$40.00	$25.00	$30.00	$33.00
2 Books	$8.00	$25.00	$52.00	$35.00	$35.00	$45.00
3 Books	$10.00	$30.00	$65.00	$40.00	$45.00	$50.00
4 Books	$12.00	$35.00	$75.00	$45.00	$55.00	$60.00
5 Books	$16.00	$38.00	$85.00	$55.00	$60.00	$66.00
6 Books	$19.00	$42.00	$95.00	$60.00	$65.00	$72.00

All payments must be in U.S. dollars and must accompany order (check, money order, or credit card). Please call (202) 828-0416 for any domestic order over 6 books. Out of U.S. orders over 6 books, please call, fax, or write for shipping costs. Orders for 5 books or more accompanied by an institutional purchased order may be invoiced.
Orders using credit cards for payment may be faxed to (202) 828-1123.

Prices are subject to change without notice. Please call 202-828-0416 for information on refunds and returns.

Shipping Information

Name:______________________

Address:______________________

City:______________________

State, Zip;______________________

Phone:______________________

Please charge my credit card:

Check one: ❑ Mastercard ❑ Visa

Card No:______________ Exp. Date:______________

Name as it appears on card:______________________

Daytime Phone No:______________________

Signature:______________________